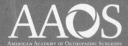

AAOS
AMERICAN ACADEMY OF ORTHOPAEDIC SURGEONS

SECOND EDITION

Anatomy & Physiology

for the Prehospital Provider

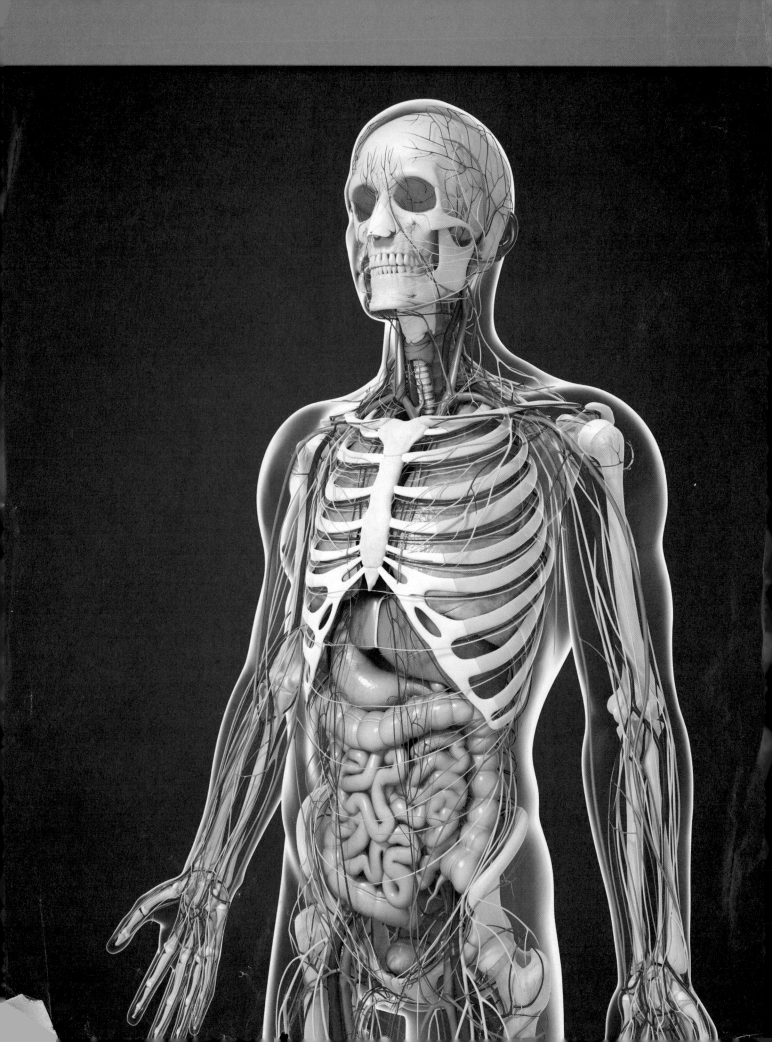

SECOND EDITION

Anatomy & Physiology

for the Prehospital Provider

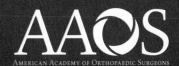

AMERICAN ACADEMY OF ORTHOPAEDIC SURGEONS

Bob Elling, MPA, EMT-P

Kirsten M. Elling, BS, EMT-P

Series Editor: Andrew N. Pollak, MD, FAAOS

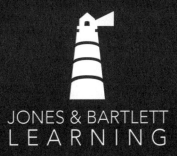

JONES & BARTLETT
LEARNING

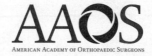
AMERICAN ACADEMY OF ORTHOPAEDIC SURGEONS

World Headquarters
Jones & Bartlett Learning
5 Wall Street
Burlington, MA 01803
978-443-5000
info@jblearning.com
www.jblearning.com

Jones & Bartlett Learning books and products are available through most bookstores and online booksellers. To contact Jones & Bartlett Learning directly, call 800-832-0034, fax 978-443-8000, or visit our website, www.jblearning.com.

Substantial discounts on bulk quantities of Jones & Bartlett Learning publications are available to corporations, professional associations, and other qualified organizations. For details and specific discount information, contact the special sales department at Jones & Bartlett Learning via the above contact information or send an email to specialsales@jblearning.com.

Production Credits
Chief Executive Officer: Ty Field
President: James Homer
Chief Product Officer: Eduardo Moura
Executive Publisher: Kimberly Brophy
Executive Editor—EMS: Christine Emerton
Senior Content Developer: Jennifer Deforge-Kling
Production Editor: Cindie Bryan
VP, Sales—Public Safety Group: Matthew Maniscalco
Director of Sales, Public Safety Group: Patricia Einstein

VP, Marketing: Alisha Weisman
VP, Manufacturing and Inventory Control: Therese Connell
Art Development Editor: Joanna Lundeen
Composition: diacriTech
Cover and Text Design: Kristin E. Parker
Photo Research and Permissions Coordinator: Lauren Miller
Cover Image: © pixologicstudio/iStock/Thinkstock
Printing and Binding: Courier Companies
Cover Printing: Courier Companies

Library of Congress Cataloging-in-Publication Data
Elling, Bob, author.
 [Paramedic]
Anatomy & physiology for the prehospital provider / American Academy of Orthopaedic Surgeons; Bob Elling, Kirsten M. Elling. —Second edition.
   p. ; cm.
Anatomy and physiology for the prehospital provider
Preceded by Paramedic: anatomy and physiology / American Academy of Orthopaedic Surgeons; Bob Elling, Kirsten M. Elling, Mikel A. Rothenberg; editor, Andrew N. Pollak. c2004.
Includes bibliographical references and index.
ISBN-13: 978-1-4496-4230-3 (pbk.)
ISBN-10: 1-4496-4230-6 (pbk.)
I. Elling, Kirsten M., author. II. American Academy of Orthopaedic Surgeons, author. III. Title. IV. Title: Anatomy and physiology for the prehospital provider.
[DNLM: 1. Anatomy—Problems and Exercises. 2. Physiology—Problems and Exercises. 3. Emergency Treatment—methods—Problems and Exercises. QS 18.2]
QM23.2
616.02'5—dc23
                        2014002815
6048

Printed in the United States of America
18 17 16 15 14 10 9 8 7 6 5 4 3 2

Brief Contents

Contents

Acknowledgments

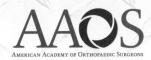

AMERICAN ACADEMY OF ORTHOPAEDIC SURGEONS

The American Academy of Orthopaedic Surgeons would like to acknowledge the reviewers of *Anatomy & Physiology for Prehospital Providers, Second Edition.*

Bruce Barry, RN, CEN, NREMT-P
Peak Paramedicine, LLC
Wilmington, New York

Lynn Browne-Wagner, MSN, RN
Northland Pioneer College
Show Low, Arizona

Amanda Creel, RN, BS, NRP
University of South Alabama
Mobile, Alabama

Kathleen Grote
Anne Arundel County Fire Department
Millersville, Maryland

Kevin Keen, AEMCA
Multi Agency Training Center: Hamilton Fire
Department
Hamilton, Ontario, Canada

Steven M. Kirschbaum, Paramedic
SwedishAmerican Health System
Rockford, Illinois

Mary Katherine Lockwood, PhD, AEMT, I/C
University of New Hampshire
Durham, New Hampshire

Vickie Martin, BA, NREMT-P, NCEE
Lancaster EMS
Millersville, Pennsylvania

Donna McHenry, MS, NREMT-P
University of New Mexico
Los Alamos, New Mexico

John E Mitchell, BS, MBA, PA(ASCP)^{CM}
Pitt Community College
Greenville, North Carolina

Daniel W. Murdock, BT, NREMT-P, CIC
SUNY Cobleskill Paramedic Program
Cobleskill, New York

Colt Patterson, FF, EMT-P, EMT-P I/C, Rescue Diver
Crossville Fire Department
Crossville, Tennessee

Jennifer Purdom, BS, FP-C
PHI Air Medical
Denton, Texas

Bryan L. Spangler, MHA, NREMT-P, EMSI, CMTE
Central Ohio Technical College
Newark, Ohio

Candice Thompson, BS, LAT, NREMT-P
Bulverde-Spring Branch EMS & the Centre for
Emergency Health Sciences
Spring Branch, Texas

Jackilyn E. Williams, RN, MSN, NRP
Portland Community College Paramedic Program
Portland, Oregon

Human Anatomy and Physiology: An Overview

Learning Objectives

1. Define the terms anatomy, physiology, pathophysiology, and homeostasis. (p 2)

2. Describe the systems of the body. (p 2-4)

3. Define the terms anatomic position, frontal plane, transverse plane, sagittal plane, and midsagittal plane. (p 3, 5)

4. Use proper terminology to describe the location of body parts with respect to one another. (p 3, 5-7)

5. Understand the basics of chemistry and their contribution to the study of anatomy and physiology. (p 9-16)

Skidplate © Photodisc; Cells © ImageSource/age fotostock

Introduction

Knowledge of anatomy and physiology is a fundamental portion of the education of any health care provider and is paramount for successful practice as an EMS provider. In every patient encounter, you will call on your knowledge of anatomy and physiology to help you understand the patient's presentation, anticipate or understand the suspected disease process, and make a decision regarding the care you will provide. A strong foundation of anatomy and physiology is also required to help you fully understand the concepts you will learn throughout your education.

Anatomy is the study of the structure and makeup of the organism. This knowledge can be divided into gross anatomy, which studies organs and their location in the body, and microscopic anatomy, which studies the tissue and cellular components that cannot be seen with the naked eye. Physiology is the study of the processes and functions of the body. These systems, operating simultaneously and relying on a great number of interactions, all work together to maintain a state of balance in which organs and systems can function effectively, known as homeostasis. Maintaining homeostasis is necessary for normal life processes to function correctly. The word pathophysiology refers to the study of the functioning of an organism in the presence of disease. When the body can no longer maintain homeostasis, disease may result. Determining the cause of the disease process often helps EMS providers identify a reasonable approach to evaluation and initial treatment of patients.

The study of human anatomy and physiology can be approached in several ways. One approach studies systemic anatomy, which focuses on the anatomy and physiology of each organ system separately. Another approach studies regional anatomy, or specific regions of the body. This textbook follows the systemic approach to the study of anatomy and physiology. Definitions and medical descriptions of various types of body movements are presented.

Individual chapters discuss the following body systems: skeletal, muscular, circulatory, lymphatic, immune, respiratory, nervous, gastrointestinal, urinary, reproductive, endocrine, and integumentary. In addition to the overall description of each system, this textbook presents both the

Case Study | PART 1

Your ambulance is responding to an assault that occurred at a local bar. On arrival near the scene, you see the police already there; they notify you that it is safe for you to proceed directly to the scene. After you have completed the scene size-up, you begin a primary assessment. Your general impression indicates a young man who has numerous cuts and bruises on his torso and extremities. He is in the Fowler position. As you complete your primary assessment, you find no immediate life threats. Your partner quickly obtains a set of baseline vital signs while you begin your rapid trauma exam. On completion of your trauma exam, your partner tells you the patient's baseline vital signs. Most of the bleeding has subsided. During your evaluation you realize that your ability to communicate with medical control and document the patient's injuries on the prehospital care report (PCR) is greatly enhanced by your knowledge of anatomic terms.

Recording Time: 0 Minutes	
Appearance	Young male with no apparent threats to life
Level of consciousness	Alert (oriented to person, place and day)
Airway	Appears patent
Breathing	Normal and regular
Circulation	No life-threatening external bleeding
Pulse	96 beats/min and regular
Blood pressure	118/70 mm Hg
Respirations	20 breaths/min
Spo₂	97%

1. On the basis of the mechanism of injury (MOI) and your findings in the primary assessment, how should you position the patient? *Semi Fowlers Position of Comfort.*

2. What body regions are assessed during the rapid trauma examination?

gross anatomy and the microscopic anatomy or histology of vital structures. How the body systems function, both individually and together as a unit, is also discussed. The basic concepts of chemistry are addressed as an essential component to your understanding of anatomy and physiology.

Clinical Tip

The human body has been studied for thousands of years. Even though some of its inner workings are well understood, new discoveries are still being made even today. Researchers frequently discover new information about physiology, particularly at the molecular level, but basic human anatomy changes only very slowly, over the course of thousands of years.

Overview of Body Systems

The human body is comprised of a series of body parts, cavities, tissues, and organ systems. From an organizational perspective, the organism (human being) is made up of many smaller components, or building blocks. Each of these building blocks is related. As you work your way through these chapters, you will see the relationship between atoms and molecules, macromolecules, organelles, cells, tissue, organs, organ systems, and, ultimately, the organism Figure 1-1.

The following body systems are discussed in detail:

- Skeletal System – is composed of 206 bones and provides the essential functions of support, movement, and protection for the structures of the body.
- Muscular System – is composed of fibers that contract, causing movement. The body contains three types of muscle: skeletal (striated), smooth, and cardiac.
- Circulatory System – consists of the heart, the blood vessels, and the blood.
- Lymphatic System – is a passive circulatory system that transports lymph, a thin plasma-like fluid formed from interstitial or extracellular fluid that bathes the tissues of the body.
- Immune System – is integrally related to the lymphatic system and is the body system that

mounts a defense against foreign substances and disease-causing agents.
- Respiratory System – includes the organs and structures associated with breathing, gas exchange, and the entrance of air into the body.
- Nervous System – is a complex array of structures that help control body activities, both voluntary and involuntary.
- Gastrointestinal System – is composed of structures and organs involved in the consumption, digestion, and elimination of food.
- Urinary System – removes waste products from the blood by a complex filtration process, producing urine.
- Reproductive System – includes the structures, both male and female, that are responsible for sexual reproduction.
- Endocrine System – consists of glands located throughout the body that secrete proteins called hormones to regulate body functions.
- Integumentary System – includes the skin, nails, hair, and sweat and oil glands.

Each of these body systems are illustrated in Figure 1-2.

Topographic Anatomy

The surface of the body has many definite visible features that serve as guides or landmarks to the structures that lie beneath them. You must be able to identify the superficial landmarks of the body—its topographic anatomy—to perform an accurate assessment. To accomplish this,

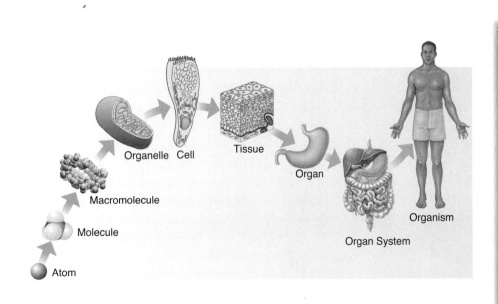

Figure 1-1 Organizational levels of the body.

Source: Adapted from Shier DN, Butler JL, Lewis R. *Hole's Essentials of Human Anatomy & Physiology*, 10th ed. New York, NY: McGraw Hill Higher Education; 2009.

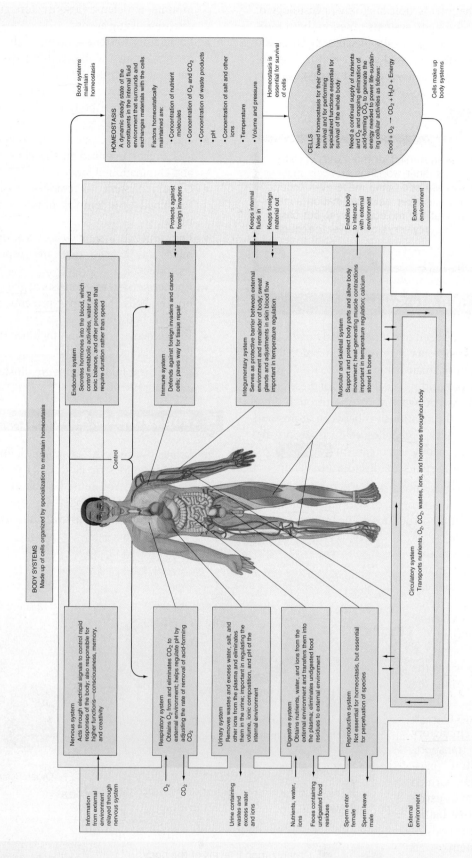

Figure 1-2 Systems of the body.

the terms that are used to describe the topographic anatomy are applied to the body when it is in the anatomic position Figure 1-3. In the anatomic position, the patient stands facing you, arms at the side, with the palms of the hands forward. Directional terms pertain to the patient's left or right as the reference point, not the observer's left or right.

The Planes of the Body

When a patient experiences an injury, the anatomic planes are often used to describe the location of the injury. For example, a patient may have received a laceration to the medial aspect of the midshaft right femur or thigh.

The anatomic planes of the body are imaginary straight lines that divide the body Figure 1-4. These are the frontal (coronal) plane, transverse (axial) plane, and sagittal (lateral) plane. The midsagittal plane (midline) is a special

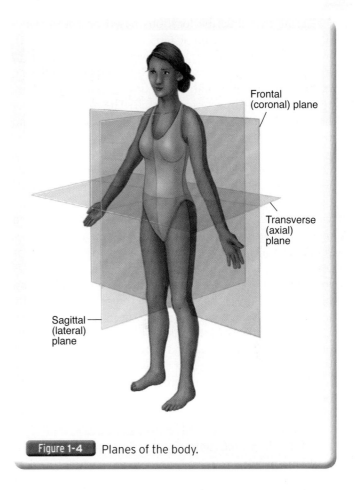

Figure 1-4   Planes of the body.

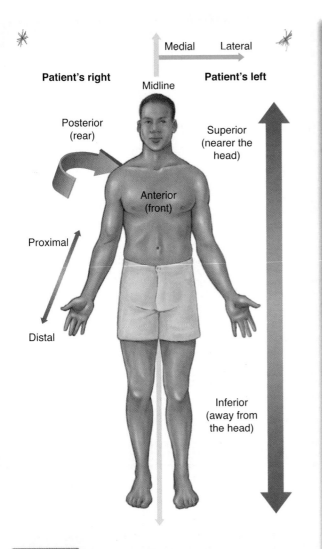

Figure 1-3   The anatomic position. Directional terms indicate the distance and direction from the midline.

Table 1-1	Planes of the Body
Plane of the Body	**Description**
Coronal	Front and back
Transverse	Top and bottom
Sagittal	Left and right
Midsagittal (midline)	Left and right–equal halves

type of sagittal plane where the body is cut in half, leaving equal left and right halves. These planes describe distinct three-dimensional frames of reference about which the location of various organs and their relation to one another may be specified Table 1-1.

Directional Terms

Directional terms used in the study of anatomy include words that describe relative positions of body parts as well as imaginary anatomic divisions. When you are discussing where an injury is located or how a pain radiates in the body, you need to know the correct directional terms.

Terms that describe locations based on the division of the body by the frontal (coronal), transverse (axial), or sagittal (lateral) planes are universally used. Table 1-2 provides these terms, which include superior, inferior, medial, lateral, proximal, distal, superficial, deep, anterior (ventral), and posterior (dorsal). The superior part of the body refers to a structure that is closer to the head from a specific reference point. The inferior part of the body refers to a structure that is closer to the feet. Medial means situated toward the midline or inner structure or organ, whereas lateral means situated away from the midline. Proximal and distal describe the relationship of any two structures on an extremity; proximal means nearer to or toward the trunk of the body, and distal means farther from the trunk and toward the free end of an extremity. For example, the knee is proximal to the ankle, and the wrist is proximal to the fingers; the toe is distal to the ankle, and the wrist is distal to the elbow. Anterior refers to the belly or front side of the body. Another term for anterior is ventral. Posterior refers to the spinal side or back of the body, including the back of the hand. Another term for posterior is dorsal.

The frontal plane runs through the body from head to toe, dividing it into anterior (or ventral) and posterior (or dorsal) sections. For example, pain in the breast area would be described as being located on the anterior, or ventral, portion of the chest wall. An injury near the buttocks, however, would be specified as being located on the posterior, or dorsal, portion of the body.

The transverse plane runs through the body parallel to the horizon. There is no specified area of the body through which this plane must pass. A body part that is closer to the head than another part in the transverse plane is described as being superior to the other part. Any body part closer to the feet than another part in the transverse plane is described as being inferior to the other part. An injury to the breast area would be described as being located superior to the navel (a possible transverse plane), whereas pain in the foot may be described as being inferior to the navel.

The midsagittal plane, also referred to as the midline, runs through the body in line with the umbilicus (navel). It is perpendicular to the frontal plane and divides the body into equal right and left halves. As discussed earlier, structures that are closer to the midline are specified as medial. Structures that are farthest from the midline are specified as lateral.

A number of imaginary lines can also be used to help describe the location of an injury or landmark on the body. A line drawn vertically through the middle portion of the clavicle (collarbone) and parallel to the midline would be the midclavicular line. The midaxillary line is a vertical line drawn through the axilla (armpit) to the waist Figure 1-5. A parallel line drawn about an inch in front of the midaxillary

Table 1-2	Common Directional Terms
Term	**Definition**
Axillary	pertaining to the armpit
Brachial	pertaining to the upper arm
Buccal	pertaining to the cheek
Cardiac	pertaining to the heart
Cervical	pertaining to the neck
Cranial	pertaining to the skull or cranium
Cutaneous	pertaining to the skin
Deltoid	pertaining to the shoulder muscle
Femoral	pertaining to the thigh
Gastric	pertaining to the stomach
Gluteal	pertaining to the buttocks
Hepatic	pertaining to the liver
Inguinal	pertaining to the groin (depressions of abdominal wall near thighs)
Lumbar	pertaining to the loin (lower back, between ribs and pelvis)
Mammary	pertaining to the breast
Nasal	pertaining to the nose
Occipital	pertaining to the inferior posterior region of the head
Orbital	pertaining to the bones surrounding the eye
Parietal	pertaining to the superior posterior region of the head
Patellar	pertaining to the front of the knee (kneecap)
Pectoral	pertaining to the chest
Perineal	pertaining to the perineum; between the sacrum and pubis
Plantar	pertaining to the sole of the foot
Popliteal	pertaining to the posterior knee
Pulmonary	pertaining to the lungs
Renal	pertaining to the kidneys
Sacral	pertaining to the inferior most portion of the spine
Temporal	pertaining to temples of the skull
Umbilical	pertaining to the navel
Volar	pertaining to the sole of the foot or palm of the hand

line would be the anterior axillary line; a parallel line drawn about an inch behind the midaxillary line would be the posterior axillary line.

The way to describe the sections of the abdominal cavity is by quadrants. Imagine two lines intersecting at the umbilicus, dividing the abdomen into four distinct quadrants: the right upper quadrant, left upper quadrant, right lower quadrant, and left lower quadrant. Specific organs are located in each of the four quadrants, and pain or injury often is described as being in a specific quadrant Figure 1-6 . An example would be the typical presentation of appendicitis—periumbilical pain that migrates to the right lower quadrant over time.

Clinical Tip

Often the lungs are auscultated for the presence of air movement in the location where the anterior axillary line intercepts the nipple level. An understanding of the imaginary lines helps the EMS provider decide exactly where to place the diaphragm of the stethoscope.

Movement and Positional Terms

All movements of the body, from the simplest grasp to the most complicated ballet or martial arts maneuvers, can be broken down into a series of simple components and described with specific terms. As with the terms for anatomic positions, an accepted set of terms describes body movements. These are particularly useful in describing how an injury occurred.

Range of motion (ROM) is the full distance that a joint can be moved. In the anatomic position, moving a distal point of an extremity closer to the trunk is called flexion. Flexion of the elbow brings the hand closer to the shoulder, flexion of the knee brings the foot up to the buttocks, and flexion of the fingers forms the hand into a fist. Extension is the motion associated with the return of a body part from a flexed position to the anatomic position. In the anatomic position, all extremities are in extension A patient's neck can be in one of several positions when the patient is found in the supine position Figure 1-7 .

The prefix hyper often is added to the terms flexion or extension to indicate a mechanism of injury. Hyper

Case Study   PART 2

After making sure that the patient has not sustained any back or neck injury and learning that the patient is feeling a little dizzy, you position him down on his back in the supine position to perform the rest of your examination.

The injuries you find include the following:

- A deep laceration to the medial aspect of the right forearm
- A superficial laceration to the right anterior chest extending from the midclavicular line to the anterior axillary line at the nipple level
- A contusion to the right upper quadrant of the abdomen
- A contusion to the lateral aspect of the left midshaft thigh (femur)

Recording Time: 5 Minutes	
Appearance	Multiple cuts and bruises
Level of consciousness	Alert (oriented to person, place and day)
Airway	Open and clear
Breathing	Normal and regular
Circulation	Pale skin, most bleeding subsided

3. Why were the patient's legs not elevated?

4. What area of the body do you think would be most commonly overlooked for injuries?

5. On the basis of the location of the injuries discovered, which injury has the potential for being the most serious?

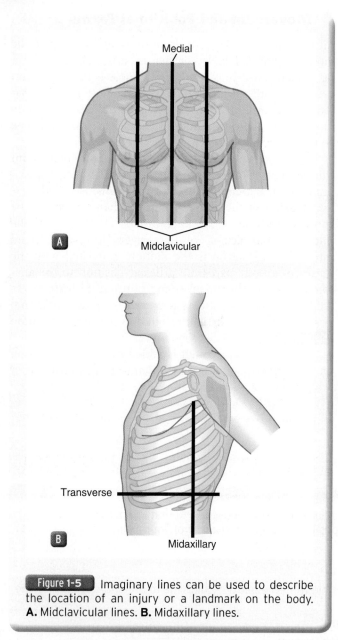

A

Medial

Midclavicular

Transverse

B

Midaxillary

Figure 1-5 Imaginary lines can be used to describe the location of an injury or a landmark on the body. **A.** Midclavicular lines. **B.** Midaxillary lines.

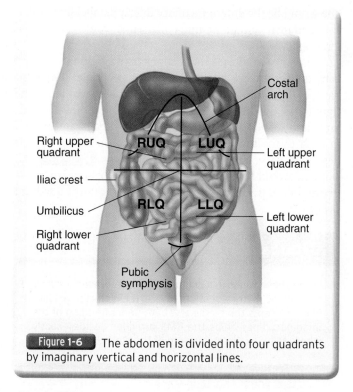

Figure 1-6 The abdomen is divided into four quadrants by imaginary vertical and horizontal lines.

Right upper quadrant — RUQ
LUQ — Left upper quadrant
Costal arch
Iliac crest
Umbilicus
RLQ
LLQ — Left lower quadrant
Right lower quadrant
Pubic symphysis

implies that the normal range of motion for the particular movement was maximized or even exceeded, potentially resulting in injury. This prefix is used commonly in clinical literature, as well as in written and verbal communication among health care providers. The term hyperflexion refers to a body part that was flexed to the maximum level or even beyond the normal ROM. A hyperflexion injury to the back can occur while bending. Hyperextension refers to a body part that was extended to the maximum level or even beyond the normal ROM. A hyperextension injury occurs when a person falls on an outstretched hand, resulting in a distal radius fracture **Figure 1-8**. Ankle injuries can also be described using the terms supination and pronation.

Internal rotation describes turning an extremity medially toward the midline. The lower extremity is internally rotated when the toes are turned inward. External rotation describes turning an extremity away from the midline. Often, when an injured extremity is compared with the uninjured extremity, rotational deformities are noted. A hip can be dislocated anteriorly or posteriorly. In an anterior hip dislocation, the foot is externally rotated and the head of the femur is palpable in the inguinal area. In the more common posterior hip dislocation, the knee and foot usually are flexed internally. The term rotation also can be applied to the spine. The spine is rotated when it twists on its axis. Placing the chin on the shoulder rotates the cervical spine. Abduction of an extremity moves it away from the midline. Adduction moves the extremity toward the midline.

Recumbent refers to any position in which the patient is lying down or leaning back. The body is in the supine position when lying face up; the body is in the prone position when lying face down. In the Trendelenburg position, the body is supine with the head lower than the feet. A patient who is sitting up with the knees bent or straight is in the Fowler position; a patient who is sitting up but with the upper body slightly leaning back is in the semi-Fowler position. The recovery position, also referred to as the left lateral recumbent position, is used to help maintain a clear airway in an unresponsive patient. A patient who has not sustained trauma to the neck or back but who needs

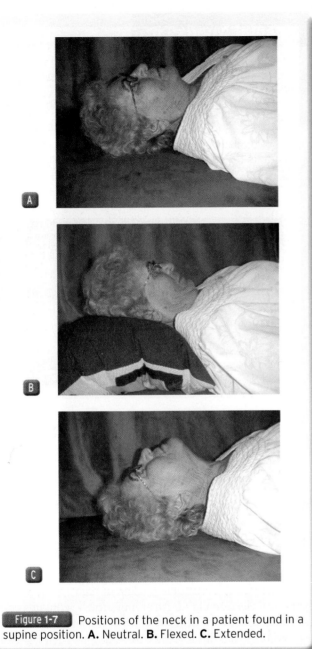

Courtesy of Rhonda Beck

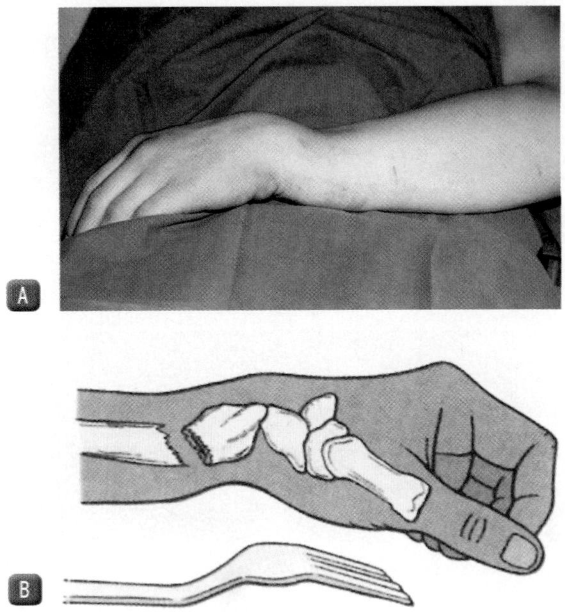

© Wellcome Photo Library/Custom Medical Stock Photo

Figure 1-7 Positions of the neck in a patient found in a supine position. **A.** Neutral. **B.** Flexed. **C.** Extended.

Figure 1-8 The range of motion of an extremity can be limited by a fracture. Fractures of the distal radius produce a characteristic silver fork deformity.

to be placed in a position where fluids can drain from the mouth should be placed in the recovery position **Figure 1-9** .

Clinical Tip

Most patients are placed in either a supine or Fowler position for transport. Unless there are extenuating circumstances, such as the presence of an impaled object, a patient should not be transported in a prone position, especially when the patient has been restrained. Patient deaths have resulted from hypoxia or asphyxia.

Basic Chemistry

If you understand the basics of chemistry, your understanding of anatomy and physiology will be improved. Chemistry is the study of matter, which is defined as anything that takes up space and has mass. Mass is a physical property that determines an object's weight, based on the earth's gravitational pull. Elements are fundamental substances that compose matter. Most living organisms need about 20 elements to survive. **Table 1-3** lists the major and trace elements required by the human body.

Atoms are tiny particles that compose elements. Atoms are the smallest complete units of an element, and vary in size, weight, and interaction with other atoms. The characteristics of living and nonliving objects result from the atoms that they contain, as well as how those atoms combine and interact. Thus, by forming chemical bonds, atoms can combine with other atoms that are not similar to them.

Atomic Structure

Atoms are composed of subatomic particles. Each atom consists of protons, neutrons, and electrons. Protons and neutrons are similar in size and mass; however, protons bear a positive electrical charge whereas neutrons are electrically neutral (uncharged). Electrons bear a negative electrical charge. An atom's mass is determined mostly by the

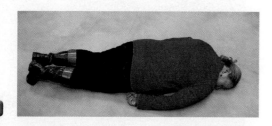

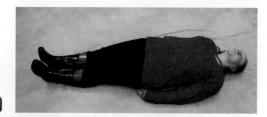

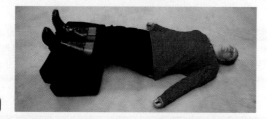

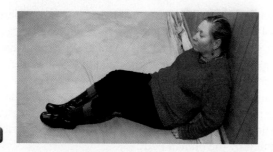

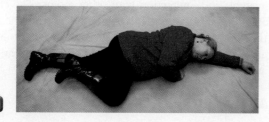

© Jones & Bartlett Learning. Courtesy of MIEMSS

Figure 1-9 Anatomic positions. **A.** Prone. **B.** Supine. **C.** Modified Trendelenburg position. **D.** Fowler position. **E.** Recovery position.

Special Needs Tip

Infants and small children should not be placed with the neck in a hyperextended position; instead, they should simply be placed with their neck extended or in a neutral position. This position prevents kinking of an infant's soft airway. It also is important to remember that the toddler has a relatively large head compared with the rest of the body, so the easiest way to open a toddler's airway is to place a small towel behind the shoulders **Figure 1-10**.

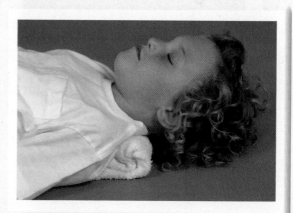

© Jones & Bartlett Learning. Courtesy of MIEMSS

Figure 1-10 Placing a small towel behind a toddler's shoulders helps to keep the neck in the neutral or extended position.

number of protons and neutrons in the nucleus. The mass of a larger object, such as the human body, is the sum of the masses of all of its atoms **Figure 1-12**.

Electrons orbit an atom's nucleus at high speed, forming a spherical electron cloud. An atom normally contains equal numbers of protons and electrons in its nucleus. The number of protons in an atom is known as its atomic number. Thus, hydrogen (H), the simplest atom, has one proton, giving it the atomic number 1, whereas magnesium, with 12 protons, has the atomic number 12.

The atomic weight of an element's atom equals the number of protons and neutrons in its nucleus. For example, oxygen has eight protons and eight neutrons, so its atomic weight is 16. An isotope is defined as when an element's atoms have nuclei containing the same number of protons, but different numbers of neutrons. Isotopes may or may not be radioactive. Radioactivity is the emission of energetic particles known as radiation, which occurs because of instability of the atomic nuclei.

The nuclei of certain isotopes (radioisotopes) spontaneously emit subatomic particles or radiation in measurable amounts. The process of emitting radiation is called

Table 1-3 Elements of the Human Body	
Major Elements (totaling 99.9%)	**Percentage in the Body**
Oxygen (O)	65%
Carbon (C)	18.5%
Hydrogen (H)	9.5%
Nitrogen (N)	3.2%
Calcium (Ca)	1.5%
Phosphorus (P)	1%
Potassium (K)	0.4%
Sulfur (S)	0.3%
Chlorine (Cl)	0.2%
Sodium (Na)	0.2%
Magnesium (Mg)	0.1%
Trace Elements (totaling 0.1%)	
Chromium (Cr)	–
Cobalt (Co)	–
Copper (Cu)	–
Fluorine (F)	–
Iodine (I)	–
Iron (Fe)	–
Manganese (Mn)	–
Zinc (Zn)	–

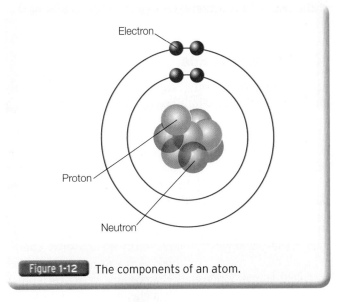

Figure 1-12 The components of an atom.

radioactive decay. Strongly radioactive isotopes are dangerous because their emissions can destroy molecules, cells, and living tissue. For diagnostic procedures, weaker radioactive isotopes are used to diagnose structural and functional characteristics of internal organs. Radiation occurs in one of three common forms: alpha, beta, or gamma. Gamma radiation is the most penetrating type, and is similar to x-ray radiation.

Molecules

The term molecule is defined as any chemical structure that consists of atoms held together by covalent bonds (involving the sharing of electrons between atoms). When two atoms

Clinical Tip

Normally, the jugular veins of the neck are not prominent when a patient is standing or sitting. However, when the patient is in the supine position, it is expected that the veins in the neck would fill with blood. The presence of jugular venous distention (JVD) in the patient who is not supine is an indication that the blood may be having difficulty flowing back into the right side of the heart, possibly because of a pericardial tamponade, tension pneumothorax, or right-sided heart failure. The medical patient is routinely assessed for JVD in the semi-Fowler position **Figure 1-11**. Generally, trauma patients are immobilized in the supine position, so an assessment for JVD may not be entirely accurate.

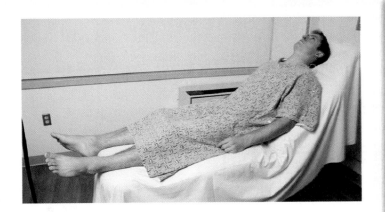

Figure 1-11 Medical patients are assessed for JVD in the semi-Fowler position. In this position, the jugular veins generally should not be distended unless there is a significant medical abnormality.

of the same element bond, they produce molecules of that element, such as hydrogen, oxygen, or nitrogen molecules.

Chemical Bonds

Atoms can bond with other atoms by using chemical bonds that result from interactions between their electrons. During this process, the atoms may gain, lose, or share electrons. Chemically inactive atoms are known as *inert* atoms. An example of a chemical that is made up of inert atoms is helium. Atoms that either gain or lose electrons are called ions. These atoms are electrically charged. An example of an electrically charged atom, or ion, is sodium.

Ionic Bonds

Ionic bonds form between ions. Ions with a positive charge (+) are called cations, and those with a negative charge (−) are called anions. Oppositely charged ions attract each other to form an ionic bond. This is a chemical bond that forms arrays (indiscreet molecules) such as crystals. An example is when sodium forms an ionic bond with chloride to create sodium chloride (table salt).

Covalent Bonds

Some atoms can complete their outer electron shells by sharing electrons to create a covalent bond. They do not gain or lose electrons. In a covalent bond, each atom achieves a stable form. An example of a covalent bond is when two hydrogen atoms bond to form a hydrogen molecule Figure 1-13 .

If a single pair of electrons is shared, the result is a single covalent bond. If two pairs are shared, the result is a double covalent bond. Some atoms can even form triple covalent bonds. Some covalent bonds do not share electrons equally, resulting in a polar molecule—one that has an uneven distribution of charges. Polar molecules have equal numbers of protons and electrons, but one end of the molecule is slightly negative while the other end is slightly positive. An example of a polar molecule is water, created by hydrogen and oxygen atoms.

When the positive hydrogen end of a polar molecule is attracted to the negative nitrogen or oxygen end of another polar molecule, the attraction is called a hydrogen bond Figure 1-14 . These bonds are weak at body temperature, and may change form, from water to ice and back again. Hydrogen bonds are important in protein and nucleic acid structure, forming between polar regions of different parts of a single, large molecule.

Molecules made up of different bonded atoms are called compounds. Examples of compounds include water (a compound of hydrogen and oxygen), table sugar, baking soda, alcohol as used in beverages, natural gas, and most medicinal drugs. A molecule of a compound has specific types

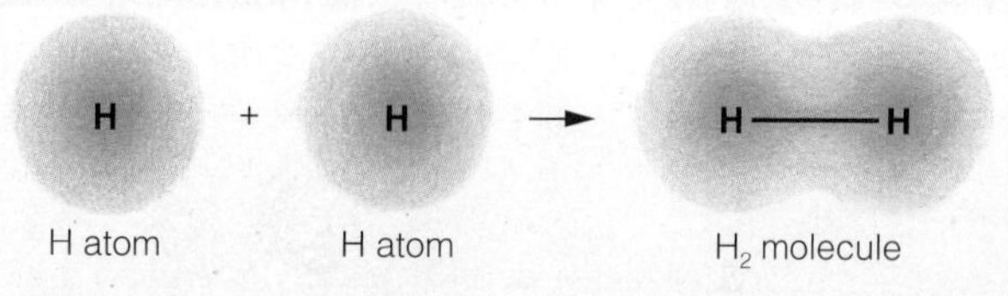

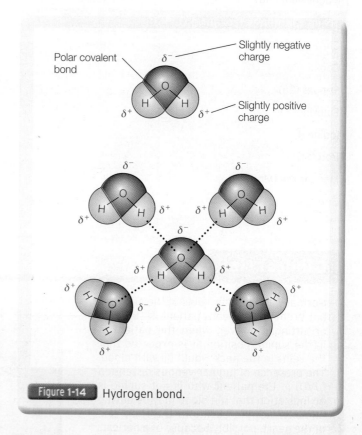

Figure 1-13 Covalent bond.

Figure 1-14 Hydrogen bond.

Case Study   PART 3

To prepare for transport, you decide to place the patient in the left lateral recumbent position because he is now nauseated but is no longer complaining of dizziness. Being comfortable using anatomic terms will help you when you describe the patient's injuries to hospital personnel and complete the PCR.

6. What should be assessed in an injured extremity?

7. What knowledge is necessary to describe the location of a patient's pain or injury?

and amounts of atoms. For example, water consists of two hydrogen atoms and one oxygen atom. When two hydrogen atoms bind with two oxygen atoms, they form hydrogen peroxide instead of water.

The numbers and types of atoms in a molecule are represented by a molecular formula. The molecular formula for water is H_2O, signifying the two atoms of hydrogen and the one atom of oxygen. Structural formulas are used to signify how atoms are joined and arranged inside molecules. Single bonds are represented by single lines, and double bonds are represented by double lines. When structural formulas are represented in three-dimensional models, different colors are used to show different types of atoms.

Types of Chemical Reactions

Four types of chemical reactions are important to the study of physiology: synthesis reactions, decomposition reactions, exchange reactions, and reversible reactions.

Synthesis Reactions

Chemical reactions change the bonds between atoms, molecules, and ions to generate new chemical combinations. A synthesis reaction is a reaction that occurs when two or more reactants (atoms) bond to form a more complex product or structure. The formation of water from hydrogen and oxygen molecules is a synthesis reaction. Synthesis always involves the formation of new chemical bonds, whether the reactants are atoms or molecules. Synthesis requires energy, and it is important for growth and the repair of tissues.

Synthesis is symbolized as follows: A + B $\longrightarrow$ AB

Decomposition Reactions

A decomposition reaction is a reaction that occurs when bonds within a reactant molecule break, forming simpler atoms, molecules, or ions. For example, a typical meal contains molecules of sugars, proteins, and fats that are too large and too complex to be absorbed and used by the body. Decomposition reactions in the digestive tract break these molecules down into smaller fragments before absorption begins.

Decomposition is symbolized as follows: AB $\longrightarrow$ A + B

Exchange Reactions

In an exchange reaction, parts of the reacting molecules are shuffled around to produce new products. An example of an exchange reaction is the reaction of an acid with a base, which forms water and a salt.

Exchange reactions are symbolized as follows:
AB + CD $\longrightarrow$ AD + CB

Reversible Reactions

A reversible reaction is one wherein the products of the reaction can change back into the reactants they originally were. These reactions can proceed in opposite directions, depending on the relative proportions of reactants and products, as well as how much energy is available.

So, if A + B $\rightleftharpoons$ AB, then AB $\rightleftharpoons$ A + B. Many important biologic reactions are freely reversible.

Enzymes

Enzymes promote chemical reactions by lowering the activation energy requirements. Activation energy is the energy that must be overcome in order for a chemical reaction to occur. Therefore, enzymes make chemical reactions possible. They belong to a class of substances called catalysts (compounds that accelerate chemical reactions without themselves being permanently changed or consumed). A cell makes an enzyme molecule to promote a specific reaction. Enzymatic reactions, which are reversible, can be written as:

enzyme
A + B $\rightleftharpoons$ AB

Acids, Bases, and the pH Scale

Electrolytes are substances that release ions in water. When they dissolve in water, the negative and positive ends of water molecules cause ions to separate and interact with water molecules instead of each other. The resulting solution contains electrically charged particles (ions) that will conduct electricity. Acids are electrolytes that release hydrogen ions in water. An example of an acid is hydrochloric acid, made up of hydrogen and chloride ions. Bases are electrolytes that release ions that bond with hydrogen ions. An example of a base is sodium hydroxide, made up of sodium, oxygen, and hydrogen ions. In body fluids, the concentrations of hydrogen and hydroxide ions greatly affect chemical reactions. These reactions control certain physiologic functions such as blood pressure and breathing rates.

Hydrogen ion concentrations can be measured by a value called pH. The hydrogen ion concentration in body fluids is vital. It is expressed in a type of mathematical shorthand based on concentrations calculated in moles per liter (with a mole representing an amount of solute in a solution). The pH of a solution is defined as the level of acidity or alkalinity. The pH scale ranges from 0 to 14, with 7 being the midpoint (meaning it has equal numbers of hydrogen and hydroxide ions). Pure water has a pH of 7, and this midpoint is considered to be neutral (neither acidic nor basic). Measurements of less than 7 pH are considered acidic, meaning that there are more hydrogen ions than hydroxide ions. Measurements of more than 7 pH are considered basic, also known as alkaline, meaning that there are more hydroxide ions than hydrogen ions.

The pH of blood usually ranges from 7.35 to 7.45. Abnormal fluctuations in pH can damage cells and tissues, change the shapes of proteins, and alter cellular functions. Acidosis is an abnormal physiologic state caused by a blood pH that is lower than 7.35. If pH falls below 7, coma may occur. Alkalosis results from a blood pH that is higher than 7.45. If pH rises above 7.8, it generally causes uncontrollable and sustained skeletal muscle contractions.

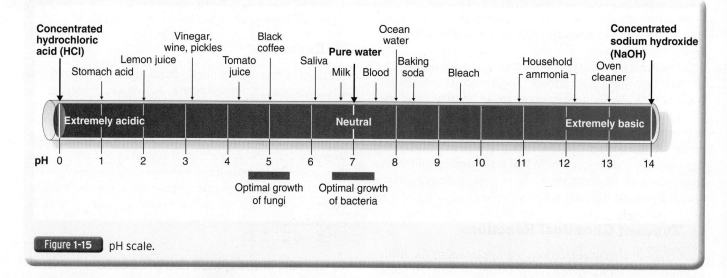

Figure 1-15 pH scale.

Chemicals that resist pH changes are called buffers. They combine with hydrogen ions when these ions are excessive and contribute hydrogen ions when these ions are reduced. **Figure 1-15** shows the pH values of various acids and bases.

Chemical Constituents of Cells

Chemicals can basically be divided into two main groups: organic and inorganic. Organic chemicals are those that always contain the elements carbon and hydrogen, and generally oxygen as well. Inorganic chemicals are any chemicals that do not. Inorganic substances release ions in water and are also called electrolytes. Though many organic substances also dissolve in water, they dissolve to greater effect in alcohol or ether. Organic substances that dissolve in water usually do not release ions and are known as nonelectrolytes.

Inorganic Substances

Inorganic substances in body cells include oxygen, carbon dioxide, compounds that are known as salts, and water. The most abundant compound in the human body is water, accounting for nearly two thirds of body weight. Any substance that dissolves in water is called a solute. Because solutes dissolved in water are more likely to react with each other as they break down into smaller particles, most metabolic reactions occur in water. In the blood, the watery (aqueous) portion carries vital substances such as oxygen, salts, sugars, and vitamins among the digestive tract, respiratory tract, and the cells.

Oxygen enters the body through the respiratory organs and is transported in the blood. The red blood cells bind and carry the largest amount of oxygen. Organelles inside the cells use oxygen for energy release from nutrients such as glucose (sugar) to drive cellular metabolic activities. Carbon dioxide is an inorganic compound produced as a waste product when some metabolic processes release energy. It is exhaled via the lungs.

Salts are compounds of oppositely charged ions that are abundant in tissues in fluids. Many ions required by the body are supplied in salts, including sodium, chloride, calcium, magnesium, phosphate, carbonate, bicarbonate, potassium, and sulfate. Salt ions are important for transporting substances to and from the cells, as well as for muscle contractions and nerve impulse conduction.

Organic Substances

Organic substances include carbohydrates, lipids, proteins, and nucleic acids. Many organic molecules are made up of long chains of carbon atoms linked by covalent bonds. The carbon atoms usually form additional covalent bonds with hydrogen or oxygen atoms and, less commonly, covalent bonds with nitrogen, phosphorus, sulfur, or other elements.

Carbohydrates

Carbohydrates provide much of the energy required by the body's cells, as well as helping to build cell structures. Carbohydrate molecules consist of carbon, hydrogen, and oxygen molecules. The carbon atoms they contain join in chains that vary with the type of carbohydrate. Carbohydrates with shorter chains are called sugars.

Simple sugars have 6 carbon atoms, 12 hydrogen atoms, and 6 oxygen atoms ($C_6H_{12}O_6$). They are also known as monosaccharides. Simple sugars include glucose, fructose, galactose, ribose, and deoxyribose. Ribose and deoxyribose differ from the others in that they each contain five atoms of carbon. Complex carbohydrates include sucrose (table sugar) and lactose (milk sugar). Some of these carbohydrates are double sugars or disaccharides. Other types of complex carbohydrates contain many simple joined sugar units, such as plant starch, and are known as polysaccharides. Humans and other animals synthesize a polysaccharide called glycogen.

Lipids

Lipids are not soluble in water. They may dissolve in other lipids, oils, ether, chloroform, or alcohol. Lipids include a variety of compounds with vital cell functions. These compounds include fats, phospholipids, and steroids. Fats are the most common type of lipids. Like carbohydrates, fat molecules also contain carbon, hydrogen, and oxygen, but they have far fewer oxygen atoms than do carbohydrates.

Fatty acids and glycerol are the building blocks of fat molecules. A single fat molecule consists of one glycerol molecule bonded to three fatty acid molecules. These fat molecules are known as triglycerides, a subcategory of lipids that includes fat and oil. These molecules are formed by the condensation of one molecule of glycerol, which is a three-carbon alcohol. Glycerol contains three fatty acid molecules. Triglycerides contain different saturated and unsaturated fatty acid combinations. Those with mostly saturated fatty acids are called saturated fats. Those with mostly unsaturated fatty acids are called unsaturated fats.

Saturated fat is defined as containing carbon atoms that are bound to as many hydrogen atoms as possible, becoming saturated with them. Fatty acid molecules with double bonds only are called unsaturated. Fatty acid molecules with many double-bonded carbon atoms are called polyunsaturated.

Similar to a fat molecule, a phospholipid consists of a glycerol portion with fatty acid chains. Phospholipids are structurally related to glycolipids. Human cells can synthesize both types of lipids, primarily from fatty acids. A phospholipid includes a phosphate group that is soluble in water and a fatty acid portion that is not. Phospholipids are an important part of cell structures.

Steroid molecules are large lipid molecules that share a distinctive carbon framework. Steroids have four connected rings of carbon atoms. All steroid molecules have the same basic structure: three 6-carbon rings joined to one 5-carbon ring. They include cholesterol, estrogen, progesterone, testosterone, cortisol, and estradiol.

Proteins

Proteins are the most abundant organic components of the human body, and in many ways the most important. Proteins are vital for many body functions, including structures and their functions, energy, enzymatic function, defense (antibodies), and hormonal requirements. On cell surfaces, some proteins combine with carbohydrates to become glycoproteins. They allow cells to respond to certain molecules that bind to them.

There are more than 200,000 types of proteins in the human body. Antibodies are proteins that detect and destroy foreign substances. All proteins contain carbon, hydrogen, oxygen, and nitrogen atoms, with small quantities of sulfur also present. Proteins always contain nitrogen atoms. Twenty-two different amino acids make up the proteins that exist in humans and most other living organisms. Protein molecules consisting of amino acids held together by peptide bonds are called peptides.

Other types of proteins include structural proteins such as collagen, which gives strength to ligaments and connective tissues, and keratin, which functions to prevent water loss through the skin. More active proteins include antibodies and enzymes. Cell membrane proteins may serve as receptors and carriers for specific molecules.

Nucleic Acids

Nucleic acids are large organic molecules (macromolecules) that carry genetic information or form structures within cells. They are composed of carbon, hydrogen, oxygen, nitrogen, and phosphorus. Nucleic acids store and process information at the molecular level, inside the cells. The two classes of nucleic acids are deoxyribonucleic acid (DNA) and ribonucleic acid (RNA). Nucleic acids are found in all living things, cells, and viruses.

The DNA in your cells determines your inherited characteristics, including hair color, eye color, and blood type. DNA affects all aspects of body structure and function. DNA molecules encode the information needed to build proteins. By directing structural protein synthesis, DNA controls the shape and physical characteristics of the human body.

Several forms of RNA cooperate to manufacture specific proteins by using the information provided by DNA. Important structural differences distinguish RNA from DNA. An RNA molecule consists of a single chain of nucleotides.

Human cells have three types of RNA:

- Messenger RNA (mRNA)
- Transfer RNA (tRNA)
- Ribosomal RNA (rRNA)

A DNA molecule consists of a pair of nucleotide chains **Figure 1-16**. The two DNA strands twist around each other in a double helix that resembles a spiral staircase.

Case Study | PART 4

While en route to the hospital, you perform a reassessment of the patient. You check your interventions by assessing the adequacy of oxygen delivery and management of bleeding and wound care. Your knowledge of anatomic definitions and positions is an important part of the assessment and management of this patient.

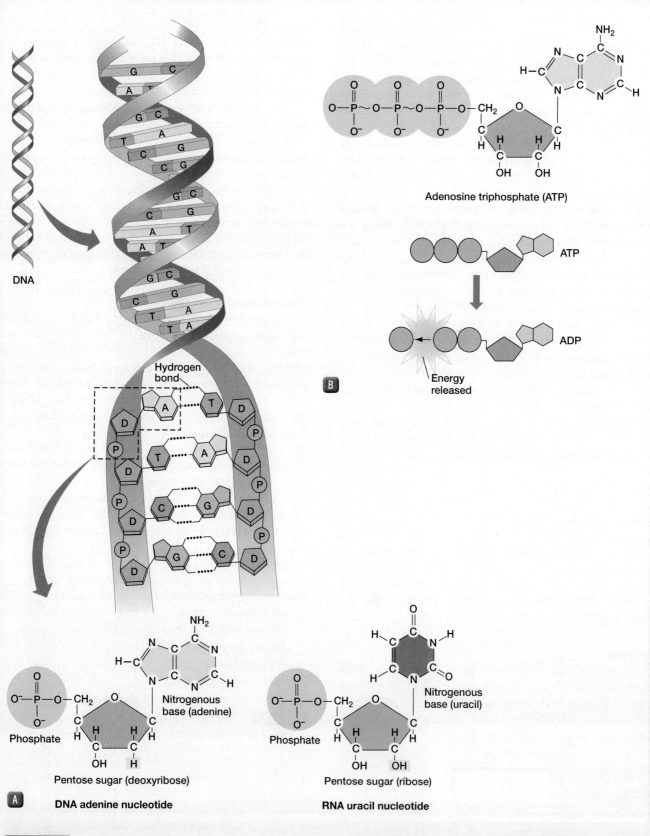

Figure 1-16   **A.** Nucleic acids, DNA, a DNA nucleotide, and an RNA nucleotide. **B.** Adenosine triphosphate (ATP).

Prep Kit

Chapter Summary

- The systemic approach to anatomy and physiology is presented.
- Topographic anatomy involves terminology used to describe the body's parts in relationship to the body surface and the anatomic position.
- Imaginary planes or flat surfaces are used as references when describing locations on the body (ie, frontal plane, transverse plane, sagittal plane, and midsagittal plane).
- The anatomic position is the position of reference in which the patient stands facing you, arms at the side, with the palms of the hands forward.
- Terms such as anterior, posterior, superior, and inferior are used to describe specific locations of injuries or abnormalities.
- Movements of body parts about joints can be described in terms of extension, flexion, rotation, abduction, and adduction.
- Gross anatomy focuses on the parts visible to the naked eye.
- Microscopic anatomy focuses on parts visible only with a microscope.
- Chemistry describes the composition of substances and how chemicals react with each other. The human body is made up of chemicals.
- Elements are composed of atoms, which are the smallest complete units of elements.
- An atom consists of one or more electrons surrounding a nucleus, which contains one or more protons and usually one or more neutrons.
- Electrons are negative, protons are positive, and neutrons are uncharged.
- When atoms combine, they gain, lose, or share electrons.
- Organic substances in cells include carbohydrates, lipids, proteins, and nucleic acids.
- Nucleic acids carry genetic information or form structures with cells, and include DNA and RNA.
- Terminology is standardized and its use is important for documentation by the EMS provider in the field.

Vital Vocabulary

abduction Motion of a limb away from the midline.

acids Electrolytes that dissociate in water to release hydrogen ions.

activation energy The amount of energy required to start a reaction.

adduction Motion of a limb toward the midline.

anatomic planes Imaginary surfaces used as references to identify parts of the body.

anatomic position The position of reference in which the patient stands facing you, arms at the side, with the palms of the hands forward.

anatomy The study of the structure of an organism and its parts.

anion An ion that contains an overall negative charge.

anterior The front surface of the body; the side facing forward in the anatomic position.

atomic number A whole number representing the number of positively charged protons in the nucleus of an atom.

atomic weight The total number of protons and neutrons in the nucleus of an atom.

atoms The smallest complete units of an element that have the element's properties; they vary in size, weight, and interaction with other atoms.

bases Electrolytes that release ions that bond with hydrogen ions.

carbohydrates Substances (including sugars and starches) that provide much of the energy required by the body's cells, as well as helping to build cell structures.

catalysts Atoms or molecules that can change the rate of a reaction without being consumed during the process.

cation An ion that contains an overall positive charge.

chemistry The study of the composition of matter and changes in its composition.

compounds Molecules made up of different bonded atoms.

covalent bond A chemical bond where atoms complete their outer electron shells by sharing electrons.

decomposition reaction A reaction that occurs when bonds with a reactant molecule break, forming simpler atoms, molecules, or ions.

distal Farther from the trunk or nearer to the free end of an extremity.

dorsal The posterior surface of the body, including the back of the hand.

electrolytes Salt or acid substances that become ionic conductors when dissolved in a solvent (ie, water); chemicals dissolved in the blood.

electrons Single, negatively charged particles that revolve around the nucleus of an atom.

elements Fundamental substances, such as carbon, hydrogen, and oxygen, that compose matter.

enzymes Substances designed to speed up the rate of specific biochemical reactions.

exchange reaction A chemical reaction where parts of the reacting molecules are shuffled around to produce new products.

extension The bending of a joint resulting in the distal segment moving away from the proximal segment. Typically results in straightening of the limb at the joint.

external rotation Rotating an extremity at its joint away from the midline.

flexion The bending of a joint resulting in the distal segment moving toward the proximal segment.

Fowler position The position in which the patient is sitting up with the knees bent or straight.

frontal (coronal) plane An imaginary plan dividing the body into anterior and posterior halves.

gross anatomy The study of body parts that are visible to the naked eye, such as bones, muscles, and organs.

homeostasis A tendency to constancy or stability in the body's internal environment.

hydrogen bond The attraction of the positive hydrogen end of a polar molecule to the negative nitrogen or oxygen end of another polar molecule.

hyperextension When a body part is extended to the maximum level or beyond the normal range of motion.

hyperflexion When a body part is flexed to the maximum level or beyond the normal range of motion.

inferior Below a body part or nearer to the feet.

inorganic Not having both carbon and hydrogen atoms.

internal rotation Rotating the segment of the extremity distal to the joint toward the midline.

ions Atoms that either gain or lose electrons.

isotope One of two (or more) forms of an element having the same number of protons and electrons, but different numbers of neutrons; they may or may not be radioactive.

lateral In anatomy, parts of the body that lie farther from the midline; also called outer structures.

lipids Fats, fat-like substances (cholesterol and phospholipids), and oils that supply energy for body processes and building of certain structures.

medial Parts of the body that lie closer to the midline; also called inner structures.

microscopic anatomy The study of tissue structure and/or cellular structure or organization, often visible only through a microscope.

midaxillary line An imaginary line drawn through the midportion of the axilla to the waist that is parallel to the midline.

midclavicular line An imaginary line drawn through the midpoint of the clavicle that is parallel to the midline.

midsagittal plane An imaginary vertical line drawn from the middle of the forehead through the nose and the umbilicus (navel) to the floor; also called the midline.

molecule Particles made up of two or more joined atoms.

neutrons Unchanged or "neutral" particles in the nucleus of an atom.

nucleic acids Large organic molecules, or macromolecules, that carry genetic information or form structures within cells, and include DNA and RNA.

organic Having both carbon and hydrogen atoms.

pathophysiology The study of body functions of a living organism in an abnormal state.

peptides Protein molecules consisting of amino acids held together by peptide bonds.

pH The measure of acidity or alkalinity of a solution.

phospholipid A type of lipid molecule that comprises the cell membrane.

physiology The study of the body functions of the living organism.

polar molecule A molecule that uses a covalent bond in which electrons are not shared equally; this results in a shape that has an uneven distribution of charges.

posterior In anatomy, the back surface of the body.

pronation Rotation of an extremity so that the palm faces downward.

prone position Lying flat, and face down.

proteins Created from amino acids, they include enzymes, plasma proteins, muscle components (actin and myosin), hormones, and antibodies.

protons Single, positively charged particles inside the nucleus of an atom.

proximal Closer to the trunk.

radioisotopes Also known as radioactive isotopes or radionuclides, they are atoms with unstable nuclei.

range of motion (ROM) The arc of movement of an extremity at a joint.

recovery position When a patient is placed on his or her side to allow the easy drainage of fluids from the mouth; also called the left lateral recumbent position.

recumbent Any position in which the patient is lying down or leaning back.

regional anatomy Study of anatomy associated with a particular body region; also called topographic anatomy.

reversible reaction A chemical reaction where the products of the reaction can change back into the reactants they originally were.

sagittal (lateral) plane An imaginary plane dividing the body into left and right parts.

steroid Molecules with four connected rings of carbon atoms, including cholesterol, estrogen, progesterone, testosterone, cortisol, and estradiol.

superior Above a body part or nearer to the head.

supination Turning the palms upward (toward the sky).

supine position The position in which the body is lying face up.

synthesis reaction A reaction that occurs when two or more reactants (atoms) bond to form a more complex product or structure.

systemic anatomy The study of anatomy associated with a particular organ system.

topographic anatomy The study of anatomy associated with a particular body region; also called regional anatomy.

transverse (axial) plane An imaginary line where the body is cut into top and bottom parts.

Trendelenburg position The position in which the body is supine with the head lower than the feet.

ventral The anterior surface of the body.

■ Case Study Answers

1. On the basis of the mechanism of injury (MOI) and your findings in the primary assessment, how should you position the patient?

   Answer: On the basis of a potentially significant MOI and the discovery of no immediate life threats during the primary assessment, you should manually stabilize the patient's head and neck while the patient remains in Fowler's position, until you are able to determine that there is no possibility of spinal injury.

2. What body regions are assessed during the trauma examination?

   Answer: The trauma examination is a quick head-to-toe physical examination to determine whether injuries have occurred to the head, neck, anterior chest, abdomen, pelvis, extremities, and posterior surface of the body. Some systems refer to this as the "rapid trauma exam."

3. Why were the patient's legs not elevated?

   Answer: The Trendelenburg position, in which the patient is supine with the lower extremities elevated and the head down, is now controversial. In many local protocols, this position is not recommended due to a lack of evidence in its effectiveness and due to the potential risk of increasing intracranial pressure.

4. What area of the body do you think would be most commonly overlooked for injuries?

   Answer: The posterior surface of the body frequently is overlooked for injuries. Often, the patient is secured on a long backboard and treatment is begun without any inspection of the back for injury.

5. On the basis of the location of the injuries discovered, which injury has the potential for being the most serious?

   Answer: The contusion in the right upper quadrant of the abdomen indicates the potential for significant internal hemorrhage. (The presence of facial injuries could indicate a possible head injury.)

6. What should be assessed in an injured extremity?

   Answer: Assess the injured extremity for deformities, contusions, abrasions, punctures, burns, tenderness, lacerations, and swelling. Also check distal pulse, motor, and sensation (PMS) functions and range of motion.

7. What knowledge is necessary to describe the location of a patient's pain or injury?

   Answer: The health care provider must understand topographic anatomy, which refers to terms that uniformly describe the position and movement of the body.

Cells

Learning Objectives

1. Discuss the relevance of understanding human body system function and structure to conditions commonly found in the field. (p 21-38)

2. Name and describe the two general classes of cells. (p 21)

3. Name the three basic parts of the cell. (p 21)

4. Describe the function of the cell membrane. (p 22-24)

5. State the arrangement of the molecules in the cell membrane. (p 22-24)

6. State the five functions of proteins in the cell membrane. (p 22)

7. Describe the different types of cell permeability. (p 23-24)

8. Define each of these cellular transport mechanisms and give an example of the role of each in the body: diffusion, osmosis, facilitated diffusion, and active transport. (p 23-24)

9. Describe the function of the nucleus and chromosomes. (p 25)

10. Describe the cytoplasm and the role of organelles and cytosol within the cytoplasm. (p 25-27)

11. Describe how the cell membrane regulates the composition of the cytoplasm. (p 25)

12. Describe what happens in mitosis/cytokinesis and meiosis and the importance of each. (p 27)

13. Describe the four types of tissues and give general characteristics of each. (p 27-32)

14. Describe the function of epithelial tissues and connective tissues and relate them to the function of the body or an organ system. (p 27-31)

15. Name some membranes of connective tissue. (p 30-31)

16. List the three types of muscle tissues and the basic differences between them. (p 31-32)

17. Discuss the function of nervous tissues. (p 32)

18. List the organs made of nervous tissues. (p 32)

19. Name the organ systems of the body. (p 33-35)

20. Name two body regions and the structures they contain. (p 33-35)

21. Name the body cavities, their membranes, and examples of organs within each cavity. (p 35-37)

22. Explain the four quadrants of the abdomen and name the organs in each quadrant. (p 36-37)

Introduction

Cells are the foundation of the human body. An entire organism like an amoeba consists of only one cell. In human beings, single cells group together to form complex systems. Billions of cells compose the human body. Some cells make hair, other cells are involved in storing memory, and others help to move your eyes as you read this page. Each cell is a minute mass of colorless substance, called protoplasm (or cytoplasm). Protoplasm is a viscous liquid matrix that supports all internal cellular structures (organelles) and provides a convenient medium for intracellular transport of various substances such as nutrients, signaling molecules, adenosine triphosphate (ATP), and proteins.

Cells with a common job grow close to each other and are called tissues. The types of tissues and components of the cells are discussed in detail. Groups of tissues that all perform interrelated jobs form organs. A series of organs working together make up the body systems that are discussed in this chapter. The functions of the organ systems, such as the respiratory or nervous or skeletal systems, are introduced; however, they are discussed in further detail within their specific chapters.

The disruption of homeostasis (the stability of the body's normal internal environment) can have a serious impact from the cellular level up to the organ systems and the entire organism. Simply said, the body likes it to be not too cold, not too hot, not too acidic, and not too alkalotic, with just the right amount of water and minerals all the time!

Structure of the Cell

The human body contains two general classes of cells: sex cells and somatic cells. Sex cells (also called germ cells or reproductive cells) are either the sperm of males or the oocytes (eggs) of females. Somatic cells (derived from the term *soma*, meaning "body") include all the other cells in the human body. This chapter focuses on somatic cells.

Case Study | PART 1

Your unit is standing by at the city's annual October marathon (26.2 mile). Approximately 18,000 runners have trained and prepared for this race for months. As you comment to your partner that the temperature is 20° warmer than is usual for this time of the year and it is severely humid, a woman stumbles into the medical tent, which is situated near the finish line. You determine that the scene continues to be safe, and you form a general impression of your patient, a woman who is staggering as she approaches you. She tells you that she feels dizzy, so from that information you can establish that symptom is likely the chief complaint.

Your primary assessment reveals that the only immediate threat to this patient is the possibility that she may soon pass out, so you quickly assist her into the Trendelenburg position because your EMS system still recommends this position for some patients, and you apply a nonrebreathing mask to deliver oxygen at a rate of 15 L/min. You next obtain a history and perform a secondary physical examination while your partner quickly obtains a set of baseline vital signs.

Recording Time: 0 Minutes	
Appearance	Young, thin adult female with wet and pale skin - *Running*
Level of consciousness	Alert (oriented to person, place, and day) _ *N/A*
Airway	Appears patent - *Normal*
Breathing	Rapid and shallow - *Exertion / Outside Temp ↑*
Circulation	Pale and very clammy — *Exertion*
Pulse	120 beats/min, weak and irregular with extra occasional beats *] Unusally High...*
Blood pressure	96/66 mm Hg
Respirations	24 breaths/min and shallow
Spo₂	96 %

1. On the basis of the scene size-up and primary assessment findings, what are the possible causes of the patient's chief complaint? *The Pt is running a marathon*

2. What organ systems have abnormal findings in the primary assessment? *The HR is high as per the Pt*

There are three basic parts to a cell: the cell membrane, the nucleus, and the cytoplasm. The cell membrane encloses the cell, its nucleus, various organelles, and its cytoplasm. The nucleus contains the cell's genetic material and controls its activities. The cytoplasm fills out the cell and its shape. Organelles are microscopic, specialized cell structures that perform specific functions required by the cell **Figure 2-1**.

Cell Membrane

The cell membrane (also called the plasma membrane) controls movement of substances both into and out of the cell. Substances outside the cell membrane are referred to as extracellular; those inside it are intracellular. The cell membrane, consisting of a complete set of neatly arranged molecules, is remarkably able to alter its structure, depending on the needs of the cell at any one time. The atoms that make up molecules are comprised of smaller particles called protons (that have a positive electrical charge), electrons (that have a negative electrical charge), and neutrons (that are uncharged). The cell membrane allows selective communication between the intracellular and extracellular compartments while aiding in cellular movement. It gives form to the cell and is also where much of the cell's biologic activities are conducted. Molecules in the cell membrane form pathways that allow the signals from outside the cell to be detected and transmitted inside. When cells form tissues, the cell membrane assists by adhering the cell to other cells. Each cell's membrane is extremely thin and delicate, able to stretch to differing degrees. There are usually tiny

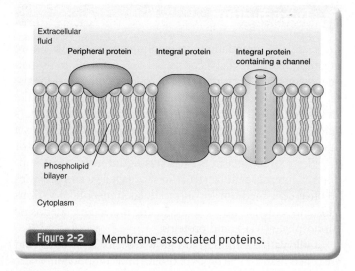

Figure 2-2 Membrane-associated proteins.

folds on the surface, which help to increase its surface area. Cell membranes can be differentially permeable or semipermeable. A semipermeable membrane allows certain elements to pass through while not allowing others to do so. Only certain substances can enter or leave each cell (a condition known as selective permeability).

Lipids and proteins are the primary substances that make up cell membranes, usually in a double layer of phospholipid molecules **Figure 2-2**. The phosphate portion forms the outer surface, with the fatty acid portion forming the inner surface. Substances such as oxygen and carbon dioxide, which are soluble in lipids, can easily pass through this double layer (also called a bilayer). Other substances, such as amino acids, proteins, nucleic acids, certain ions, and sugars cannot pass through this layer. Cholesterol in the inner cell membrane helps to keep the membrane stable.

Proteins periodically interrupt the lipid bilayer by acting as doorways, called channels, which allow certain molecules to enter or exit the cell. These proteins in the cell membrane serve various functions. They are essential to the structure and function of the body. Structures such as cell walls, various membranes, connective tissue, and muscles are mainly protein. They serve as transporters for various molecules (as in facilitated and active transport), signal receptors (binding sites for drugs and body chemicals, such as epinephrine), and ion channels (to allow the movement of charged molecules, such as sodium) between cells.

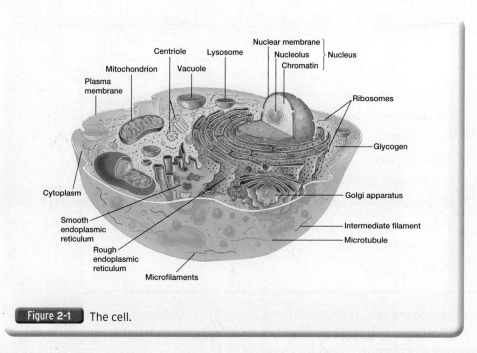

Figure 2-1 The cell.

A membrane consists of a sheet of epithelium and its underlying connective tissue. Membranes usually are kept moist by mucus or serous fluid. These membranes often are known as either mucous membranes or serous membranes. Mucus lubricates the tissues in mucous membranes and also helps immune function by trapping foreign matter. In addition to lining the tubular organs of the body, mucous membranes line the oral and nasal cavities, sinuses, respiratory tract, and urinary tract.

In the resting state, the concentration of sodium is greater outside the cell than inside. The reverse is true for potassium. A sodium-potassium exchange pump moves sodium out of cells and potassium into cells via active transport. Certain drugs, such as digitalis preparations, affect the pump's ability to work in the heart. In toxic doses, potassium may then accumulate to an abnormally high level outside of the cell, resulting in hyperkalemia. Hyperkalemia may cause dysrhythmias, life-threatening rhythm disturbances of the heart.

The cell membrane consists mostly of fats. Chemically, fatty compounds are neutral (uncharged). Electrolytes (sodium and potassium) are water-based (charged). It is a well-known principle that "oil and water do not mix." Fats are soluble in oil, but are not soluble in water. Thus, for a charged molecule to enter through a cell membrane, some type of special pathway must be present. Cells have various types of transport channels, or ion channels, to allow electrolyte movements among them. Local anesthetics, such as lidocaine, and antidysrhythmic drugs, such as amiodarone, exert their effects by blocking ion channels. Hereditary abnormalities of ion channel proteins explain many of the inherited prolonged QT syndromes that predispose persons to sudden death. Approximately 2% of deaths caused by sudden infant death syndrome (SIDS) are now known to be due to a hereditary abnormality of sodium channel proteins.

Permeability of the Cell Membrane

The cell membrane is described as being selectively permeable, which means that it allows some substances to pass through it, but not others Figure 2-3 . It is important for you to understand how materials enter and exit the cell because this relates to fluid administration.

Selective permeability allows normal differences in concentrations between intracellular and extracellular environ-

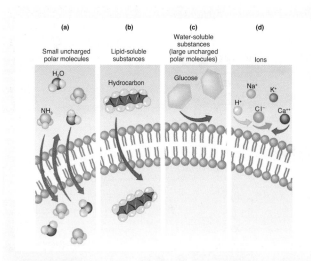

Figure 2-3 A selectively permeable membrane maintains homeostasis by allowing some molecules to pass through while others may not.

ments to be maintained. The separation of the extracellular and intracellular areas by a selectively permeable membrane helps to maintain homeostasis. Various enzymes, sugar molecules, and electrolytes freely pass in and out of the cell. Electrolytes are chemicals that are dissolved in the blood and are made up of salt or acid substances that become ionic conductors when dissolved in a solvent such as water.

Several mechanisms, such as diffusion, osmosis, facilitated diffusion, and active transport, allow material to pass through the cell wall Figure 2-4 .

■ **Diffusion.** Cell particles such as molecules and ions live in water, which creates a solution. Water is the most common solvent or substance, in which other substances or solutes will dissolve. Diffusion is the movement of solutes, particles such as salts that are dissolved in a solvent, from an area of high concentration to one of low concentration, to produce an even distribution of particles in the space available. The degree of diffusion across a membrane depends on the permeability of the membrane to that substance and the concentration gradient, which is the difference in concentrations of the substance on either side of the membrane. Small molecules diffuse more easily than large ones. Watery solutions diffuse more rapidly than thicker, viscous solutions. Many of the cell's nutrients, such as oxygen, enter the cell by diffusion.

■ **Osmosis.** Osmosis is the movement of a solvent, such as water, from an area of low solute concentration to one of high concentration through a selectively permeable membrane. The membrane is permeable to the solvent but not to the solute. Movement generally continues until the concentrations of the solute equalize on both sides of the membrane.

Osmotic pressure is a measure of the tendency of water to move by osmosis across a membrane. If too much

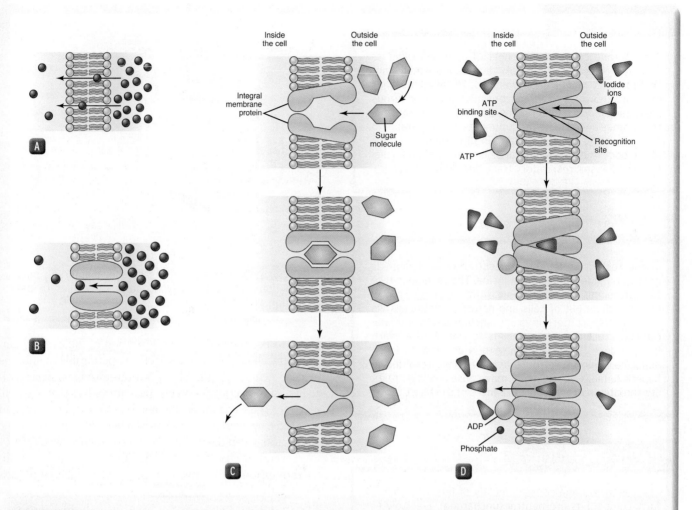

Figure 2-4 Methods of material transport through the cell wall. **A.** Simple diffusion. **B.** Diffusion through protein pores. **C.** Facilitated diffusion. **D.** Active transport.

water moves out of a cell, the cell shrinks abnormally, a process known as crenation. If too much water enters a cell, it will swell and burst, a process known as lysis.

- **Facilitated Diffusion.** Facilitated diffusion is the process in which a carrier molecule moves substances in or out of cells from areas of high concentration to areas of lower concentration. Energy is not required; the number of molecules transported is directly proportional to the concentration of the molecules.

- **Active Transport.** Active transport is the movement of a substance against a concentration or gradient such as the cell membrane. Active transport requires energy as well as some type of carrier mechanism and is a movement opposite that of the normal movement of diffusion. Both glucose and amino acids are absorbed via active transport. At times, the active transport mechanism may exchange one substance for another. Endocytosis and exocytosis both use energy from the cell to move substances into or out of the cell without crossing the cell membrane. Endocytosis is the uptake of material

through the cell membrane by a membrane-bound droplet or vesicle that forms within the protoplasm of the cell. The cell membrane surrounds the material, engulfing it within the cell. When endocytosis involves solid particles, the process is called phagocytosis, which means "cell eating." A phagocyte is any cell that ingests microorganisms or other cells and foreign particles. Phagocytosis occurs commonly when infection-fighting white blood cells consume bacteria and foreign particles. In certain disease states, these cells lose their ability to phagocytize, resulting in life-threatening infections. Endocytosis of liquids, or "cell drinking," is called pinocytosis. Exocytosis is the release of secretions from the cells. These secretions accumulate within vesicles, which then move to the cell membrane. The vesicles bond or fuse to the membrane, and the content of the vesicle is eliminated from the cell. Examples of exocytosis include secretion of digestive enzymes by the pancreas, mucus secretion by the salivary glands, and secretion of milk from the mammary glands.

Pathophysiology

The term serum osmolality refers to the number of osmotically active particles in a liter of serum, the clear straw-colored, liquid portion of the plasma that remains after the solid elements have been separated out. Osmolality refers to the number of osmotically active particles in a kilogram of solvent. Abnormal elevations of blood glucose and sodium concentrations may result in an increase in serum osmolality. When this occurs, movement of the blood is impeded and tissue oxygenation decreases. A condition known as hyperosmolar hyperglycemic nonketotic coma (HHNC) may result. HHNC is a diabetic emergency that occurs when a relative insulin deficiency results in marked hyperglycemia but with the absence of ketones and acidosis.

Pathophysiology

The transport of glucose in and out of most cells occurs by facilitated diffusion. If glucose accumulates within the cell to a concentration that is as high as the concentration outside the cell, the process would stop. Thus, when glucose enters the cell, it is rapidly converted to other molecules. If the cell's ability to convert glucose is hindered, such as in severe shock, low glucose concentrations or hypoglycemia will occur within the cell.

Nucleus

The nucleus is usually the largest, most visible structure inside a cell. The nucleus serves as the control center for cellular operations. It contains deoxyribonucleic acid (DNA), or genetic material, that controls cell activities. A single nucleus stores all required information that directs the synthesis of the 100,000 proteins in the human body. A cell without a nucleus cannot repair itself. It will disintegrate within 3 to 4 months. The nucleus contains the genetic instructions needed to synthesize the proteins that determine cell structures and functions. These instructions are stored in the chromosomes. These structures consist of DNA and various proteins that control and access genetic information. Most cells contain a single nucleus, with the exception of skeletal muscle cells (with numerous nuclei) and mature red blood cells (with no nuclei).

The nucleus of a cell is usually round, and is enclosed in a double nuclear envelope, with inner and outer lipid membranes. This envelope also has a protein lining, allowing certain molecules to exit the nucleus. Inside the nucleus is a fluid called nucleoplasm, which suspends the following structures:

- A "mini nucleus" called a nucleolus, made up mostly of ribonucleic acid (RNA) and protein molecules, with no surrounding membrane. Ribosomes form in the nucleolus and migrate out to the cell's cytoplasm.

- Loosely coiled DNA and protein fibers called chromatin that condense, forming chromosomes. The DNA controls protein synthesis, and when the cell starts to divide, the chromatin fibers coil tightly to form the chromosomes.

Clinical Tip

Many recent advances in medicine have centered on the genetic code, carried on DNA in the chromosomes. In essence, genes are made up of molecules of DNA that code for various proteins. The process of making specific proteins based on the genetic code in DNA is fascinating and extremely complex. The following information presents the process in a straightforward manner:

- Genes carry the DNA, the genetic code for each protein.
- Messenger RNA (mRNA) is made or transcribed in the nucleus, using DNA as the guide or template.
- Messenger RNA moves from the nucleus to the protoplasm, where it attaches to a group of ribosomes (polyribosome complex).
- Another form of RNA, transfer RNA (tRNA), carries amino acids to the ribosomes.
- Using the information on the mRNA as a guide, the ribosomes assemble the amino acids into a chain, forming a protein (also called a polypeptide). This process is known as translation of RNA.
- The protein detaches from the ribosomes and is transported to the Golgi apparatus.
- In the Golgi apparatus, the protein is "packaged" and undergoes final biochemical modifications prior to becoming functional, either in the cell of origin or another cell.
- DNA is transcribed to mRNA, which is then translated to proteins.

Cytoplasm

Cytoplasm is the substance that contains all the cellular contents between the cell membrane and the nucleus. It serves as a matrix substance in which chemical reactions occur. Cytoplasm makes up most of each cell's volume, and is a gel-like material suspending the cell's organelles, which perform most of the tasks that keep the cell alive and functioning normally. Cytoplasm usually appears clear with scattered "specks," though more powerful magnification reveals that it contains membranous networks, protein frameworks, and a cytoskeleton (cell skeleton). Cytoplasm consists of organelles (excluding the nucleus) and cytosol.

Organelles

Organelles are internal cellular structures within the cells that carry out the functions needed for the human body to function. Each organelle accomplishes specific tasks related to cell structure, growth, maintenance, and metabolism. The organelles operate in a cooperative and organized manner to maintain the life of the cell. They include the following components:

- Centrioles, which are important in the formation of the spindle apparatus, and spindle fibers, microtubules radiating from the centrioles, are essential in the process of cell division. During cell division, the centrioles form the spindle-shaped structure needed for movement of DNA strands.
- Cilia and flagella are structures that extend from certain cell surfaces. Cilia are hair-like, moving in a coordinated sweeping motion to move fluids over the surface of tissues. They are found on cells lining the respiratory tract and on cells lining the reproductive tract. The motion of the cilia in the trachea and bronchi continuously move a layer of mucus from the lower portions of the lung to the throat. Cigarette smoking paralyzes the motion of the cilia, resulting in an accumulation of foreign substances in the lungs. Flagella are longer than cilia, and often exist as only a single flagellum (an example of which is the flagellum that appears as the "tail" of a sperm cell. One cause of male infertility is an abnormality of sperm flagellum, which makes sperm unable to propel itself through the vagina and into the uterus for fertilization.
- Ribosomes contain ribonucleic acid (RNA) and protein. RNA is responsible for controlling cellular activities. Ribosomes interact with RNA from other parts of the cell, joining amino acids together to form proteins. This interaction takes place on the endoplasmic reticulum, a series of membranes in which specific proteins and fats (lipids) are manufactured.
- The endoplasmic reticulum is a network of tubules, vesicles, and sacs. Rough endoplasmic reticulum is involved in building proteins. Smooth endoplasmic reticulum is involved in building lipids (fats), such as those found in the cell membranes.
- The Golgi apparatus, which is also called the Golgi complex, is located near the nucleus of the cell. It is involved in the formation of various carbohydrates (sugars) and complex protein molecules, such as enzymes.
- Lysosomes are membrane-bound vesicles that contain digestive enzymes. These enzymes function as an intracellular digestive system, breaking down organic debris, such as bacteria, that has been taken into the cell.
- Similar to lysosomes, peroxisomes are found in high concentrations in the liver and neutralize toxins such as alcohol.
- Mitochondria are small rod-like or spherical organelles. They function as the metabolic center of the cell, and produce adenosine triphosphate (ATP), the major energy source for all chemical reactions in the body. ATP is the primary molecule used by cells to store and transfer energy.

- The nucleus contains two different types of genetic material. Deoxyribonucleic acid (DNA) is contained in the chromosomes, which are long and thin in the non-dividing cell and cannot be identified as distinct structures. Instead, they appear as a network of granules called nuclear chromatin. RNA is contained in spherical intranuclear structures called nucleoli. The nucleus is surrounded by a membrane called the nuclear envelope; the nucleus itself is embedded in the cytoplasm.

Clinical Tip

The key core concepts of cellular metabolism are simple: When you breathe, you take in oxygen. Through various metabolic processes, the oxygen, water, and nutritional molecules (eg, glucose) are metabolized to produce energy in the form of adenosine triphosphate (ATP) and heat. Water and carbon dioxide are also formed as by-products. Incredibly, the heart alone uses approximately 35 kg (more than 70 lb) of ATP each day!

Cytosol

Cytosol is the fluid portion of cytoplasm, containing mostly water, as well as glucose, amino acids, fatty acids, ions, lipids, proteins, adenosine triphosphate (ATP), and waste

Pathophysiology

Sodium and potassium are two of the most important electrolytes (dissolved chemicals) in the blood. Most of the body's supply of potassium is contained in fluid within the cells, known as the intracellular fluid (ICF). Conversely, most of the body's supply of sodium resides in the fluid outside of cells, known as the extracellular fluid (ECF). Both fluids and electrolytes may move between the ICF and ECF, depending on many factors. Abnormal concentrations of either sodium or potassium in the ECF may result in life-threatening conditions. Measured levels of sodium or potassium may be normal, high, or low. The most common causes of electrolyte abnormalities are abnormalities in the body's fluid balance such as caused by dehydration, overhydration, or drugs. Failure to recognize and promptly treat any of these abnormalities may result in harm to the patient. Hyponatremia is an abnormally low sodium level in the blood; an abnormally high sodium level is referred to as hypernatremia. Either condition may result in altered levels of consciousness, seizures, and, often, coma. Hyperkalemia, an abnormal elevation of potassium levels in the blood, is relatively common both in kidney failure and as a complication of certain medications. Untreated hyperkalemia results in abnormalities in the electrical system of the heart, resulting in dysrhythmias and, possibly, cardiac arrest. Similarly, hypokalemia, or abnormally decreased potassium levels in the blood, also affects the heart and may cause life-threatening cardiac rhythm problems.

products. Cytosol is the site of many chemical reactions that are required for cells to exist. It is the part of the cytoplasm that cannot be removed by centrifugation.

Cell Division

Many cells actively divide during life. Others die and are replaced by new cells. This ongoing process of cell renewal is called remodeling and is a normal process of life. Interphase describes this period of preparation to divide. During interphase, the cell manufactures new living material, duplicating membranes, lysosomes, mitochondria, and ribosomes. It also replaces its own genetic material. There are two types of cell division: meiosis and mitosis/cytokinesis. Meiosis is a specialized form of cell division that occurs only in the production of mature sperm and ova. Normally, cells contain 46 chromosomes. Meiosis reduces by half the number of chromosomes, from 46 to 23, in eggs and sperm so that when they unite, the fertilized egg will have the proper total of 46 chromosomes.

In the rest of the body, cell numbers are increased by mitosis, the division of the nucleus of a cell, and cytokinesis, the division of the cytoplasm of a cell. All cells except egg and sperm cells can be divided by mitosis. When the nucleus divides, it must be precise so that an accurate copy of the DNA information can be made by the new cell Figure 2-5 . During mitosis, division of the cell nucleus and protoplasm (including the organelles) occurs in the following four stages: prophase, metaphase, anaphase, and telophase.

In the first stage, prophase, two new centriole pairs move to opposite ends of the cell. In the second stage, metaphase, the chromosomes align near the middle portion (equatorial plane) between the centrioles, and spindle fibers attach to them. During the third stage, anaphase, the centromere sections of each chromosome are pulled apart to become individual chromosomes, and move toward opposite ends of the cell. In the last stage, telophase, chromosomes arrive at each pole, and new nuclear membranes form.

Cytoplasmic division (cytokinesis) begins during anaphase, when the cell membrane constricts down the middle portion of the cell. This continues through telophase (the last stage) to divide the cytoplasm. The two newly formed nuclei are then separated and nearly half of the organelles are distributed into each new cell.

Types of Tissue

Groups of cells that work together are called tissues. There are four types of tissues: epithelial tissues, connective tissues, muscle tissues, and nervous tissues.

Epithelial Tissues

Epithelial tissues cover body surfaces (such as the skin), cover and line internal organs (such as the gallbladder), and make up the glands (enabling secretion and absorption to occur throughout the body). Most epithelial tissues have a basement membrane, a noncellular layer that secures the overlying tissues. Epithelial tissue is classified according to the number of cell layers and the shape of each epithelial cell. Cell shapes include flat sheets (squamous epithelium),

Case Study | PART 2

After obtaining a SAMPLE history from the patient, you discover that she did not hydrate well before the race and did not make many water stops. She said she did not have much to drink because her stomach was bothering her. The patient has no significant past medical history, no known allergies, and takes an antihistamine only for seasonal allergies.

Recording Time: 5 Minutes	
Appearance	Still very pale
Level of consciousness	Alert (oriented to person, place, and day)
Airway	Still open and clear
Breathing	Unchanged
Circulation	Still very pale, no external bleeding

3. What is the pathophysiology of dehydration in this patient?

4. What electrolyte abnormalities should be considered in this patient?

5. Where should you focus your secondary assessment next?

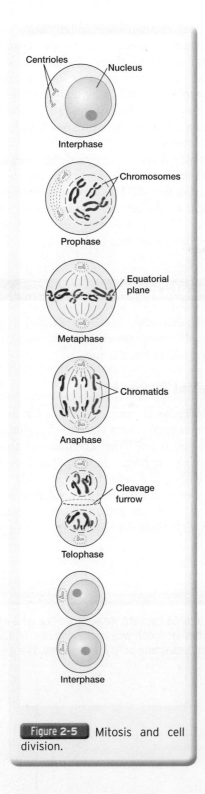

Figure 2-5 Mitosis and cell division.

Type	Location	Function
Simple squamous epithelium	Air sacs of lungs, capillary walls, linings of lymph, and blood vessels	Diffusion, filtration, osmosis, covering of surfaces
Simple cuboidal epithelium	Ovary surfaces, kidney tubule linings, linings of ducts of certain glands	Absorption, secretion
Simple columnar epithelium	Intestine, stomach, and uterus linings	Absorption, protection, secretion
Pseudostratified columnar epithelium	Respiratory passage linings	Movement of mucus, protection, secretion
Stratified squamous epithelium	Outer layer of skin, linings of anal canal, oral cavity, throat, and vagina	Protection
Stratified cuboidal epithelium	Linings of larger mammary gland ducts, pancreas, salivary glands, sweat glands	Protection
Stratified columnar epithelium	Part of male urethra and parts of the pharynx	Protection, secretion
Transitional epithelium	Inner urinary bladder lining, linings of ureters, and part of urethra	Distensibility, protection
Glandular epithelium	Endocrine, salivary, and sweat glands	Secretion

Table 2-1   Types of Epithelial Tissues

rows of square-shaped cells (cuboidal epithelium), or rows of tall, thin cells (columnar epithelium). A comparison of different types of epithelial cells and their markedly different functions is shown in Table 2-1.

Simple epithelium consists of a single layer of cells, all of which are in contact with the basement membrane. Stratified epithelium consists of more than one layer of cells, only one of which is in contact with the basement membrane. Pseudostratified epithelium contains a single layer of cells of varying heights. All cells attach to the basement membrane, but some fail to reach the free surface, giving the appearance of multiple layers. Transitional epithelium consists of layers of stratified cells that change shape from cuboidal to squamous when the organ is stretched Figure 2-6.

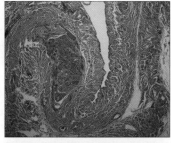

Simple squamous epithelium

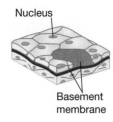

Nucleus

Basement membrane

Stratified squamous epithelium

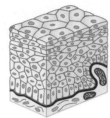

Non-cornified

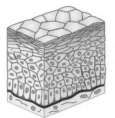

Cornified

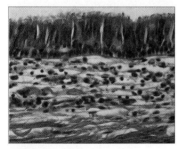

Pseudostratified columnar epithelium

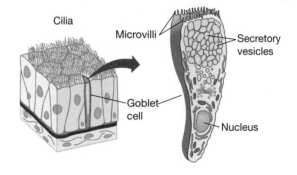

Cilia

Microvilli

Secretory vesicles

Goblet cell

Nucleus

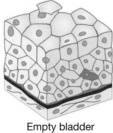

Transitional epithelium

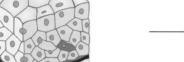

Empty bladder

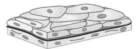

Full bladder

Figure 2-6 Organizational arrangement and surface modification of epithelial cells.

Clinical Tip

Transitional epithelial cells line body cavities that can expand, such as the urinary bladder. These cells change from a cuboidal to squamous shape when the bladder is full of urine and the wall of the organ is stretched.

Connective Tissues

Connective tissues bind other types of tissue together. Connective tissues are classified based on their physical properties. The three general categories of connective tissue are connective tissue proper, supporting connective tissues, and fluid connective tissues Figure 2-7 .

- Connective tissue proper includes those connective tissues with many types of cells and extracellular fibers in a syrup-like ground substance. They are divided into dense connective tissue, which contains many collagenous fibers and appears white, and loose connective tissue, which includes adipose (fat) tissue, areolar tissue, and reticular connective tissue. Adipose tissue lies beneath the skin, between muscles, around the kidneys, behind the eyes, in certain membranes of the abdomen, on the heart's surface, and around some of the body's joints. Areolar tissue binds skin to underlying organs and fills in spaces between muscles. Reticular connective tissue helps to create a framework inside internal organs such as the spleen and liver.

- Supporting connective tissue differs from connective tissue proper because it has a less diverse cell population and a matrix that contains many more densely packed fibers. Supporting connective tissue protects soft tissues and carries most of or all of the body's weight. The two types of supporting connective tissue

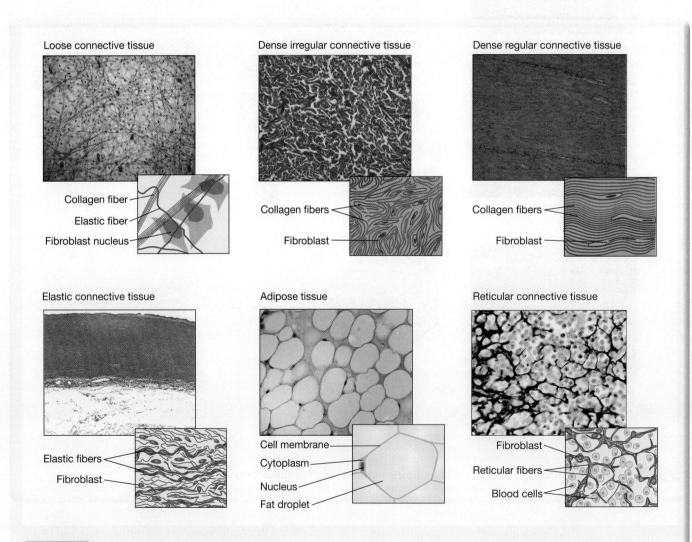

Figure 2-7 Types of typical connective tissues.

are cartilage and bone. Cartilage is a rigid connective tissue with a gelatinous matrix that contains an abundance of fibers. It supports, frames, and attaches to many underlying tissues and bones. Bone is the most rigid type of connective tissue, with a high mineral content that makes it harder than other types. Bone tissue establishes the framework of the body. Bones attach to muscles and protect as well as support vital body structures.

- Fluid connective tissues have distinctive populations of cells suspended in a water matrix that contains dissolved proteins and may be of two types: either blood or lymph. These tissues transport many materials between interior body cells and other cells that exchange substances with the environment, maintaining a stable internal environment. Blood contains formed elements (red blood cells, white blood cells, and platelets), which are suspended in a liquid extracellular matrix known as blood plasma. Together, the formed elements and blood plasma make up the blood. Most blood cells are formed in the red bone marrow. Lymph forms as interstitial fluid enters the lymphatic vessels, which return the lymph to the cardiovascular system.

Muscle Tissues

Muscle tissues are located within the substance of the body and invariably enclosed by connective tissue. Muscles overlie the framework of the skeleton and are classified by both structure and function. Structurally, muscle tissue is either striated (skeletal or cardiac), in which microscopic bands or striations can be seen, or nonstriated (smooth) **Figure 2-8**.

Functionally, muscle movement is either voluntary (consciously controlled) or involuntary (not normally under conscious control). The three types of muscle tissue are skeletal muscle tissue (striated voluntary), cardiac muscle tissue (striated involuntary), and smooth muscle tissue (nonstriated involuntary).

- Skeletal muscle tissue is known as voluntar muscle tissue because it is found in the muscles controlled by conscious effort; it attaches to bones and is composed of long thread-like cells that have light and dark markings called striations **Figure 2-9**. Skeletal muscle tissue moves the head, trunk, and limbs, allowing all voluntary movements in these body areas.
- Cardiac muscle tissue is also called myocardium; it is a thick contractile middle layer of the heart wall. The contractile tissue of the myocardium is composed of fibers with the characteristic cross-striations of muscular tissue. Myocardial muscle contains less

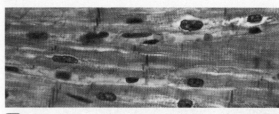

Nuclei   Muscle fiber

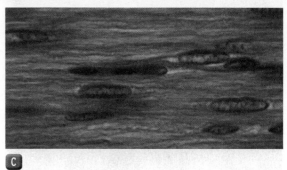

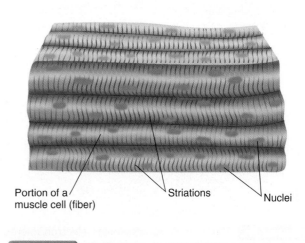

© John D. Cunningham/Visuals Unlimited

© R. Calentine/Visuals Unlimited

Figure 2-8   Types of muscle tissue. **A.** Skeletal. **B.** Cardiac. **C.** Smooth.

Figure 2-9   Skeletal muscle with striations.

Portion of a muscle cell (fiber)   Striations   Nuclei

connective tissue than skeletal muscle. Cardiac muscle is involuntary, and makes up most of the heart. Cardiac muscles rely on pacemaker cells or nodes of tissue in the conduction system for regular contraction. Under the right circumstances each cardiac tissue has the ability to generate an impulse. This property is known as automaticity and may be caused by hypoxia or electrolyte imbalance in the cardiac cells. It primarily affects the cells in the conduction system but can affect other cardiac cells to generate impulses.

- Smooth muscle tissue is composed of elongated, spindle-shaped cells in muscles not under voluntary control. They are also called nonstriated involuntary muscles or unstriated muscles. Because smooth muscle cells can divide, they regenerate after being injured. Smooth muscle tissue composes hollow internal organ walls (such as the intestines and stomach). Smooth muscle cannot, in most cases, be controlled by conscious effort. This type of tissue moves food through the digestive tract, empties the urinary bladder, and constricts blood vessels.

Nervous Tissues

Nervous tissues are specialized for the conduction of electrical impulses from one region of the body to another. Nervous tissues contain two basic types of cells: (1) neurons, and (2) several kinds of supporting cells, collectively called neuroglia, or glial cells. Nervous tissues are found in the brain, spinal cord, cranial nerves, and peripheral nerves. Peripheral nerves include all of the nerves that extend from the brain and spinal cord, exiting from between the vertebrae to various parts of the body. Neurons are the main conducting cells of nervous tissue. They coordinate, integrate, and regulate a wide variety of functions in the body.

Two projections typically extend from the neuron: dendrites and axons. Dendrites receive electrical impulses from the axons of other neurons and conduct them toward the cell body. Axons typically conduct electrical impulses away from the cell body. Each neuron has only one axon but may have several dendrites **Figure 2-10**.

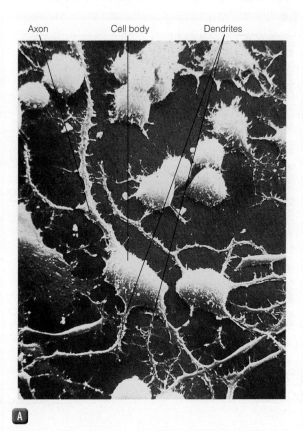

Axon   Cell body   Dendrites

© David M. Phillips/Visuals Unlimited

A

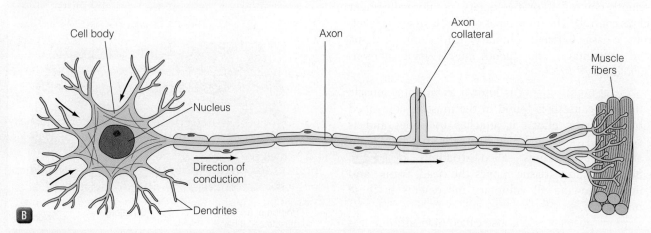

Cell body   Axon   Axon collateral   Muscle fibers

Nucleus

Direction of conduction

Dendrites

B

Figure 2-10 The neuron. **A.** A scanning electron micrograph of the cell body and dendrites of a multipolar neuron, which resides in the central nervous system. **B.** Collateral branches may occur along the length of the axon. When the axon terminates, it branches many times, ending on individual muscle fibers.

Pathophysiology

Communication among cells is vital to the body's function. Various messengers or transmitters travel among cells, carrying information. A well-known example of this process is the stimulus to contract transmitted from a nerve to a muscle. Chemically, the process takes place by the movement of neurotransmitters across the nerve synapse, causing depolarization of the muscle. Depolarization represents the change in electrical potential between the inside and the outside of a cell from the potential when the cell is at rest. It occurs as a result of the movement of sodium (Na^+), potassium (K^+), and calcium (Ca^{++}) in and out of cells. The movement of these ions occurs through anatomically proven channels or pathways. Often, cells communicate by using a G-protein, which is an intermediate compound that is released. This protein binds to a receptor, causing the cell to produce another chemical, called a "second messenger," that instructs the final target cell (effector) to carry out a certain task.

Potassium channels in the pancreas regulate insulin secretion, whereas other types of potassium channels in the heart maintain the normal heart rhythm. Disordered function of these cardiac potassium channels can be the basis of dysrhythmias and may cause sudden death. Potassium channels in the central nervous system, in conjunction with G-proteins, play important roles at various receptor sites in the transmission of nerve impulses. Deficiencies in these central nervous system channels have been linked to some rare genetic diseases.

Organs

Various tissues work together in organs to perform tasks. Together, these components serve to pump blood throughout the arteries and veins of the circulatory system. The skin, or integument, contains all four types of tissues and is the largest organ in the body. It preserves heat, prevents fluid loss (dehydration), and protects against invasion of the body's surface by infection-causing bacteria. Other organs include the liver, spleen, pancreas, digestive organs, reproductive organs, and the organs of special sense. These organs will be discussed in detail in later chapters.

Organ Systems

In each organ system of the body, organs work together to maintain homeostasis. Organ systems of the human body include the skeletal, muscular, respiratory, circulatory, lymphatic, nervous, integumentary, digestive, endocrine, urinary, and genital systems **Figure 2-11**. Combined, the various organ systems form an organism, any individual living thing. The human organism is very complex, consisting of mutually dependent organs and organ systems that carry out vital functions. The anatomy and physiology of each organ system are described in detail in the following chapters.

Body Regions

The body is divided into several regions. The appendicular region includes the extremities and their associated girdles, the bony structures that attach the limbs to the body. The upper extremity is divided into the arm, forearm, wrist, and hand and attaches to the body at the shoulder girdle. The region inferior to the shoulder, or armpit, is referred to as the axilla. The bend or crook of the elbow is known as the antecubital fossa. The lower extremity is divided into the thigh, leg, ankle, and foot and is attached to the body by the hip or pelvic girdle. The space behind the knee is known as the popliteal fossa.

The axial region consists of the head, neck, and trunk, that is, the body excluding the bony girdles and limbs. The scalp is the skin layer of the head, excluding the face and ears, that normally is covered with hair. The scalp consists of five layers, from the external surface moving inward. These layers are the skin, subcutaneous tissue, muscle, loose connective tissue, and the periosteum **Figure 2-12**. The scalp is highly vascular and tends to bleed freely when cut. The three layers of the meninges, the dura mater, arachnoid, and pia mater, lie within the skull and provide protection for the brain. Covering the outside of the skull and all bones is a membrane called the periosteum.

The skull houses the brain and is composed of two main parts: the cranium and the facial bones. The bones of the skull are connected together at special joints known as sutures. Fibrous tissues called fontanelles, which soften and expand during childbirth, link the sutures **Figure 2-13**. The tissue felt through the fontanelles are layers of the scalp and thick membranes overlying the brain. Under normal conditions, the brain may not be felt through the fontanelle. By the time a child reaches age 18 months, the sutures should have solidified and the fontanelles closed.

Three major triangles lie within the neck: the anterior triangle, carotid triangle, and posterior triangle. The anterior triangle is bounded by the sternocleidomastoid muscle, anterior midline of the neck, and inferior border of the mandible. The carotid triangle lies within the anterior triangle and contains the carotid artery and internal jugular vein. The posterior triangle runs from the posterior portion of the sternocleidomastoid muscle to the posterior midline of the neck and the base of the skull. It contains numerous lymph nodes, the brachial plexus, spinal accessory nerve, and a portion of the subclavian artery.

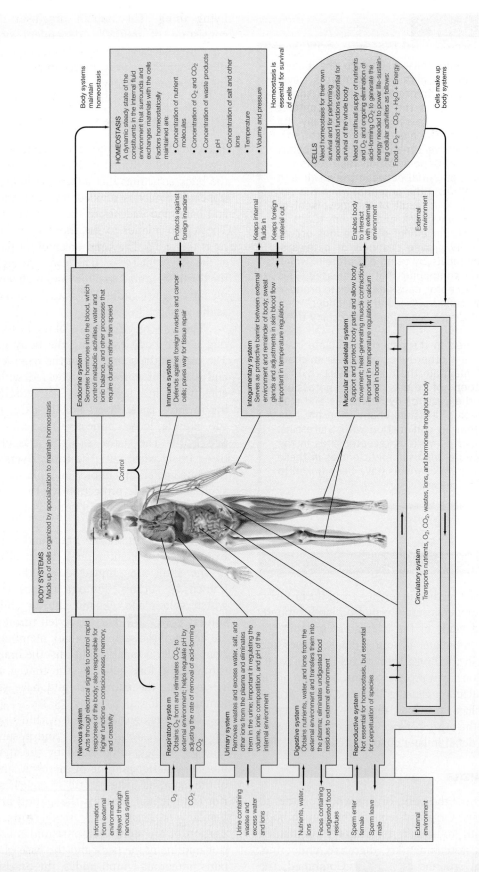

Figure 2-11 Systems of the body.

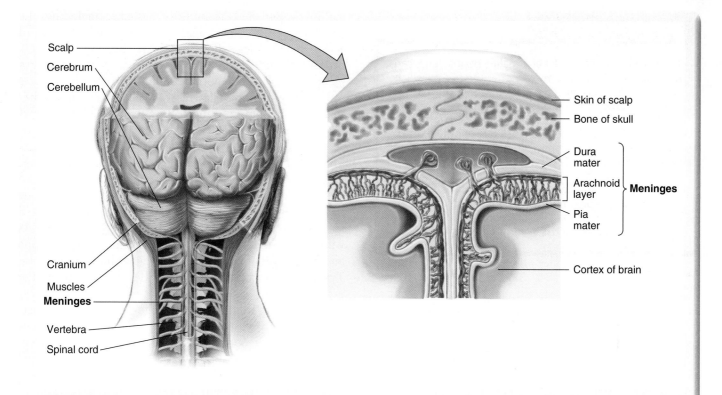

Scalp
Cerebrum
Cerebellum

Skin of scalp
Bone of skull
Dura mater
Arachnoid layer ⎱ **Meninges**
Pia mater

Cranium
Muscles
Meninges
Vertebra
Spinal cord

Cortex of brain

Figure 2-12 In addition to the layers of protection the scalp affords the brain, the three layers of the meninges are connective tissue covering the brain.

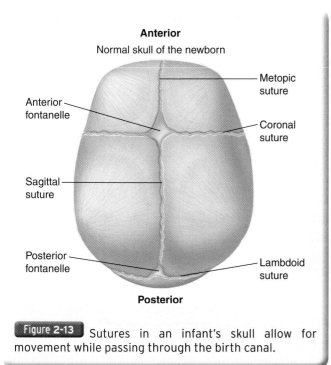

Anterior
Normal skull of the newborn

Metopic suture
Anterior fontanelle
Coronal suture
Sagittal suture
Posterior fontanelle
Lambdoid suture

Posterior

Figure 2-13 Sutures in an infant's skull allow for movement while passing through the birth canal.

The trunk is further subdivided into the thorax, abdomen, and the pelvis **Figure 2-14**. The anterior thorax is often studied separately from the posterior thorax.

Body Cavities

Body cavities are hollow areas within the body that contain organs and organ systems. The skull and vertebral column contain the brain and spinal cord. The cranial cavity has a domed top, a bony base, a hollow interior, and contains the brain. The spinal cavity is connected to the cranial cavity and travels down the vertebrae in the spine, also called the vertebral column. The spinal cord is located in the hollow spinal cavity. Both the brain and the spinal cord are part of the nervous system and special sensory system.

The muscular diaphragm divides the trunk into the thoracic and abdominal cavities **Figure 2-15**.

The cavities of the trunk are lined by serous membranes, a specialized form of thin connective tissue. Each membrane has two portions. The parietal portion of a serous membrane lines the wall of the cavity. The visceral portion covers the internal organs. The serous membranes secrete fluid that

Pathophysiology

Trauma or a congenital abnormality of the lung can result in a condition known as a pneumothorax, which is an abnormal accumulation of air within the pleural space or between the layers of pleura. Strictly speaking, any amount of air in the pleural space constitutes a pneumothorax. Clinically, a small pneumothorax may not be evident without specialized radiographic studies obtained in the hospital. Remember, it is the patient's symptoms, not the size of the pneumothorax, that matter. An anatomically small pneumothorax can still result in a tension pneumothorax, an ongoing accumulation of air in the pleural space that progressively increases pressure in the chest and is a life-threatening condition.

fills the space between the visceral and parietal membranes. The membranes and fluid protect the internal organs from friction. The amount of lubricating fluid present depends on the specific cavity.

The thoracic cavity, or thorax, is bound by the rib cage, the base of the neck, and the diaphragm. The thoracic cavity contains major organs of both the cardiovascular and respiratory systems, including the heart and lungs. The lungs are surrounded by a set of serous membranes called the pleura. Between the layers of visceral and parietal pleura is a space known as the pleural space. Under normal circumstances, this cavity is only a potential space; it rarely contains anything other than a small amount of lubricating fluid called the pleural fluid.

The mediastinum is a large space between the lungs. The mediastinum holds the heart, major large blood vessels, part of the esophagus, trachea, and the mainstem bronchi. The heart is surrounded by a set of serous membranes known as the pericardium. The potential space between the membranes is the pericardial sac. As with the pleural space, the pericardial sac rarely contains anything other than a small amount of lubricating fluid. The region surrounding the heart is referred to as the pericardial cavity.

Extending from the diaphragm above to the pelvic brim below is the abdominal cavity. The spine and abdominal wall border the abdominal cavity anteriorly and posteriorly. The abdominal wall is lined with a serous membrane known as the peritoneum. Abdominal organs are attached to the abdominal wall and receive their blood

Case Study PART 3

The physical examination reveals that the patient's mental status and ABCs are still stable, her lung sounds are clear, and her heart rate has decreased, although the rate is still slightly irregular, sustaining a tachycardic rate with premature atrial contractions. You take the patient's blood pressure and measure her oxygen saturation by pulse oximetry (SpO_2). Her blood glucose level is 90 mg/dL, which is in the normal range.

The patient states that the dizziness has decreased while lying down, but now she is beginning to shiver and is experiencing muscle cramping in her legs.

Recording Time: 10 Minutes	
Appearance	Some color coming back to her face
Level of consciousness	Alert (oriented to person, place and day)
Airway	Open and clear
Breathing	No obvious distress
Circulation	Pale, but skin remains dry after being toweled off
Pulse	110 beats/min, fewer extra occasional beats
Blood pressure	100/66 mm Hg
Respirations	20 breaths/min and regular
SpO_2	98%

6. To help replace some of the fluids lost, what type of solution should you infuse?

7. Which two electrolytes, found in blood, are most likely to be out of normal range because of the patient's apparent dehydration?

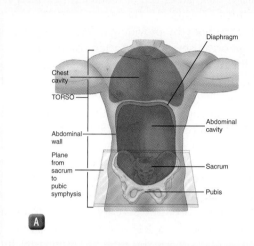

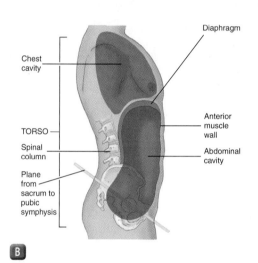

Figure 2-14 The thorax, abdomen, and pelvic cavities.
A. Anterior view. **B.** Lateral view.

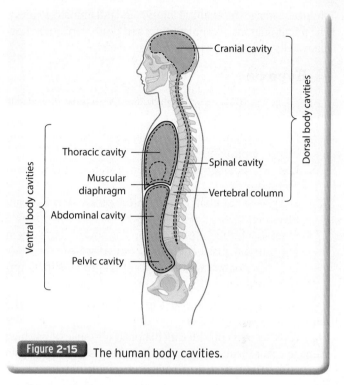

Figure 2-15 The human body cavities.

Pathophysiology

An abnormal accumulation of fluid within the pericardial sac is called a pericardial effusion. At times, and particularly following trauma, fluid rapidly accumulates in the sac, preventing the heart from filling adequately with blood and restricting stroke volume. The heart then is unable to maintain adequate circulation, and a life-threatening condition known as pericardial tamponade develops.

Pathophysiology

An abnormal accumulation of fluid within the pleural space is known as a pleural effusion. The four most common causes of a pleural effusion are heart failure, infection, cancer, and trauma. In each case, the contents of the fluid reflect the underlying disease process. For example, the accumulated fluid following trauma usually is bloody and is referred to as a hemothorax, indicating the presence of blood in the pleural space. It is difficult, if not impossible, to prove the existence of a pleural effusion without radiographic studies. Clinically, a large effusion causes decreased breath sounds and dullness to chest percussion, as do several other common conditions, such as pneumonia or hemothorax.

Cellular Injury

supply through a membranous double fold of tissue in the abdomen, the mesentery. The abdomen is divided into four quadrants—the right upper quadrant, right lower quadrant, left upper quadrant, and left lower quadrant—by two imaginary perpendicular lines crossing at the umbilicus (navel).

The retroperitoneal space is the area located posterior to the parietal peritoneum that contains the retroperitoneal organs: the pancreas, kidneys, duodenum, and major blood vessels.

The lower portion of the abdominal area is the pelvic cavity. The pelvic cavity contains the urinary, reproductive organ, and part of the gastrointestinal systems. The pelvic girdle supports the pelvic cavity with the pubis, ischium, coccyx, ilium, and sacrum bones. These bones also provide protection to the intra-pelvic organs.

Cellular injury may result from various causes, such as hypoxia (lack of oxygen), ischemia (lack of blood supply), chemical injury, infectious injury, immunologic (hypersensitivity) injury, physical damage (mechanical injury), and inflammatory injury. The manifestations of cellular injury and death depend on how many cells and which types of cells are damaged.

Hypoxia

Hypoxia is a common—and often deadly—cause of cellular injury. It may result from:

- Decreased amounts of oxygen in the air (such as in carbon monoxide poisoning)
- Loss of hemoglobin function (such as in carbon monoxide poisoning)
- Decreased number of red blood cells (such as from bleeding)
- Disease of the respiratory or cardiovascular system (eg, chronic obstructive pulmonary disease)
- Loss of cytochromes (mitochondrial proteins that convert oxygen to ATP; such as in cyanide poisoning)

Although hypoxia has deleterious effects on cells, the damage does not stop there. Cells that are hypoxic for more than a few seconds produce mediators (substances) that may damage other local or distant body locations. The result is a positive feedback cycle in which mediators lead to more cell damage, which leads to more hypoxia, which leads to further mediator production, and so forth. The result is widespread and potentially deadly tissue damage.

Chemical Injury

A variety of chemicals, including poisons, lead, carbon monoxide, ethanol, and pharmacologic agents, may injure and ultimately destroy cells. Common poisons include cyanide and pesticides. Cyanide induces cell hypoxia by blocking oxidative phosphorylation in the mitochondria and preventing the metabolism of oxygen. Pesticides block an enzyme, acetylcholinesterase, thereby preventing proper transmission of nerve impulses.

Infectious Injury

Infectious injury to cells occurs as a result of an invasion of bacteria, fungi, or viruses. Bacteria may cause injury by direct action on cells or by the production of toxins. Viruses often initiate an inflammatory response that leads to cell damage and patient symptoms.

Immunologic and Inflammatory Injury

Inflammation is a protective response that can occur without bacterial invasion. Infection is the invasion of microorganisms that causes cell or tissue injury, which leads to the inflammatory response. The immune system provides protection for the body by providing defenses to attack and remove foreign organisms such as bacteria or viruses.

The cellular membranes may be injured by direct contact with the cellular and chemical components of the immune or inflammatory process, such as phagocytes (lymphocytes and macrophages), histamine, antibodies, and lymphokines. When cell membranes are altered, potassium leaks out of the cells and water flows inward. The result is swelling of the cell. The nuclear envelope, organelle membranes, and the cell membrane may all rupture, leading to death of the cell. The degree of the swelling and membrane rupture depends on the severity of the immune and inflammatory response.

Pathophysiology

Severe inflammation or infection within the abdominal cavity results in irritation of the peritoneum, a condition known as peritonitis. Clinically, it is difficult to differentiate between inflammation of organs in the peritoneal cavity, such as the stomach, and the retroperitoneal organs, such as the kidneys. Signs of peritoneal inflammation include decreased bowel sounds, rebound tenderness, and abdominal rigidity and may be noted in either source.

Additional Factors

Genetic factors, nutritional imbalances, and physical agents can also cause cell injury and death. Genetic factors include chromosomal disorders, such as Down syndrome. There are two ways an abnormal gene may develop in a person: (1) by mutation of a gene during meiosis, which affects the newly formed fetus, or (2) by heredity.

Good nutrition is required to maintain good health and assist the cells in fighting off disease. Examples of nutritional disorders that can injure cells and the organism as a whole include obesity, malnutrition, vitamin excess or deficiency, and mineral excess or deficiency. Any of these conditions can lead to alterations in physical growth, mental and intellectual deficiencies, and even death.

Physical agents, such as heat, cold, and radiation, may cause cell injury. Examples include burns, frostbite, sickness, and tumors. The degree of cell injury that results is determined by both the strength of the agent and the length of exposure.

Case Study PART 4

Management of this patient will involve administering oxygen, monitoring her heart rhythm, administering IV fluid, proper positioning, and prompt transport to the hospital.

Prep Kit

■ Chapter Summary

- Cells are the foundation of the human body.
- Each cell is a minute mass of colorless substance called protoplasm or cytoplasm.
- The cell membrane consists of fatty substances arranged in a double layer called a lipid bilayer, which separates the intracellular material from the extracellular material.
- Permeability of the cell membrane involves selectivity in allowing some, but not all, substances to pass through.
- The methods by which material can pass through the cell include simple diffusion, osmosis, facilitated diffusion, and active transport.
- The structure of the cell includes internal structures called organelles, which are supported by the protoplasm.
- The nucleus of the cell is the nerve center of the cell and contains the DNA.
- Microtubules are the hollow filamentous structures that make up various components of a cell and provide movement of the cell, such as flagella and cilia.
- Meiosis is the specialized cell division that produces the sperm and egg.
- Tissues are classified as epithelial, connective, muscle, or nervous, and each type has a specific function.
- Mitosis is the division of the nucleus of a cell, and cytokinesis is the division of the cytoplasm of a cell. All cells except egg and sperm cells can be divided by mitosis.
- Different types of tissues that are working together for a particular function are known as an organ.
- An organ system is a group of organs with a common purpose.
- The body cavities are hollow areas of the body that contain organs and organ systems.
- Cellular injury may result from various causes, such as hypoxia, chemical injury, infectious injury, and inflammatory injury.

■ Vital Vocabulary

active transport A method used to move compounds across a cell membrane to create or maintain an imbalance of charges, usually against a concentration gradient and requiring the expenditure of energy.

adenosine triphosphate (ATP) The major source of energy for all chemical reactions of the body.

adipose (fat) tissue A type of connective tissue that contains large amounts of fat.

antecubital fossa The anterior surface at the bend of the elbow.

anterior triangle The area of the neck that is bordered by the sternocleidomastoid muscle, the anterior midline of the neck, and the inferior border of the mandible.

appendicular region A division of the skeletal system that includes the extremities and their attachments to the body.

axial region A division of the skeletal system that includes the head, neck, and trunk.

axilla The armpit.

axons Components of the nerve cell that conduct impulses to adjacent cells.

basement membrane The noncellular layer in an epithelial cell that anchors the overlying epithelial tissues.

body cavities Hollow areas within the body that contain organs and organ systems.

cardiac muscle tissue Striated involuntary muscle that has the capacity to generate and conduct electrical impulses.

carotid triangle Area of the anterior triangle of the neck that contains the carotid artery and internal jugular vein.

cell membrane The cell wall; a selectively permeable layer of cells that surrounds intracellular contents and controls movement of substances into and out of the cell.

cells The basic building blocks of life, made up of protoplasm (cytoplasm); specialized for particular functions.

centrioles Organelles that are essential in cell division.

chromosomes Structures containing DNA within the cell's nucleus; human cells contain 23 pairs of chromosomes.

cilia The hair-like microtubule projections on the surface of a cell that can move materials over the cell surface.

columnar epithelium Rows of tall, thin epithelial cells.

concentration gradient The natural tendency for substances to flow from an area of higher concentration to an area of lower concentration, within or outside the cell.

cranial cavity The hollow portion of the skull.

crenation Shrinkage of a cell that results when too much water leaves the cell through osmosis.

cuboidal epithelium Rows of square-shaped epithelial cells.

cytoplasm The gel-like material inside a cell. It makes up most of the cell's volume, and suspends the cell's organelles; also called protoplasm.

cytosol The clear liquid portion of the cytoplasm.

dendrites Components of the neurons that receive impulses from the axon and contain vesicles for release of neurotransmitters.

deoxyribonucleic acid (DNA) The genetic material found on the chromosomes in the cell's nucleus.

diffusion A process where molecules move from an area of higher concentration to an area of lower concentration.

dysrhythmias Disturbances in cardiac rhythm.

electrolytes Salt or acid substances that become ionic conductors when dissolved in a solvent (ie, water); chemicals dissolved in the blood.

electrons Negatively charged particles that revolve around the nucleus of an atom.

endocytosis The uptake of material through the cell membrane by a membrane-bound droplet or vesicle formed within the cell's protoplasm.

endoplasmic reticulum A series of membranes in which proteins and fats are manufactured.

exocytosis The release of secretions from cells that have been accumulated in vesicles.

extracellular Substances located outside of the cell membrane.

extracellular fluid (ECF) Fluid outside of the cell, in which most of the body's supply of sodium is contained.

facilitated diffusion The process whereby a carrier molecule moves substances in or out of cells from areas of higher to lower concentration.

flagella Tail-like microtubule structures capable of motion to propel the cell.

fontanelles Areas in the infant's skull where the sutures between the skull bones have not yet closed.

girdles Bony structures that attach the limbs to the body (hip and shoulder).

Golgi apparatus A set of membranes in the protoplasm involved in the formation of sugars and complex proteins.

hemothorax An abnormal accumulation of bloody fluid within the pleural space following trauma.

hyperkalemia An excessive amount of potassium in the blood.

hypernatremia A serum sodium level of greater than 145 mEq/L.

hyperosmolar hyperglycemic nonketotic coma (HHNC) A diabetic emergency that occurs from a relative insulin deficiency, resulting in hyperglycemia, hyperosmolarity, and an absence of significant ketosis.

hypoglycemia Abnormally low blood glucose level.

hypokalemia A low concentration of potassium in the blood.

hyponatremia A serum sodium level that is less than 135 mEq/L.

hypoxia A dangerous condition in which the supply of oxygen to the tissues is reduced.

integument Skin, the covering of the body surface.

intracellular Substances, such as the organelles, that are found inside the cell membrane.

intracellular fluid (ICF) Fluid within cells in which most of the body's supply of potassium is contained.

ion channels Protein-lined pores or transport channels, specifically sized for each substance, which allow electrolyte movements among the cells.

lysis The process of disintegration or breakdown of cells that occurs when excess water enters the cell through osmosis.

lysosomes Membrane-bound vesicles that contain a variety of enzymes functioning as a cell's digestive system.

mediastinum The space between the lungs, in the center of the chest, that contains the heart, trachea, mainstem bronchi, part of the esophagus, and large blood vessels.

meiosis A specialized form of cell division that results in the production of mature sperm and ova.

microtubules Hollow filamentous structures that make up various components of the cell.

mitochondria Small, rod-like organelles that function as the metabolic center of the cell and produce adenosine triphosphate (ATP).

mitosis The division of chromosomes in a cell nucleus.

nervous tissues Neurons and neuroglia.

neuroglia Collectively, the name for the connective and supporting tissues of the nervous tissue.

neurons The main functional unit of the nervous system.

neutrons Uncharged or "neutral" particles in the nucleus of an atom.

nonstriated Smooth muscle tissue.

nuclear envelope The membrane that surrounds the nucleus of the cell.

nucleoli Rounded, dense structures in the protoplasm that contain RNA and synthesize proteins.

nucleus The nerve center, or central body, of the cell, embedded within the protoplasm.

organ system A group of organs that have a common purpose, such as the skeleton and muscles.

organelles The internal structures within the cell that carry out specific functions for the cell.

organism Any individual living thing; made up of various organ systems.

organs Different types of tissues working together to perform a particular function.

osmosis The movement of a solvent, such as water, from an area of low solute concentration to one of high concentration through a selectively permeable membrane to equalize concentrations of a solute on both sides of the membrane.

osmotic pressure The measure of the tendency of water to move by osmosis across a membrane.

parietal portion The portion of the serous membrane that lines the walls of the trunk cavities.

pericardial cavity The region around the heart.

pericardial effusion An abnormal accumulation of fluid within the pericardial sac.

pericardial sac The lubricated potential space between the layers of the pericardium.

pericardial tamponade A condition that occurs as fluid accumulates around the heart, which restricts the heart's stroke volume.

pericardium The serous membranes that surround the heart.

peripheral nerves The nerves that extend from the brain and spinal cord to various parts of the body by exiting between the vertebrae of the spine.

peritonitis Inflammation of the peritoneum, the protective membrane that lines the abdominal and pelvic cavities.

phagocytosis The process in which one cell "eats" or engulfs a foreign substance to destroy it.

pinocytosis A process by which cells ingest the extracellular fluid and its contents.

pleura The serous membranes covering the lungs and lining of the thoracic cavity.

pleural space The potential space between the visceral and parietal pleura.

pleural effusion Excessive accumulation of fluid within the pleural space.

pleural fluid The small amount of lubricating fluid that fills the pleural space.

pneumothorax An abnormal accumulation of air within the pleural space.

popliteal fossa The space behind the knee.

posterior triangle The area of the neck containing the lymph nodes, brachial plexus, spinal accessory nerve, and a portion of the subclavian artery.

protons Single, positively charged particles inside the nucleus of an atom.

protoplasm A viscous liquid matrix that supports all internal cellular structures and provides a medium for intracellular transport; also called cytoplasm.

pseudostratified epithelium A single layer of epithelial cells of varying heights, all of which attach to the basement membrane, but all do not reach the free surface.

remodeling The ongoing process of cell renewal where some cells actively divide during life and others die and are replaced by new cells.

retroperitoneal organs The organs (kidneys, pancreas, and duodenum) and major blood vessels located in the retroperitoneal space.

retroperitoneal space The area located posterior to the parietal peritoneum that contains the kidneys, pancreas, reproductive organs, duodenum, and major blood vessels.

ribonucleic acid (RNA) A nucleic acid associated with controlling cellular activities.

ribosomes Organelles that contain RNA and protein.

selective permeability The ability of the cell membrane to selectively allow compounds into the cell based on the cell's current needs.

semipermeable The property of the cell membrane that describes the ability to allow certain elements to pass through while not allowing others to do so.

serous membranes Membranes that line body cavities that lack openings to the outside.

serum osmolality The number of osmotically active particles in serum.

sex cells Germ (reproductive) cells; in males they are known as sperm and in females they are known as oocytes (eggs).

simple epithelium A single layer of cells, all of which are in contact with the basement membrane of the epithelial cell.

skeletal muscle tissue Voluntary muscle tissue attached to bones and composed of long thread-like cells that have light and dark striations.

skull The protective vault that houses the brain and is composed of the cranium and facial bones.

smooth muscle tissue Nonstriated, involuntary muscle tissue found in vessel walls, glands, and the gastrointestinal tract.

sodium-potassium exchange pump A mechanism that uses active transport to move sodium out of the cells and potassium into the cells.

solutes Dissolved particles, such as salts, contained in a solvent.

somatic cells All of the other cells in the human body besides the sex cells.

spinal cavity The spinal column or vertebral canal, housing the spinal cord.

spindle fibers Microtubules radiating from the centrioles.

squamous epithelium Flat sheets of epithelial cells.

stratified epithelium More than one layer of cells, only one of which is in contact with the basement membrane of the epithelial cell.

striated Muscle tissue that has microscopic bands and may be either voluntary, such as leg muscles, or involuntary, such as cardiac muscle.

tachycardia A rapid pulse rate.

tachypnea A rapid respiratory rate.

tissues Groups of similar cells that work together.

transitional epithelium Tissue that changes in appearance due to tension; it lines the urinary bladder, ureters, and superior urethra.

umbilicus The navel.

vertebral column The spine or primary support structure of the body that houses the spinal cord and the peripheral nerves.

visceral portion The portion of a serous membrane that covers the outside of an internal organ.

■ Case Study Answers

1. On the basis of the scene size-up and primary assessment findings, what are the possible causes of the patient's chief complaint?

Answer: The scene size-up reveals a marathon that is being held in unseasonably warm temperatures and high humidity, and the primary assessment findings reveal a 35-year-old woman who is staggering, dizzy, pale, clammy, with vital signs that indicate shock. The most probable cause of the patient's chief complaint is shock resulting from excessive fluid loss. Additional immediate causes to be considered include cardiac problems, hypoglycemia, and exposure to heat.

2. What organ systems have abnormal findings in the primary assessment?

Answer: The circulatory, muscular, and integumentary systems have abnormal findings in the primary assessment.

3. What is the pathophysiology of dehydration in this patient?

Answer: The impact of inadequate fluid intake and the warm temperature is the loss of large amounts of salt and water resulting from sweating. Inadequate intake of fluid and electrolytes and excessive sweating can result in hypovolemic shock from dehydration.

Water leaves the extracellular fluid compartment, but some of the intracellular water passes into the extracellular compartment by osmosis, keeping the osmolality of the extracellular and intracellular fluids equal to each other. The result is dehydration.

4. What electrolyte abnormalities should be considered in this patient?

Answer: The excessive salt loss is called hyponatremia, and it can produce serious symptoms such as muscular weakness, dizziness, headache, hypotension, tachycardia, and shock. Severe sodium loss can result in mental confusion, stupor, and coma. Also potassium and glucose abnormalities should be considered.

5. Where should you focus your secondary assessment next?

Answer: The most common causes for electrolyte abnormalities are abnormalities in the body's fluid balance (eg, dehydration or overhydration) and consumption of drugs. Failure to recognize and promptly treat any of these abnormalities may result in harm to the patient.

Continuously reassess the patient's mental status, airway, breathing, and circulation, and obtain an electrocardiogram, blood glucose reading, and serial vital signs. Be alert for altered mental status, rhythm disturbances, nausea, and vomiting.

6. To help replace some of the fluids lost, what type of solution should you infuse?

Answer: An isotonic solution (ie, 0.9% normal saline) is appropriate for the prehospital care of this patient. An isotonic solution has the same osmolarity as the cells and body fluids, so the cells will neither shrink nor swell.

7. Which two electrolytes, found in blood, are most likely to be out of normal range because of the patient's apparent dehydration?

Answer: One of the most common causes of electrolyte abnormalities in relation to the body's fluid balance is due to the patient's dehydration. Sodium and potassium are two important electrolytes to consider for abnormalities in such conditions as dehydration or overhydration.

The Skeletal System

Learning Objectives

1. Describe the function of the skeleton. (p 44)
2. Explain how bones are classified and give an example of each. (p 45-47)
3. Explain how joints are classified; give an example of each and describe the movements possible. (p 47-49)
4. Describe how the embryonic skeleton is replaced by bone. (p 50-51)
5. State the nutrients necessary for bone growth. (p 51)
6. Name the hormones involved in bone growth and maintenance. (p 51)
7. Explain what is meant by exercise for bones and explain its importance. (p 51)
8. Identify the two major subdivisions of the skeleton and list the bones in each area. (p 54-68)

■ Introduction

The skeleton gives us our recognizable human form. The skeletal system is composed of 206 bones and provides the essential functions of support, movement, and protection for the structures of the body. The body's support framework consists of bones and their associated connective tissues: cartilage, tendons, and ligaments. Virtually every muscle in the body attaches to bones. Muscle contraction results in the movement of the bones at the joints. Bony structures provide protection for the most vital organs of the body such as the skull, which covers the brain, and the rib cage, which surrounds the heart, lungs, and mediastinum. Finally, the skeletal system serves several vital metabolic functions such as the production of blood cells, platelets, and regulation of serum levels of the essential mineral calcium.

Special Needs Tip

Fractures are more common in older persons because of a decrease in bone mineral density. The result is weaker bones.

■ Cartilage, Tendons, and Ligaments

Cartilage, tendons, and ligaments are important connective tissues that work with bones to provide the support framework of the skeleton. Shiny connective tissue called cartilage is lubricated by a transparent viscous joint fluid (synovial fluid) that is secreted by the synovial membrane in an articulation to provide a slippery surface over which the bones may

Case Study | PART 1

You and your partner respond to a call in a residential community where a homeowner working on his roof fell onto the driveway. A neighbor heard the man scream before seeing him slide off the second-story roof, landing feet first. The neighbor stated that the man did not strike his head or lose consciousness. On arrival, you determine that the scene is safe. Your general impression is that the man is in severe pain and is bleeding from his legs. You are careful to take standard precautions because of the presence of body fluids.

Your primary assessment reveals that the only immediate life threat to the patient is bleeding from open fractures in the lower legs. You are able to control the bleeding easily with direct pressure and a bandage. You apply a cervical collar and a nonrebreathing mask set at 15 L/min. You ask a police officer at the scene to assist you by maintaining manual stabilization of the patient's head and neck while you prepare to begin the rapid trauma examination. Because of the significant mechanism of injury (MOI) and the pain that the patient is experiencing, you consider the patient to be high priority and your partner notifies an additional medic unit to continue their response to the scene.

Your partner obtains the first set of baseline vital signs.

Recording Time: 0 minutes	
Appearance	Middle-aged male in obvious pain from leg injuries
Level of consciousness	Alert (oriented to person, place, and day)
Airway	Appears patent
Breathing	Normal
Circulation	Pale, cool, and clammy skin, bleeding from both legs
Pulse	110 beats/min and thready
Blood pressure	112/70 mm Hg
Respirations	20 breaths/min and regular
Spo$_2$	96%

1. What are the probable skeletal injuries in this patient?

2. What would be your next steps in assessing the patient?

move freely. In addition to lubricating the joint, synovial fluid contains white blood cells to fight infections and provides nourishment to the cartilage covering the bone. Synovial fluid is found in the joint cavity, the space between the joint capsule (a connective tissue capsule that surrounds the bones) and the bones. Although there are several different types of cartilage, hyaline cartilage is the type most commonly associated with joints. A double-layered connective tissue membrane known as the perichondrium surrounds the cartilage.

Tendons are specialized tough cords or bands of dense white connective tissue that are continuous with the periosteum of the bone, the double-layer membrane that covers all bones except the articular surfaces. Tendons connect muscles to bones. Ligaments are tough white bands of tissue that bind bones together. Tendons and ligaments are composed of densely packed fibers of collagen, a twisted rope-like protein. The collagen fibrils in ligaments often are less compact than those in tendons. Ligaments usually are more flattened than tendons, forming sheets or bands of tissue. A sprain occurs when the bone ends partially or temporarily dislocate and the supporting ligaments are partially stretched or torn. Following a sprain, the joint surfaces generally fall back into alignment.

When a muscle contracts, tendon pulls on bone, resulting in motion at a joint, a point where two or more bones come together, allowing movement to occur. A strain, or muscle pull, occurs when a muscle is stretched or torn, resulting in pain, swelling, and bruising of surrounding soft tissues. No ligament or joint damage occurs with a strain. Sprains and strains are graded based on their severity and physical findings during examination Table 3-1.

Classifications of Bones

Bones are classified according to their shape Figure 3-1. Long bones are longer than they are wide and include most bones of the upper and lower extremities, including the femur, tibia, fibula, ulna, radius, and humerus. Short bones are approximately as broad as they are long and often are cube-shaped or round, as exemplified by the bones of the wrist or of the foot. Flat bones are relatively thin and flattened and include certain skull bones, ribs, the sternum (breastbone), and the scapulae (shoulder blades).

Table 3-1	**Types of Strains and Sprains**	
Grade Strains	**Degree of Damage**	**Clinical Findings and Implications**
Grade I	Minimal damage or disruption	Tender without swelling No bruising or palpable defect Active contraction and passive stretch are painful Prognosis is good with minimal impairment
Grade II	Moderate damage	Tender with swelling Mild to moderate bruising Passive movement and attempted active movement are painful Joint ROM limited Prognosis usually is good with minimal impairment but requires a longer healing/rehabilitation period
Grade III	Complete disruption of the muscle, tendon, or both	Extreme tenderness with swelling Palpable defect may be present Complete loss of muscle function No increase in pain with passive stretch (nerve fibers are completely torn) Prognosis is variable (injury may require surgery) Requires a prolonged healing/rehabilitation period
Sprains		
Grade I	Minimal damage or disruption	Tender without swelling No bruising Active and passive range of motion are painful Prognosis is good with no expectation of instability or functional loss
Grade II	Moderate damage	Moderate swelling and bruising Very tender with more diffuse tenderness than grade I Range of motion is very painful and restricted Joint may be unstable, and functional loss may result
Grade III	Complete disruption of the ligament	Severe swelling and bruising Structural instability with abnormal increase in range of motion (due to a complete tear of ligament) Pain on passive range of motion may be less than lower grades (nerve fibers are completely torn) Significant functional loss that may require surgery to restore

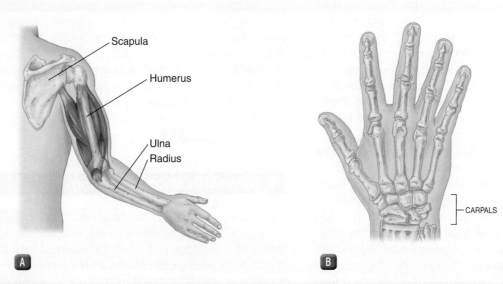

Figure 3-1 Bones are classified according to their shape. **A.** The scapula is a flat bone, and the humerus, ulna, and radius are long bones. **B.** The carpals, or wrist bones, are short bones.

Long bones consist of a shaft, the diaphysis; the ends, or epiphyses; and the physis (growth plate or epiphyseal plate), which is the major site of bone elongation during growth **Figure 3-2** . The physis closes at the termination of skeletal growth, which leaves a scar known as a physeal scar which is present in some adult bones. The physis (epiphyseal plate) is located next to the epiphysis. The metaphysis is the flared region of a long bone between the diaphysis and epiphysis. The periosteum, which consists of a double layer of connective tissue, lines the outer surface of the bone, and the inner surfaces are lined with endosteum.

The diaphysis of many bones includes the medullary cavity, an internal cavity that contains a substance known as bone marrow. In adults, most bone marrow in the long bones in the extremities contains adipose (fat) tissue and is, therefore, called yellow marrow. The bones of the axial skeleton and girdles contain red marrow, where most red blood cells are manufactured.

The two main types of bone are compact bone and cancellous bone. Compact bone is mostly solid, with few spaces; cancellous bone consists of a lacy network of bony rods called trabeculae. The trabeculae are oriented along the lines of stress to increase the weight-bearing capacity of the long bones.

Blood vessels typically do not penetrate trabeculae. Thus, cancellous bone receives its nutrients via canaliculi. However, blood vessels do directly penetrate compact bone. The lamellae are oriented around these blood vessels in units called osteons or haversian systems. The blood vessels of the haversian canals are interconnected by a series of vessels called perforating canals **Figure 3-3** .

Bones grow in two ways: appositional growth, the formation of new bone on the surface of a bone, or endochondral growth, the growth of cartilage in the physis

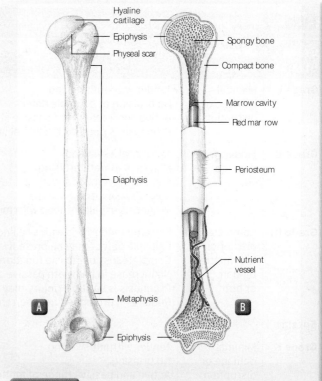

Figure 3-2 The components of the long bone. **A.** Drawing of the humerus. Notice the long shaft and dilated ends. **B.** Longitudinal section of the humerus showing compact bone, spongy bone, and marrow.

(epiphyseal plate) and its eventual replacement by bone. As a person grows, old bone is removed by osteoclasts and new bone is deposited by osteoblasts, resulting in changes in the bone's shape, a process known as bone remodeling.

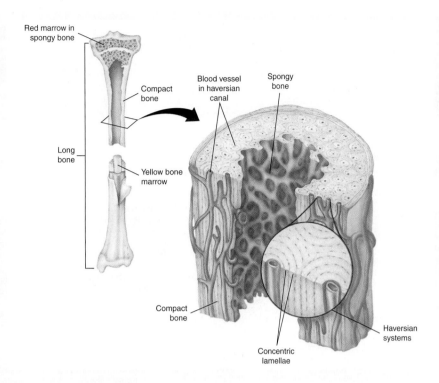

Red marrow in spongy bone

Compact bone

Long bone

Yellow bone marrow

Blood vessel in haversian canal

Spongy bone

Compact bone

Concentric lamellae

Haversian systems

Figure 3-3 The shaft of the bone, shown at three levels of detail. The shaft is dense and compact, giving the bone strength. The ends of the bone and lining of the cavity within the long bone are spongy, with more open lattice areas. Blood cells are formed within red bone marrow that fills the lattice at the ends of the bone. Inset shows a magnified haversian system with its concentric lamellae. Yellow bone marrow fills the cavity in the shaft of the long bone.

Clinical Tip

Dysfunction or suppression of the bone marrow may develop in persons who have adverse reactions to certain drugs, such as nonsteroidal anti-inflammatory drugs (NSAIDs), or who receive chemotherapy for cancer. Use of chemotherapy and NSAIDs can result in anemia caused by a decrease in the number of cells produced by the marrow, increased susceptibility to infection caused by a decrease in the number of infection-fighting white blood cells, and a tendency for internal or external bleeding caused by a decrease in the number of platelets (blood-clotting cells).

■ Joints

Joints are also referred to as articulations. They act as junctions between bones, and vary widely in structure and function **Figure 3-4**. They are classified both as to how they move and according to the types of tissue that binds bones together at the joint.

Joints are classified as immovable (synarthrotic), slightly movable (amphiarthrotic), or freely movable (diarthrotic). They can also be grouped according to the type of tissue binding them at their junctions. These groups include

fibrous, cartilaginous, and synovial joints. **Table 3-2** shows the functional classification of joints.

The 230 joints in the human body are summarized as follows:

- Fibrous joints. Lying between bones that closely contact each other, they are joined by thin, dense connective tissue. An example of a fibrous joint is a suture between flat bones of the skull. No real movement takes place in most fibrous joints, making them synarthrotic in classification. Those with limited movement (amphiarthrotic) include the joint between the distal tibia and fibula.
- Cartilaginous joints. Connected by hyaline cartilage, or fibrocartilage, these joints include those that separate the vertebrae. Each intervertebral disk is an example of a cartilaginous joint, and has slight flexibility.
- Synovial joints. These joints allow free movement (diarthrotic) and are more complex than other types of joints. They have an outer layer of ligaments (the joint capsule) and an inner lining of synovial membrane that secretes synovial fluid, which lubricates the joint. Some synovial joints have shock-absorbing fibrocartilage pads called menisci. They may also have fluid-filled sacs (bursae), commonly located between tendons and underlying bony prominences such as in the knee or elbow.

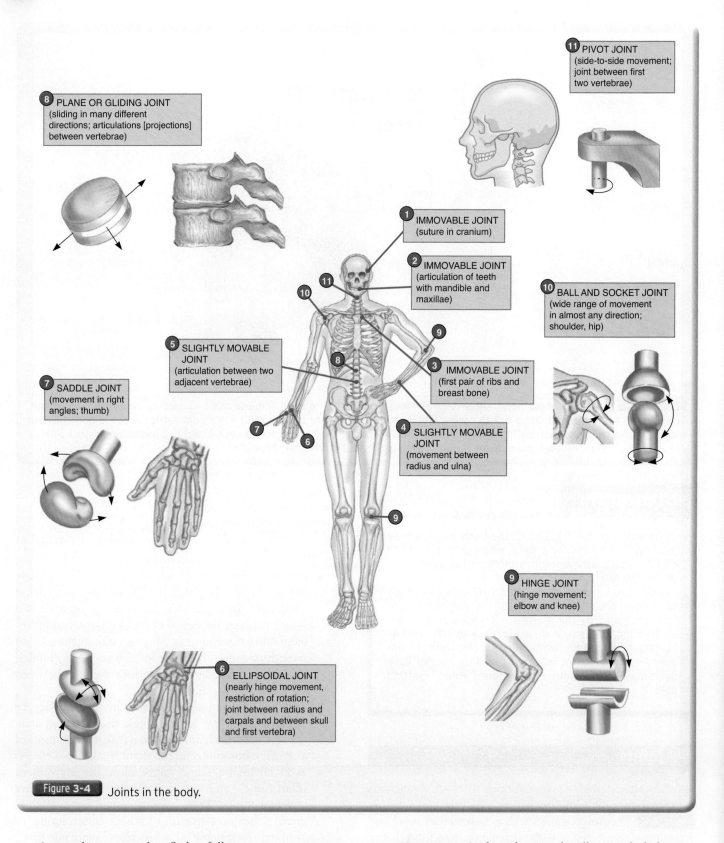

11 PIVOT JOINT (side-to-side movement; joint between first two vertebrae)

8 PLANE OR GLIDING JOINT (sliding in many different directions; articulations [projections] between vertebrae)

1 IMMOVABLE JOINT (suture in cranium)

2 IMMOVABLE JOINT (articulation of teeth with mandible and maxillae)

10 BALL AND SOCKET JOINT (wide range of movement in almost any direction; shoulder, hip)

5 SLIGHTLY MOVABLE JOINT (articulation between two adjacent vertebrae)

7 SADDLE JOINT (movement in right angles; thumb)

3 IMMOVABLE JOINT (first pair of ribs and breast bone)

4 SLIGHTLY MOVABLE JOINT (movement between radius and ulna)

9 HINGE JOINT (hinge movement; elbow and knee)

6 ELLIPSOIDAL JOINT (nearly hinge movement, restriction of rotation; joint between radius and carpals and between skull and first vertebra)

Figure 3-4   Joints in the body.

Synovial joints are classified as follows:

- *Ball-and-socket joints.* Such as in the shoulders and hips
- *Condyloid (ellipsoidal) joints.* Such as those between the metacarpals and phalanges
- *Gliding (plane) joints.* Such as in the wrists and ankles

- *Hinge joints.* Such as those in the elbow and phalanges
- *Pivot joints.* Such as between the proximal ends of the radius and ulna
- *Saddle joints.* Such as between the carpal and metacarpal bones of the thumb

Table 3-2 Functional Classification of Joints

Category and Type	Description	Example
Amphiarthrosis (little movement)		
Fibrous: Suture	Fibrous connections and interlocking projections	Between skull bones
Fibrous: Gomphosis	Fibrous connections and insertion in alveolar process	Between teeth and jaws
Cartilaginous: Synchondrosis	Cartilage plate interposed	Epiphyseal cartilages
Bony fusion: Synostosis	Conversion of other joint forms to a solid bone mass	Parts of skull, epiphyseal lines
Diarthrosis (free movement)		
Fibrous: Syndesmosis	Connections of ligaments	Between tibia and fibula
Cartilaginous: Symphysis	Connections via a fibrocartilage pad	Between pubic bones of pelvis; between vertebrae
Synarthrosis (no movement)		
Synovial	Complex joint in a joint capsule with synovial fluid	Numerous; subdivided according to range of movement
Monaxial	Allows movement in one plane	Elbows and ankles
Biaxial	Allows movement in two planes	Ribs and waist
Triaxial	Allows movement in all three planes	Shoulders and hips

Pathophysiology

Bursitis is a relatively common irritation or inflammation of a bursa. However, the fluid within a bursa as well as within a joint can become infected with bacteria, resulting in a much more serious condition that requires hospitalization for antibiotics and potentially surgery. The most common shoulder disorder is supraspinatus tendinitis, which is associated with subacromial bursitis. The subacromial bursa is located immediately superior to the shoulder joint and below the acromion process. The supraspinatus tendon runs beneath the floor of the bursa. Irritation of the tendon (tendinitis) results in concomitant inflammation in the overlying bursa, and significant and potentially disabling shoulder pain may occur.

Frozen shoulder, or adhesive capsulitis, results in a decreased ability to move the upper arm at the shoulder joint. Persons older than age 40 years who have sustained trauma are most often affected by frozen shoulder. Tendinitis of the biceps or rotator cuff tendons also may irritate the overlying shoulder bursa. In both frozen shoulder and tendinitis, excess scar tissue may form at the articulation of the proximal humerus and glenoid fossa, leading to restriction of movement about the shoulder joint. Patients often seek medical care because of the pain and stiffness associated with these conditions; however, these symptoms often occur only after much range of motion has already been lost. At this point, the pain may be quite severe, interfering with sleep. Prevention of restriction of movement is the best treatment and is achieved by minimizing the time of immobilization for relatively minor shoulder injuries and encouraging early range-of-motion exercises, especially in elderly patients. Elderly patients often have frozen shoulder because the injured extremity is immobilized in a sling for a long period of time, limiting shoulder motion. Corticosteroids injected into the shoulder joint may offer some benefit, but the course of this condition is quite variable. Frozen shoulder may subside after several months or may result in disability and permanent restriction of movement.

Shoulder dislocation occurs when a traumatic disruption of the ligaments of the shoulder joint allows the humeral head to slip out of the glenoid fossa in an anterior, posterior, or inferior direction. Most commonly, dislocation of the shoulder occurs anteriorly and is the result of a fall. Dislocations of the shoulder are among the most common joint dislocations seen in emergency care, and complications can occur. Prompt recognition and treatment of the dislocation are essential. The shoulder joint has great freedom of movement, but it is inherently unstable. The glenoid fossa is relatively shallow. The rotator cuff tendons, as well as the long head of the biceps, prevent anterior-superior dislocation. The rotator cuff, however, does not extend inferiorly, which leaves only the capsular ligaments to hold the humeral head in place. The strongest of these ligaments is the inferior glenohumeral ligament. As the arm moves overhead, the acromion process limits abduction and external rotation of the humerus. When the shaft of the humerus reaches the acromion, a fulcrum is created. Any further attempt to abduct the arm forces the humeral head out of the glenoid fossa against the inferior glenohumeral ligament. If the tolerance of the ligament is exceeded, anterior-inferior dislocation of the shoulder occurs Figure 3-5 .

The typical mechanism of an anterior shoulder dislocation places significant stress on the rotator cuff, particularly on the supraspinatus tendon, glenoid rim, joint capsule, stabilizing ligaments, and humeral head. Additional stresses are placed on the neurovascular structures that course through the axilla.

Posterior dislocations result in a posteriorly displaced humeral head. In a posterior dislocation, the anteriorly placed subscapularis muscle and tendon place significant stress on the humeral head, resulting in an internally rotated humeral head with marked loss of external rotation that is noted on clinical examination. The usual mechanism of injury is internal rotation and adduction. A direct

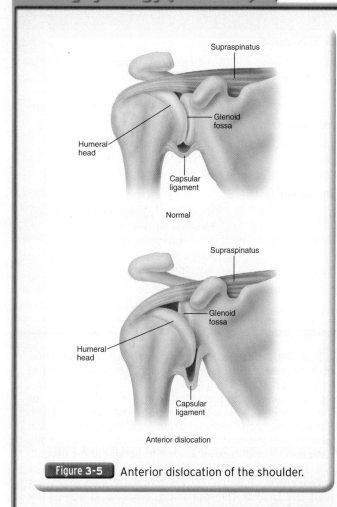

Figure 3-5   Anterior dislocation of the shoulder.

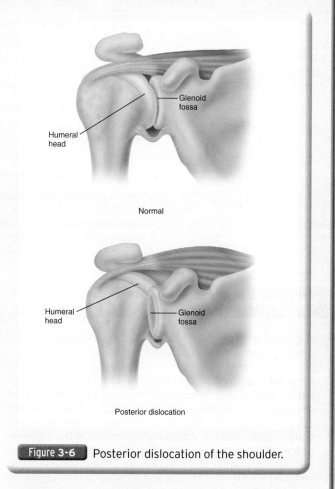

Figure 3-6   Posterior dislocation of the shoulder.

force also may result in posterior dislocation **Figure 3-6**. Occasionally posterior dislocations occur as a consequence of seizures. Posterior dislocations are far less common than anterior shoulder dislocations.

Complications associated with either anterior or posterior shoulder dislocations include vascular injury, nerve injury, recurrence, missed diagnosis, and dislocation arthropathy (arthritis). A high rate of recurrent dislocation has been noted in young patients who have been managed with immobilization with or without rehabilitation, which is the standard nonsurgical treatment. Anterior dislocation has a higher risk of recurrence than posterior dislocation. The risk of recurrence in young male patients who sustain a dislocation as a result of participation in athletics can be as high as 90% and younger patients often require surgery to prevent future recurrences. Older patients have a lower risk of recurrence.

Growth and Development of Bones

Bones are a living substance with cells requiring a blood supply. Bones begin to form in utero during the first 6 weeks after fertilization. Intramembranous bones originate between layers of connective tissues that are sheet-like in appearance. Examples of intramembranous bones are the flat, broad bones of the skull. These bones begin development when unspecialized connective tissues form at the sites where future bones will be developed. Bone-forming cells (osteoblasts) develop, depositing bony matrix around them. When extracellular matrix has surrounded the osteoblasts, they are termed osteocytes. The surrounding membranous tissues begin to form the periosteum of a bone. Inside the periosteum, the osteoblasts form a compact bone layer over the new spongy bone.

Endochondral bones begin as cartilaginous masses that are eventually replaced by bone tissue. These bones develop from hyaline cartilage that is shaped similarly to the bones they will become **Figure 3-7**. They grow rapidly at first, and then begin to change in appearance. When spongy bone begins to replace the original cartilage, a primary ossification center is created, with bone tissue developing outward toward the ends of the structure. Eventually, secondary ossification centers will appear in the epiphyses, forming more spongy bone.

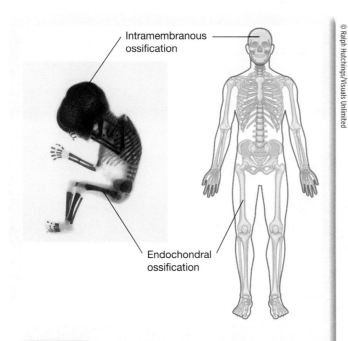

Intramembranous ossification

Endochondral ossification

Figure 3-7 Intramembranous ossification results in the development of flat bones. Endochondral ossification results in the production of long bones.

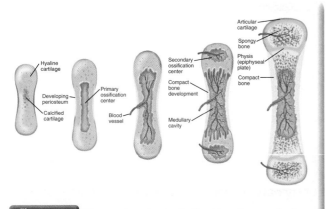

Hyaline cartilage

Developing periosteum

Calcified cartilage

Primary ossification center

Blood vessel

Secondary ossification center

Compact bone development

Medullary cavity

Articular cartilage

Spongy bone

Physis (epiphyseal plate)

Compact bone

Figure 3-8 The major stages in the development of an endochondral bone.

Source: Adapted from Shier, D. N., Butler, J. L., and Lewis, R. *Hole's Essentials of Human Anatomy & Physiology*, 10th ed. New York, NY. McGraw-Hill Higher Education, 2009.

During the first 6 weeks of development, the skeleton is cartilaginous. The bones increase greatly in size as the fetus develops, and throughout childhood **Figure 3-8**. Bone growth continues through adolescence. The process of replacing other tissues with bone is called ossification, which involves the deposition of calcium salts.

Osteogenesis is defined as the formation of bone. Long bones are first formed of hyaline cartilage, and later replaced by bony tissue that becomes compact bone. This process begins with the diaphysis and ends with the epiphyses of each long bone. This process of bone formation is called endochondral ossification.

Flat bones are not formed in this manner. These bones develop from connective tissue membranes that are replaced by spongy bone, and then compact bone. This process is called intramembranous ossification.

When the bones are growing, the diaphyses meet the epiphyses at a structure called the physis (epiphyseal plate). It is made up of four cartilage layers: reserve cartilage, proliferating (hyperplastic) cartilage, hypertrophic cartilage, and the calcified matrix. Growth of long bones depends on good nutrition and several hormones, including human growth hormone (hGH). Human growth hormone increases the rate of growth of the skeleton by causing cartilage cells and bone cells to reproduce and lay down their intercellular matrix, as well as stimulating the deposition of mineral within this matrix. The hormone also stimulates muscles to grow. The other hormones involved in long bone growth include thyroid hormone, estrogen, and testosterone. Once the physis (epiphyseal plate) experiences closure, the long bones can no longer grow **Figure 3-9**. Increased length of bone is balanced by increased bone width. Osteoblast and osteoclast activity is balanced in the body so that the bones grow uniformly and proportionately.

Bone development, growth, and repair are influenced by nutrition, hormones, and exercise. Bone also serves as a storage site for minerals, particularly calcium, and has a role in the formation of blood cells and platelets. Bones consist of collagen and the mineral hydroxyapatite, a compound that contains calcium and phosphate. The collagen fibers in bone act much like reinforcing rods in a concrete structure, lending flexible strength to the bone. The mineral components of the bone supply strength for bearing weight, much like concrete does in a structure. Bone without the necessary amount of mineral is very flexible; bone without enough collagen is extremely brittle. Vitamin D is required for the absorption of calcium in the small intestine. Without it, calcium is not absorbed well, softening bones and potentially causing deformity. Growth hormone from the pituitary gland stimulates cell division in the physis (epiphyseal plate) and sex hormones stimulate ossification of these plates. Exercise stresses the bones, stimulating them to become thickened and strong. Decreased activity or sedentary periods lead to decreased bone thickness. Calcium-rich foods, vitamin D, and exercise all help to maintain good bone health and prevent osteoporosis in women and men.

In postmenopausal women especially, weight-bearing activities and efficient maintenance of estrogen and calcium levels are significant factors in slowing bone deterioration and osteoporosis.

Fractures

A fracture is a broken bone. More precisely, it is a break in the continuity of bone. When a bone is fractured, damaged blood vessels release blood, which forms a blood clot. Within days, cells known as fibroblasts secrete

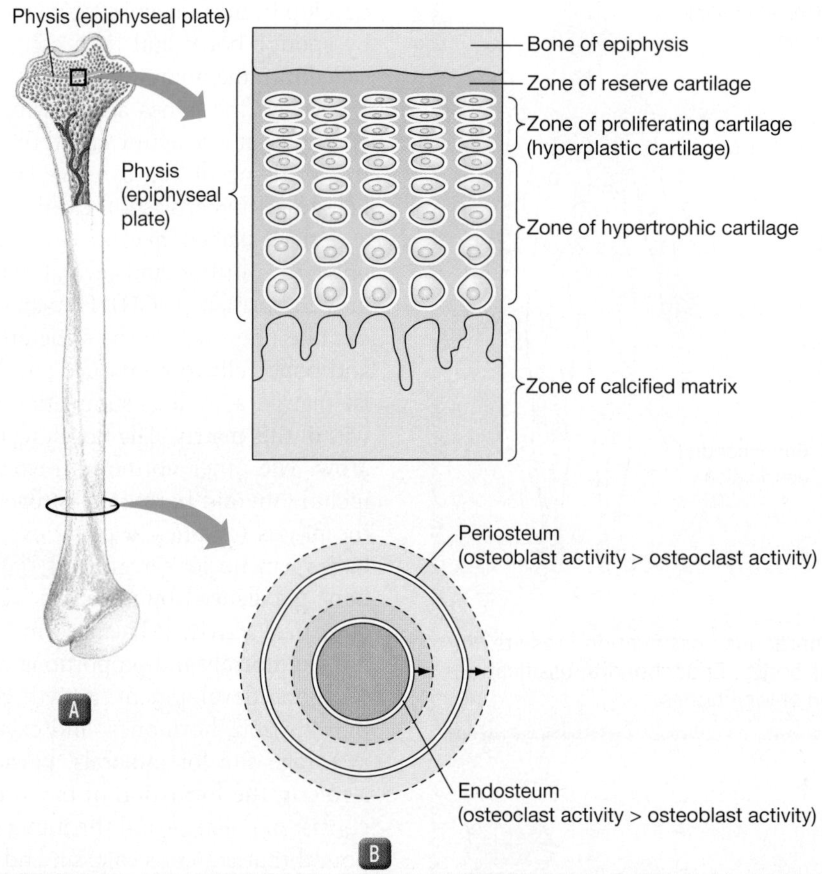

Physis (epiphyseal plate)

Bone of epiphysis

Zone of reserve cartilage

Zone of proliferating cartilage
(hyperplastic cartilage)

Physis
(epiphyseal
plate)

Zone of hypertrophic cartilage

Zone of calcified matrix

Periosteum
(osteoblast activity > osteoclast activity)

A

Endosteum
(osteoclast activity > osteoblast activity)

B

Figure 3-9   **A.** Lengthwise growth occurs in the physis (epiphyseal plate) until puberty when the physis (epiphyseal plate) closes, becoming the physeal scar. **B.** Growth in diameter involves altered rates of osteoclast and osteoblast activity at the periosteum and endosteum.

proteins and collagen to form a network of connective tissue between the broken bone ends. Other cells, chondroblasts, produce cartilage within the network. The zone of repair that results is called a callus, in which a mass of exudates and connective tissue form around a break in a bone, converting to bone during the healing process. Osteoblasts from surrounding normal bone then invade the area to form cancellous bone trabeculae. As time passes, bone remodeling occurs and cancellous bone is replaced by compact bone. At this point, depending on the location and severity of the fracture, healing is complete, usually 4 to 6 weeks following the initial injury.

Fractures are classified as either closed or open. A closed fracture occurs when a bone is fractured but the bony ends have not penetrated through the skin. An open fracture occurs when the skin over the fracture is penetrated. An open fracture may occur from the inside out, when the bone ends protrude through the skin, or from the outside in, when an object penetrates the skin, secondarily fracturing the underlying bone. Fractures also may be described by whether the bone is moved from its normal position, either as a nondisplaced fracture or a displaced fracture **Figure 3-10**. Open fractures are susceptible to infection and often must be surgically débrided.

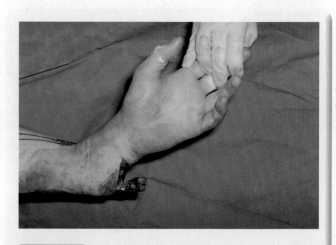

© Medical-on-Line/Alamy Images

Figure 3-10   An open fracture in which the bone ends have protruded through the skin.

Medical personnel often use the following special terms to describe particular types of fractures **Figure 3-11** :

- Greenstick. An incomplete fracture that passes only partway through the shaft of a bone but may still cause substantial angulation; occurs in children.
- Comminuted. A fracture in which the bone is broken into more than two fragments.
- Pathologic. A fracture of weakened or diseased bone, seen in patients with osteoporosis or cancer, generally produced by minimal force.
- Epiphyseal. A fracture that occurs in a growth section of a child's bone and may lead to growth abnormalities.
- Oblique. A fracture in which the bone is broken at an angle across the bone. This is usually the result of a sharp angled blow to the bone.
- Transverse. A fracture that occurs straight across the bone. This is usually the result of a direct blow or stress fracture caused by prolonged running.

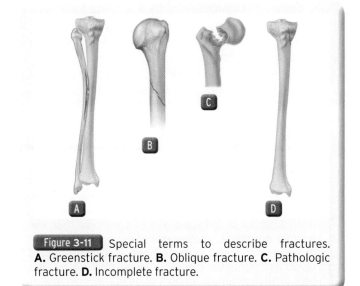

Figure 3-11 Special terms to describe fractures. **A.** Greenstick fracture. **B.** Oblique fracture. **C.** Pathologic fracture. **D.** Incomplete fracture.

Case Study | PART 2

As you perform a rapid exam, you discover the following significant findings:

- Head: The patient did not sustain any apparent injury to the head.
- Neck: Although there was no obvious neck injury, the patient is experiencing pain and soreness at the cervical spine.
- Chest: The patient's breath sounds are equal bilaterally, and he does not report any pain or tenderness in his ribs or sternum.
- Abdomen: Examination of the four quadrants does not elicit a response of pain.
- Pelvis: Although there is no obvious swelling or deformity, the patient reports pain in the pelvic girdle.
- Extremities: The patient has open fractures in both lower extremities. Abrasions are present on the upper extremities, but there is no evidence of more serious injury to the upper extremities. Distal pulses, motor, and sensory functions are present in all four extremities.
- Back and buttocks: By carefully reaching around the patient with a minimum of movement, you determine that except for tenderness in the patient's lumbar spine, there is no evidence of deformity to the patient's back and buttocks.

The additional EMS unit has arrived, and you now have more hands to help prepare the patient for transport. Because of the severity of the patient's injuries and the potential for shock from the loss of blood, you and your crew carefully apply splints to the patient's lower extremities, and then place the patient onto a long backboard. Although the patient is experiencing a significant amount of pain, he remains alert. Your partner is preparing to start two large-bore IV lines while you are en route to the hospital.

Recording Time: 5 minutes	
Appearance	Still in severe pain
Level of consciousness	Alert (oriented to person, place, and day)
Airway	Open and secure
Breathing	Normal
Circulation	Still very pale and clammy, bleeding from legs is controlled

3. Describe the components of the spine.

4. What are the potential injuries to the spine for this patient?

- Spiral. A fracture caused by a twisting force, causing an oblique fracture around the bone and through the bone. This is sometimes associated with abuse in very young children.
- Incomplete. A fracture that does not extend completely through the bone; a nondisplaced partial crack.

Pathophysiology

Most fractures heal uneventfully, but complications can occur. Complications that may be a direct result of the fracture include infection, osteomyelitis, osteonecrosis, and malunion. Infection may occur following an open fracture or following a closed fracture that was treated surgically. Osteomyelitis is an infection that involves the bone. Complications involving delayed union and nonunion can occur when fractures do not heal in an appropriate amount of time. Osteonecrosis is a condition in which portions of the bone die because of inadequate blood supply. Malunion is a condition that results when bones heal in less than perfect alignment.

Complications that can be attributed to an associated injury, rather than as a direct result of the fracture itself, include injury to major blood vessels, nerves, viscera, and tendons, or to posttraumatic arthritis or fat embolism.

Clinical Tip

In open fractures, sharp bone ends may protrude through the skin and bleeding control may be necessary. During management of these injuries, in addition to the use of standard precautions for blood exposure, the EMS provider must use caution to avoid personal injury from the sharp or jagged bone ends.

Pathophysiology

Various disorders other than fractures may affect bones. Abnormalities of bone growth may result in gigantism, a state of bony overgrowth, or dwarfism, a state of abnormally small bones. Osteogenesis imperfecta is a genetic disorder in which the patient lacks sufficient collagen for proper strength of the bones, resulting in brittle bones and frequent fractures. Osteomyelitis is an infection of the bone usually caused by a bacterial organism, most commonly *Staphylococcus aureus*.

Tumors of the bone may be primary, originating in the bone tissue itself, or metastatic, originating from some other site. The most common tumors to metastasize to bone are breast, prostate, and lung tumors.

Osteomalacia is an abnormal softening of bones because of a loss of calcium. Causes of osteomalacia include inadequate nutrition, vitamin D deficiency (rickets), or an inability of the intestine to absorb calcium and phosphorus. Osteoporosis is a reduction in the actual quantity of bony tissue, most commonly in postmenopausal women, sedentary or immobilized persons, and patients on long-term corticosteroid therapy. Fractures, especially of the hips and the vertebrae, are common in these persons.

As people age, they begin to lose bone tissue. In most people, this process is slow and gradual. Bone tissue begins to disappear between ages 30 and 40 years and continues throughout life. However, bone loss varies greatly among persons, and some elderly persons show no sign of bone loss. Several factors influence both the loss of bone mass with age and the formation of bone mass in a person who is growing. The single most important factor associated with reduced bone mass is the loss of the female sex hormone, estrogen. Tobacco smoking, lack of exercise, and low dietary calcium levels also reduce bone density.

Skeletal Organization

The skeleton is divided into two major portions: the axial skeleton Figure 3-12 and the appendicular skeleton. Including the bones of the middle ear, there are 206 bones in the human body.

The Axial Skeleton

The axial skeleton supports and protects the head, neck, and trunk. It includes the skull, hyoid bone (a single bone in the neck that supports the tongue and its muscles), vertebral column, and thoracic cage.

The Skull

The human skull is made up of 28 bones in three anatomic groups. These are divided into the cranium (brain case), the face, and the auditory ossicles. The cranium is made up of 8 bones, and the face is made up of 14. The six auditory ossicles function in hearing and are located deep within cavities of the temporal bone. The lines where the bones of the skull lock together are called sutures. The only movable bone in the skull is the mandible (lower jaw), which is attached to the cranium by ligaments. The cranium houses and protects the brain. Air-filled spaces inside the cranial bones called paranasal sinuses help the voice to resonate and also reduce the weight of the skull. Figure 3-13 shows various views of the human skull and its bones.

The bones of the cranium are as follows:

- Frontal bone. This bone forms the anterior skull above the eyes, with each eye orbit (the eye socket) having a supraorbital foramen or notch. Blood vessels and nerves pass through this structure to the forehead tissues. The frontal bone contains two frontal sinuses above the central part of the eyes.

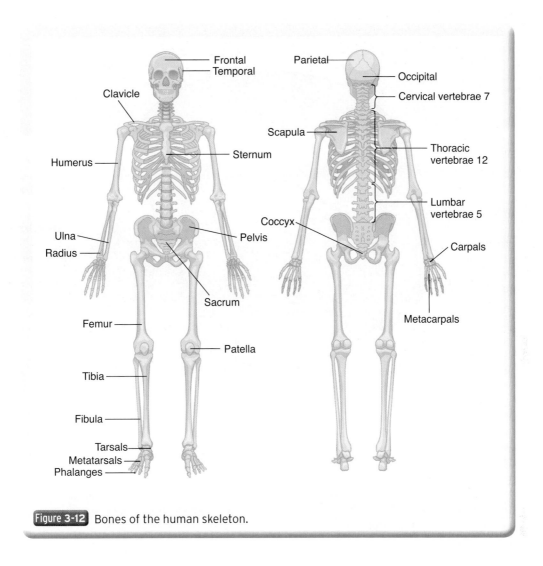

Figure 3-12 Bones of the human skeleton.

- Parietal bones. These bones are located on each side of the skull behind the frontal bone. These two bones form the sides and roof of the cranium and are fused in the middle along the sagittal suture. They meet the frontal bone along the coronal suture.
- Occipital bone. Joining the parietal bones along the lambdoid suture, the occipital bone forms the back of the skull and base of the cranium. A large opening at the lower portion of this bone (the foramen magnum) allows nerve fibers to pass through from the brain into the spinal cord. Rounded occipital condyles on each side of the foramen magnum articulate with the first vertebra of the spine.
- Temporal bones. These two bones join the parietal bone on each side of the skull, along the squamous suture, and form parts of the sides and base of the cranium. An opening called the external acoustic meatus leads through each temporal bone to the ossicles (the three small bones in the middle ear: the malleus, incus, and stapes) and to the inner ear structures. The

mandibular fossae are depressions that articulate with the mandible. Two projections below each external acoustic meatus (the mastoid process and the styloid process) provide points of attachment. The mastoid process attaches to certain neck muscles, and the styloid process attaches to muscles of the tongue and pharynx. The zygomatic process projects from the temporal bone to join the zygomatic bone, helping to form the cheek.
- Sphenoid bone. This bone forms part of the base of the cranium, sides of the skull, and floors and sides of the eye orbits. A portion of the sphenoid bone has an indentation that forms the sella turcica, which contains the pituitary gland. Two sphenoidal sinuses are also housed within the sphenoid bone.
- Ethmoid bone. Located in front of the sphenoid bone, the ethmoid bone forms a mass on each side of the nasal cavity that is joined by thin cribriform plates that partially form the roof of the nasal cavity. These horizontal bones are perforated with numerous foramina

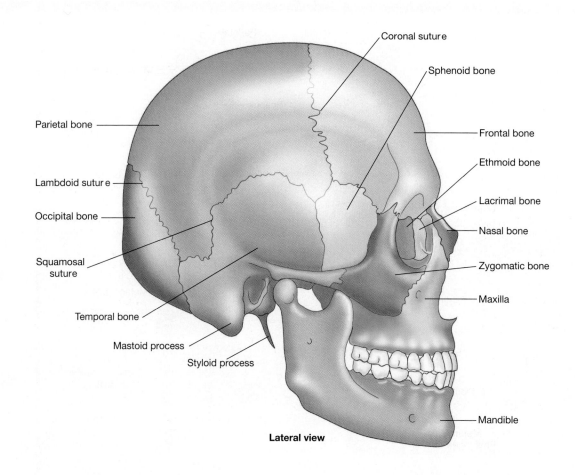

Coronal suture
Sphenoid bone
Parietal bone
Frontal bone
Ethmoid bone
Lambdoid suture
Lacrimal bone
Occipital bone
Nasal bone
Squamosal suture
Zygomatic bone
Maxilla
Temporal bone
Mastoid process
Styloid process
Mandible

Lateral view

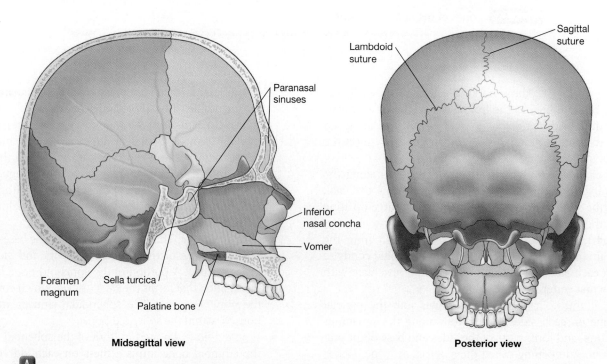

Paranasal sinuses
Lambdoid suture
Sagittal suture
Inferior nasal concha
Vomer
Foramen magnum
Sella turcica
Palatine bone

Midsagittal view

Posterior view

A

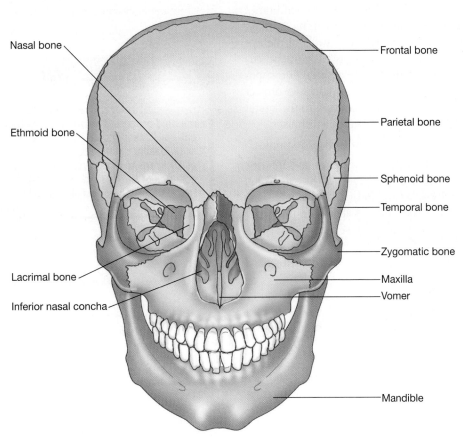

Nasal bone

Ethmoid bone

Lacrimal bone

Inferior nasal concha

Frontal bone

Parietal bone

Sphenoid bone

Temporal bone

Zygomatic bone

Maxilla

Vomer

Mandible

Anterior view

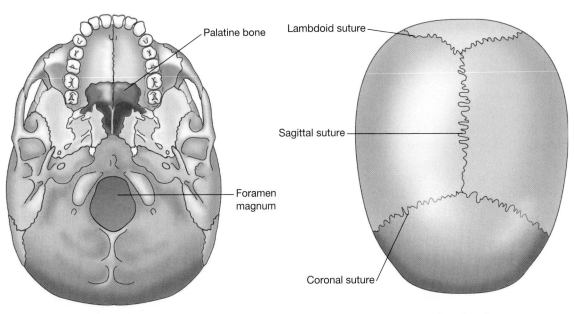

Palatine bone

Foramen magnum

Inferior view

Lambdoid suture

Sagittal suture

Coronal suture

Superior view

B

Figure 3-13 Bones of the skull.

for the passage of the olfactory nerve filaments from the nasal cavity. Between the cribriform plates, a triangular process (the crista galli) attaches to membranes (meninges) that enclose the brain. Parts of the ethmoid bone form pieces of the cranial floor, walls of the eye orbits, and walls of the nasal cavity. A perpendicular plate forms most of the nasal septum. The superior nasal conchae and middle nasal conchae project inward toward the perpendicular plate, with the lateral ethmoid bone containing many ethmoidal sinuses.

The facial skeleton consists of the following 14 bones:

- Maxillae. These two bones form the upper jaw, anterior roof of the mouth (hard palate), floors of the eye orbits, and the nasal cavity sides and floor. The maxillae contain the upper teeth sockets as well as the maxillary sinuses, which are the largest sinuses in the skull. As the human body grows, palatine processes of the maxillae grow together and fuse to form the anterior hard palate. Along with the alveolar process, the alveolar arch (dental arch) is formed, where the teeth are bound via dense connective tissue.
- Zygomatic bones. These two bones form the cheek prominences below the eyes as well as the lateral walls and floors of the eye orbits. A temporal process extends from the zygomatic bones to form a zygomatic arch.
- Nasal bones. These two long, thin bones lie side by side, fusing at the midline to form the bridge of the nose.
- Vomer bone. This thin, flat bone is found along the midline of the nasal cavity, joining the ethmoid bone to form the nasal septum.
- Inferior nasal conchae. These two bones are scroll-shaped, attached to the lateral nasal cavity walls, and support the mucous membranes of the cavity.
- Lacrimal bones. These two thin structures are located in the medial wall of each eye orbit between the maxillae and ethmoid bone.
- Palatine bones. Located behind the maxillae, the two L-shaped palatine bones form the posterior hard palate and nasal cavity floor, as well as the nasal cavity lateral walls.
- Mandible. This horseshoe-shaped bone projects upward at each end with the mandibular condyle and coronoid process. It articulates with the temporal bone and provides attachments for the muscles needed for chewing. The curved alveolar arch contains the hollow sockets for the lower teeth. The mandible is the only movable bone of the facial skeleton.

In infants, the cranial bones are connected by fibrous membranes through fontanelles (soft spots) that allow the cranium to slightly change shape. When the infant is born, the cranium compresses somewhat to facilitate passage through the birth canal. The fontanelles eventually close as the cranium ossifies and the bones grow together. The skull of an infant fractures less easily than that of an adult.

The two fontanelles are termed anterior and posterior. The anterior fontanelle closes at age 18 months, and the posterior fontanelle closes at age 2 months.

Pathophysiology

Battle sign refers to bruising behind the ear, over the mastoid process. The presence of Battle sign in a trauma patient is likely caused by a fracture at the base of the skull. Basilar skull fractures require special studies such as CT scans to aid in an accurate diagnosis. However, the absence of Battle sign does not eliminate the possibility that a patient has a basilar skull fracture.

Pathophysiology

Fractures of the cribriform plate result in leakage of cerebrospinal fluid (CSF) into the nose. CSF is the fluid that bathes and provides hydraulic cushioning to the brain and spinal cord. Leakage of clear, watery fluid from the nose suggests leakage of CSF.

Pathophysiology

The temporomandibular joint (TMJ) is the joint between the temporal bone and the posterior condyle of the mandible that allows for movements of the jaw. Temporomandibular joint (TMJ) syndrome is an abnormal condition that is characterized by pain in the jaw and difficulty chewing and talking. Although dental malocclusion is regarded as the primary cause of TMJ syndrome, multiple factors, including head trauma, systemic disease, and stress, also may cause the syndrome. A genetic or acquired predisposition to TMJ syndrome may result in underlying alterations of the bones and soft tissues of the joint.

Patients with TMJ syndrome report pain in and around the joint itself, although it also may radiate to the back and shoulders. Often, the pain is severe, resulting in headaches, and there may be clicking and popping of the joint, a grinding sensation (crepitus), or spasm in the muscles of chewing (trismus) that results in difficulty talking and chewing. Problems such as ringing in the ears (tinnitus) and dizziness also may occur.

No single treatment method appears to be uniformly successful. Physical therapy is helpful, especially in patients who have sustained trauma. Intraoral appliances to adjust malocclusion and prevent bruxism (grinding together of the upper and lower teeth) help many patients, along with stress management techniques. Surgery is a last resort.

Pathophysiology

Sinusitis is an inflammation of the paranasal sinuses that is relatively common. Sinusitis may range in severity from a simple upper respiratory infection consisting of a headache and nasal drainage to a potentially life-threatening brain infection, depending on the extent of the infection and which sinuses are affected.

The Spine

The vertical axis of the human skeleton is formed by the vertebral column (backbone), which extends from the skull to the pelvis. It is made up of 24 bony vertebrae separated by intervertebral disks made of cushioning cartilage, connected by ligaments Figure 3-14 . Each vertebra has a drum-shaped body, making up the thick anterior portion of the bone. Between each vertebral body is the intervertebral disk, a mass of fibrocartilage consisting of an exterior fibrous ring, the anulus fibrosus, and the internal gelatinous nucleus pulposus Figure 3-15 .

The head and trunk are supported by the vertebral column, which also protects the spinal cord. The spinal cord passes through a vertebral canal created by openings in the vertebrae. At the bottom of the backbone, some vertebrae are fused to form the sacrum (a part of the pelvis) and the coccyx (tailbone), which is attached to the end of the sacrum.

Two short stalks (pedicles) project from each drum-shaped vertebra, with two plates called laminae that fuse to become a spinous process. These structures collectively form a bony vertebral arch around the vertebral foramen, through which the spinal cord passes. A transverse process projects posteriorly and laterally on each side attaching to ligaments and muscles. Superior and inferior articular processes project upward and downward with cartilage coverings, joined to the vertebra above and below. Notches align with adjacent vertebrae forming openings (intervertebral foramina) through which the spinal nerves pass.

The vertebrae that make up the spine are listed below, beginning with those located at the top of the spine, with the others listed sequentially (moving down the spine).

Case Study PART 3

Serial vital signs obtained while you are en route to the hospital reveal signs consistent with compensated shock, and reassessment of the extremities shows that distal pulses, motor function, and sensory function are still present. Each time the ambulance hits a bump in the road, the patient cries out in pain. The patient reports that the pain is intense in his low back and hips. Further examination of the hips and lower extremities reveals no obvious swelling or deformity and no shortening or rotation of either leg. Your paramedic partner is discussing an analgesic for the pain in light of the patient's BP.

Recording Time: 10 minutes	
Appearance	Starting to calm down
Level of consciousness	Alert (oriented to person, place, and day)
Airway	Open and clear
Breathing	Normal and regular
Circulation	Bleeding is controlled at this point
Pulse	100 and stronger
Blood pressure	110/70 mm Hg
Respirations	20 breaths/min and regular
Spo$_2$	98%

5. Describe the bones of the pelvic girdle and the potential injuries associated with a pelvic injury.

6. Describe the bones of the hip joint and possible injuries associated with the hip.

7. Which of the patient's musculoskeletal injuries discovered in the physical examination is potentially the most serious?

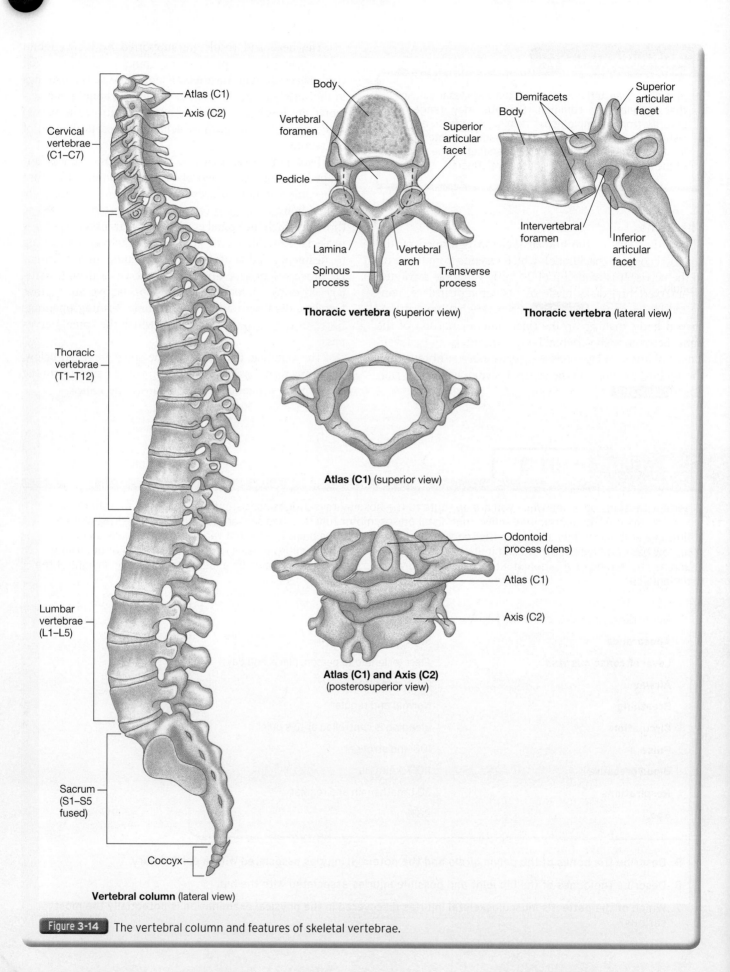

Vertebral column (lateral view)

Thoracic vertebra (superior view)

Thoracic vertebra (lateral view)

Atlas (C1) (superior view)

Atlas (C1) and Axis (C2)
(posterosuperior view)

Figure 3-14   The vertebral column and features of skeletal vertebrae.

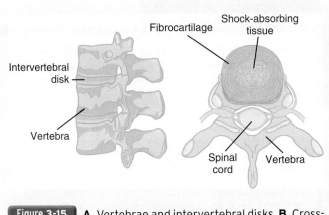

Figure 3-15 **A.** Vertebrae and intervertebral disks. **B.** Cross-section of intervertebral disk showing the fibrocartilaginous anulus fibrosus and the shock-absorbing nucleus pulposus.

through which nerves and blood vessels pass. The sacral canal continues through the sacrum to an opening called the sacral hiatus, where four pairs of anterior sacral foramina allow nerves and blood vessels to pass.

■ Coccyx. Also known as the tailbone, the coccyx is the lowest part of the vertebral column and is composed of four fused vertebrae. It is attached to the sacral hiatus by ligaments.

The Thorax

The thorax is composed of the thoracic cage, which includes 12 pairs of ribs (connected posteriorly to the thoracic vertebrae); the sternum (breastbone); and the costal cartilages, which attach the ribs to the sternum anteriorly **Figure 3-16**. The thoracic cage supports the pectoral girdle and upper limbs. It also protects the visceral organs inside the thoracic and upper abdominal cavities.

■ Sternum. Also known as the breastbone, the sternum is located in the middle anterior thoracic cage. It is

■ Cervical vertebrae. These seven structures comprise the neck, with distinctive transverse processes and transverse foramina, which allow the arteries leading to the brain to pass through. The forked processes of the second through fifth cervical vertebrae provide attachments for muscles. The atlas (first vertebra) supports the head with two kidney-shaped facets articulating with the occipital condyles. The axis (second vertebra) has a process (the dens) that projects upward into the ring of the atlas. When the head turns side to side, the atlas pivots around the dens.

■ Thoracic vertebrae. These 12 structures are larger than the cervical vertebrae and have long transverse processes that slope downward to articulate with the ribs. The thoracic vertebrae increase in size down the spine, to bear increasing loads of body weight.

■ Lumbar vertebrae. These five structures in the lower back are even larger than the thoracic vertebrae, supporting more body weight.

■ Sacrum. This triangular structure containing five fused vertebrae forms the vertebral column's base. A ridge of tubercles project outward with rows of openings (the posterior sacral foramina)

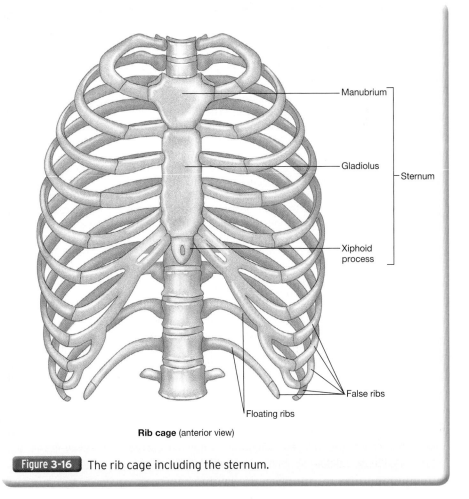

Rib cage (anterior view)

Figure 3-16 The rib cage including the sternum.

composed of an upper manubrium, a middle body (gladiolus), and a lower xiphoid process. The manubrium attaches to the clavicles.

- Ribs. One pair of ribs is attached to each of the 12 thoracic vertebrae, totaling 24 in all. The first seven pairs are true ribs (vertebrosternal ribs), attached to the sternum via costal cartilages. The last five pairs are false ribs (meaning their cartilages do not reach the sternum directly). The cartilages of the upper three false rib pairs join the cartilages of the seventh true ribs. The final two false rib pairs are called floating ribs (vertebral ribs) because they do not attach to the sternum via cartilage at all. Ribs are curved with enlarged ends (heads) allowing them to attach to the sternum via facets (surfaces where bones meet). The transverse process of the vertebrae articulates with a tubercle (projection) close to the rib's head.

Special Needs Tip

Intervertebral disks become compressed with age. The space between vertebral bodies decreases as a normal part of aging, resulting in a decrease in the overall height of a person.

Pathophysiology

An exaggeration of the lumbar curve is called lordosis, or hollow back. An excessively concave thoracic curve is known as kyphosis, or hump back. Scoliosis is an abnormal curve of the spine in the coronal plane and often is accompanied by other abnormal curvatures in the sagittal plane, such as kyphosis.

Pathophysiology

As a result of trauma, aging, and other forms of acute and chronic musculoskeletal stress, various diseases may involve the spine. A compression fracture usually results from a fall in which the trunk flexes sharply forward. The force of the impact causes the anterior portion of the vertebral body to collapse, resulting in a wedge-shaped appearance on radiographs. Minimal trauma may result in injury in a patient with severe underlying bone disease, such as osteoporosis. Compression fractures commonly accompany degenerative disk disease as well. The lower thoracic and upper lumbar vertebrae are most commonly involved, and neurologic deficit is rare. Although most compression fractures respond to rest, pain medication, and, sometimes, the use of back braces, some patients require more aggressive intervention to achieve adequate pain control.

Degenerative disk disease is a progressive form of arthritis in which the anulus fibrosus becomes stressed from chronic movements. The amount of water in the nucleus pulposus decreases, making it less gel-like. These changes interfere, to one degree or another, with the interrelationships of the vertebral bodies and their connecting ligaments. As a result, the irritated bone forms osteophytes, or spurs. Essentially, osteophytes represent "scar bone" formed in response to irritation. Localized degenerative disk disease, such as from trauma, will be present only in the injured area. More diffuse disease of the cervical spine, lumbosacral spine, or both, is more common in patients with no history of specific injury. Osteophytes are commonly seen in radiographs of the backs of persons older than age 40 years who usually have no symptoms. Because many healthy patients have abnormal radiographs of the back, it is likely that the abnormality preexists in a trauma patient. Therefore, plain radiographs may not be helpful in determining whether a given radiographic finding occurred as a result of a person's injury. Management consisting of exercise and nonsteroidal anti-inflammatory drugs (NSAIDs) is sufficient for most people with degenerative disk disease. Surgery is only rarely indicated.

A herniated disk occurs when there is a tear in the anulus fibrosus that results in leakage of some or all of the nucleus pulposus. The herniation, or rupture, is most commonly problematic if it occurs posterolaterally, where the gelatinous material can cause pressure against the exiting nerve roots. However, herniation may occur anywhere about the circumference of the disk. The degree and type of symptoms depend on the location of the herniation; 95% of disk herniations occur at the L4-L5 or L5-S1 levels. Sometimes, the nerve root is directly irritated. Often, there is no direct impingement on or irritation of a nerve. Pain is believed to occur because nearby ligaments and muscles become irritated and, as a result, release inflammatory substances, irritating tissues in the area. A central disk herniation occurs when the nuclear material protrudes straight back into the vertebral canal. In severe instances, it may cause compression of the lower portion of the spinal cord and lead to permanent loss of bowel and bladder control. Loss of bowel or bladder function indicates the need for immediate surgical consultation.

Treatment initially includes rest and pain medications, and surgery is rarely necessary unless the patient has prolonged intractable pain, bowel or bladder dysfunction, or progressive neurologic deficit.

Anatomically, a bulging disk is different from a herniated disk. A tear in the anulus fibrosus results in a herniated disk; with a bulging disk, the anulus is intact but there is a circumferential ballooning of the intact disk. Recent data suggest that bulging disks and herniated disks are present on MRIs in many persons with no symptoms and can therefore be "normal variants." Disk herniation is seen most commonly in the lumbar spine region but frequently occurs in the cervical region also.

▇ The Appendicular Skeleton

The appendicular skeleton contains the upper and lower limb bones, as well as the bones anchoring the limbs to the axial skeleton. The appendicular skeleton includes the pectoral girdle, upper limbs, pelvic girdle, and lower limbs.

The Pectoral Girdle

Also known as the shoulder girdle, the pectoral girdle is made up of a clavicle (collarbone) and a scapula (shoulder blade) on each side of the body **Figure 3-17**. These structures aid in the movements of the arms. The pectoral girdle is actually an incomplete ring that opens in the back between the scapulae. It connects the upper limb bones to the axial skeleton. The sternum separates the bones of the pectoral girdle in the front. The pectoral girdle supports the upper limbs and is where the muscles that move the upper limbs originate.

- Clavicles. The collarbones are shaped like rods with an elongated S-shape. They are located at the base of the neck, running horizontally between the manubrium and the scapulae. These bones brace the scapulae to hold the shoulders in place and provide muscle origination points for the upper limbs, chest, and back.
- Scapulae. The shoulder blades are somewhat triangular bones on either side of the upper back. Each scapula is divided by a spine that leads to an acromion process (forming the tip of the shoulder) and a coracoid process (that curves to the clavicle). The acromion process provides muscle attachments for the upper limbs and chest. The coracoid process provides similar attachments. The glenoid fossa is a depression that articulates with the head of the humerus bone in the arm.

The Upper Limbs

The bones of the upper limbs include those of the arms, forearms, and hands. They provide muscle attachments and function to move limb parts. The following lists the bones of the upper limbs **Figure 3-18**:

- Humerus. The upper arm bone, extending from the scapula to the elbow. It has a smooth upper head that fits into the glenoid fossa, with two tubercles providing muscle attachment points. The lower portion of the humerus has two smooth condyles that articulate with the ulna and radius. The narrow depression in the proximal portion of the humerus that separates it from the tubercles is the anatomic neck. Distally, structures called epicondyles attach to the muscles and ligaments of the elbow. The olecranon fossa is a depression on the posterior surface of the humerus

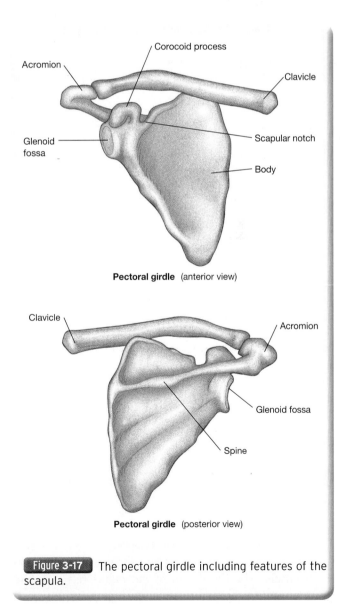

Pectoral girdle (anterior view)

Pectoral girdle (posterior view)

Figure 3-17 The pectoral girdle including features of the scapula.

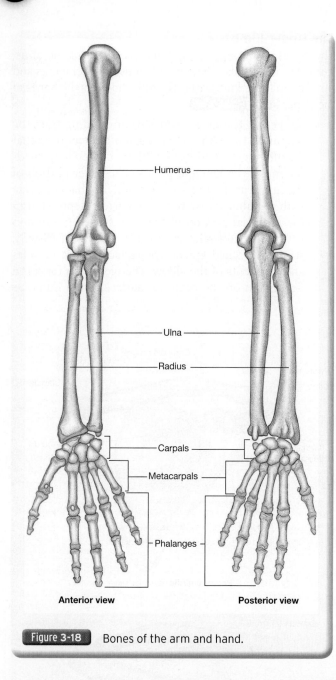

Anterior view   **Posterior view**

Figure 3-18 Bones of the arm and hand.

- **Ulna**. Longer than the radius, the ulna overlaps the end of the humerus and has a trochlear notch at its proximal end that articulates with the humerus. The olecranon and coronoid processes, located on each side of this notch, provide attachments for muscles. The distal end of the ulna has a head that articulates with the notch of the radius. A disk of fibrocartilage joins the triquetrum bone of the wrist.
- **Hand**. This part of the upper limb consists of the wrist, palm, and fingers. The wrist contains eight bones called carpals, in two rows of four bones each. This mass (the carpus) articulates with radius, ulna, and metacarpal bones. Five bones called metacarpals form the palm (metacarpus) of the hand. The distal rounded ends of these bones form the knuckles and are numbered from one to five, beginning with the thumb. The metacarpals articulate with the carpals and phalanges (finger bones). Each finger except the thumb has three phalanges (a proximal, middle, and distal phalanx). The thumb has only two phalanges because it lacks a middle phalanx.

Pathophysiology

Acromioclavicular (AC) separation, also called a separated shoulder, occurs when any of the four ligaments of the acromioclavicular (AC) joint are partially or completely torn. In partial tears, no deformity is noted unless the patient attempts to hold a weight with the arm directed downward. In this case, the weakened joint is transiently widened, a finding visible on radiographs. In cases of complete separation, in which all four ligaments are severely damaged, the clavicle essentially lies above the acromion, causing a visible deformity in the patient's shoulder area.

Pathophysiology

Olecranon bursitis is a painful condition resulting from inflammation of the bursa that overlies the olecranon process posteriorly. Normally, the bursa contains a small amount of fluid that facilitates movement at the elbow joint. Inflammation commonly develops because of underlying arthritis in the elbow joint. Primary bursa infection can result from an abrasion of the elbow area against a dirty surface, especially when the skin overlying the bursa is tightened and thinned because the arm is bent. Bacteria entering the bursa through the wound thrive in the fluid.

Generally, olecranon bursitis responds well to treatment, regardless of its etiology. Recurrent or refractory swelling may occur in noninfectious cases, which is more of a bother than an actual disability and requires frequent aspirations of the fluid from the bursa.

that receives an ulnar olecranon process when the upper limb straightens at the elbow. At the lower end of the humerus are two smooth condyles (round projections) that articulate with the radius and ulna at the elbow joint.

- Radius. Located on the thumb side of the forearm, this bone extends from the elbow to the wrist, crossing over the ulna when the hand is turned. Its upper end articulates with the humerus and a notch in the ulna. A process called the radial tuberosity serves as an attachment for the biceps brachii muscle. The distal end of the radius has a styloid process providing ligament attachments to the wrist.

Pathophysiology

Epicondylitis, which is better known as tennis elbow, is inflammation and pain at the origin of the flexor (medial epicondyle) or extensor (lateral epicondyle) muscle of the forearm. The lateral epicondyle is involved more often, and the irritation comes from repeated flexion and extension. Minor tears in muscle tendons often are present. Clinically, the patient reports the gradual onset of a dull ache over the affected area that is worse when the affected muscles are used. Rotation and grasping, such as opening a jar, cause the pain to become worse and radiate into the forearm.

Pressure over the involved epicondyle causes significant discomfort. Radiographic findings usually are normal.

Any activity that causes the pain should be avoided. In addition, heat, ultrasound, and other forms of physical therapy offer some relief, as does the use of nonsteroidal anti-inflammatory drugs. Corticosteroid injections often provide permanent relief, but they may need to be repeated for several months prior to full recovery. Some patients benefit from the use of braces or casts. Surgery is reserved for resistant cases only.

Pathophysiology

Irritation of structures, particularly the median nerve, within the carpal tunnel results in a painful condition known as carpal tunnel syndrome (CTS). CTS results when swelling and inflammation in the carpal tunnel result in compression of the median nerve between the flexor retinaculum and the flexor tendons. CTS is bilateral in up to 50% of patients and is most prevalent in women between 30 and 60 years of age.

CTS can have numerous causes, but repetitive hand motions (using a computer keyboard, cooking, knitting, screwdriver use, weed-trimmer use, or painting) most often are the cause, especially in terms of workers' compensation claims. Other medical conditions that may be associated with CTS include hypothyroidism, rheumatoid and gouty arthritis, pregnancy (especially in the third trimester), vitamin B6 deficiency, complications of fracture healing (malaligned Colles fracture), infection, tumor, and diabetes.

Clinically, patients have gradually worsening wrist and hand pain, more commonly at night. Pain may radiate up the forearm to the elbow and the shoulder. On examination, atrophy of the thenar eminence (thumb side of the palm) is a late finding. Either the Tinel sign (reproduction of pain and tingling with tapping of the medial nerve at the carpal tunnel) or the Phalen test (reproduction of symptoms with 1 minute or less of bilateral wrist flexion, holding the hands together dorsum to dorsum) may be positive; however, both of these signs can be unreliable.

Treatment consists of eliminating the cause of CTS, if possible. Patients are advised to avoid extremes of wrist positions and to use job-specific wrist-splints and take nonsteroidal anti-inflammatory drugs. Corticosteroid injections into the carpal canal offer temporary relief for many patients. Many times, in fact, the signs and symptoms resolve with nonsurgical management alone. With severe symptoms that do not respond to nonsurgical management, such as pain or weakness of the hand, surgery to cut the transverse carpal ligament can result in resolution of symptoms. Typically, improvement may take weeks to months following surgery. Motor function returns last.

The Pelvic Girdle

Two hip bones, which articulate with each other and the sacrum, make up the pelvic girdle **Figure 3-19**. The pelvic girdle attaches the lower limbs to the axial skeleton. Together, the sacrum, coccyx, and pelvic girdle form the pelvis.

The pelvis of females is usually wider in all diameters than that of males. The pelvic girdle supports, protects, and/or articulates with the trunk, lower limbs, urinary bladder, large intestine, and reproductive organs. The hip bones each have three parts (the ilium, ischium, and pubis) fused together into an acetabulum, which articulates with the rounded head of the femur (thigh bone).

- Ilium. The largest portion of the hip bone, it forms the prominence of the pelvis. The margin of the prominence is called the iliac crest. The ilium joins the sacrum at the sacroiliac joint. A projection from the ilium provides attachments for ligaments and muscles.
- Ischium. The lowest portion of the hip bone, it is L-shaped. It supports the weight of the body when sitting. Its angle, the ischial tuberosity, points downward and posteriorly.
- Pubis. The anterior portion of the hip bone, it forms an angle known as the pubic arch. The two pubic bones join at the symphysis pubis, the upper margin of which (the pelvic brim) separates the lower pelvis from the upper portion. A large opening, known as the obturator foramen, lies between the pubis and the ischium.

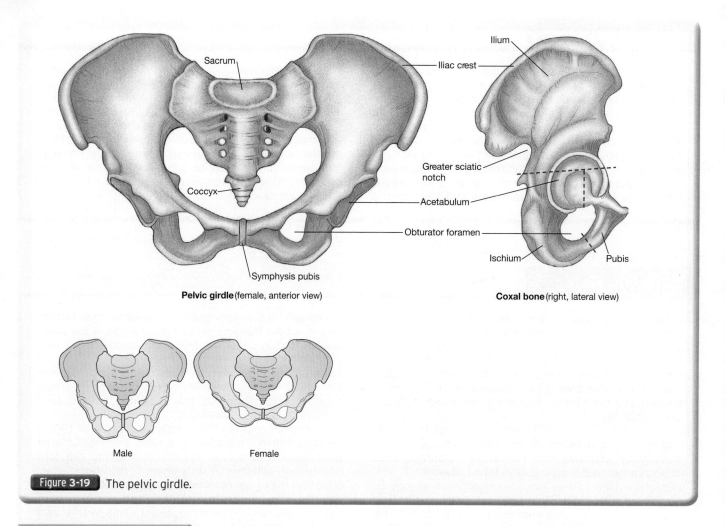

Figure 3-19 The pelvic girdle.

Pathophysiology

Hip fractures actually are fractures of the proximal portion of the femur near or at the site of articulation with the acetabulum. These fractures are classified based on the structures of the femur involved. Fractures between the femoral head and the trochanteric region are termed femoral neck fractures. These include subcapital, midcervical, and basicervical variants. Fractures between trochanters are described as intertrochanteric and fractures extending below the lesser trochanter are described as subtrochanteric **Figure 3-20**.

Hip fractures account for 350,000 hospital admissions each year in the United States. Approximately 70% of hip fractures occur in women. Results often are disabling because many patients are elderly and have underlying cardiac disease, osteoporosis, and senility. Mortality from all causes for elderly patients who sustain a hip fracture is 25% in the first year following injury. Treatment depends on the portion of the proximal femur that is injured.

Dislocations of the hip joint commonly occur from a fall or during a motor vehicle crash in which the knee impacts the dashboard. The force of the impact is transmitted posteriorly to the hip, resulting in posterior dislocation. Anterior hip dislocations are less common.

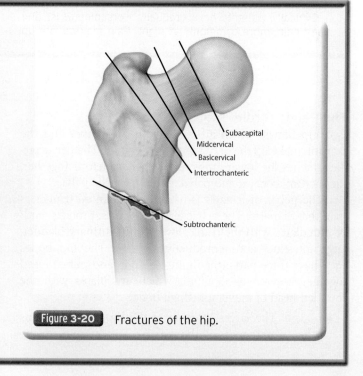

Figure 3-20 Fractures of the hip.

The Lower Limbs

The lower limbs consist of the bones of the thigh, leg, and foot **Figure 3-21**.

- **Femur.** The thigh is the part of the extremity that extends from the hip to the knee and contains the femur, the longest bone in the body. Various processes from the femur provide attachments for muscles of the lower limbs and buttocks. A pit on the head of the femur capitis marks the point of attachment of the ligamentum capitis. Just below the head is a neck (constriction) and the large processes known as the lateral greater trochanter and the medial lesser trochanter, where muscles are also attached. The kneecap (patella) articulates with the femur and is located in a tendon passing over the knee. The femur articulates with the tibia via the lateral and medial condyles (processes).

- **Tibia.** The shinbone is the larger of the two leg bones, located on the medial side of the leg. Proximally, the tibial tuberosity is the process where the patellar ligament attaches. The distal end of the tibia has an inner prominence (the medial malleolus) where ligaments attach. A depression on its lateral side articulates with the fibula.

- **Fibula.** A slender bone located on the lateral side of the tibia, it does not enter into the knee joint and does not bear any body weight. The fibula has slightly enlarged ends, a proximal head and a distal lateral malleolus. The fibula plays a critical role in maintaining stability around the knee and the ankle.

- **Foot.** This part of the lower limb consists of the ankle, instep, and toes. The

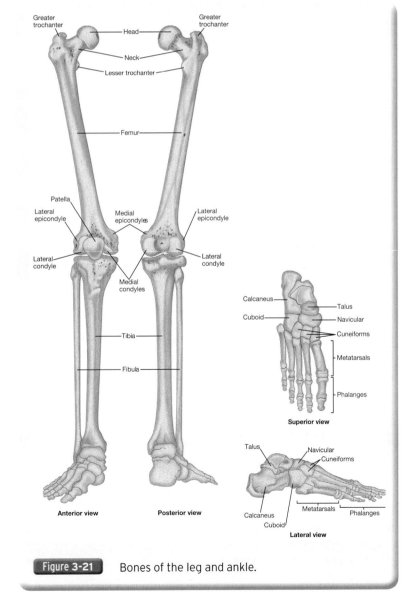

Figure 3-21   Bones of the leg and ankle.

ankle (tarsus) is made up of seven bones called tar-sals that are arranged so that the talus bone moves freely where it joins the leg bones. The tarsal bones connect the tibia and fibula to the foot. The other tarsal bones are firmly bound in a mass supporting the talus. The largest tarsal bone is the calcaneus (heel bone), which helps support body weight and

provides muscle attachment for foot movement. The instep (metatarsus) is made up of five bones called metatarsals numbered one through five, beginning with the medial side. The phalanges of the toes, similar to those of the fingers, are aligned with the metatarsals. Each toe has three phalanges except the great toe, which has only two.

Pathophysiology

Chondromalacia patella refers to a softening and fraying of cartilage and often occurs on the posterior (articular) surface of the patella. Although some patients may be asymptomatic, others, especially young adults, may experience knee pain. Typically, pain is felt beneath or near the patella and is worse with stair climbing, squatting, or following prolonged sitting. Active extension of the leg at the knee worsens pain. Often, chondromalacia is bilateral and may be confused with other cartilage problems. Radiographs usually are normal, and there is no correlation between the degree of crepitus and severity of the condition or pain. In most patients, nonsurgical management, including heat, nonsteroidal anti-inflammatory drugs, and quadriceps exercises, is effective. Surgery is reserved for resistant cases and is associated with variable outcomes.

Patellar dislocations commonly occur in teenagers and young athletes. Dislocations may be recurrent, and minor twisting of the knee may be enough to cause a dislocation in particularly susceptible people. The patella usually dislocates to the lateral side and produces a significant deformity with the knee locked in a moderately flexed position Figure 3-22. This type of injury is very painful. Treatment includes splinting the extremity in the position it is found and analgesia for the pain.

Cartilage and ligament injuries of the knee are relatively common. The C-shaped lateral and medial menisci function as cartilagenous cushions between the femur and tibia. The anterior and posterior cruciate ligaments prevent abnormal motion of the knee from front to back, and the medial and lateral collateral ligaments stabilize the joint against abnormal side-to-side motions.

A common knee injury involves the medial meniscus and can occur when the knee is twisted while the foot remains planted in place, bearing weight. The meniscus may be

partially or completely torn. Often, there is a popping or tearing sensation, followed by severe, poorly localized pain. Swelling develops over several hours. After the acute injury, patients may report intermittent locking, buckling, giving out, and swelling of the involved knee. Both stair walking and squatting are painful. Pain becomes more localized with time. The McMurray test results may be positive, involving the presence of a clicking or popping sensation over the involved cartilage when the leg is held in flexion and gently rotated from side to side and flexed. MRI may be diagnostic, although false-negative and false-positive results are possible.

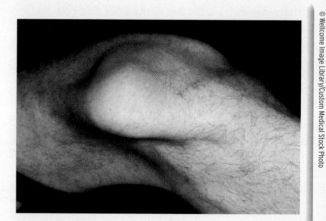

© Wellcome Image Library/Custom Medical Stock Photo

Figure 3-22   A dislocated patella will typically appear with the patella displaced lateral to the knee and the knee moderately flexed.

Pathophysiology

The tibial plateau is the anatomic region between and including the medial and lateral condyles. Fractures in the tibial plateau can be very serious and may require surgery.

Pathophysiology

Twisting injuries can often result in ankle sprains. An ankle sprain usually occurs from forceful inversion (turning inward) of the foot resulting in partial or complete tearing of the ligaments or tendons.

Pathophysiology

Plantar fasciitis is an irritation of the plantar fascia (the tough band of connective tissue extending from the calcaneus to the proximal phalange of each toe). The plantar fascia is the same tissue that supports the arch of the foot. Repetitive strain may cause irritation or inflammation of the plantar fascia, resulting in heel pain that radiates along the medial or lateral side of the foot. Plantar fasciitis frequently is bilateral. Heel pain also may be an early indication of ankylosing spondylitis, rheumatoid arthritis, or gout. On examination, the patient exhibits point tenderness over the bottom of the heel as well as pain with dorsiflexion of the foot. Radiographs often are normal, but may show an associated calcaneal (heel) spur. The heel spur is an outgrowth of "scar bone" at the plantar fascia's attachment site, resulting from chronic irritation. Management consisting of a combination of orthotic shoe inserts, nonsteroidal anti-inflammatory drugs, and stretching usually is effective. Generally, the response to treatment is good.

Case Study PART 4

The patient has remained alert during transport to the hospital, and his blood pressure has remained steady. While en route, your paramedic partner obtains permission from medical control to administer a dose of pain medication, and this helps the patient considerably during transport.

Prep Kit

Chapter Summary

- The skeletal system provides the framework and support of the body. The tissues of the skeletal system include the bones, cartilage, tendons, and ligaments.
- Cartilage is shiny connective tissue that provides a slippery surface over which the bones may move freely.
- Tendons connect muscles to bones and consist of densely packed fibers of collagen.
- Ligaments are tough white bands of tissue that bind together connecting bones to one another at joints.
- Wherever two long bones come in contact, a joint is formed.
- Joints are classified as slightly moveable, freely movable, or immovable.
- Joints can also be grouped according to the type of tissue binding them at their junctions. These groups include fibrous, cartilaginous, and synovial joints.
- Bones protect the internal organs and, with the assistance of the muscles, enable movement.
- The bones are classified by their shape (eg, long, short, and flat). There are two main types of bone: compact, which is mostly solid, and cancellous, which consists of a lacy network of bony rods called trabeculae.
- Clinically, fractures are either closed or open. A closed fracture occurs when a bone is broken but there is no penetration of the skin with the bone end. An open fracture occurs when there is a break through the skin.
- The skeleton is divided into two major components: the axial skeleton and appendicular skeleton.
- The axial skeleton runs the length of the torso.
- The axial skeleton includes the skull, hyoid bone, vertebral column, and thoracic cage.
- The skull is made up of 28 firmly interlocked bones, which are divided into the cranium (brain case), the facial bones, and the auditory ossicles.
- The facial bones include the maxillae, zygomatic bones, nasal bones, vomer bone, inferior nasal conchae, lacrimal bones, palatine bones, and mandible.
- The spine is organized into five sections: cervical vertebrae, thoracic vertebrae, lumbar vertebrae, sacrum, and coccyx.

- The remainder of the axillary skeleton includes the rib cage. There are 12 pairs of ribs. Ten pair are attached either directly or indirectly to the sternum by costal cartilages, two pair are free floating.
- The sternum is divided into three portions: the manubrium, the gladiolus, and the xiphoid process.
- The appendicular skeleton contains the upper and lower limb bones, as well as the bones anchoring the limbs to the axial skeleton.
- The appendicular skeleton includes the pectoral girdle (or shoulder girdle), upper limbs, pelvic girdle, and lower limbs.
- The pectoral girdle includes the clavicle and scapula.
- The shoulder joint is a ball-and-socket joint.
- The upper extremities include the arms, forearms, and hands. The humerus is in the upper arm, and the ulna and radius are in the forearm. The hand and wrist consist of the carpals, metacarpals and phalanges.
- The pelvic girdle is the attachment point for the lower extremities and consists of the ilium, ischium, and pubis. The hip joint is a ball-and-socket joint.
- The lower extremities include the bones of the thigh, leg, and foot, consisting of the femur in the upper leg, and the tibia and fibula in the lower leg. The foot includes the tarsals, metatarsals, and phalanges. The knee joint is traditionally classified as a hinge joint and is unusual because ligaments are contained within the joint.
- The talus articulates with the tibia and fibula to form the ankle joint. The calcaneus is inferior and lateral to the talus and provides support for standing.

Vital Vocabulary

acetabulum The depression on the lateral pelvis where its three component bones join, articulates with the femoral head.

acromioclavicular (AC) joint The point at which the clavicle attaches to the acromion process.

acromioclavicular (AC) separation An injury caused by distraction of the clavicle away from the acromion process of the scapula.

acromion process The tip of the shoulder and the site of attachment for both the clavicle and shoulder musculature.

alveolar arch The ridges between the teeth, which are covered with thickened connective tissue and epithelium; also called alveolar ridges.

anulus fibrosus A ring of fibrous or fibrocartilaginous tissue that is part of the intervertebral disk.

appendicular skeleton The portion of the skeletal system that comprises the arms, legs, pelvis, and shoulder girdle.

appositional growth The formation of new bone on the surface of a bone.

atlas The first cervical vertebra (C1), which provides support for the head.

axial skeleton The part of the skeleton comprising the skull, spinal column, and rib cage.

axis The second cervical vertebra, the point that allows the head to turn.

Battle sign Bruising over the mastoid process, usually from a basilar skull fracture.

bone marrow Specialized tissue found within bone that manufactures most erythrocytes.

bruxism Grinding together of the upper and lower teeth.

bulging disk A ballooning of an intervertebral disk without frank herniation.

bursae Small fluid-filled sacs located between a tendon and a bone help lubricate two surfaces that are rubbing against each other.

calcaneus The heel bone.

callus The zone of repair in which a mass of exudates and connective tissue forms around a break in a bone and converts to bone during healing.

canaliculi A minute canal in a bone.

cancellous bone Bone that is made up of a lacy network of bony rods called trabeculae.

carpal tunnel syndrome (CTS) Compression of the median nerve within the carpal canal at the wrist.

carpals The bones of the wrist; they include the scaphoid, lunate, triquetrum, pisiform, trapezium, trapezoid, capitate, and hamate bones.

cartilage The support structure of the skeletal system that provides cushioning between bones; also forms the nasal septum and portions of the outer ear.

central disk herniation The most serious disk rupture that occurs when nuclear material protrudes straight back into the spinal canal, potentially compressing neurologic elements and causing neurologic injury.

cerebrospinal fluid (CSF) Fluid produced in the ventricles of the brain that flows in the subarachnoid space and bathes the meninges.

cervical vertebrae The seven smallest vertebrae, found in the neck.

chondroblasts Cells that produce cartilage.

clavicle The collarbone; it is lateral to the sternum and anterior to the scapula.

closed fracture A fracture in which the bone ends have not been exposed by a break through the skin.

coccyx The tailbone.

compact bone Bone that is mostly solid, with few spaces.

compression fracture A fracture of a vertebral body associated with collapse of the body.

coronal suture The point where the parietal bones join together with the frontal bone.

costochondritis Inflammation of the costal cartilage, which attaches the ribs to the sternum.

cranium The bones that encase and protect the brain, including the parietal, temporal, frontal, occipital, sphenoid, and ethmoid bones.

crepitus A grinding sound or sensation.

cribriform plates Horizontal bones perforated with numerous foramina for the passage of the olfactory nerve filaments from the nasal cavity.

crista galli A prominent bony ridge in the center of the anterior fossa to which the meninges are attached.

degenerative disk disease A progressive form of arthritis that causes deterioration of the intervertebral disk.

diaphysis The shaft of a long bone.

displaced fracture A fracture in which bone fragments are separated from one another and are not in anatomic alignment.

dwarfism A state of abnormally small bones.

endochondral growth The growth of cartilage in the physis (epiphyseal plate) which is eventually replaced by bone.

endosteum A layer that lines the inner surfaces of bone.

epicondylitis An inflammation of the muscles of the elbow joint; more commonly known as tennis elbow.

epiphyses The growth plate of a long bone.

ethmoid bone The main supporting structure of the nasal cavities; it also forms part of the eye orbits.

external acoustic meatus An opening in the temporal bone that contains the ear canal.

facial skeleton The maxillae, zygomatic bones, nasal bones, vomer, inferior nasal conchae, lacrimal bones, palatine bones, and mandible.

femur The thighbone; the longest and one of the strongest bones in the body.

fibroblasts Cells that secrete proteins and collagen to form connective tissue between broken bone ends and at other sites of injury throughout the body.

fibula The long bone on the lateral aspect of the lower leg.

flat bones Types of bone that are relatively thin and flattened.

foramen magnum The large opening at the bottom of the skull through which the brain connects with the spinal cord.

foramina Small openings, perforations, or orifices in the bones of the cranial vault.

fracture A break in the continuity of a bone.

frontal bone The bone that forms the forehead and part of the roof of the nasal cavity.

gigantism A state of bony overgrowth.

girdles The bony belts that attach the extremities to the axial skeleton.

glenoid fossa The part of the scapula that forms the socket in the ball-and-socket joint of the shoulder.

haversian systems Units of compact bone consisting of a tube (haversian canal) with the laminae of bone that surrounds them.

herniated disk A tear in the anulus fibrosus that results in leakage of the nucleus pulposus, most commonly against exiting nerve roots.

humerus The supporting bone of the upper arm.

hydroxyapatite A mineral compound containing calcium and phosphate that, along with collagen, comprises the structural element of bone.

hyoid bone The bone that supports the tongue and its muscles.

ilium One of three bones that fuse to form the pelvic ring.

inferior nasal conchae Scroll-shaped bones attached to the lateral nasal cavity walls that support the mucous membranes.

intervertebral disk A mass of fibrocartilage between each vertebral body of the spine, composed of the anulus fibrosus and the nucleus pulposus.

intervertebral foramina The opening between each vertebra through which the spinal (peripheral) nerves pass from the spinal cord.

ischium One of the three bones that fuse to form the pelvic ring.

joint The point where two or more bones come together, allowing movement to occur.

kyphosis Outward curve of the thoracic spine.

lacrimal bones Bones that make up part of the eye orbits and contain the tear sacs.

lambdoid suture The point where the occipital bones attach to the parietal bones.

lamellae Thin sheets or layers into which bone tissue is organized.

lateral malleolus An enlargement of the distal end of the fibula, which forms the lateral wall of the ankle joint.

ligaments Bands of fibrous tissue that connect bones to bones; they support and strengthen a joint.

long bones Type of bone that is longer than it is wide.

lordosis Inward curve of the lumbar spine just above the buttocks; an exaggerated form of lordosis results in the condition known as swayback.

lower limbs The femurs, tibias, fibulas, patellae, tarsals, metatarsals, and phalanges.

lumbar vertebrae The five vertebrae of the lower back.

mandible The bone of the lower jaw; the only moveable bone in the face.

mastoid process A prominent bony mass at the base of the skull behind the ear.

maxillae The bones that make up the upper jaw.

medial malleolus The distal end of the tibia, which forms the medial side of the ankle joint.

medullary cavity The internal cavity of the diaphysis of a long bone that contains bone marrow.

meninges The three layers of membranes, the dura, mater arachnoid, and pia mater, that surround the brain.

menisci Shock-absorbing fibrocartilage pads within some synovial joints.

metacarpals The bones of the palms of the hand.

metaphysis The area of a long bone where the diaphysis and epiphysis converge; where the physis (epiphyseal plate) is located.

metatarsals The bones on the soles of the feet; they form the foot arches.

nasal bones The thin, delicate bones that join to form the bridge of the nose.

nasal cavity The chamber inside the nose that lies between the floor of the cranium and the roof of the mouth.

nasal septum The rigid partition composed of bone and cartilage that separates the right and left nostrils.

nondisplaced fracture A fractured bone that has not moved from its normal position.

nucleus pulposus The gelatinous mass that makes up the center of each intervertebral disk.

oblique fracture A fracture that forms an angle to the shaft of the bone.

occipital bone The bone that forms the back and base of the cranium.

occipital condyles Articular surface on the occipital bone where the skull articulates with the atlas on the vertebral column.

open fracture A fracture in which a bone end has penetrated the skin; also called a compound fracture.

orbits Bony cavities in the frontal skull that enclose and protect the eyes.

ossicles The three small bones in the middle ear: the malleus, incus, and stapes.

ossification The formation of bone by osteoblasts.

osteoblasts Bone-forming cells.

osteoclasts Large, multinucleated cells that dissolve bone tissue and play a major role in bone remodeling.

osteocyte An osteoblast that becomes surrounded by bony matrix; a mature bone cell.

osteogenesis imperfecta A genetic bone disease that results in fragile bones.

osteomalacia An abnormal softening of bones because of a loss of calcium.

osteomyelitis Inflammation of the bone and muscle caused by infection.

osteons Units within a compact bone in which blood vessels are located; also called the haversian system.

osteoporosis A reduction in the quantity of bony tissue.

palatine bones Irregularly shaped bones found in the posterior part of the nasal cavity.

paranasal sinuses The sinuses, or hollowed sections of bone in the front of the head, that are lined with mucous membrane and drain into the nasal cavity; the frontal and maxillary sinuses.

parietal bones Bones that form the upper sides and roof of the cranium.

patella The kneecap.

pectoral girdle The scalpulae and clavicles.

pedicles The feet of each vertebra in the vertebral arch.

pelvic girdle The hip bones.

pelvis The attachment of the lower extremities to the body, consisting of the sacrum and two pelvic bones.

periosteum A double layer of connective tissue that lines the outer surface of the bone.

phalanges The small bones of the digits of the fingers and toes.

physis The major site of bone elongation, located at each end of a long bone between the epiphysis and metaphysis; also called the growth plate.

pituitary gland An endocrine gland, located in the sella turcica of the brain, responsible for directly or indirectly affecting all bodily functions.

plantar fasciitis An irritation of the tough band of connective tissue extending from the calcaneus to the metatarsal head of each toe.

pubic arch An angle formed by the anterior portion of the hip bone (pubis).

pubis One of three bones that fuse to form the pelvic ring.

radius The shorter, lateral bone of the forearm.

ribs The 12 pairs of bones that primarily make up the thoracic cage, connecting posteriorly to the thoracic vertebrae.

rickets A disease caused by vitamin D deficiency.

sacrum One of three bones (sacrum and two pelvic bones) that make up the pelvic ring; consists of five fused sacral vertebrae.

saddle joint Two saddle-shaped articulating surfaces oriented at right angles to each other so that complementary surfaces articulate with each other, such as is the case with the thumb.

sagittal suture The point of the skull where the parietal bones join together.

scapula The triangular-shaped bone that comprises the shoulder blade, which is an integral component of the shoulder girdle.

scoliosis Sideways curvature of the spine.

sella turcica A depression in the middle of the sphenoid bone where the pituitary gland is located.

short bones Types of bone that are as broad as they are long.

shoulder joint A ball-and-socket joint consisting of the head of the humerus and the glenoid fossa.

sinusitis Inflammation of the paranasal sinuses.

skull The structure at the top of the axial skeleton that houses the brain and consists of the 28 bones that comprise the auditory ossicles, the cranium, and the face.

sphenoid bone The anterior portion of the base of the cranium.

sternum The breastbone in the center of the anterior chest.

sutures Attachment points in the skull where the cranial bones join together.

synovial fluid The small amount of liquid within a joint used as lubrication.

talus A bone that articulates with the tibia, calcaneus, and navicular bones to form the lower part of the ankle joint.

tarsals The bones of the ankles; they include the medial cuneiform, intermediate cuneiform, lateral cuneiform, navicular, cuboid, talus, and calcaneus.

temporal bones Bones that form the lower sides and base of the cranium.

temporomandibular joint (TMJ) The joint between the temporal bone and the posterior condyle of the mandible that allows for movements of the jaw.

tendons Fibrous connective tissue that attaches muscles to bones.

thoracic cage The ribs, thoracic vertebrae, and sternum.

thoracic vertebrae The 12 vertebrae located in the center of the vertebral column that (mostly) connect with the ribs.

tibia The shin bone; the larger of the two bones of the lower leg.

tinnitus The perception of sound in the inner ear with no external environmental cause; often reported as "ringing" in the ears, but may be roaring, buzzing, or clicking.

trabeculae Bony rods that make up a lacy network of cancellous bones and are oriented to increase weight-bearing capacity of long bones.

trismus Involuntary contraction of the mouth resulting in clenched teeth; occurs during seizures and head injuries.

ulna The longer, medial bone of the forearm.

upper limbs The humerus bones, radius bones, ulna bones, carpals, metacarpals, and phalanges.

vertebral arch The posterior portion of a vertebra, which contains the bony processes, facets, and pedicles.

vertebral column The spine, or primary support structure of the body, which houses the spinal cord and the peripheral nerves.

vertebral foramen A hole through which spinal nerves pass from the spinal cord.

vomer bone The flat bone making up the lower posterior nasal septum.

zygomatic bones Also known as the malar bones; they form the prominence of each cheek.

■ Case Study Answers

1. What are the probable skeletal injuries in this patient?

   Answer: The mechanism of injury (MOI) was a fall from the second story and landing on both feet; therefore, the potential for injury begins with the feet and ankles. As the energy from the fall is transferred up the body, other skeletal injuries may include injury to the knees, hips, pelvis, and spine.

2. What would be your next steps in assessing the patient?

   Answer: You must maintain manual stabilization of the head and neck while you quickly obtain a history and perform a rapid trauma examination. Considering the potential for so many skeletal injuries, you should keep the patient in a supine position until you can secure him to a long backboard.

3. Describe the components of the spine.

   Answer: The spine is composed of 24 vertebrae and is organized into five sections: the cervical, thoracic, and lumbar spines and the sacrum and coccyx. The sacrum and coccyx are fused together to form the posterior pelvis and tailbone. Each vertebra is composed of the vertebral foramen, transverse process, spinous process, and intervertebral disks.

4. What are the potential injuries to the spine for this patient?

   Answer: Traumatic injury occurs most commonly in the cervical and lumbar spines. Potential injuries to the spine as a result of the fall include compression fracture, herniated disk, or bulging disk. In a compression fracture, the force of the impact causes the anterior portion of the vertebral body to collapse, resulting in a wedge-shaped appearance on radiographs. In a herniated disk, some or all of the nucleus pulposus leaks from a tear in the anulus fibrosus. In a bulging disk, the disk bulges but has no tear or leakage. All of these injuries can impinge on the spinal cord or nerve roots, causing further injury.

5. Describe the bones of the pelvic girdle and the potential injuries associated with a pelvic injury.

   Answer: The pelvic girdle consists of the ilium, ischium, pubis, sacrum, and coccyx and is the attachment point for the lower extremities. It takes a severe trauma to fracture the pelvis, and patients who sustain fractures of the pelvis are likely to have any of a number of serious complications, including nerve damage, hemorrhagic shock, bladder or urethra rupture, and rectal or vaginal injuries.

6. Describe the bones of the hip joint and possible injuries associated with the hip.

   Answer: The hip joint is a ball-and-socket joint made up of the acetabulum (socket) and the femoral head (ball). Fractures and dislocation injuries are associated with the hip joint. Hip fractures actually are fractures of the proximal portion of the femur near or at the site of articulation with the acetabulum. Dislocations can be anterior or posterior.

7. Which of the patient's musculoskeletal injuries discovered in the physical examination is potentially the most serious?

   Answer: The mechanism of injury (MOI), as well as pain and tenderness, indicates that the patient may have sustained a pelvic injury. Pelvic injury would be the most serious injury and could result in nerve damage, hemorrhagic shock, bladder or urethra rupture, and rectal or vaginal injuries. Injury to the lumbosacral nerves occurs in up to half of patients with the most severe pelvic fractures. Hemorrhage following pelvic fracture may be life threatening, resulting in substantial blood loss. Hemorrhagic shock is the cause of death in many patients who die following pelvic fractures.

The Musculoskeletal System

Learning Objectives

1. Describe muscle structure in terms of muscle cells, tendons, and bones. (p 76-82)

2. Describe the neuromuscular junction and explain the function(s) for each part. (p 77-78)

3. Describe the structure of a sarcomere. (p 77)

4. Describe the sliding filament theory of muscle contraction. (p 78-80)

5. Explain polarization, depolarization, and repolarization in terms of ions and charges. (p 79-80)

6. Name the energy sources for muscle contraction. (p 80-81)

7. Explain the importance of hemoglobin, myoglobin, oxygen debt, and lactic acid. (p 81)

8. Describe the difference between antagonistic and synergistic muscles. (p 82)

9. State the major muscles of the body and their functions. (p 83-92)

Introduction

The human body is a well-designed system whose form, upright posture, and movement are provided by the musculoskeletal system. The term musculoskeletal refers to the bones and voluntary muscles of the body. The musculoskeletal system also protects the vital internal organs of the body. Muscle is composed of fibers that contract, causing movement. The body contains three types of muscle: skeletal muscle (striated), smooth muscle, and cardiac muscle. Muscles are a form of tissue that causes body movement. The understanding of muscle tissue is very important to your clinical field practice. Whether the patient is an injured athlete, a victim of a motor vehicle crash, or has runaway tachycardia caused by irritable cardiac muscle tissue, you need to be familiar with how muscles work.

Skeletal Muscle

Skeletal muscle, so named because it attaches to the bones of the skeleton, forms the major muscle mass of the body. It is also called voluntary muscle because skeletal muscle can be consciously controlled by the brain **Figure 4-1**. The body contains more than 350 skeletal muscles.

Movement of the body, like waving or walking, results from skeletal muscle contraction or relaxation. Usually a specific motion is the result of several muscles contracting and relaxing simultaneously. Individual skeletal muscles are separated from other muscles and held in position by layers of fibrous connective tissue known as fascia.

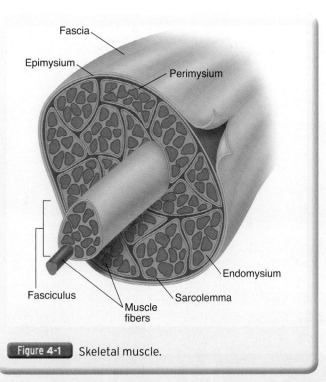

Figure 4-1 Skeletal muscle.

Coverings of Connective Tissue

Fascia surrounds every muscle and may form cordlike tendons beyond each muscle's end. Tendon fibers may intertwine with bone fibers to attach muscles to bones. Broad sheets of fibers that may attach to bones or to the coverings of other muscles are known as aponeuroses.

Skeletal muscles are closely surrounded by a layer of connective tissue known as an epimysium. The muscle is separated into small compartments by another layer known as the perimysium. Inside these compartments are muscle fascicles (muscle fasciculus), which are bundles of skeletal muscle cells bound together by connective tissue and forming one of the constituent elements of a muscle fibers. These layers form a thin covering (endomysium). The many layers of connective tissue that enclose and separate skeletal muscles allow a great deal of independent movement.

Pathophysiology

Tendon lacerations, especially in the hand, may result in long-term impairment unless they are properly treated. Unless a tendon is completely transected, the patient often will retain some motion of the finger. The examiner must test for pain against resistance to motion rather than simply motion itself. A partially torn or lacerated tendon will allow motion but also causes pain against resistance to motion. If a partially torn tendon is missed and the hand is improperly immobilized, the tear may become complete. If repair is delayed in such a situation, the surgical procedure becomes much more complicated and the results are not as good.

Pathophysiology

The median nerve passes through a strong band of connective tissue in the wrist, the carpal tunnel. Many conditions, including glandular diseases, pregnancy, and overuse, can result in irritation and compression of the nerve, or carpal tunnel syndrome. Carpal tunnel syndrome is a common source of occupational disability claims.

Structure of Skeletal Muscle Fibers

A single cell that contracts in response to stimulation and relaxes when the stimulation ceases is known as a skeletal muscle fiber. These fibers are thin, elongated cylinders with rounded ends. The cell membrane (sarcolemma) lies above the cytoplasm (also known as sarcoplasm), with many small, oval-shaped mitochondria and nuclei. The sarcoplasm is made up of many threadlike myofibrils arranged parallel to each other.

Myofibrils have thick protein filaments composed of myosin, and thin protein filaments mostly composed of actin Figure 4-2 . These filaments are organized so that they appear as striations—areas of alternating colored bands of skeletal muscle fiber. The repeating patterns of striation units that appear along each muscle fiber are referred to as sarcomeres. Muscles are basically considered to be collections of sarcomeres.

There are two main parts of the striation pattern of skeletal muscle fibers. The light bands (I bands) are made up of thin filaments of actin attached to Z lines. The dark bands (A bands) are made up of thick filaments of myosin that overlap thin filaments of actin. There is a central region (H zone) of thick filaments, with a thickened area (the M line) that consists of proteins holding them in place. Sarcomeres extend from one Z line to another Z line, as shown in Figure 4-2.

Inside the sarcoplasm of a muscle fiber, a network of channels surrounds each myofibril Figure 4-3 . These membranous channels form the sarcoplasmic reticulum. Transverse tubules (T-tubules) are other membranous channels extending inward and passing through the fiber. These tubules open to the outside of the muscle fiber and contain extracellular fluid. Each tubule lies between enlarged structures called cisternae, near the point where actin and myosin filaments overlap. Together, the sarcoplasmic reticulum and T-tubules activate muscle contraction when stimulated.

Neurologic Structures

Neurons (nerve cells) conduct nerve impulses. Motor neurons control effectors, which include skeletal muscle. Each skeletal muscle fiber is connected in a functional manner to the axon of a motor neuron. These pass outward from the brain or spinal cord. Each functional connection is called a synapse. At the synapses, neurons communicate with other cells by releasing neurotransmitters (chemicals that enable communication). Skeletal muscle fibers usually contract when stimulated by motor neurons.

A neuromuscular junction is the connection between a motor neuron and a muscle fiber Figure 4-4 . A motor

---

Case Study PART 1

Your unit is standing by at the local high school's regional soccer tournament. Four games have been playing simultaneously for the past 4 hours and there are 2 more hours to go. Suddenly, you notice a commotion over on field 4 and find a girl has been injured and is lying on the field. Witnesses say that she was running after the ball and came to a sudden stop while attempting to make a turn. You determine that the scene is safe, and your general impression of this patient reveals a girl whose right knee is flexed and swollen. The patient did not strike her head or lose consciousness. She is crying in apparent pain and is attempting to hold her knee still.

You take standard precautions and determine that there are no immediate life-threats. Examination reveals that the patient has no injuries to the spine, head, or body parts other than the knee. The patient states that she heard a pop and now feels that the knee joint is unstable and she cannot bear any weight on the leg.

Recording Time: 0 Minutes	
Appearance	Adolescent female in pain with a swollen knee
Level of consciousness	Alert (oriented to person, place, and day)
Airway	Appears patent
Breathing	Normal
Circulation	Normal pulse detected distal to injury, skin flushed with diaphoresis
Pulse	90 beats/min, regular
Blood pressure	110/70 mm Hg
Respirations	22 breaths/min, regular
Spo$_2$	98%

1. What type of muscle is involved in the function of a joint such as the knee?

2. What is the primary function of the type of muscle found around the knee?

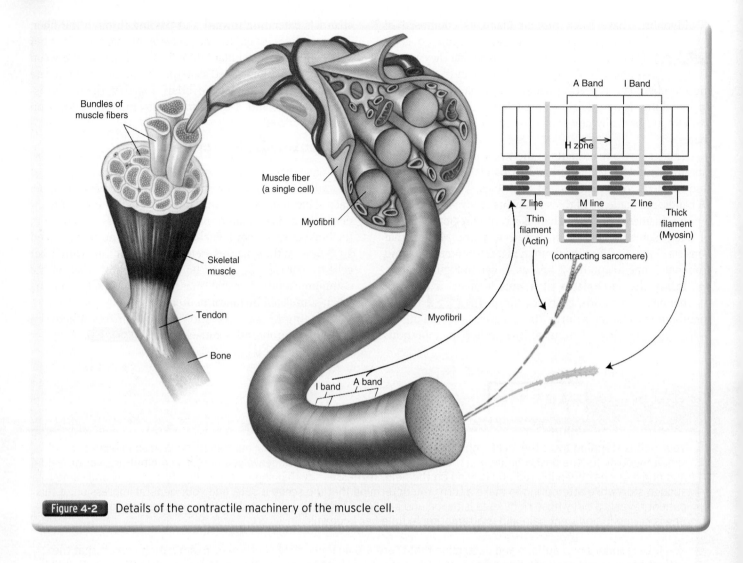

Figure 4-2   Details of the contractile machinery of the muscle cell.

end plate is formed by specialized muscle fiber membranes. Motor end plates have abundant mitochondria and nuclei, with greatly folded sarcolemmas.

Motor neurons branch out and project into muscle fiber membrane recesses. Cytoplasm at these distal ends have many mitochondria and tiny synaptic vesicles that contain neurotransmitters. On receiving impulses, the vesicles release neurotransmitters into the synaptic cleft between the neuron and motor end plate, stimulating muscle contraction.

Pathophysiology

Certain types of nerve gas, as well as ingredients in certain pesticides, bind to acetylcholinesterase and inhibit its function. Thus, acetylcholine is not degraded in the synaptic cleft and continues to constantly stimulate the muscle fiber, resulting in spastic paralysis, a condition in which muscles fire spontaneously but cannot relax, resulting in paralysis, an inability to respond to voluntary stimuli.

Motor Units

Most muscle fibers have a single motor end plate, though motor neuron axons have many branches connecting the motor neuron to various muscle fibers. When an impulse is transmitted, all of the connected muscle fibers contract at the same time. A motor unit is therefore made up of a motor neuron and the muscle fibers that it controls **Figure 4-5**.

Contraction of Skeletal Muscles

Skeletal muscles contract when organelles and molecules bind myosin to actin to cause a pulling action. The myofibrils then move as the actin and myosin filaments slide, shortening the muscle fiber and pulling on its attachments.

Required Chemicals

Myosin molecules are made up of two protein strands with globe-shaped cross-bridges that project outward. Groups of many myosin molecules make up a myosin (thick) filament.

Actin molecules are globe-shaped with a binding site that attaches to myosin cross-bridges. Groups of many

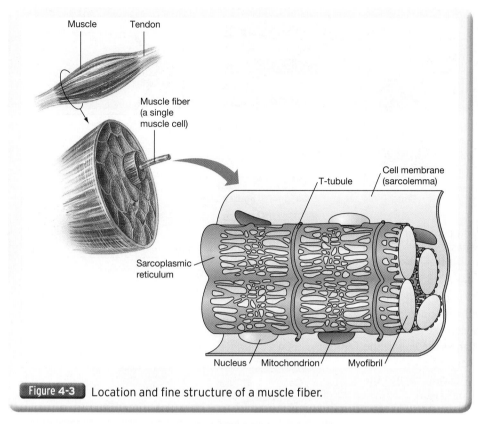

Muscle

Tendon

Muscle fiber
(a single
muscle cell)

T-tubule

Cell membrane
(sarcolemma)

Sarcoplasmic
reticulum

Nucleus   Mitochondrion   Myofibril

Figure 4-3 Location and fine structure of a muscle fiber.

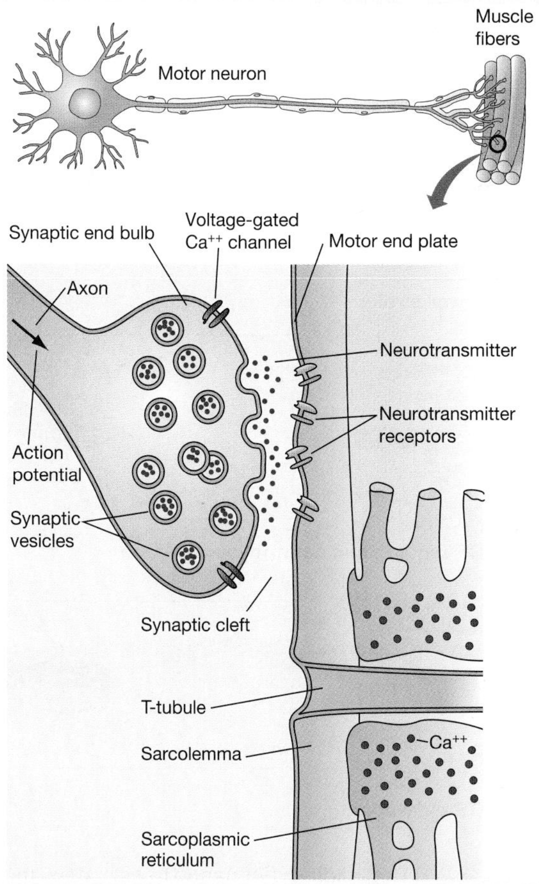

Muscle
fibers

Motor neuron

Synaptic end bulb

Voltage-gated
Ca++ channel

Motor end plate

Axon

Neurotransmitter

Neurotransmitter
receptors

Action
potential

Synaptic
vesicles

Synaptic cleft

T-tubule

Sarcolemma

Ca++

Sarcoplasmic
reticulum

Figure 4-4 A synapse or neuroeffector junction.

actin molecules twist in double strands (helixes) to form an actin (thin) filament, which includes the proteins known as troponin and tropomyosin Figure 4-6.

Strands of tropomyosin prevent actin–myosin interaction. One subunit of the troponin molecule binds to tropomyosin, forming the troponin–tropomyosin complex. Another subunit binds to G actin to hold the complex in position. A third subunit has a receptor binding a calcium ion. When the muscle is at rest, intracellular calcium is very low, and the binding site is empty. Contractions cannot occur unless the position of the troponin–tropomyosin complex changes to expose the active sites on F actin. The position change occurs when calcium ions bind to receptors on the troponin molecules. This binding causes a change in the structure of the actin molecule that allows actin and myosin to react with each other, forming a troponin-tropomyosin complex, resulting in muscle contraction.

The functional unit of skeletal muscle is the sarcomere. When sarcomeres shorten within a skeletal muscle fiber, a skeletal muscle contracts. This occurs because of the cross-bridges pulling on the thin filaments of actin. The sliding filament model is so named because of the way sarcomeres shorten, with thick and thin filaments sliding past each other toward the center of the sarcomere, from both ends.

Myosin filaments contain the enzyme adenosine triphosphatase (ATPase) in their globe-shaped portions. This enzyme catalyzes the breakdown of adenosine triphosphate (ATP) to both adenosine diphosphate (ADP) and phosphate, releasing energy. The myosin cross-bridges assume a "cocked" position, binding to actin to pull on the thin filament. After the pulling occurs, the cross-bridge is released from actin before the ATP splits. The cycle repeats as long as there is enough ATP for energy and muscular stimulation occurs.

Contraction Stimulus

The impulse that causes contraction of skeletal muscle is transmitted through motor neurons as a nerve impulse. These impulses are also known as action potentials, and are transmitted from one cell to another in the nervous system, causing each successive cell in the chain to "fire." The process by which cells activate in response to the action potential is known as depolarization. When the cell is at rest, ions are actively transported into and out of the cell to create an electrochemical gradient across the cell membrane. This is known

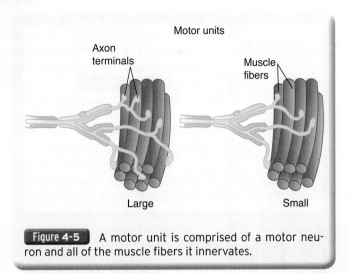

Figure 4-5 A motor unit is comprised of a motor neuron and all of the muscle fibers it innervates.

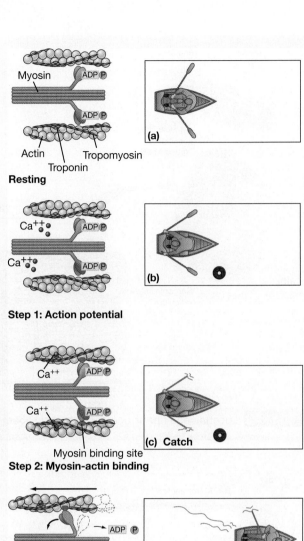

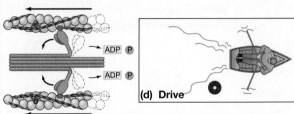

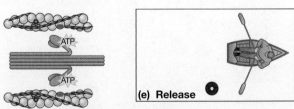

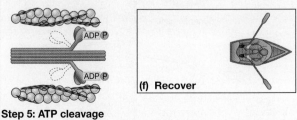

Figure 4-6 The sliding filament theory: how muscle fibers contract.

as being polarized. When the cell is activated by the release of a neurotransmitter, proteins in the cell wall open rapidly, allowing a rapid influx of ions that equalizes the charges on either side of the cell wall. When the charges are equal, the cell has depolarized, and the protein channels close. Then the process of repolarization begins, which again creates the electrochemical gradient so the cell can "fire" again.

The neurotransmitter that stimulates skeletal muscle to contract is acetylcholine. Synthesized in the cytoplasm of motor neurons, acetylcholine is released into the synaptic clefts between motor neuron axons and motor end plates. It rapidly diffuses, binding to certain protein receptors in the muscle fiber membrane, increasing permeability to sodium. These charged particles stimulate a muscle impulse that passes in many directions over the muscle fiber membrane. This impulse eventually reaches the sarcoplasmic reticulum.

The sarcoplasmic reticulum has a high calcium ion concentration, and it responds to the muscle impulse by becoming more permeable to calcium. Calcium is then released into the cytoplasm where it binds to troponin, initiating a contraction cycle in which troponin and tropomyosin interact to form linkages between actin and myosin filaments. The muscular contraction also requires ATP and continues as long as acetylcholine is released.

Muscle relaxation is caused by the decomposition of acetylcholine via the enzyme acetylcholinesterase. It prevents a single nerve impulse from stimulating the muscle fiber continuously. When the stimulus ceases, calcium ions are transported back to the sarcoplasmic reticulum. The actin and myosin linkages break, and the muscle relaxes.

Energy Sources

Muscle contraction, regardless of type, requires energy. Muscle fibers have just enough ATP for short-term contraction. ATP must be regenerated when fibers are active, using existing ATP molecules in the cells. ATP is regenerated from ADP and phosphate. Creatine phosphate enables this with high-energy phosphate bonds. It is between four and six times more abundant in muscle fibers than ATP; however, it does not directly supply energy. It stores excess energy from the mitochondria in the phosphate bonds.

When ATP breaks down, energy from creatine phosphate is transferred to ADP molecules to convert them back into ATP. Creatine phosphate stores are exhausted rapidly when muscles are active; therefore, the muscles use cellular respiration of glucose as energy to synthesize ATP.

Clinical Tip

Many cardiac drugs influence the passage of calcium, sodium, or both across cell membranes. These drugs include standard anti-dysrhythmic agents, such as lidocaine or procainamide, and calcium channel blockers, such as verapamil, diltiazem, and amiodarone.

Oxygen Use and Debt

Oxygen is required for the breakdown of glucose in the mitochondria. Red blood cells carry oxygen, bound to hemoglobin molecules. Hemoglobin is the pigment that makes blood appear red. The pigment myoglobin is synthesized in the muscles to give skeletal muscles their reddish-brown color. Myoglobin can also combine with oxygen and temporarily store it in order to reduce muscular requirements for continuous blood supply during contraction.

When skeletal muscles are used for a more than a minute or two, anaerobic respiration is required for energy. In one type of anaerobic respiration, glucose is broken down via glycolysis to yield pyruvic acid, which is converted to lactic acid. Lactic acid can accumulate in muscles, but often diffuses in the bloodstream, reaching the liver, where it is converted back into glucose.

When a person is exercising strenuously, oxygen is used mostly to synthesize ATP. As lactic acid increases, an oxygen debt develops. Oxygen debt is equivalent to the amount of oxygen that liver cells require to convert the lactic acid into glucose, as well as the amount needed by muscle cells to restore ATP and creatine phosphate levels.

It may take several hours for the body to convert lactic acid back into glucose. Muscles may experience a change in their metabolic activity as exercise levels change. Increased exercise raises the muscles' capacity for glycolysis. Aerobic exercise increases the muscles' capacity for aerobic respiration.

Muscle Fatigue

Prolonged exercise may cause a muscle to become unable to contract. This condition is called fatigue, and it may also occur because of interruption of muscular blood supply, or occasionally a lack of acetylcholine in the motor neuron axons. Lactic acid accumulation is the usual cause of muscular fatigue. As lactic acid lowers pH levels, muscle fibers become progressively less able to respond to stimulation.

When a muscle becomes fatigued and cramps, it experiences a sustained, involuntary contraction. Though not fully understood, muscle cramps appear to be caused by changes in the extracellular fluid surrounding muscle fibers and motor neurons.

Production of Heat

Most of the energy released in cellular respiration becomes heat. Muscle tissue generates a large amount of heat because muscles form so much of the total body mass. Body temperature is partially maintained by the blood transporting heat generated by the muscle to other body tissues.

Muscle Responses

Muscle contractions can be observed by using a myogram to "see" muscle twitches. This requires electrical signals that can cause various strengths and frequencies of responses. A muscle fiber will remain unresponsive until a certain strength of stimulation (the threshold stimulus) is applied. An action potential is then generated that results in an impulse that spreads throughout the fiber, releasing calcium and activating cross-bridge binding. This causes contraction.

The contractile response of a fiber to an impulse is called a twitch, and it consists of a period of contraction followed by a period of relaxation. A myogram records this pattern of events. There is a brief delay between the stimulation time and the beginning of contraction. This is known as the latent period, and may last less than 2 milliseconds. A myogram results from the combined twitches of muscle fibers taking part in contraction. There are two types of twitches: the fatigue-resistant slow twitch and the fatigable fast twitch.

The force of individual twitches combines via the process of summation. When sustained contractions have no relaxation at all, they are referred to as either tetanic contractions or the condition known as tetany. High intensities of stimulation can activate many motor units (recruitment).

Actions of Skeletal Muscles

Skeletal muscles cause unique movements based on the type of joint they attach to and where the attachment points are. When a muscle appears to be at rest, its fibers still undergo some sustained contraction, known as muscle tone or tonus.

Origins and Insertions

One end of a skeletal muscle usually is fastened to a relatively immovable part (origin) at a moveable joint. The other end connects to a one side of a movable joint (insertion) on the other side of the joint. As contraction occurs, the insertion is pulled toward the origin. There may be more than one origin or insertion, such as in the biceps brachii muscle of the arm. When this muscle contracts, the insertion being pulled toward its origin causes the forearm to flex and supinate at the elbow Figure 4-7.

The head of a muscle is the part closest to its origin. The term flexion describes a decrease in the angle of a joint; for example, a movement of the forearm that causes it to bend

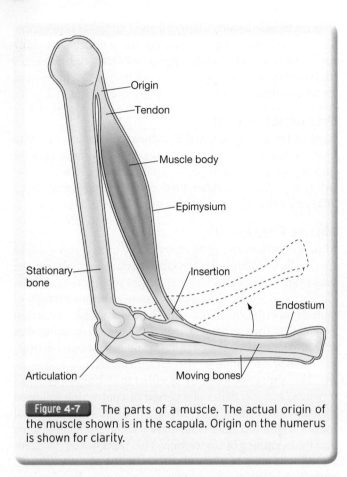

Figure 4-7 The parts of a muscle. The actual origin of the muscle shown is in the scapula. Origin on the humerus is shown for clarity.

at the elbow. The term extension describes an increase in the angle of a joint; for example, a movement of the forearm that straightens the elbow.

Skeletal Muscle Interactions

Skeletal muscles usually function in groups, with the nervous system stimulating the desired muscles to perform the intended function. A muscle that contracts to provide most of a desired movement is called a prime mover or agonist. Other muscles, known as synergists, work with a prime mover to make its action more effective. For example, when you bend your forearm, the agonist muscles are the biceps, whereas the synergists are the brachialis.

Other muscles act as antagonists to prime movers. They cause movement in the opposite direction. In the above example, the triceps would be the antagonists to the biceps. Smooth body movement depends on antagonists relaxing while prime movers contract. Muscles may work opposite to each other or together in order to control various movements.

Smooth Muscle

Smooth muscle cells are smaller than those of skeletal muscle. They are spindle-shaped with a single nucleus. Smooth muscle cells contain fewer actin and myosin myofilaments than do skeletal muscle cells. The myofilaments of smooth muscle are not organized into sarcomeres; therefore, smooth muscle is considered to be nonstriated muscle.

The two types of smooth muscle are visceral and multiunit smooth muscle. Visceral smooth muscle is the more common of the two types and normally is made up of sheets of muscle that form the layers of the digestive, reproductive, and urinary tracts. Electrochemical signals travel quickly from one cell to another because numerous conduction areas, or gap junctions, interconnect the individual cells. Multiple sheets of smooth muscle tend to function as a single unit because of rapid transmission of the action potential. Sometimes, contraction of muscles in this fashion is referred to as a functional syncytium.

Multiunit smooth muscle may be found in sheets (as in the walls of blood vessels), in small bundles (as in the iris of the eye), or as single cells (as in the capsule of the spleen). This form of smooth muscle has few gap junctions; each cell contracts as an independent unit when stimulated by nerves. Thus, the rate of contraction is somewhat slower than that of visceral smooth muscle.

The autonomic nervous system innervates smooth muscle. Because the autonomic nervous system is not under conscious control, smooth muscle contraction is involuntary. Unlike skeletal muscle, smooth muscle has very little sarcoplasmic reticulum. The calcium required for contraction diffuses into the cell from the surrounding fluid (extracellular fluid). Calcium binds to an intracellular protein, calmodulin, resulting in muscle contraction. Whether or not actin and myosin filaments actually form cross-bridges between each other is unknown. In general, contraction of smooth muscle occurs at a slower rate than that of skeletal muscle.

In addition to electrochemical stimulation that the autonomic nervous system provides to smooth muscle, various hormones released by the glands also affect smooth muscle contraction. For example, the hormone oxytocin stimulates contractions of uterine smooth muscle.

Cardiac Muscle

Cardiac muscle is striated like skeletal muscle, and muscle cells contain only one nucleus. Intercalated disks are branching fibers between cells and protein-lined ion channels that allow action potentials to pass from cell to cell. For an action potential (an electrochemical cell signal or impulse) to occur, the process needs a polarized cell, which is a cell at rest, waiting to react to a stimulus. Depolarization of the polarized cell requires a trigger or minimum energy level. Depolarization opens channels into the cell, allowing sodium to rush in. When enough sodium is inside the awaiting cell, an action potential fires stimulating surrounding cells. Repolarization is the recovery phase that follows depolarization. During this phase sodium leaves the cell via active transport, allowing the cell to return to a polarized state awaiting the next stimulus.

Cardiac muscle has the property of intrinsic automaticity, meaning that, to an extent, it is able to generate its own electrical activity. Depolarization of cardiac muscle results from the influx of both sodium and calcium ions across the cell membrane. Under the right conditions (electrolyte abnormality, sodium, potassium or calcium abnormalities, or hypoxemia), any cell in the heart can become irritable and begin giving off extrasystoles. It is these extrasystoles that can precede ventricular fibrillation.

Muscular Anatomy

It is important for you to know the muscle groups, their locations, and their functions. Names of muscles often describe their sizes, shapes, locations, actions, number of attachments, or direction of fibers. For example, the word pectoralis means "chest" in Latin. The major muscle of the chest wall is the pectoralis major. The word "angina" means pain, thus angina pectoralis is "pain in the chest." The word brevis means "short" in Latin; and the word

longus means "long." The adductor brevis muscle is a short muscle that adducts the thigh. One of its synergists, the adductor longus, is a long muscle that performs the same task.

In Greek, the word deltoid translates as "triangular." The deltoid muscle is a large triangular muscle of the arm and shoulder. In Latin, the term rectus means "straight," and the linear muscle of the abdomen is the rectus abdominis. The sternocleidomastoid muscle originates at the sternum and travels over the clavicle and then inserts into the mastoid process. The biceps muscle of the arm has two heads.

The anterior and posterior views of the superficial skeletal muscles are shown in Figure 4-8 and Figure 4-9.

The Head, Trunk, and Upper Extremity

The Head

The muscles that enable head movement are located in the anterior, posterior, and lateral aspects of the skull. As a rule, most of these muscles originate at the upper cervical vertebrae and insert in the skull, most often the occipital bone Figure 4-10. Innervation is provided by cervical roots C1 and C2, as well as the spinal accessory nerve.

Case Study | PART 2

You suspect that the patient has sustained an injury to the ligaments that hold the knee joint together. You ask the patient and her father, who has been at her side since moments after the injury occurred, about her history, revealing that the patient is a 14-year-old girl who weighs 49 kg. Her SAMPLE history shows the following:

- **S**igns and symptoms: Swelling, pain, tenderness, and distal muscular motor weakness secondary to pain in the injured extremity
- **A**llergies to medications: No known drug allergies
- **M**edications taken: Ibuprofen, vitamin C
- **P**ast pertinent medical history: Previously injured right knee while alpine skiing and fractured right wrist while skateboarding
- **L**ast food/fluid intake: A few orange slices during the last break, otherwise no food since breakfast
- **E**vents prior to onset: Noncontact injury involving rapid deceleration and rotation of the right knee

Recording Time: 5 Minutes	
Appearance	Still in pain but calming down
Level of consciousness	Alert (oriented to person, place, and day)
Airway	Open and clear
Breathing	20 breaths/min, regular
Circulation	Color returning yet still diaphoretic

3. In addition to tendons, what other structures in and around the knee may have been injured?

4. What types of knee injuries are most common in this situation?

5. What are your concerns for management of this injury?

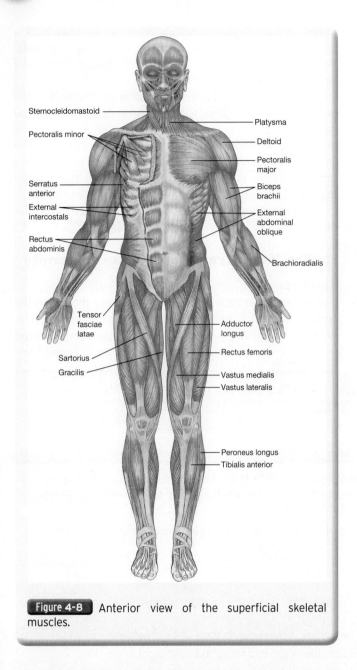

Figure 4-8 Anterior view of the superficial skeletal muscles.

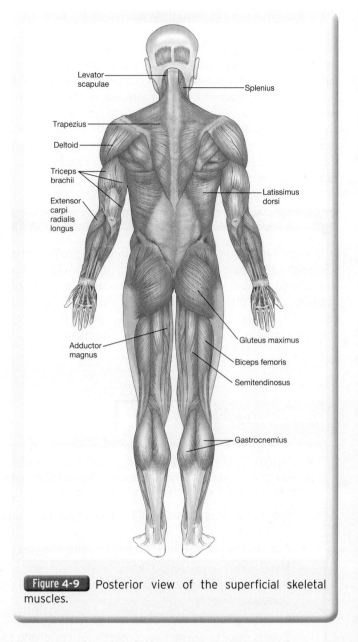

Figure 4-9 Posterior view of the superficial skeletal muscles.

Located anteriorly, both the longus capitis and rectus capitis muscles rotate and flex the head. Numerous posterior muscles assist in rotation and extension of the head. Laterally, the sternocleidomastoid muscles rotate and extend the head, whereas the rectus capitis lateralis abducts it.

The Face

The skeletal muscles of the face are superficial and attach to the skin. They originate on various facial bones and, with one exception, are innervated by the seventh cranial nerve, the facial nerve. The exception, the levator palpebrae superioris, is innervated by the third cranial nerve, the oculomotor nerve **Figure 4-11**.

Six muscles attach to the eyeball, allowing it to rotate within the orbit in many directions. These muscles are innervated by the oculomotor nerve. The motions of muscles of both eyeballs coordinate, so that eye movements occur in synchrony.

Muscles of mastication (chewing) are innervated by the fifth cranial nerve. The temporalis muscle elevates and retracts the mandible, as does the masseter. The lateral and medial pterygoid muscles perform the opposite action, depressing the mandible. The tongue contains several muscles that also are very important in both chewing and speech **Figure 4-12**.

Swallowing is a complex process that involves coordinated contraction of numerous muscles of the palate, pharynx, and larynx. Many of these muscles are innervated by the recurrent laryngeal nerve.

The Shoulder and Back

The muscles of the posterior thorax form the first layer of back muscles. These include the trapezius, deltoids, rhomboids,

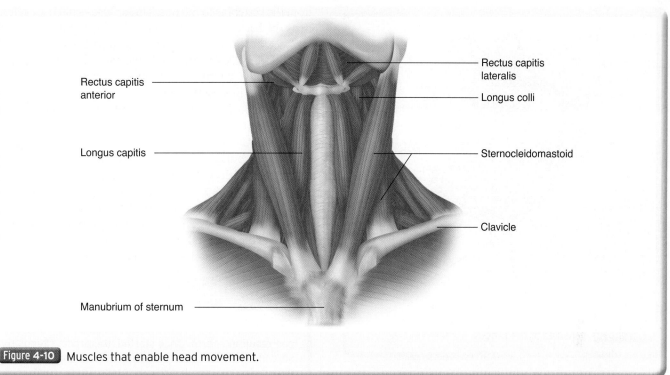

Figure 4-10 Muscles that enable head movement.

Pathophysiology

The term <u>whiplash</u> describes a neck injury associated with sudden flexion or extension and resulting in pain or other evidence of injury. Typically, a hyperextension-hyperflexion injury of the cervical spine occurs as a result of a rear-end collision. The patient reports neck and head pain, which may radiate down either arm. At times, concomitant stimulation of the sympathetic nervous system may result in dizziness, blurred vision, or pain behind the eyeballs. In the absence of fracture, dislocation, or neurologic injury, symptoms typically resolve spontaneously within 6 to 8 weeks, and long-term impairment is rare.

Pathophysiology

<u>Bell palsy</u> is a condition that results from dysfunction of the facial nerve, as a result of either trauma or infection. The patient becomes unable to move the facial muscles on the affected side, and the lip sags during speech and attempts at smiling. The most significant problem that results from Bell palsy is that the patient often is unable to close his or her eyelid and loses the protective blinking reflex. To protect the eye, patients can instill artificial tears or keep the eyelid taped shut. Nerve function returns in most persons, at least to a degree, within a few weeks.

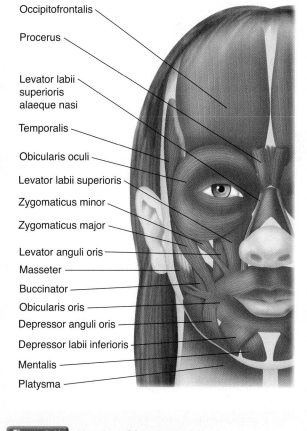

Figure 4-11 Muscles of facial expression.

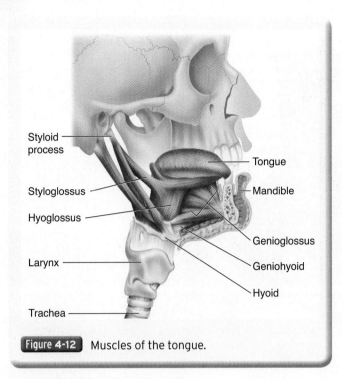

Figure 4-12 Muscles of the tongue.

Labels: Styloid process, Styloglossus, Hyoglossus, Larynx, Trachea, Tongue, Mandible, Genioglossus, Geniohyoid, Hyoid

from the vertebrae to the ribs. These muscles often are referred to as the back muscles. Various spinal nerves innervate all of the back muscles, depending on the muscle's location.

Collectively, the erector spinae form the largest group of superficial back muscles. This group is subdivided into three groups: the iliocostalis, longissimus, and spinalis muscles. The longissimus group provides the greatest muscle mass and strength in the back.

Deep muscles of the back include the interspinales muscles, which connect the spinous processes of all vertebrae; the intertransversarii muscles, which connect the transverse processes; the multifidus muscles, which help erect and rotate the spine; the rotatores, which lie deep in the groove between the spinous and transverse processes of the vertebrae and extend and rotate the vertebral column toward the opposite side; and the semispinalis muscles, which help to rotate the spine.

Clinical Tip

Injury to even one of the smallest deep back muscles can result in spasm. Once started, the process tends to spread and involve surrounding tissues. Inflammation also is common with muscle spasm. These conditions often are treated with a combination of pain medications and anti-inflammatory and anti-spasm (muscle relaxing) agents. Nonsteroidal anti-inflammatory drugs such as ibuprofen are the most common type of anti-inflammatory agents used for back pain and spasm. Depending on local protocols, severe muscle spasm in the prehospital setting may be treated with a combination of pain medication (such as morphine) and muscle relaxants (such as diazepam).

Pathophysiology

Laryngeal spasm (spasm of the muscles of the larynx) can occur following severe allergic reactions. If swelling is severe enough, it can block passage of air into the trachea. Unless this condition is promptly corrected, hypoxia can cause brain damage or death.

Clinical Tip

Sprains and strains of the lower back are often sustained by EMS providers and usually are caused by repetitive lifting or straining of the lower back muscles, tendons, and ligaments. Sprains and strains sometimes can occur after a single attempt at trying to lift an object that is too heavy, or they can occur because of poor posture or lifting techniques. In a business in which the EMS provider has to lift and move people who can and will be found in the most unusual places and positions, it is essential that good lifting mechanics are used at all times to help prevent back injuries from occurring.

The pain from sprains and strains of the lower back sometimes is described as soreness and aching and is localized over the lower part of the back. The pain often is severe and, at times, a sharp pain may occur with sudden movements such as twisting or bending to pick something up. The pain sometimes is relieved by lying flat on the back or with the use of heat or ice. The pain from back spasm alone does not travel down the leg or cause numbness or weakness. The pain may last for several weeks or longer.

Clinical Tip

Clinically, oculomotor nerve function is evaluated by having the patient move the eyes in various directions—right, left, up, down, and at 45° angle combinations (eg, up and to the right, down and to the left). These are called the extraocular movements. The easiest way to evaluate the extraocular movements is to ask the patient to follow a fingertip or flashlight with his or her eyes. Normally, both eyes should move the same amount in each direction.

and latissimus dorsi. All of these muscles are involved in motion of the upper thorax and shoulder girdle (see Figures 4-8 and 4-9).

Two groups of muscles move the spine: deep muscles and superficial muscles. The deep muscles originate and insert from vertebra to vertebra, whereas the superficial muscles run

The Thorax

During breathing, the major movement is produced by contraction of the diaphragm, a flattened dome-shaped muscle located at the base of the thoracic cavity. The phrenic nerve innervates the diaphragm. Damage to this nerve can result in difficulty breathing. Other muscles of respiration include the scalene muscles, which elevate the first two ribs during inspiration, and the external and internal intercostal muscles Figure 4-13 .

Pathophysiology

Hiccups occur when there is irritation of the phrenic nerve, resulting in sudden and unpredictable contractions of the diaphragm.

The Abdomen

The abdominal muscles, which consist of both superficial and deep layers of muscles, flex and rotate the spine. A tendinous area known as the linea alba lies in the midline. The muscles originate along the pelvic bones and the ribs and insert in the same areas, depending on which muscle is involved. Spinal nerves provide innervation to the abdominal muscles.

The Upper Extremity

Six muscle groups hold the scapula firmly against the body when the muscles of the arm contract. All originate on the upper vertebrae and ribs and insert onto various portions of the scapula. Except for the trapezius muscle, all are innervated by spinal nerves. The trapezius muscle receives innervation from the 11th cranial nerve, the spinal accessory nerve.

The pectoralis major and latissimus dorsi muscles attach the arm to the thorax. The rotator cuff is a special group of four muscles that forms a cuff or cap over the proximal humerus, attaches the humerus to the scapula, and provides for rotation of the arm.

Numerous other muscles are involved in movements of the arm. Major flexors include the deltoid and biceps brachii muscles. The triceps brachii and deltoid muscles are primarily responsible for extension of the arm. Abduction, adduction, and medial and lateral rotation are caused by actions of the triceps brachii and deltoid muscles, as well as several other accessory muscles Figure 4-14 .

Muscles acting on the forearm include those of the arm, as noted above, as well as intrinsic muscles of the forearm. The anconeus muscle stabilizes the elbow in extension; the brachioradialis flexes it. Both the pronator quadratus and pronator teres muscles pronate the forearm, whereas the supinator muscle supinates the forearm.

Hand, wrist, and finger movements are primarily mediated by muscles in the forearm. These muscles are divided into extensor muscles, groups of muscles that cause extension, and flexor muscles, groups of muscles that cause flexion when contracted. For example, the flexor digitorum superficialis causes flexion of the fingers. As a rule,

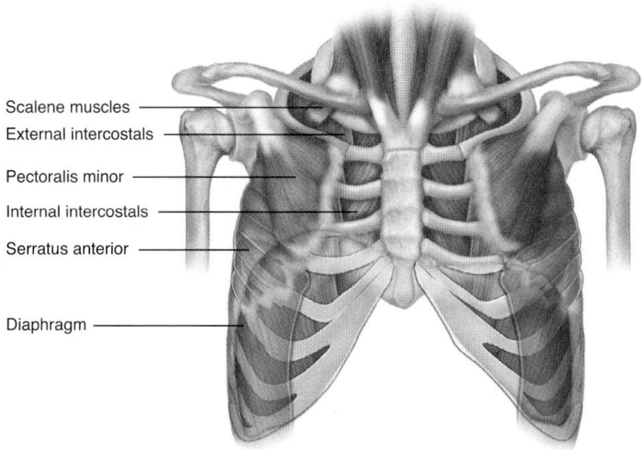

Scalene muscles
External intercostals
Pectoralis minor
Internal intercostals
Serratus anterior
Diaphragm

Figure 4-13 The muscles of respiration.

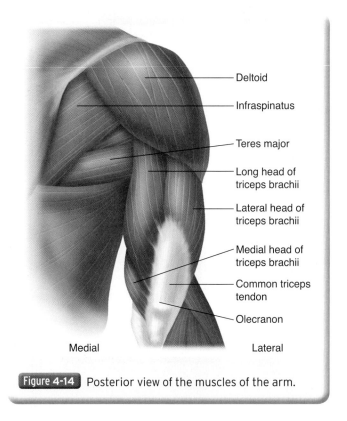

Deltoid
Infraspinatus
Teres major
Long head of triceps brachii
Lateral head of triceps brachii
Medial head of triceps brachii
Common triceps tendon
Olecranon

Medial   Lateral

Figure 4-14 Posterior view of the muscles of the arm.

the extensor muscles originate on the lateral aspect of the elbow, and the flexor muscles originate on the medial side **Figure 4-15** .

Movement is also affected by the intrinsic muscles of the hand, the lumbricales and the interossei, as well as the muscles of the thenar and hypothenar eminences, fleshy prominences at the base of the thumb (thenar) and fifth finger (hypothenar). These small muscles are located entirely within the hand **Figure 4-16** . All muscles that cause motion of the hand and fingers are innervated by the median, ulnar, or radial nerve.

The Pelvis and Lower Extremity

The Pelvic Floor and Perineum

The coccygeus muscle and the levator ani muscle form the floor of the pelvis. The area below these muscles is the perineum. The structures of the urogenital system (sometimes called the urogenital triangle) lie anteriorly; the structures of the anus, or anal triangle, lie posteriorly.

Pathophysiology

Rotator cuff injuries are a common source of shoulder pain and often occur as a result of tendon degeneration from age and repeated trauma. As the tendons weaken, thickening and chronic inflammation occur in the overlying shoulder bursa. Complete ruptures occasionally occur during athletic events involving heavy lifting or a fall on an outstretched hand, but they occur far more frequently as a result of chronic degeneration. Patients typically report pain and tenderness over the shoulder, which is worsened by abduction of the arm. In the absence of complete tendon rupture, some strength is maintained. With rupture, severe weakness and variable pain are both common. Radiographs often are normal; magnetic resonance imaging can help diagnose complete and partial tears. Strains of the rotator cuff or tendinitis respond well to rest and treatment with nonsteroidal anti-inflammatory drugs. Tears may require surgical repair.

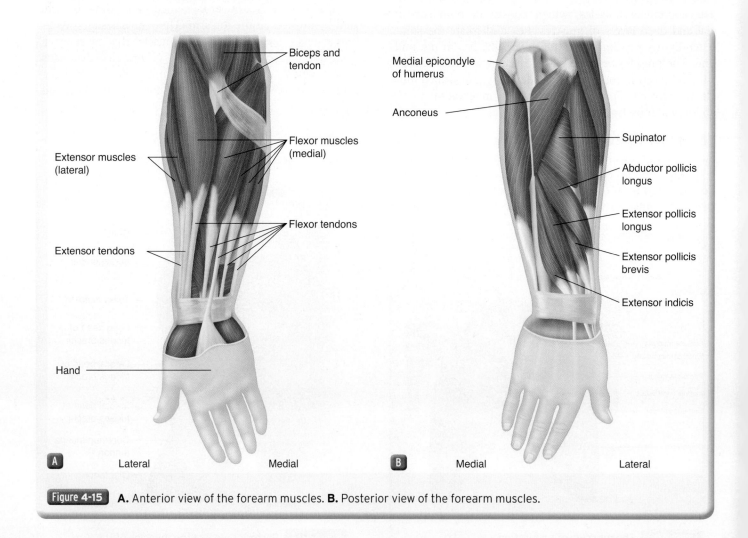

Figure 4-15   **A.** Anterior view of the forearm muscles. **B.** Posterior view of the forearm muscles.

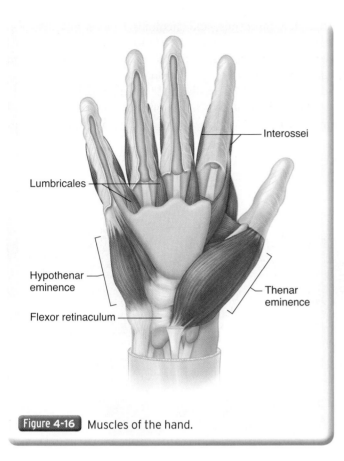

Figure 4-16 Muscles of the hand.

Labels: Interossei, Lumbricales, Hypothenar eminence, Flexor retinaculum, Thenar eminence

Pathophysiology

Bicipital tendinitis is a common cause of shoulder pain in adults older than 40 years; however, it also may occur in younger athletes who use repeated throwing motions. The common denominator is inflammation of the biceps tendon, as well as its sheath, in the bicipital groove. Patients have pain over the anterolateral aspect of the shoulder, which often radiates down the arm. Palpation reveals tenderness in the bicipital groove of the humerus, and a positive Yergason test, supported by pain in the bicipital groove on supination of the forearm against resistance. Radiographic studies most often are normal. Treatment consists of rest, heat, range-of-motion exercises, and nonsteroidal anti-inflammatory drugs. Sometimes, corticosteroids are injected into the shoulder. Surgery is a last resort.

In males, the bulbospongiosus muscle constricts the urethra and aids in the erection of the penis; in females, it results in erection of the clitoris. The orifice of the anal canal is kept closed by the sphincter ani externus, whereas the urethral sphincter muscle constricts the urethra Figure 4-17.

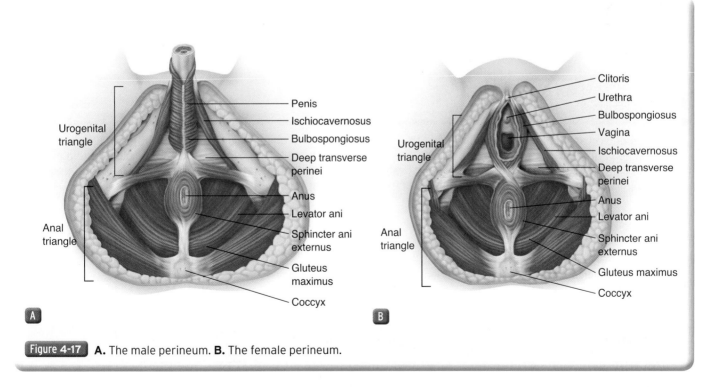

Figure 4-17 **A.** The male perineum. **B.** The female perineum.

The Lower Extremity

The muscles of the hip cause movement of the thigh at the hip joint. Many of these muscles originate in the pelvis and insert on the femur. Various lumbar and sacral spinal nerves innervate this area.

Flexion of the hip occurs when the iliopsoas muscle contracts. Posterolaterally, the gluteal muscles (the gluteus minimus, medius, and maximus) and the tensor fasciae latae extend and rotate the hip. Deeper muscles, the gemellus, obturator, piriformis, and quadratis femoris muscles, also cause flexion and rotation at the hip. Muscles of the medial compartment, the adductor brevis, adductor longus, and adductor magnus, the gracilis, and the pectineus muscles— adduct, flex, and internally rotate the thigh   Figure 4-18 .

Movements at the knee joint are effected by sets of muscles located in two compartments of the thigh, anatomic spaces that are enclosed by fascia. The anterior compartment contains the quadriceps femoris and sartorius

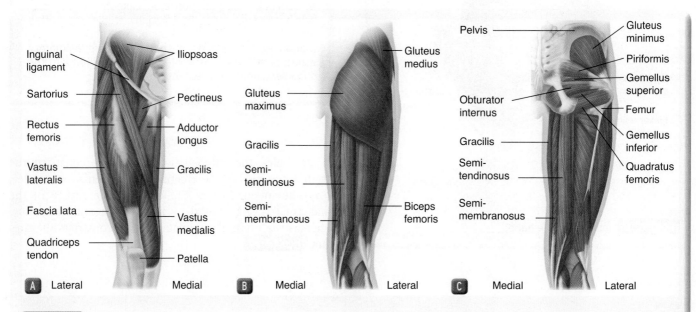

Figure 4-18   **A.** Anterior view of the hip and thigh muscles. **B.** Superficial, posterior view of the hip and thigh muscles. **C.** Deep, posterior view of the hip and thigh muscles.

Case Study | PART 3

At this point, you and your team carefully splint the injury, making sure to apply ice to help control the swelling, and prepare the patient for transport to the hospital. The patient is alert and talking with her father. As you roll the patient off the field on your stretcher, all the parents and bystanders applaud. You can see on her face that she appreciates their support, while at the same time, she appears anxious about her injury.

Recording Time: 10 Minutes

Appearance	Less pain now that the splint is applied
Level of consciousness	Alert (oriented to person, place, and day)
Airway	Open and clear
Breathing	Normal and regular
Circulation	Color returning and starting to dry off

6. What would be your next steps in assessing the patient?

muscles. The <u>quadriceps femoris</u> muscle primarily extends the knee when it contracts. (Because portions of the quadriceps femoris also cross the hip, a secondary function of this muscle is flexion of the hip joint.) The <u>sartorius muscle</u> is the longest muscle in the body, and it flexes the knee and the hip when it contracts. In the posterior compartment, the <u>biceps femoris</u> muscle flexes and laterally rotates the knee and extends the hip. The semimembranosus and semitendinosus muscles flex and medially rotate the knee. Together, the biceps, semimembranosus, and semitendinosus muscles are referred to as the hamstrings.

Muscles located in the leg act on the ankle and foot. These muscles typically originate on the tibia and fibula and insert into the foot **Figure 4-19**. The tibial and peroneal nerves, terminal divisions of the sciatic nerve, innervate these muscles.

Anatomically and functionally, the leg contains four compartments: the anterior, the superficial posterior, the deep posterior, and the lateral compartments. The anterior compartment contains muscles that extend (or dorsiflex) the ankle and toes. The superficial posterior compartment contains the gastrocnemius, plantaris, and soleus muscles, which are superficial muscles that plantar flex the ankle. The <u>Achilles tendon</u> is the strong tendon that attaches these muscles to the calcaneus. The deep posterior compartment contains muscles that flex the toes and invert the foot and ankle. The lateral compartment contains muscles that primarily evert the foot.

The intrinsic foot muscles are located within the foot itself and are arranged similarly to the intrinsic muscles of the hand. They flex, extend, abduct, and adduct the toes **Figure 4-20**.

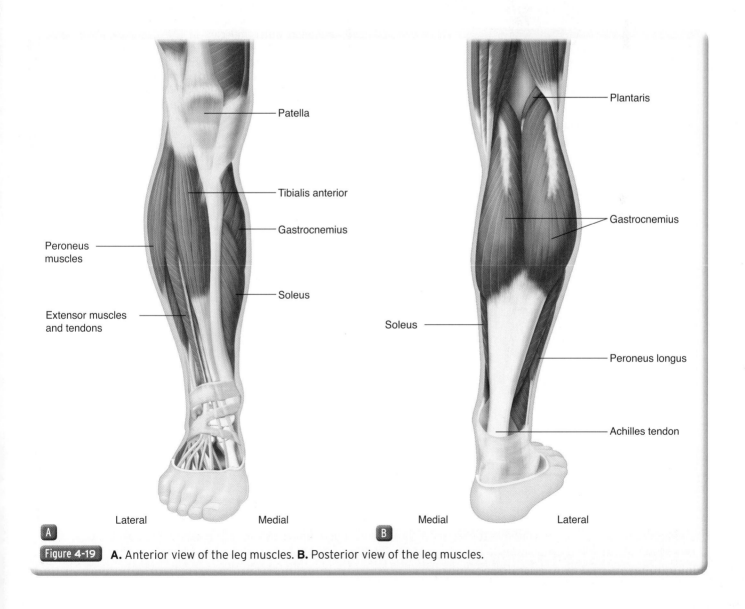

— Patella

— Tibialis anterior

— Gastrocnemius

Peroneus muscles —

— Soleus

Extensor muscles and tendons —

Lateral   Medial

A

— Plantaris

— Gastrocnemius

Soleus —

— Peroneus longus

— Achilles tendon

Medial   Lateral

B

Figure 4-19   **A.** Anterior view of the leg muscles. **B.** Posterior view of the leg muscles.

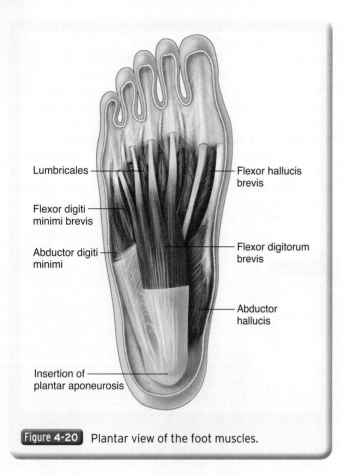

Lumbricales

Flexor digiti minimi brevis

Abductor digiti minimi

Insertion of plantar aponeurosis

Flexor hallucis brevis

Flexor digitorum brevis

Abductor hallucis

Figure 4-20 Plantar view of the foot muscles.

Pathophysiology

Each anatomic compartment of the leg is enclosed by fascia and is essentially a closed space. Following trauma, blood or fluid can accumulate within a compartment, resulting in compression of the blood vessels and tissue damage secondary to ischemia, a condition known as compartment syndrome. If not recognized and promptly treated, compartment syndrome can cause death of muscle and loss of the limb.

Pathophysiology

The Achilles tendon can be ruptured, usually following jumping or overstretching activities such as racquetball. Spontaneous rupture is rare. Following the injury, the patient walks flat-footed and is unable to stand on the ball of the foot. Active plantar flexion is lost, although other muscles in the calf may allow some motion to remain. The Thompson test is a test that is used to evaluate the integrity of the Achilles tendon for possible rupture; in the uninjured foot, the test normally is positive—squeezing the calf results in plantar flexion at the ankle. With a complete tear, the foot remains stationary. Treatment is occasionally surgical.

Case Study | PART 4

En route to the hospital, you continue to take serial vital signs, which remain stable. You reassess the splint and reevaluate the patient's distal pulse, motor, and sensory function. The application of ice has helped diminish the patient's pain somewhat. You find out from the patient's father that he tore his anterior cruciate ligament about 10 years ago at work and had it reconstructed, so he is very familiar with this type of injury.

Prep Kit

■ Chapter Summary

- Muscles are classified as skeletal muscle (voluntary), smooth muscle (involuntary), or cardiac muscle.

- Muscle fibers, as well as connective tissue, blood vessels, and nerves, comprise the more than 350 voluntary skeletal muscles in the body.

- Myofibrils, which are threadlike structures that extend from one end of the muscle fiber to the other, are located within individual muscle cells.

- A cell membrane surrounds each muscle fiber. As several muscle fibers are bundled with connective tissue, they form a muscle fasciculus. A complete muscle consists of many fasciculi grouped together, surrounded by the perimysium.

- One end of a skeletal muscle usually is fastened to a relatively immovable part (origin) at a movable joint. The other end connects to one side of a movable joint (insertion) on the other side of the joint.

- Calcium and energy, from ATP, are important to the contraction of muscles.

- There are two types of smooth muscle: visceral and multiunit. Smooth muscles are nonstriated and are involuntary. The smooth muscles are located in the digestive, reproductive, and urinary tracts, as well as in the linings of blood vessels.

- The autonomic nervous system innervates smooth muscle throughout the body.

- The study of muscular anatomy involves understanding the placement of muscles and their function in moving bones.

- Synergists are muscles that work together to accomplish a particular movement; antagonists are muscles that work in opposition to one another.

- Specific muscles are key to the movement of the head, face and eyes, back, thorax, abdomen, pelvis, and the upper and lower extremities.

■ Vital Vocabulary

acetylcholine A chemical neurotransmitter that serves as a mediator in both the sympathetic and parasympathetic nervous system.

acetylcholinesterase The enzyme that causes muscle relaxation by helping to break down acetylcholine.

Achilles tendon The strong tendon that joins the muscles in the posterior leg to the calcaneus.

actin The component that makes up most of the thin protein filaments of the myofibrils.

action potentials Changes in electrical potential that occur when a cell or tissue has been activated by a stimulus.

adductor brevis The short muscle that adducts the thigh.

adductor longus The long muscle that adducts the hip.

agonist A prime mover; a muscle that contracts to provide most of a desired movement.

anal triangle The area within the pelvis that contains the anus.

antagonists Muscles working in opposition to each other.

aponeuroses Broad sheets of fibers that may attach to bones or to the coverings of other muscles.

Bell palsy A condition caused by damage, either through trauma or infection, to the facial nerve, resulting in an inability to move the facial muscles on the affected side.

biceps femoris Located in the posterior compartment of the leg; flexes and laterally rotates the knee and extends the hip.

calmodulin An intracellular protein to which calcium binds, resulting in muscle contraction.

cardiac muscle Muscle that is found only in the heart, providing the contractions needed to propel the blood through the circulatory system.

compartment syndrome Accumulation of blood or fluid in a fascial compartment, typically following trauma, resulting in compression of blood vessels and tissue damage secondary to ischemia and, if not recognized and promptly treated, death of muscle and loss of the limb.

compartments Anatomic spaces within the body that are enclosed by fascia.

creatine phosphate An organic compound in muscle tissue that can store and provide energy for muscle contraction.

depolarization The rapid movement of electrolytes across a cell membrane that changes the cell's overall charge. This rapid shifting of electrolytes and cellular charges is the main catalyst for muscle contractions and neural transmissions.

diaphragm A muscular dome that forms the undersurface of the thorax, separating the chest from the abdominal cavity. Contraction of the diaphragm (and the chest wall muscles) brings air into the lungs. Relaxation allows air to be expelled from the lungs.

endomysium The delicate connective tissue surrounding individual muscular fibers.

epimysium A layer of connective tissue that closely surrounds skeletal muscles.

extensor muscles Groups of muscles that cause extension.

extracellular fluid Fluid outside of the cells, in which most of the body's supply of sodium in contained; accounts for 15% of body weight.

extraocular movements Movement of the eyes in various directions.

fascia A layer of fibrous connective tissue outside the epimysium that separates individual muscles and individual muscle groups.

flexor muscles Groups of muscles that cause flexion when contracted.

gap junctions Conduction areas between cells (eg, in visceral smooth muscle) that interconnect individual muscle cells.

hemoglobin An iron-containing protein within red blood cells that has the ability to bind to oxygen.

insertion A moveable part of the body to which a skeletal muscle is fastened at a moveable joint.

intercalated disks Branching fibers in cardiac muscle that allow action potentials to pass from cell to cell.

intrinsic automaticity The ability of a muscle to generate its own electrical activity.

lactic acid A metabolic end product of the breakdown of glucose that accumulates when metabolism proceeds in the absence of oxygen.

motor end plate The flattened end of a motor neuron that transmits neural impulses to a muscle.

motor neurons Specialized nerve cells that deliver an impulse to muscle cells, causing them to contract.

motor unit A motor neuron and the muscle fibers that it controls.

multiunit smooth muscle One of the two types of smooth muscle, it is formed into sheets of muscle (as in the walls of blood vessels), small bundles of muscles (as in the iris of the eye), or single cells (as in the capsule of the spleen).

muscle Fibers that contract causing movement; three types of muscle are present in the body: skeletal muscle, smooth muscle, and cardiac muscle.

muscle fasciculus A bundle of skeletal muscle cells bound together by connective tissue and forming one of the constituent elements of a muscle.

muscle impulse One that passes in many directions over a muscle fiber membrane after stimulation by acetylcholine.

musculoskeletal system The bones and voluntary muscles of the body.

myofibrils Threadlike structures that extend from one end of the muscle fiber to the other.

myoglobin An iron-containing red pigment, similar to hemoglobin, that is found in muscle fibers.

myosin The component that makes up most of the thick protein filaments of the myofibrils.

nerve impulse Electrochemical changes transmitted by neurons to other neurons and to cells outside the nervous system.

neuromuscular junction The junction between a motor neuron and a muscle fiber; one type of a synapse.

neurotransmitters Chemical substances that transmit nerve impulses across a synapse.

origin A relatively immovable part of the body where a skeletal muscle is fastened at a moveable joint.

oxygen debt The amount of oxygen that liver cells need to convert lactic acid into glucose, as well as the amount needed by muscle cells to restore adenosine triphosphate and creatine phosphate levels.

pectineus muscles Deep muscles of the medial compartment that adduct, flex, and internally rotate the thigh.

pectoralis major The largest muscle of the chest wall; it adducts and internally rotates the shoulder.

perimysium The connective tissue sheath that surrounds a muscle and forms sheaths for the bundles of muscle fibers.

perineum The area below the coccygeus and levator ani muscles, which forms the floor of the pelvis.

polarized When a cell is at rest, ions are actively transported into and out of the cell to create an electrochemical gradient across the cell membrane.

prime mover The muscle in a group of muscles that has the major role in movement.

quadriceps femoris Muscle contained in the anterior compartment of the thigh that extends the knee when contracted.

rectus abdominis The linear muscle of the midline of the abdomen.

repolarization The process by which ions are moved across the cell wall to return to a polarized state.

rotator cuff A special group of four muscles that forms a cap over the proximal humerus and ties the humerus to the scapula; it controls rotation at the shoulder joint.

sarcolemma The thin transparent sheath surrounding a striated muscle fiber.

sarcomeres The repeating patterns of striation units that appear along each skeletal muscle fiber.

sarcoplasmic reticulum A system of membranes that transport materials in muscle cells.

sartorius muscle The longest muscle in the human body, it is located in the anterior compartment of the thigh and flexes both the hip and knee when it contracts.

scalene muscles Muscles of respiration that elevate the first two ribs during inspiration.

skeletal muscle Striated muscles that are under direct volitional control of the brain; also called voluntary muscle.

sliding filament model A method of action of muscle contraction involving how sarcomeres shorten, with thick and thin filaments sliding past each other toward the center of the sarcomere from both ends.

smooth muscle Nonstriated muscle that carries out much of the automatic work of the body, such as moving food through the digestive tract and dilating and constricting the pupils of the eye; also called involuntary muscle.

striations Areas of alternating, colored bands of skeletal muscle fiber.

synapse A functional connection where neurons communicate with other cells.

synaptic cleft The space between neurons.

synergists Muscles that work together to accomplish a particular movement.

tendons Tough, ropelike cords of fibrous tissue that attach muscles to bones.

Thompson test A test used to evaluate the integrity of the Achilles tendon for possible rupture.

transverse tubules T-tubules; membranous channels extending inward and passing through muscle fibers.

tropomyosin An actin-binding protein that regulates muscle contraction and other actin-related mechanical function of the body.

troponin A regulatory protein in the actin filaments of skeletal and cardiac muscle that attaches to tropomyosin.

urogenital triangle The region within the pelvis that contains the structures of the urogenital system.

visceral smooth muscle Sheets of muscle found in the digestive, reproductive, and urinary tracts.

whiplash A layman's term for traumatic soft-tissue injury to the structures of the neck, associated with sudden flexion or extension.

Yergason test Supination of the forearm against resistance to evaluate whether a patient has bicipital tendinitis.

■ Case Study Answers

1. What type of muscle is involved in the function of a joint such as the knee?

   Answer: Striated or skeletal muscle produces motion around a joint such as the knee. These voluntary muscles are composed of muscle fibers, connective tissue, blood vessels, and nerves.

2. What is the primary function of the type of muscle found around the knee?

Answer: Skeletal muscle comprises 40% of the body's weight and is responsible for most voluntary body movements. The body contains more than 350 skeletal muscles.

3. In addition to tendons, what other structures in and around the knee may have been injured?

   Answer: The knee is unusual in that it contains ligaments within the joint. It is traditionally classified as a hinge joint. The knee is surrounded by several fluid-filled bursae. The distal end of the femur articulates with the condyles of the proximal tibia. The C-shaped lateral and medial menisci are cartilage pads that act as cushions between the femur and tibia. The patella, a flat triangular movable bone, covers the anterior surface of the joint.

4. What types of knee injuries are most common in this situation?

   Answer: Cartilage and ligament injuries of the knee are relatively common. The anterior and posterior cruciate ligaments prevent abnormal motion of the knee from front to back, while the medial and lateral collateral ligaments stabilize the joint against abnormal side-to-side motions. When these structures are injured, abnormal motions can occur.

5. What are your concerns for management of this injury?

   Answer: An injury to the knee joint is potentially serious. Bleeding, swelling, and nerve impingement can occur, and if the injury is not managed properly, the joint may be permanently damaged. Proper positioning, with elevation if possible, and the immediate application of ice to help reduce bleeding, swelling, and pain are the important initial steps in managing an injury to the knee.

6. What would be your next steps in assessing the patient?

   Answer: The patient's condition is stable, with an isolated extremity injury; therefore, your reassessment should include repeating the primary assessment, repeating and recording the patient's vital signs every 15 minutes, and reassessing the splint and distal pulse, motor, and sensory function (PMS) of the injured extremity.

The Respiratory System

Learning Objectives

1. Discuss the relevance of understanding the function and structure of the respiratory system to conditions commonly found in the field. (p 97-108)
2. State the primary functions of the respiratory system. (p 97)
3. Identify the organs of the respiratory system and describe their functions. (p 97-101)
4. Describe the structure and function of the larynx and the speaking mechanism. (p 97-99)
5. State the roles of the visceral pleura and parietal pleura in respiration. (p 101)
6. State the changes in air pressure within the thoracic cavity during respiration. (p 101-104)

7. Describe the factors that influence the respiration rate. (p 104)
8. Identify the respiratory areas of the brain that control inspiration as well as exhalation. (p 105)
9. Explain the diffusion of gases in external and internal respiration. (p 105-106)
10. Explain how respiration affects the pH of certain body fluids. (p 106)
11. Describe how oxygen and carbon dioxide are transported in the blood. (p 107-108)

Introduction

The respiratory system includes the organs and structures associated with breathing, gas exchange, and the entrance of air into the body. These structures are divided into two groups: the upper airway, which includes the mouth, nasal cavity, and oral cavity, and the lower airway, which includes the larynx, trachea, bronchi, bronchioles, and alveoli **Figure 5-1**. The functions of the respiratory system include the intake of oxygen and the removal of carbon dioxide. Cells need oxygen to break down nutrients so that they can release energy and produce adenosine triphosphate (ATP). Carbon dioxide results from this process, and it must be excreted. The respiratory system includes tubes that filter incoming air while transporting it into and out of the lungs. Respiratory organs entrap incoming air particles, control temperature and water content in the air, produce vocal sounds, regulate blood pH, and are essential for the sense of smell.

The Respiratory System

The Upper Airway

The structures of the upper airway are located anteriorly and at the midline. The upper airway includes the nose, mouth, tongue, jaw, oral cavity, larynx, and pharynx. Inspired air flows into the body through either the nose or the mouth. The nasal cavity is referred to as the nasopharynx, and the oral cavity is referred to as the oropharynx. These two cavities connect posteriorly to form a common cavity called the pharynx (throat). The pharynx is behind the oral cavity, nasal cavity, and larynx. The larynx (commonly called the voice box) is a rigid, hollow structure made of cartilage.

The pharynx is composed of the nasopharynx, oropharynx, and the laryngopharynx. The nasopharynx and the nasal passages, which include the turbinates, warm, filter, and humidify air as a person breathes. The nasal mucosa is the mucous membrane that lines the nasal cavity. Olfactory

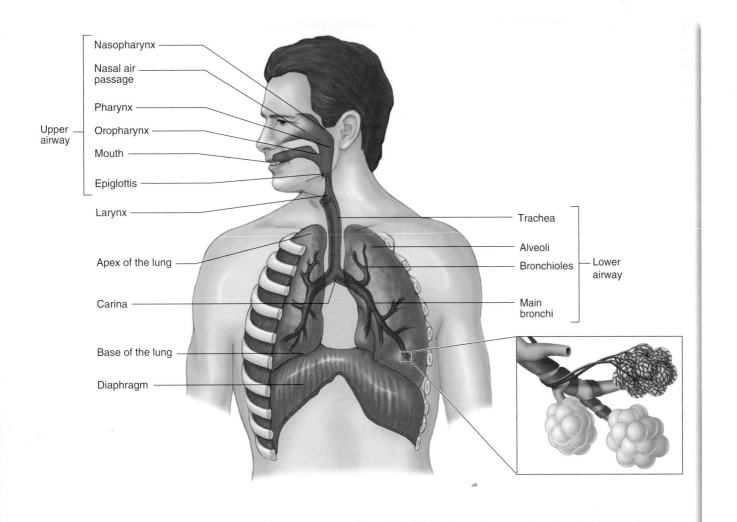

Figure 5-1   The respiratory system consists of all structures of the body that contribute to the process of breathing.

receptors located in the epithelium in the nasal cavity are responsible for recognizing odors. Air enters through the mouth more rapidly and directly. As a result, it is less moist than air that enters through the nose. Air inhaled through the mouth passes through the oropharynx, which is separated from the nasopharynx by the hard palate anteriorly and the soft palate posteriorly. Once through the nasopharynx and oropharynx, air then enters the laryngopharynx, also known as the hypopharynx because it is the inferior most passage of the upper airway.

The nasopharynx extends from the internal nares to the uvula (a small fleshy mass that hangs from the soft palate). The oropharynx extends from the uvula to the epiglottis, the thin plate of cartilage that closes over the glottis during swallowing. Inferiorly, the pharynx leads to the separate openings of the respiratory system (larynx) and the digestive system (esophagus). When swallowing, the larynx rises and the epiglottis presses downward, partially covering the opening into the larynx to help prevent foods and liquids from entering the lower airway.

The external openings of the nasopharynx are the external nares, or nostrils. The interior nares comprise the posterior opening from the nasopharynx into the pharynx. The nasal septum separates the nasopharynx into two parts. The floor of the nasal cavity is the hard palate. The lateral walls of the nasopharynx contain three bony ridges, the conchae. Together, the conchae form a set of bony convolutions, called the turbinates, that help to maintain laminar (smooth) airflow. Below each turbinate is a passageway called a meatus. Each meatus contains the drainage opening from the sinus and the nasolacrimal ducts (the ducts that drain tears from the lacrimal sac).

◼ The Lower Airway

The Adam's apple, or thyroid cartilage, is easily seen in the middle of the front of the neck. The thyroid cartilage is actually the anterior part of the larynx. The larynx consists of several sections of cartilage held together by ligaments **Figure 5-2**. Tiny muscles open and close the vocal cords and control tension on them. The superior portion of the vocal cords forms the vestibular

Case Study PART 1

At 10:30 PM, your unit is dispatched to an adult housing facility just outside of town where health care providers are not on hand during the evening and overnight hours. The patient is a 68-year-old man with increasing shortness of breath. As you enter the patient's apartment, your general impression is an elderly man who is in respiratory distress. The patient is alert, but he is having trouble speaking in full sentences. His radial pulse is strong and rapid and he is somewhat cyanotic. One of his friends tells you that he has not been feeling well the past few days and his breathing has become more labored over time. The friend also tells you that the patient has a long history of chronic obstructive pulmonary disease (COPD). You quickly place a nonrebreathing mask on the patient. While you are listening to lung sounds, you note that the patient's skin is hot, and assessment reveals an elevated temperature. You also note some audible wheezes as he breathes. You place electrodes on the patient as your partner starts an IV line. You then prepare an albuterol treatment to dilate the bronchial tree and make it easier for the patient to breathe. Your partner carefully copies down the names of the medications that the patient has been taking.

Recording Time: 0 Minutes	
Appearance	Cyanotic; struggling to breathe
Level of consciousness	Alert (oriented to person, place, and day)
Airway	Appears patent
Breathing	Shortness of breath, unable to speak in full sentences
Circulation	Cyanotic, rapid strong radial pulse, hot skin
Pulse	120 beats/min, regular
Blood pressure	142/90 mm Hg
Respirations	28 breaths/min, labored
Spo$_2$	92%

1. Describe the primary function of the respiratory system.

2. What are some of the possible causes of pulmonary dysfunction?

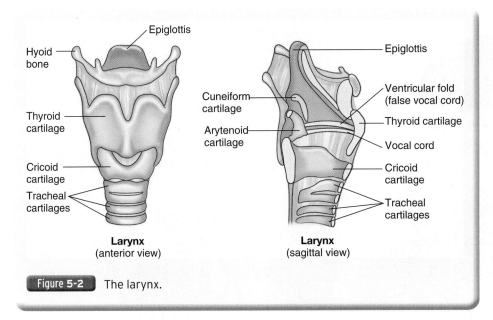

Figure 5-2   The larynx.

the right and left mainstem bronchi at the carina, a projection of the lowest portion of the tracheal cartilage. Beyond the carina, air enters the lungs through the mainstem bronchi. The point of entry for the bronchi, vessels, and nerves into each lung is called the hilum. The mainstem bronchi divide into the secondary bronchi, each one going to a separate lobe of the lung **Figure 5-4**.

Secondary bronchi branch into tertiary bronchi, which continue to branch several times. After several generations of successive branching, bronchioles, very small subdivisions of the bronchi, are formed. Respiratory bronchioles develop from the final branching of the bronchiole. Each respiratory bronchiole divides to form alveolar ducts. Each alveolar duct ends in clusters known as alveoli, tiny sacs of lung tissue in which gas exchange takes place (see Figure 5-4). The lung contains approximately 300 million alveoli; each alveolus is about 0.33 mm in diameter. Capillaries cover the alveoli. The alveolocapillary membrane lies between the alveolus and the capillary and is very thin, consisting of only one cell layer. Respiratory exchange between the lung and blood vessels occurs in the alveoli at the alveolocapillary membrane.

folds, or false vocal cords; the inferior portion forms the true vocal cords. The upper folds are called false vocal cords because they do not create sounds; they help close the airway during swallowing. The lower folds are called true vocal cords because they actually create sounds when air is forced between them, causing them to vibrate from side to side. The true vocal cords plus the opening between them is called the glottis **Figure 5-3**. When food or liquid is swallowed, the glottis closes to prevent it from entering the trachea.

As mentioned earlier, immediately below the thyroid cartilage is the palpable cricoid cartilage. Between the thyroid and cricoid cartilage lies the cricothyroid membrane, which can be felt as a depression in the midline of the neck just inferior to the thyroid cartilage.

Below the cricoid cartilage is the trachea (windpipe), which is approximately 5 inches long. The trachea extends downward anterior to the esophagus into the thoracic cavity, where it splits into right and left mainstem bronchi. Cartilage forms the anterior and lateral sides of the trachea, providing both protection and an open passageway for air.

Branched airways leading from the trachea to the alveoli make up the bronchial tree. These branches begin with the right and left primary bronchi, near the level of the fifth thoracic vertebra. Each primary bronchus divides into a secondary bronchus, tertiary bronchi, and even finer tubes.

At the level of the fifth thoracic vertebra, the trachea branches into

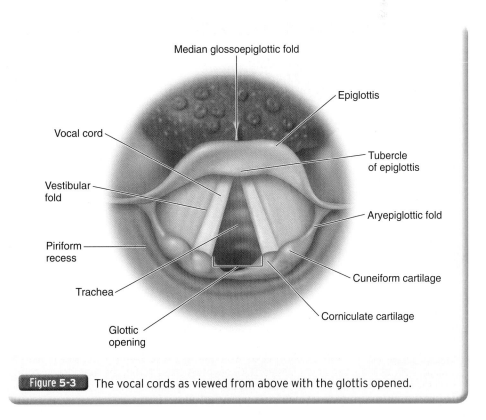

Figure 5-3   The vocal cords as viewed from above with the glottis opened.

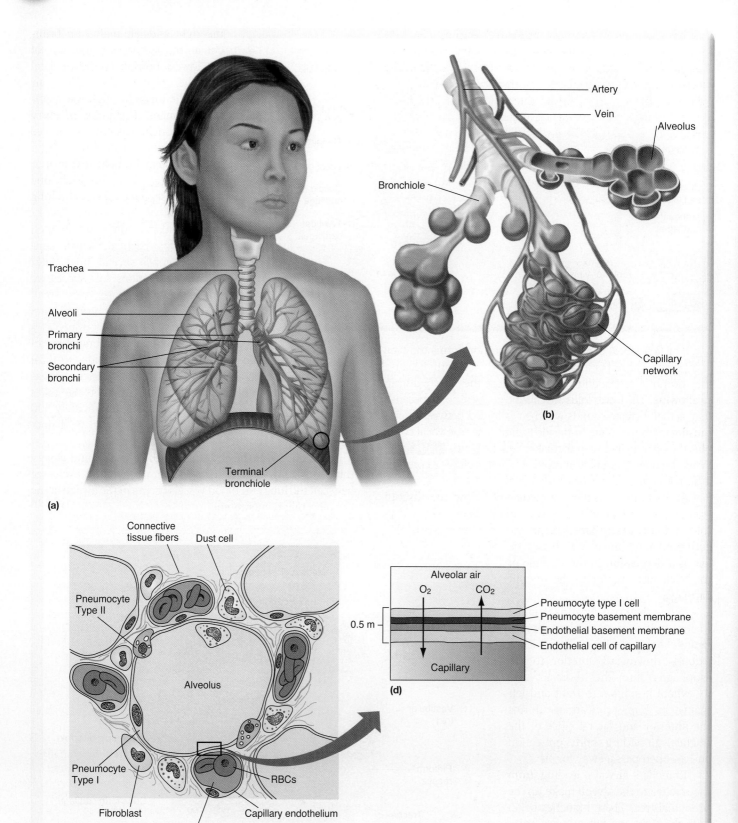

Figure 5-4 **A.** The trachea conveys air from the larynx to the bronchi, which distribute air through the lungs. **B.** The alveolar wall. **C.** Cells of the alveolar capillaries. **D.** Gases must cross within the membrane, composed of pneumocyte type I cells and their basement membrane, and endothelial cells and their basement membrane, to diffuse between the blood and the alveolar wall.

The lungs are the primary organs of breathing. They are located in the thoracic cavity and consist of soft, spongy, cone-shaped tissue. The right and left lungs are separated medially by the mediastinum and enclosed by the thoracic cage and diaphragm. The right lung contains three lobes (the upper, middle, and lower lobes), and the left lung contains two lobes (the upper and lower lobes). In the left lung, a portion known as the lingula forms the equivalent of the middle lobe in the right lung. The lungs are enveloped by a membrane of connective tissue known as pleura. A second pleural membrane lines the inner borders of the rib cage, or pleural cavity.

The pleural membrane that covers the lungs is referred to as the visceral pleura, and the pleural membrane that lines the pleural cavity is the parietal pleura. A potential space known as the pleural space exists between the visceral and parietal pleura. Normally, the two membranes are close together and a space does not exist. Both layers of pleura work together to help maintain normal expansion and contraction of the lung. Under certain disease conditions or following trauma, fluid and/or air may accumulate in the pleural space, resulting in hemothorax (a collection of blood in the pleural space) or hemopneumothorax (a collection of blood and air in the pleural space), potentially causing respiratory problems **Figure 5-5**.

The lungs receive blood in two ways. Deoxygenated blood flows from the right ventricle via the pulmonary arteries. This blood flows through pulmonary capillaries, is reoxygenated at the alveoli, and then returns to the heart via the pulmonary veins.

In addition, bronchial arteries branch off of the thoracic aorta and supply the lung tissues themselves with blood. Deoxygenated blood returns to the heart via the bron chial veins and the azygos system. Peripherally in the lungs, venous blood from the bronchi enters the pulmonary veins, returning with oxygenated blood from the alveoli.

■ Respiratory Physiology

▼ Respiration

Respiration consists of ventilation, which is the movement of air from outside of the body into and out of the bronchial tree and alveoli. Inhalation is also known as

Pathophysiology

Acute asthma is a recurring condition of reversible acute airflow obstruction in the lower airway. About 25 million people in the United States have asthma (ref: http://www.cdc.gov/vitalsigns/asthma/), and thousands with asthma die each year. It is among the most common chronic diseases of childhood. Four distinct events occur in an asthma attack. Smooth muscle spasm occurs when the muscle layers around the airways constrict (bronchospasm), resulting in narrowing of the airway diameter. Increased secretion of mucus causes mucus plugging, further decreasing the airway diameter, and, finally, inflammatory cell proliferation occurs. White blood cells accumulate in the airway and secrete substances that worsen the muscle spasm and increase mucus production.

The most common cause of an asthma attack is an upper respiratory infection, such as bronchitis or a cold. Other causes include changes in environmental conditions; emotions, especially stress; allergic reactions to pollens, foods (chocolate, shellfish, milk, nuts) or drugs (penicillin, local anesthetics); and occupational exposures.

The severity of asthma attacks varies among patients. In very severe cases (status asthmaticus), the patient may die as a result of respiratory failure. In other cases, treatment may produce rapid improvement and resolution of the asthmatic crisis. The patient's level of compliance and degree of ambulatory control may be a strong mitigating factor in the development of complications. Patients with potentially fatal asthma have a greater likelihood of a shorter duration of premonitory symptoms, worse lung function, and medication noncompliance.

Understanding the underlying pathophysiology has had a radical impact on the long-term drug therapy of asthma. Inhaled corticosteroids are now considered a mainstay of preventive therapy primarily for their anti-inflammatory effect. Oral and IV corticosteroids have been used for the same purpose in acute attacks for many years. In addition, drugs are constantly being developed that block other inflammatory compounds involved in an acute attack. One newly available drug, zileuton (Zyflo), inhibits 5-lipoxygenase, an enzyme that catalyzes formation of leukotrienes, known inflammatory mediators in asthma. Another drug, zafirlukast (Accolate), blocks leukotriene receptors. A promising combination of drugs for long-term therapy is an inhaled long-acting beta-2 agonist combined with an inhaled corticosteroid.

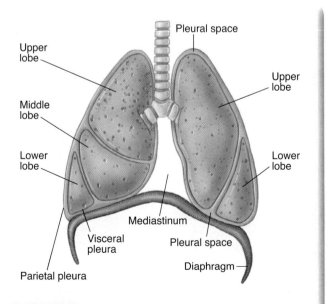

Upper lobe

Middle lobe

Lower lobe

Parietal pleura

Visceral pleura

Mediastinum

Pleural space

Upper lobe

Upper lobe

Lower lobe

Pleural space

Diaphragm

Figure 5-5 The pleura lining the chest wall and covering the lungs is an essential part of the breathing mechanism. The pleural space is not an actual space until blood or air leaks into it, causing the pleural surfaces to separate.

inspiration, and exhalation is also known as expiration. The force that moves air into the lungs is atmospheric pressure. Normal air pressure is equal to 760 millimeters of mercury (mm Hg). It is exerted on every surface that is in contact with the air. The pressure on the inside of the lungs and alveoli is almost equal to outside air pressure.

During normal inspiration, when inside pressure decreases, atmospheric pressure pushes outside air into the airways. Phrenic nerve impulses stimulate the diaphragm to contract, moving downward. The thoracic cavity then enlarges, internal pressure falls, and atmospheric pressure forces air into the airways **Figure 5-6**.

As the diaphragm contracts, the external (inspiratory) intercostal muscles between the ribs are stimulated to contract. The ribs raise and the sternum elevates, enlarging the thoracic cavity further. The lungs expand in response to these movements, as well as those of the pleural membranes. When the external intercostal muscles move the thoracic wall upward (and outward), the parietal pleura also moves, as does the visceral pleura. The lungs then expand in all directions.

In the alveoli, there is an opposing effect. The attraction of water molecules creates surface tension that makes it difficult for the alveoli to inflate. A mixture of lipids and proteins known as surfactant is synthesized, reducing the tendency of

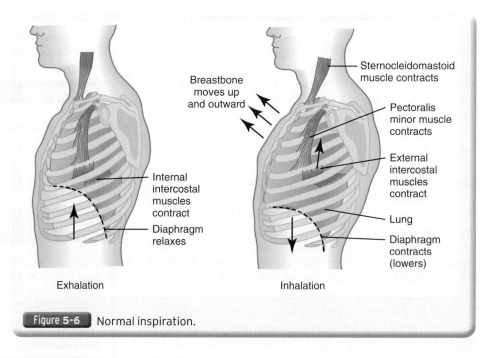

Figure 5-6   Normal inspiration.

the alveoli to collapse and easing inflation of the alveoli. When a deeper breath is required, muscles contract more forcefully than usual, and other muscles help pull the thoracic cage further upward and outward, decreasing internal pressure. The number of alveoli allows an extremely large surface area for respiratory exchange to occur in the context of a relatively limited size of the thoracic cavity **Figure 5-7**.

Expiration occurs because of the elastic recoil of tissues, as well as surface tension. As the diaphragm lowers, it compresses the abdominal organs below it. The elastic tissues cause the lungs and thoracic cage to return to their original shapes, and the abdominal organs move back into their

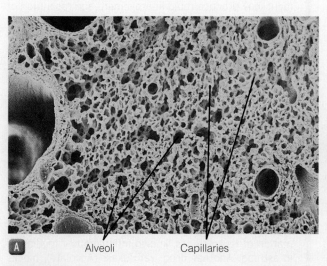

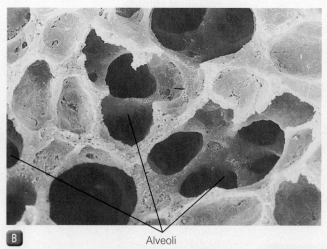

© David M.L. Phillips/Visuals Unlimited

Figure 5-7   **A.** A scanning electron micrograph of the lung showing many alveoli. The smallest openings are capillaries surrounding the alveoli. **B.** A higher magnification scanning electron micrograph of lung tissue showing alveoli.

previous shapes to push the diaphragm upward Figure 5-8A . Surface tension decreases the diameters of the alveoli, increasing alveolar air pressure. Air inside the lungs is forced out, meaning that normal resting expiration is a passive process. If more forceful exhalation is required, the posterior internal (expiratory) intercostal muscles contract Figure 5-8B . This pulls the ribs and sternum downward and inward to increase the pressure in the lungs. The abdominal wall muscles squeeze the abdominal organs inward, forcing the diaphragm even higher against the lungs.

Respiratory Volumes and Capacities

Only a small amount of the air in the lungs is exchanged during a single "quiet" respiratory cycle (which is when the diaphragm relaxes). The total volume of the lungs can be divided into volumes and capacities. These various values are useful for diagnosing problems with pulmonary ventilation. On average, adult females have smaller bodies and lung volumes than do adult males. As a result, gender-related differences exist regarding respiratory volumes and capacities.

Case Study | PART 2

Once you have started an IV line of saline at a keep open rate and have administered the bronchodilator, you reevaluate the lung sounds. You and your partner look at the monitor and recognize the rhythm shows tachycardia with no ventricular ectopy. Reevaluation of the vital signs and lung sounds indicates that there is a small improvement in the patient's breathing, and his vital signs are stable. You consider administering a second bronchodilator treatment as the patient is transferred to the stretcher.

The patient history reveals a 68-year-old man who weighs 65 kg. The SAMPLE history shows:

- **S**igns and symptoms: Hot skin, wheezes, short of breath, and cyanotic
- **A**llergies to medications: No known allergies
- **M**edications taken: Albuterol, Combivent
- **P**ast pertinent medical history: Chronic obstructive pulmonary disease
- **L**ast oral intake: Inhalers twice in the past hour, decreased appetite today
- **E**vents prior to onset: Patient experienced increasing shortness of breath over the past 12 hours

The OPQRST history shows:

- **O**nset of symptoms: The patient had difficulty speaking full sentences but was trying to avoid a trip to the hospital.
- **P**rovoking/palliative factors: A worsening upper respiratory infection
- **Q**uality of discomfort: The patient states that the discomfort is similar to the time last year that he was admitted and "tubed" in the hospital.
- **R**adiating/related signs and symptoms: The patient reports no pain associated with his dyspnea. The only position that seems to help the patient's breathing is sitting upright in the tripod position. The condition has been persistent and progressively worsening over several days.
- **S**everity: On a scale of 1 to 10, the patient states the severity would be about an 8, especially when compared with prior episodes of shortness of breath.
- **T**ime: The patient states that he is always somewhat short of breath but this deterioration in his baseline condition has occurred over the past 6 to 8 hours.

Recording Time: 10 Minutes	
Appearance	Weak and in obvious respiratory distress
Level of consciousness	Alert (oriented to person, place, and day)
Airway	Open and clear
Breathing	Rapid and labored
Circulation	Cyanotic with hot skin

3. What is the function of a spirometer, and how would it be useful?

4. Which part of the respiratory system does COPD directly affect?

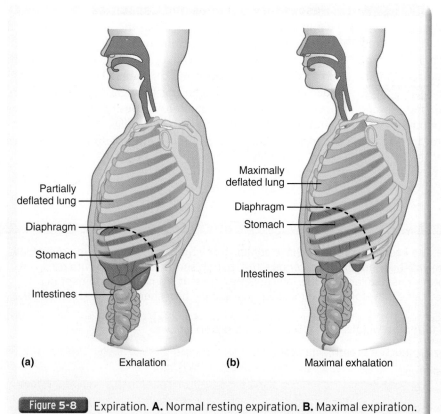

Partially deflated lung
Diaphragm
Stomach
Intestines

(a)   Exhalation

Maximally deflated lung
Diaphragm
Stomach
Intestines

(b)   Maximal exhalation

Figure 5-8 Expiration. **A.** Normal resting expiration. **B.** Maximal expiration.

expiration, meaning that the resting tidal volume is also about 500 mL.

Forced inspiration causes additional air to enter the lungs. This inspiratory reserve volume is also known as complemental air, which may be as much as 3,000 mL. Forced expiration causes the lungs to expel up to 1,100 mL of additional air beyond the resting tidal volume. This expiratory reserve volume, or forced expiratory vital capacity, is also known as supplemental air. Regardless of the level of expiration, about 1,200 mL of air remains in the lungs (residual volume).

Newly inhaled air mixes with the air already inside the lungs to prevent oxygen and carbon dioxide concentrations from fluctuating greatly. The combination of two or more of the respiratory volumes creates four respiratory capacities. Combining the inspiratory reserve volume with the tidal volume and expiratory reserve volume creates the vital capacity, which is 4,600 mL. After taking the deepest possible breath, this is the maximum volume of air a person can exhale.

The tidal volume plus the inspiratory reserve volume create the inspiratory capacity. This is the maximum volume of air a person can inhale following a resting expiration (3,500 mL). The functional residual capacity is made up of the expiratory reserve volume plus the residual volume. The vital capacity plus the residual volume create the total lung capacity, which is approximately 5,800 mL, varying with age, body size, and gender.

Remaining air that does not reach the alveoli can be found in the trachea, bronchi, and bronchioles. This air is said to occupy anatomic dead space because gas is not exchanged via these passages.

Pathophysiology

Persons with reversible restrictive lower airway disease, such as asthma, or progressive, irreversible airway disease resulting from emphysema (destruction of alveolar walls), black lung disease (consistent inhalation of coal dust), asbestosis (inhalation of asbestos particles), or chronic bronchitis (excess mucus production that blocks the airway) demonstrate typical abnormalities on pulmonary function testing. Residual volume often is increased, and the forced expiration volume is decreased. Abnormalities of these parameters indicate chronic obstructive lung disease. Often, the technician measures lung function before and following administration of a bronchodilator, medication that is designed to decrease airway resistance and thereby improve lung function. People with black lung disease, asbestosis, or other forms of lung scarring may demonstrate a significant decrease in the vital capacity, indicating restrictive lung disease.

A spirometer is used to measure air volumes during breathing. There are four distinct respiratory volumes. A respiratory cycle consists of one inspiration and a following expiration. The tidal volume is the volume of air that enters or leaves during a single respiratory cycle, usually about 500 mL. Nearly the same volume leaves during a normal, resting

Pathophysiology

Chronic obstructive pulmonary disease (COPD) is a progressive and irreversible disease of the airway marked by decreased inspiratory and expiratory capacity of the lungs. COPD may result from chronic bronchitis (excess mucus production) or emphysema (lung tissue damage with loss of elastic recoil of the lungs). Patients with COPD usually have a combination of both problems and generally function at a certain baseline level until an event occurs that causes decompensation and an acute COPD episode (or acute exacerbation). As with asthma, inflammation recently has been shown to play a significant role in COPD.

Chronic bronchitis results from overgrowth of the airway mucous glands and excess secretion of mucus, which blocks the airway. Patients have a chronic, productive cough. Emphysema results from destruction of the alveolar walls, which creates resistance to expiratory airflow. The major cause of COPD is cigarette smoking. Industrial inhalants (such as asbestos and coal dust), air pollution, and tuberculosis can also lead to COPD. The patient experiencing an acute COPD episode will report shortness of breath with gradually increasing symptoms over a period of days.

Control of Breathing

Respiratory control has both involuntary and voluntary components. The involuntary centers of the brain regulate the respiratory muscles. They control respiratory minute volume by adjusting the depth and frequency of pulmonary ventilation. This occurs in response to sensory information that arrives from the lungs, various portions of the respiratory tract, and a variety of other sites. The respiratory areas of the brain control inspiration as well as exhalation. The voluntary control of respiration reflects activity in the cerebral cortex that affects either the output of the respiratory center in the medulla oblongata and pons or the output of motor neurons in the spinal cord that control respiratory muscles. The most important parts make up the medullary respiratory center, which consists of the dorsal and ventral respiratory groups and the respiratory group of the pons.

The dorsal respiratory group is important in stimulating the muscles of inspiration. Increased impulses result in more forceful muscle contractions and deeper breathing. Decreased impulses result in passive expiration. The ventral respiratory group controls other respiratory muscles (mostly the intercostal and abdominal muscles) to increase the force of expiration and sometimes to increase inspiratory efforts. The basic rhythm of breathing may also be controlled by the pontine respiratory group in the pons.

Certain chemicals also affect breathing rate and depth. Other factors include emotional states, lung stretching capability, and levels of physical activity. Chemosensitive areas known as central chemoreceptors, located in the medulla oblongata, sense carbon dioxide and hydrogen ion changes in the cerebrospinal fluid (CSF). When these levels change, respiratory rate and tidal volume are signaled to increase. More carbon dioxide is exhaled, and both the blood and CSF levels of these chemicals fall, decreasing the breathing rate. Carbon dioxide is the most important chemical regulator of respiration. Peripheral chemoreceptors in the carotid bodies and aortic bodies sense changes in blood oxygen levels **Figure 5-9**. They then increase the

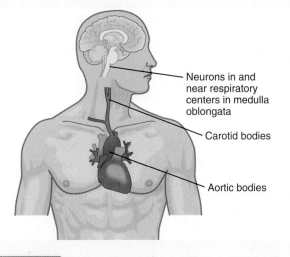

Neurons in and near respiratory centers in medulla oblongata

Carotid bodies

Aortic bodies

Figure 5-9 Decreased blood oxygen concentration stimulating peripheral chemoreceptors in the carotid and aortic bodies.

breathing rate, but this action requires extremely low levels of blood oxygen to occur.

The depth of breathing is regulated by the inflation reflex, which occurs when stretched lung tissues stimulate stretch receptors in the visceral pleura, bronchioles, and alveoli. The duration of inspiratory movements is shortened, preventing overinflation of the lungs during forceful breathing. Emotional upset, such as that caused by fear and pain, usually increases the breathing rate. If breathing stops, even for a short time, blood levels of carbon dioxide and hydrogen ions rise while oxygen levels fall. Chemoreceptors are stimulated, and the urge to inhale increases, overcoming high carbon dioxide levels.

Hyperventilation consists of deep, rapid breathing that lowers blood carbon dioxide levels. After hyperventilation, it takes longer for carbon dioxide to rise back up to levels that produce the need to breathe in. Prolonged breath holding causes abnormally low blood oxygen levels. Hyperventilation should never be used to help hold the breath during swimming. It may cause a loss of consciousness while under water.

Gas Exchange

The alveoli in the lungs carry on the exchange of gases between air and the blood. The alveoli are microscopic air sacs clustered around the distal ends of the narrowest respiratory tubes (the alveolar ducts). Each alveolus consists of a tiny space inside a thin wall, separating it from adjacent alveoli. The inner lining is made up of simple squamous epithelium. Dense networks of capillaries are found near each alveolus. At least two thicknesses of epithelial cells and a fused basement membrane layer separate the air in an alveolus from the blood in a capillary. These layers make up the respiratory membrane (also known as the alveolocapillary membrane or the pulmonary capillary membrane). It is here where blood and alveolar air exchange gases.

Air exchanges across the respiratory membrane occur by the diffusion process, the process by which a gas dissolves in a liquid. Diffusion occurs from regions of higher pressure toward regions of lower pressure. The pressure of a gas determines how it diffuses from one region to another. Ordinary air consists of mostly nitrogen (78%), with lesser quantities of oxygen (21%), carbon dioxide (0.04%), and traces of other gases. The amount of pressure each gas contributes is called the partial pressure of that gas. Air is 21% oxygen, so oxygen accounts for 21% of the atmospheric pressure (equivalent to 160 mm Hg of the atmospheric pressure of 760 mm Hg).

The resulting concentration of each gas is proportional to its partial pressure. Each gas diffuses between areas of higher partial pressure and areas of lower partial pressure, until the two areas reach equilibrium. Carbon dioxide diffuses from blood, due to higher partial pressure, across the respiratory membrane and into alveolar air. Oxygen diffuses from alveolar air into blood. Because of the large volume of air that is always in the lungs, as long as breathing continues, alveolar partial oxygen pressure stays relatively constant, at 104 mm Hg. The partial pressure of oxygen is symbolized as Pa_{O_2}, and the partial pressure of carbon dioxide is symbolized as Pa_{CO_2}.

Pathophysiology

Arterial blood gas tests measure the partial pressure of oxygen (Pa_{O_2}) and the partial pressure of carbon dioxide (Pa_{CO_2}) in the blood, as well as the pH, (the degree of acidity or alkalinity). Deviations from normal values occur in many different disease states. Essentially, Pa_{CO_2} acts as "respiratory acid." Changes in the Pa_{CO_2} value rapidly change the pH levels, either making them more basic (increased) or more acidic (decreased). Changes in the Pa_{CO_2} can be the result of diseases such as asthma, COPD exacerbation, or drug overdose or secondary to a change in the blood pH because of a metabolic problem. A decrease in the pH of the arterial blood that is caused by an elevation in the Pa_{CO_2} is called primary respiratory acidosis, whereas an increase in the pH of the blood that is caused by excessive exhalation of CO_2 is called primary respiratory alkalosis. Conversely, changes in the Pa_{CO_2} that occur in response to primary metabolic problems (alkalosis or acidosis) are called compensatory changes.

Case Study PART 3

You discover that the patient has previously had acute exacerbations of COPD brought on by upper respiratory infections. He has smoked cigarettes for 53 years. He has a productive cough with green sputum and is running a low-grade fever (101.5°F). The first nebulizer treatment is working so another is administered.

Recording Time: 15 Minutes	
Appearance	Improved, cyanosis is gone
Level of consciousness	Alert (oriented to person, place, and day), less distressed
Airway	Clear, but the patient is coughing and producing green sputum
Breathing	Improved effort
Circulation	Rapid, strong radial pulse
Pulse	118 beats/min, strong and regular
Blood pressure	138/86 mm Hg
Respirations	24 breaths/min, decreased wheezing
Sp_{O_2}	96%

5. Would you expect the patient's condition to be immediately life threatening? Why or why not?

6. How does an exacerbation of COPD affect diffusion?

Gas Transport

As oxygen from the lungs and carbon dioxide from the cells enter the blood, they dissolve in the plasma or combine with blood components. About 98% of the oxygen transported by the blood binds the iron-containing protein hemoglobin in red blood cells. The remainder dissolves in the plasma. In the lungs, oxygen dissolves in blood and combines rapidly with the iron atoms of hemoglobin to form oxyhemoglobin. These bonds are unstable. As Pa_{O_2} decreases, oxyhemoglobin molecules release oxygen, diffusing into nearby cells that have depleted their oxygen supplies in cellular respiration Figure 5-10.

As blood becomes more acidic, or blood temperature rises, carbon dioxide levels increase in the blood, causing more release of oxygen. Therefore, during physical exercise, more oxygen is released to skeletal muscles. This increases carbon dioxide concentration, decreases pH, and raises temperature. Hypoxia describes a deficiency of oxygen reaching the tissues, which may be caused by decreased arterial oxygen partial pressure (hypoxemia), anemic hypoxia, inadequate blood flow, or cellular defects.

Blood transports carbon dioxide to the lungs either as carbon dioxide dissolved in plasma, as part of a compound formed by bonding to hemoglobin, or as a bicarbonate ion. The amount of dissolved carbon dioxide in the plasma is determined by its partial pressure. The higher the partial pressure of carbon dioxide in the tissues, the more of it that will go into solution. Only about 7% of carbon dioxide transported by the blood is in this form.

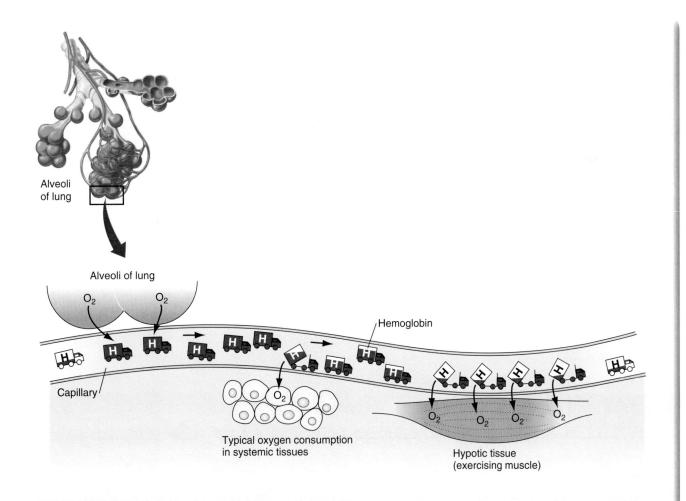

Alveoli of lung

Alveoli of lung

O_2　O_2

Hemoglobin

Capillary

Typical oxygen consumption in systemic tissues

Hypotic tissue (exercising muscle)

Figure 5-10　Blood transports oxygen molecules by entering capillaries from the alveolus and bonding to hemoglobin, forming oxyhemoglobin. Near cells and tissues, oxyhemoglobin releases oxygen.

Carbon dioxide differs from oxygen in that it bonds with the amino groups of the "globin" or protein portion of these molecules. Oxygen and carbon dioxide do not compete for binding sites. Hemoglobin can transport both molecules at the same time. Carbon dioxide loosely bonds with hemoglobin to slowly form carbaminohemoglobin, which decomposes readily in regions of low carbon dioxide partial pressure.

The most important carbon dioxide transport mechanism forms bicarbonate ions. Carbon dioxide reacts with water to form carbonic acid. In red blood cells, the enzyme carbonic anhydrase speeds the reaction of carbon dioxide and water, resulting in carbonic acid that releases hydrogen and bicarbonate ions. Nearly 70% of carbon dioxide transported by the blood is in this form.

Carbon dioxide diffuses into the alveoli in response to relatively low partial pressure of carbon dioxide in alveolar air. Hydrogen and bicarbonate ions in red blood cells simultaneously recombine to form carbonic acid, quickly yielding carbon dioxide and water.

Case Study   PART 4

En route to the hospital, a second and third albuterol treatment is given and the patient's breathing continues to improve. The focused physical exam reveals findings consistent with the patient's history: abnormal lung sounds that are improving with each treatment, except for some consolidation in the right lower lobe; a temperature of 101.5°F; a productive cough with sputum of a thick and greenish consistency; clubbing of the fingertips, a finding associated with advanced COPD; and an oxygen saturation level that has increased from 92% at baseline to 96%. On arrival at the emergency department, the patient will most likely have a chest radiograph to determine the extent of infection (ie, pneumonia), that most likely will be treated with antibiotics.

Prep Kit

Chapter Summary

- The primary functions of the respiratory system are the intake of oxygen and the removal of carbon dioxide.

- The respiratory system consists of the following structures associated with breathing, gas exchange, and gas transport: mouth, nasopharynx, oropharynx, larynx, trachea, bronchi, bronchioles, and lungs (alveoli).

- Inspired air flows into the body through either the nasopharynx or the oropharynx.

- The upper airway consists of the mouth, nasopharynx, and oropharynx.

- The nasopharynx extends from the internal nares to the uvula; the oropharynx extends from the uvula to the epiglottis.

- The lower airway starts at the larynx and includes the glottis, the vestibular folds (false vocal cords), the true vocal cords, the bronchi, and the bronchioles.

- The trachea is a tube made up of cartilage and other connective tissue, which provides an open passageway for air. At the carina, the trachea branches into the right and left mainstem bronchi, which divide into secondary and tertiary bronchi that continue branching into very small bronchioles and respiratory bronchioles. Each respiratory bronchiole divides to form alveolar ducts and ultimately ends in clusters known as alveoli, where gas exchange takes place.

- The alveoli are microscopic air sacs inside capillary networks of the lungs. They provide a large surface of epithelial cells that allow easy exchange of gases. Oxygen diffuses from the alveoli into the capillaries, and carbon dioxide diffuses from the blood into the alveoli.

- External respiration is defined as gas exchange between air in the lungs and the blood. Internal respiration is defined as gas exchange between the blood and the cells.

- The lungs are the primary organs of breathing. The right lung has three lobes (the upper, middle, and lower lobes), and the left lung has two lobes (the upper and lower lobes).

- The lungs are covered with two membranes of connective tissue known as the visceral and parietal pleura. The visceral pleura envelops each lung, and the parietal pleura lines the inner borders of the rib cage (the pleural cavity).

- There is a potential space between the visceral and parietal pleura, known as the pleural space. Both layers of pleura work together to help maintain normal expansion and contraction of the lung.

- The lungs receive blood from two sources: the right ventricle via the pulmonary arteries, and the bronchial arteries, which branch from the thoracic aorta and supply the lung tissue with blood.

- The primary function of the respiratory system is the exchange of gases at the alveolocapillary membrane. Ventilation is the process of moving oxygen in and carbon dioxide out of the lungs.

- A device called a spirometer is used to assess volumes of air that move into and out of the lungs. The commonly measured parameters include tidal volume, residual volume, vital capacity, and expiratory reserve volume (forced expiratory vital capacity).

- The respiratory areas of the brain (brainstem, pons, and medulla oblongata) control the process of respiration. The main respiratory stimulus is accumulation of CO_2 in the blood. Low blood oxygen levels also stimulate breathing, but normally have much less of an effect than does the Pa_{CO_2}.

- The medulla respiratory center consists of the dorsal and ventral respiratory groups, and the respiratory group of the pons.

- The dorsal group is important in stimulating the muscles of inspiration. The ventral group controls mostly the intercostal and abdominal muscles to increase the force of expiration, and sometimes to increase inspiratory efforts. The basic rhythm of breathing may also be controlled by the pontine respiratory group in the pons.

- Air exchanges across the respiratory membrane occur by the diffusion process.

- As oxygen from the lungs enters the blood, it (along with carbon dioxide from the cells) dissolves in the plasma or combines with blood components.

- About 98% of the oxygen transported by the blood binds the iron-containing protein hemoglobin in red blood cells. The remainder dissolves in the plasma.

- In the lungs, oxygen dissolves in blood and combines rapidly with the iron atoms of hemoglobin to form oxyhemoglobin.

Vital Vocabulary

alveolar ducts Ducts formed from division of the respiratory bronchioles in the lower airway; each duct ends in clusters known as alveoli.

alveoli Tiny sacs of lung tissue in which gas exchange takes place.

alveolocapillary membrane The very thin membrane, consisting of only one cell layer, that lies between the alveolus and capillary, through which respiratory exchange between the alveolus and the blood vessels occurs. Also known as the pulmonary capillary membrane.

asbestosis A disease of the lungs caused by inhalation of asbestos particles.

asthma A chronic inflammatory lower airway condition resulting in intermittent wheezing and excess mucus production.

bicarbonate ions Ions related to carbonic acid; they are formed from carbon dioxide transport mechanisms.

black lung disease A disease of the lung caused by consistent inhalation of coal dust.

bronchial arteries Arteries that branch off of the thoracic aorta and supply the lung tissues with blood.

bronchial veins Veins that return deoxygenated blood to the heart from the lungs.

bronchioles Fine subdivisions of the bronchi that give rise to the alveolar ducts; made of smooth muscle and dilate or constrict in response to various stimuli.

bronchodilator Medication that is designed to improve lung function by widening the bronchial tubes.

bronchospasm Severe constriction of the bronchial tree.

carbaminohemoglobin The bonding of carbon dioxide with hemoglobin.

carbonic anhydrase An enzyme in red blood cells that speeds reaction of carbon dioxide and water, resulting in carbonic acid.

carina A ridgelike projection of tracheal cartilage located where the trachea bifurcates into the right and left mainstem bronchi.

chronic bronchitis A chronic inflammatory condition affecting the bronchi that is associated with excess mucus production that results from overgrowth of the mucous glands in the airways.

chronic obstructive pulmonary disease (COPD) A progressive and irreversible disease of the airway marked by decreased inspiratory and expiratory capacity of the lungs.

conchae Three bony ridges contained within the lateral walls of the nasopharynx.

diffusion The process in which molecules move from an area of higher concentration to an area of lower concentration.

emphysema The infiltration of any tissue by air or gas; a chronic obstructive pulmonary disease characterized by distention of the alveoli and destructive changes in the lung parenchyma.

epiglottis A leaf-shaped cartilaginous structure that closes over the trachea during swallowing.

esophagus A collapsible tube that extends from the pharynx to the stomach; contractions of the muscle in the wall of the esophagus propel food and liquids to the stomach.

expiration Exhalation.

expiratory reserve volume Supplemental air; additional air that is expelled from the lungs due to forced exhalation.

external nares The external openings to the nasal cavity; also called the nostrils.

forced expiratory vital capacity The volume of air exhaled from the lung following a forceful exhalation.

functional residual capacity Expiratory reserve volume plus residual volume.

glottis The vocal cords and the opening between them.

hard palate The floor of the nasal cavity.

hemoglobin The iron-containing protein in red blood cells.

hilum The point of entry for the bronchi, vessels, and nerves into each lung.

hyperventilation Deep, rapid breathing; it lowers blood carbon dioxide levels.

hypoxia A deficiency of oxygen reaching the tissues.

inspiration Inhalation.

inspiratory capacity Tidal volume plus inspiratory reserve volume.

inspiratory reserve volume Additional air that enters the lungs due to forced inspiration.

interior nares The posterior opening from the nasopharynx into the pharynx.

larynx A complete structure formed by the epiglottis, thyroid cartilage, cricoid cartilage, arytenoid cartilage, corniculate cartilage, and cuneiform cartilage; the voice box.

lingula A small portion of the left lung that is the equivalent of the middle lobe in the right lung.

lungs The two primary organs of breathing.

mainstem bronchi The part of the lower airway below the larynx through which air enters the lungs.

meatus A passage located below each turbinate.

medullary respiratory center The dorsal and ventral respiratory groups in the medulla oblongata as well as the respiratory group of the pons.

nasal septum The rigid partition composed of bone and cartilage that separates the right and left nostrils.

nasolacrimal ducts The passage through which tears drain from the lacrimal sacs into the nasal cavity.

nasopharynx The nasal cavity (the portion of the pharynx that lies above the level of the roof of the mouth); formed by the union of the facial bones.

oropharynx A tubular structure that forms the posterior portion of the oral cavity, extending vertically from the back of the mouth to the esophagus and trachea.

oxyhemoglobin The combination of oxygen that diffuses into the blood and the hemoglobin molecule.

parietal pleura The membrane that lines the walls of the pleural cavity.

partial pressure The amount of pressure each gas contributes to diffusion.

partial pressure of carbon dioxide (Pa_{CO_2}) A measurement of the percentage of carbon dioxide in the blood.

partial pressure of oxygen (Pa_{O_2}) A measurement of the percentage of oxygen in the blood.

pH The measure of acidity or alkalinity of a solution.

pharynx The cavity lying posterior to the mouth, connecting to the esophagus; the throat.

pleura The serous membranes covering the lungs and lining the thoracic cavity, completely enclosing a potential space known as the pleural space.

pleural cavity The cavity formed by the inner borders of the rib cage and the diaphragm.

pleural space A potential space between the visceral pleura and parietal pleura; it is described as "potential" because under normal conditions, the space does not exist.

primary respiratory acidosis A decrease in the blood pH secondary to insufficient exhalation of CO_2.

primary respiratory alkalosis An increase in the blood pH secondary to excessive exhalation of CO_2.

residual volume The volume of air remaining in the respiratory passages and lungs after maximal expiration.

respiratory areas Parts of the brain that control inspiration and expiration.

respiratory bronchioles Structures formed by the final branching of the bronchioles.

respiratory capacities The four capacities created by the combination of two or more of the respiratory volumes.

respiratory cycle One cycle of inspiration followed by expiration.

respiratory membrane Layers of an alveolus that separate air from blood in a capillary; it is where blood and alveolar air exchange gases. Also known as the pulmonary capillary membrane or the alveolar capillary membrane.

respiratory system All the structures of the body that contribute to the process of breathing, including the upper and lower airways and their component parts.

respiratory volumes Four distinct volumes involved in respiration: tidal volume, inspiratory reserve volume, expiratory reserve volume, and residual volume.

resting tidal volume The volume that leaves during a normal, resting expiration (about 500 mL).

restrictive lung disease Diseases that limit the ability of the lungs to expand appropriately.

secondary bronchi Airway passages in the lungs that are formed from the division of the right and left mainstem bronchi.

spirometer A device used in pulmonary function testing that measures air entering and leaving the lungs over a specific period of time.

surface tension An effect that makes it difficult for the alveoli to inflate; it is caused by attraction of water molecules.

surfactant A mixture of lipids and proteins synthesized to reduce the tendency of alveolar collapse and to ease alveolar inflation.

tertiary bronchi Airway passages in the lungs that are formed from branching of the secondary bronchi.

tidal volume A measure of the depth of breathing; the volume of air that is inhaled or exhaled during a single respiratory cycle.

total lung capacity Vital capacity plus residual volume.

trachea The conduit for all entry into the lungs; a tubular structure that is approximately 10 to 12 cm long and composed of a series of C-shaped cartilaginous rings; also called the windpipe.

true vocal cords The inferior portion of the vocal cords that vibrate to produce sound.

turbinates A set of bony convolutions formed by the conchae in the nasopharynx that help to maintain smooth airflow.

uvula A soft-tissue structure that resembles a punching bag; located in the posterior aspect of the oral cavity, at the base of the tongue.

ventilation The process of exchanging air between the lungs and the environment; includes inhalation and exhalation.

vestibular folds The superior portion of the vocal cords; also called the false vocal cords.

visceral pleura The pleural membrane that covers the lungs.

vital capacity The amount of air moved in and out of the lungs with maximum inspiration and exhalation.

■ Case Study Answers

1. Describe the primary function of the respiratory system.

   Answer: The primary function of the respiratory system is to exchange gases at the alveolocapillary membrane. Through ventilation, oxygen is brought into the lungs and carbon dioxide is removed.

2. What are some of the possible causes of pulmonary dysfunction?

Answer: Pulmonary dysfunction can be acute or chronic. Any disease process or trauma that affects breathing, gas exchange, and the entrance of air into the body can be the cause of pulmonary dysfunction.

3. What is the function of a spirometer, and how would it be useful?

Answer: A spirometer can be used in pulmonary function testing to measure various parameters of air movement into and out of the lungs. For the patient with a restrictive airway disease, the testing can be used to establish a baseline measurement prior to treatment and then a comparison measurement after treatment. The measurement obtained is an objective assessment of the response to treatment.

4. Which part of the respiratory system does COPD directly affect?

Answer: Chronic obstructive pulmonary disease is an irreversible and progressive disease of the lower airways, which results in excess mucus production, tissue damage, and impaired pulmonary function.

5. Would you expect the patient's condition to be immediately life threatening? Why or why not?

Answer: The patient's underlying condition is that of a chronic, progressive, irreversible airway disease and the present problem is an exacerbation (worsening) brought on by an infection. It is not uncommon for this type of patient to wait until the last minute to call for help. Left untreated, the patient's condition could rapidly deteriorate.

6. How does an exacerbation of COPD affect diffusion?

Answer: Diffusion (the process in which molecules move from an area of higher concentration to an area of lower concentration) is directly affected by excess mucus production and inflammation blocking the surface, thus hindering normal exchange of gases. Carbon dioxide is retained, and an insufficient oxygen supply results in hypoxemia.

The Circulatory System

Learning Objectives

1. Describe the location of the heart and its relationship to other structures in the body. (p 114)
2. Name the chambers of the heart and the vessels that enter or leave each chamber. (p 115-119)
3. Trace the pathway of a blood cell throughout the body. (p 115-119)
4. Name the valves of the heart and their function. (p 116-119)
5. State how heart sounds are created. (p 119-120)
6. Define blood pressure and state the normal ranges for the systolic and diastolic indices. (p 120-121)
7. Describe the cardiac cycle. (p 120-124)
8. Describe the cardiac conduction system and how an electrocardiogram records electrical heart activities. (p 121-124)
9. Explain stroke volume, cardiac output, and the Starling's law of the heart. (p 121)
10. Explain how the nervous system regulates the function of the heart. (p 122)
11. List the structure and function of each of the blood vessels: arteries, veins, and capillaries. (p 124-126)
12. Describe the exchange of gases that occurs at the capillary level. (p 125)
13. Name the major systemic arteries and the parts of the body they nourish. (p 127-131)
14. Name the major systemic veins and the parts of the body they drain of blood. (p 132-133)
15. Describe the primary functions of blood. (p 133-134)
16. List the formed elements of blood and state the primary functions of each. (p 134-138)
17. Describe what happens to red blood cells at the end of their life span, including the state of hemoglobin. (p 134-136)
18. Explain the ABO and Rh blood types. (p 136)
19. Name the five kinds of white blood cells and the functions of each. (p 136)
20. Describe the function of platelets and explain how they are involved in hemostasis. (p 137-138)
21. Describe the formation of a blood clot. (p 137-138)
22. Explain how abnormal clotting is prevented in the vascular system. (p 137-138)

◾ Introduction

The circulatory system includes the heart and a complex arrangement of connected tubes, including the arteries, arterioles, capillaries, venules, and veins Figure 6-1. Another name for this system is the cardiovascular system. The human heart pumps blood through the arteries, which connect to smaller arterioles, and then even smaller capillaries. It is here that nutrients, electrolytes, dissolved gases, and waste products are exchanged between the blood and surrounding tissues. The capillaries are thin-walled vessels interconnected with the smallest arteries and smallest veins. Approximately 7,000 liters of blood are pumped by the heart every day. In an average person's life, their heart will contract about 2.5 billion times.

Blood flow throughout the body begins its return to the heart when the capillaries return blood to the venules, and then the larger veins. The cardiovascular system therefore consists of a closed circuit. The venules and veins are part of the pulmonary circuit because they send deoxygenated blood to the lungs to receive oxygen and unload carbon dioxide. The arteries and arterioles are part of the systemic circuit because they send oxygenated blood and nutrients to the body cells while removing wastes. All body tissues require circulation to survive. Cardiovascular disease accounts for a significant number of EMS calls.

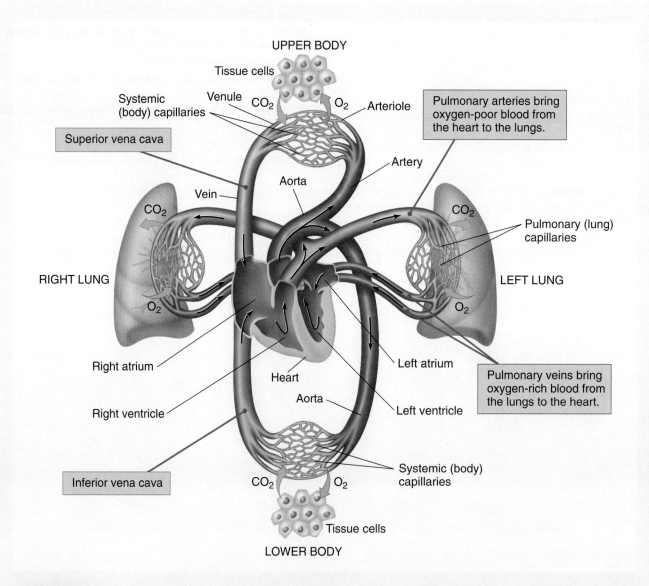

Figure 6-1 The circulatory system includes the heart, arteries, veins, and interconnecting capillaries. The capillaries are the smallest vessels and connect venules and arterioles. At the center of the system, and providing its driving force, is the heart. Blood circulates through the body under pressure generated by the two sides of the heart.

The Heart

Structures of the Heart

The heart is a muscular organ that pumps blood throughout the body. The heart lies inside the thoracic cavity, resting on the diaphragm Figure 6-2 . It is hollow and cone-shaped and varies in size but is roughly the size of a closed fist. The heart lies within the mediastinum between the lungs. Roughly two thirds of the heart mass is on the left side of the human body.

The heart muscle is referred to as the myocardium. The pericardium, also called the pericardial sac, is a thick, fibrous membrane that surrounds the heart. The pericardium anchors the heart within the mediastinum and prevents overdistention of the heart. The inner membrane of the pericardium is the serous pericardium. This inner membrane contains two layers: the visceral layer and the parietal layer. The visceral layer of the pericardium lies closely against the heart and is also called the epicardium. The second layer of the pericardium, the parietal layer, is separated from the visceral layer by a small amount of pericardial fluid that reduces friction within the pericardial sac.

The inside of the heart is divided into four hollow chambers, with two on the left and two on the right Figure 6-3 . The upper chambers are called atria and receive blood returning to the heart. They have auricles, which are small projections that extend anteriorly. The lower chambers are called ventricles and receive blood from the atria, which they pump out to the arteries. Each side of the heart contains one atrium and one ventricle. The left atrium and ventricle are separated from the right atrium and ventricle by a solid wall-like structure called a septum. Each atrium receives blood that is returned to the heart from other parts of the body; each ventricle pumps blood out of the heart. The upper

Case Study PART 1

Your unit is dispatched to a suburban residence at 1:00 AM. An elderly woman meets you at the front door, stating, "My husband very serious ... please come quickly!" After you establish scene safety, you follow the woman into the house and upstairs to their bedroom. You find a 60-year-old man sitting on the edge of his bed soaked from sweat. Your general impression is an overweight man who is clutching his chest in pain. The patient is alert, has an open airway, is having difficulty catching his breath, and has a strong, rapid and irregular radial pulse.

You immediately have your partner apply oxygen via a nonrebreathing mask as you start gathering a history. In the meantime, a second unit with a paramedic has arrived to help. You find out from the patient that the onset of his "crushing sensation" occurred suddenly about an hour earlier after he came in from shoveling the snow off the front walk. He figured it would go away if he took a warm shower since it was so cold out but it has just gotten worse. The pain is located under the mid-sternum and radiates into his left arm. He denies any aspirin allergy so you have him chew four (4) baby aspirin per protocol.

Recording Time: 0 minutes	
Appearance	60-year-old man in severe distress
Level of consciousness	Alert (oriented to person, place, and day)
Airway	Appears patent
Breathing	Speaking in short choppy sentences
Circulation	Pale and clammy, no external bleeding
Pulse	110 beats/min, irregular, strong
Blood pressure	156/90 mm Hg
Respirations	24 breaths/min, labored
Spo$_2$	94%

1. What is cardiac output?
2. How does a heart attack affect the patient's cardiac output?
3. Which blood vessels supply oxygen and nutrients to the myocardium and are the location for partial or full occlusion(s) that can result in a heart attack?

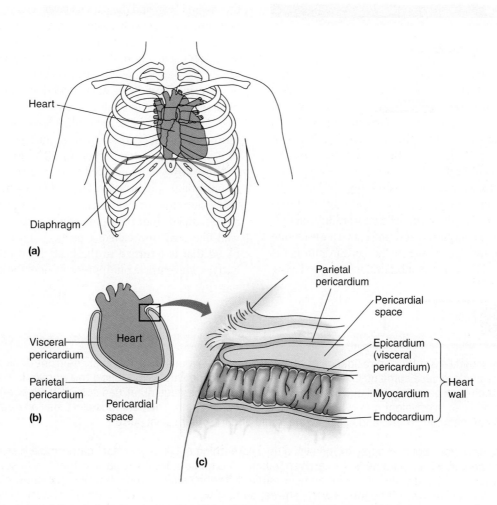

(a)

(b)

(c)

Figure 6-2 The heart. **A.** The heart within the thoracic cavity. **B.** The heart and proximal ends of the large blood vessels enclosed within the pericardium—a serous membrane that surrounds the heart. **C.** The three layers composing the wall of the heart: the epicardium, myocardium, and endocardium.

and lower portions of the heart are separated by the atrioventricular valves, which prevent backward flow of blood. Similar valves, the semilunar valves, are located between the ventricles and the arteries into which they pump blood.

The right atrium receives blood from two large veins called the superior vena cava and the inferior vena cava, as well as a smaller vein (the coronary sinus) that drains blood into the right atrium from the heart's myocardium **Figure 6-4**. Between the right and left atria is a depression, the fossa ovalis, that represents the former location of the foramen ovale, an opening between the two atria that is present in the fetus. The tricuspid valve has projections (cusps) and lies between the right atrium and ventricle. This valve allows blood to move from the right atrium into the right ventricle while preventing backflow. The cusps of the tricuspid valve are attached to strong fibers called chordae tendineae, which originate from small papillary muscles that project inward from the ventricle walls. These muscles contract as the ventricle contracts. When the tricuspid valve

closes, the papillary muscles pull on the chordae tendineae to prevent the cusps from swinging back into the atrium.

The right ventricle's muscular wall is thinner than that of the left ventricle because it only pumps blood to the lungs, which normally have a relatively low resistance to blood flow. The left ventricle is thicker because it must force blood to all body parts, which have a much higher resistance to blood flow. As the right ventricle contracts, its blood increases in pressure to passively close the tricuspid valve. Therefore, this blood can only exit through the pulmonary trunk, which divides into the left and right pulmonary arteries that supply the lungs. At the trunk's base is a pulmonary valve that allows blood to leave the right ventricle while preventing backflow into the ventricular chamber. The pulmonary valve contains three cusps.

Four pulmonary veins (two from each of the lungs) supply the left atrium with blood. The blood passes from the left atrium into the left ventricle through the mitral valve (bicuspid valve), which prevents it from flowing back into

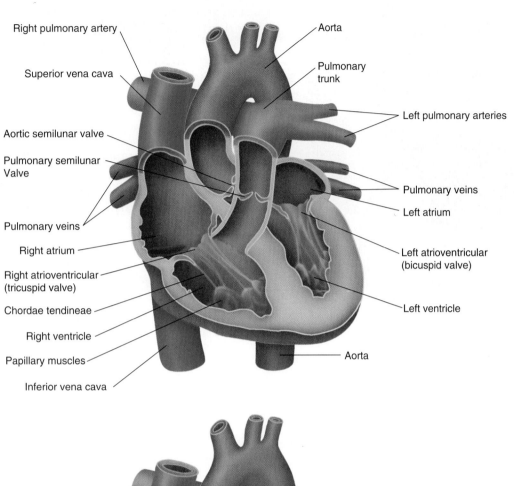

Right pulmonary artery

Superior vena cava

Aortic semilunar valve

Pulmonary semilunar
Valve

Pulmonary veins

Right atrium

Right atrioventricular
(tricuspid valve)

Chordae tendineae

Right ventricle

Papillary muscles

Inferior vena cava

Aorta

Pulmonary
trunk

Left pulmonary arteries

Pulmonary veins

Left atrium

Left atrioventricular
(bicuspid valve)

Left ventricle

Aorta

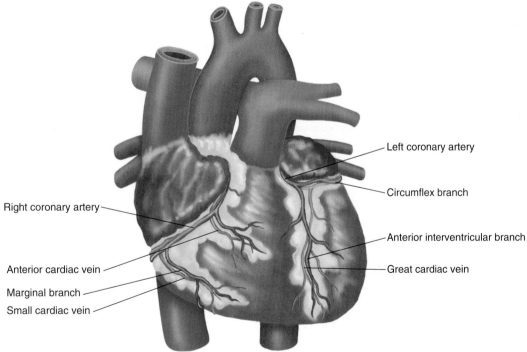

Right coronary artery

Anterior cardiac vein

Marginal branch

Small cardiac vein

Left coronary artery

Circumflex branch

Anterior interventricular branch

Great cardiac vein

Figure 6-3   Anatomy of the heart.

The right atrium receives low-oxygen blood through the venae cavae and the coronary sinus. As the right atrium contracts, the blood passes through the tricuspid valve into the right ventricle **Figure 6-5**. As the right ventricle contracts, the tricuspid valve closes. Blood moves through the pulmonary valve into the pulmonary trunk and pulmonary arteries. It then enters the capillaries of the alveoli of the lungs, where gas exchanges occur. This freshly oxygenated blood then returns to the heart through the pulmonary veins, into the left atrium.

The left atrium contracts, moving blood through the mitral valve into the left ventricle. When the left ventricle contracts, the mitral valve closes. Blood moves through the aortic valve into the aorta and its branches. The first two aortic branches are called the right and left <u>coronary arteries</u>. They supply blood to the heart tissues, with openings lying just beyond the aortic valve.

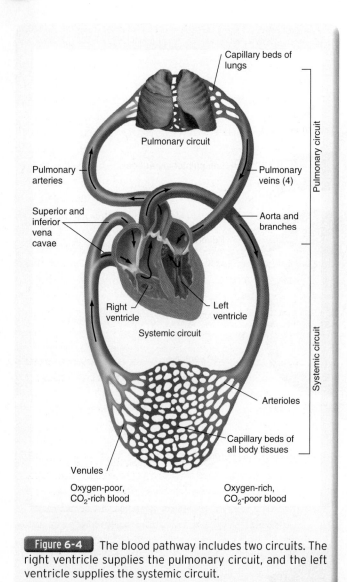

Figure 6-4   The blood pathway includes two circuits. The right ventricle supplies the pulmonary circuit, and the left ventricle supplies the systemic circuit.

the left atrium from the ventricle. Like the tricuspid valve, the papillary muscles and chordae tendineae prevent the mitral valve's cusps from swinging back into the left atrium when the ventricle contracts. The mitral valve closes passively, directing blood through the large artery known as the <u>aorta</u>.

At the base of the aorta is the <u>aortic valve</u>, which has three cusps. This valve opens to allow blood to leave the left ventricle during contraction. When the ventricle relaxes, the valve closes to prevent blood from backing up into the ventricle. The mitral and tricuspid valves are known as <u>atrioventricular valves</u> because they lie between the atria and ventricles. The pulmonary and aortic valves have half-moon shapes and are therefore referred to as <u>semilunar valves</u>.

Connective tissue that is arranged in "rings" surrounds the proximal ends of the pulmonary trunk and aorta, providing firm attachments for heart valves and muscle fibers. They prevent the outlets of the atria and ventricles from dilating during contraction. These rings, as well as other dense connective tissue masses, form the heart's "skeleton."

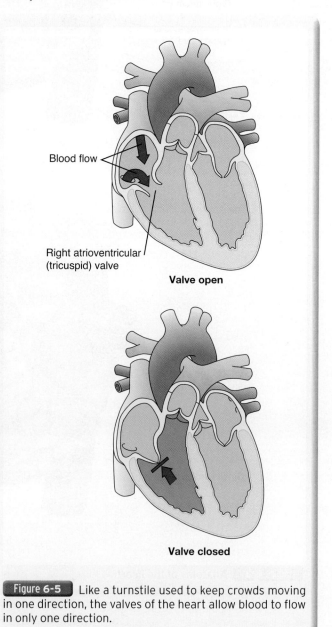

Figure 6-5   Like a turnstile used to keep crowds moving in one direction, the valves of the heart allow blood to flow in only one direction.

The body tissues require continual beating of the heart because they need freshly oxygenated blood to survive. Coronary artery branches supply many capillaries in the myocardium. These arteries have smaller branches with connections called anastomoses between vessels providing alternate blood pathways (collateral circulation). These pathways may supply oxygen and nutrients to the myocardium when blockage of a coronary artery occurs. Branches of the cardiac veins drain blood from the myocardial capillaries, joining an enlarged vein, the coronary sinus, which empties into the right atrium.

Pathophysiology

A clot can cause complete blockage of an artery that supplies oxygen to the heart resulting in death to a portion of the myocardium, or a myocardial infarction.

Pathophysiology

Infection or inflammation of the pericardial membranes causes severe chest pain, a condition known as pericarditis.

Pathophysiology

If the pericardial sac fills with too much fluid (pericardial effusion), the heart's ability to expand and contract properly is hampered significantly. A common cause of a pericardial effusion is trauma. When sufficient fluid is present in the pericardial sac to restrict filling of the heart, a condition called cardiac tamponade can develop and life-threatening shock rapidly results. A needle must be placed immediately into the pericardial sac (pericardiocentesis), to remove the fluid Figure 6-6.

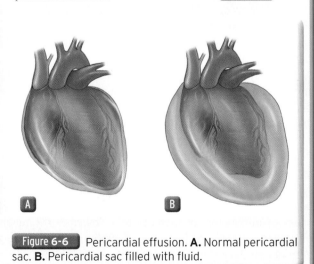

Figure 6-6 Pericardial effusion. **A.** Normal pericardial sac. **B.** Pericardial sac filled with fluid.

Blood Flow Within the Heart

Two large veins, the superior vena cava and the inferior vena cava, return deoxygenated blood from the body to the right atrium. Blood from the upper part of the body returns to the heart through the superior vena cava, and blood from the lower part of the body returns through the inferior vena cava. The inferior vena cava is the larger of the two veins. From the right atrium, blood passes through the tricuspid valve into the right ventricle. Blood is then pumped by the right ventricle through the pulmonic valve into the pulmonary artery and to the lungs. In the lungs, various processes take place that return oxygen to the blood, and at the same time, remove carbon dioxide and other waste products. These processes are discussed in greater detail in the Respiratory System chapter.

Freshly oxygenated blood is returned to the left atrium through the pulmonary veins. Blood then flows through the mitral valve into the left ventricle, which pumps the oxygenated blood through the aortic valve, into the aorta, the body's largest artery, and then to the entire body. The left ventricle is the strongest and largest of the four cardiac chambers because it is responsible for pumping blood through blood vessels throughout the body.

Heart sounds are often described as sounding like "lub-DUB, lub-DUB, lub-DUB" when the heart is listened to with a stethoscope. These sounds are caused by the contraction and relaxation of the heart, the flow of blood, and the movement of the heart valves. There are two normal heart sounds. The first, termed S1 ("lub"), results from sudden closure of the mitral and tricuspid valves at the start of ventricular contraction (systole). The second and normally louder heart sound, S2 ("DUB"), is caused by closure of the pulmonic and aortic valves at the end of systole Figure 6-7. Both S1 and S2 are normal and should always be present.

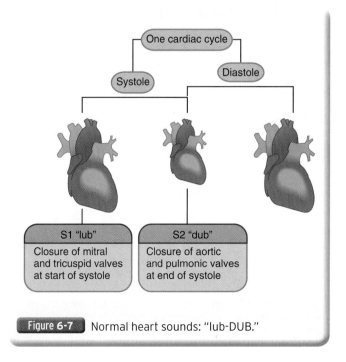

Figure 6-7 Normal heart sounds: "lub-DUB."

Two other heart sounds (S3 and S4) are usually abnormal and not heard in people with normal heart sounds. An S3 heart sound is soft and low-pitched. If present, it occurs about one third of the way through ventricular relaxation (diastole). This leads the heart cycle to sound like "lub-DUB-da." The "da" sound is rapid ventricular filling due to an inrush of blood. An S3 heart sound is sometimes present in young, healthy people. However, in the majority of people, it indicates increased left atrial filling pressure secondary to heart failure. The S4 heart sound occurs prior to S1. It is moderately pitched and causes the heart cycle to sound like "bla-lub-DUB." An S4 heart sound is almost always abnormal and results either from increased atrial pressure or decreased compliance of the left ventricle **Figure 6-8**.

There are four more abnormal heart sounds. A murmur indicates turbulent blood flow within the heart and causes a "whooshing" sound. Many murmurs are benign and go away with age. Several types indicate heart disease. A bruit is a whooshing sound indicating turbulent blood flow in a major blood vessel. Hardening of the arteries often causes bruits. Clicks and snaps, the other abnormal heart sounds, are caused by abnormal heart valve function. These sounds are brief and may be intermittent, making them difficult to hear.

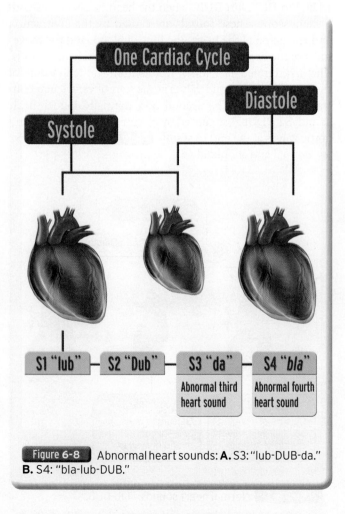

Figure 6-8 Abnormal heart sounds: **A.** S3: "lub-DUB-da." **B.** S4: "bla-lub-DUB."

Pathophysiology

Disease processes may involve any of the heart valves. Rheumatic fever is an acute condition that affects children and young adults and can cause permanent damage to the aortic and mitral valves. In rheumatic fever, the valve cusps (leaflets) become rigid, failing to open and close properly. If the valve becomes limited in its ability to open, the amount of forward blood flow is decreased, resulting in valvular stenosis. If the valve fails to close properly, blood leaks between the leaflets during cardiac contraction, resulting in valvular regurgitation. Ischemia to or rupture of a papillary muscle during a myocardial infarction is another common cause of mitral regurgitation. Ischemia occurs when arterial blood flow to a localized tissue site is decreased, resulting in a lack of oxygen to that site. An infection of a heart valve is called endocarditis.

Pathophysiology

In most people, the foramen ovale closes shortly after birth. In some people, it remains open, resulting in a patent foramen ovale. This condition is one of the most common forms of congenital heart disease. It may be asymptomatic or may result in severe symptoms, requiring surgery.

The Cardiac Cycle

The contraction of the heart leads to pressure changes in the cardiac chambers. This results in blood movement from areas of high pressure to areas of low pressure. The pumping process begins with the onset of myocardial contraction and ends with the beginning of the next contraction. This repetitive process is termed the cardiac cycle.

The pumping of blood into the systemic and pulmonary circulation during ventricular contraction is known as systole. During systole, a pressure is created within the arteries that can be recorded and is known as the systolic blood pressure. A normal systolic blood pressure in an adult is between 110 and 130 mm Hg. A pressure also exists in the vessels during diastole, the relaxation phase of the heart cycle, and is called the diastolic blood pressure. A normal diastolic blood pressure in an adult is between 70 and 90 mm Hg.

Blood pressure is noted as a fraction, and the systolic reading is placed above the diastolic reading (for example, a systolic reading of 130 and a diastolic reading of 70 would be noted as 130/70 mm Hg). The unit of measure mm Hg refers to millimeters of mercury and describes the height, in millimeters, to which the blood pressure elevates a column of liquid mercury in a glass tube. Although many blood pressure measurement devices now use dials, blood pressure is still described in millimeters of mercury.

The pressure in the aorta against which the left ventricle must pump blood is called the afterload. The greater the afterload, the harder it is for the ventricle to eject blood into the aorta, reducing the stroke volume, or the amount of blood ejected per contraction. To a large degree, afterload is governed by arterial blood pressure. Afterload is greater with vasoconstriction and less with vasodilation.

Expressed as liters per minute, the cardiac output is the amount of blood pumped through the circulatory system in 1 minute. Mathematically, the cardiac output equals the heart rate multiplied by the stroke volume (the amount of blood pumped out of the left ventricle during each contraction).

Cardiac Output = Stroke Volume × Heart Rate

Anything the affects the heart rate or stroke volume will affect the cardiac output and tissue perfusion.

To a point, increased venous return to the heart stretches the ventricles, resulting in increased cardiac contractility. This relationship was first described by the British physiologist Dr. Ernest Henry Starling and has become known as the Starling's law. Starling noted that if a muscle is stretched slightly, prior to stimulating it to contract, it would contract harder. So, if the heart is stretched, the muscle contracts harder. This is a normal defense mechanism. The amount of blood returning to the right atrium may vary somewhat from minute to minute, yet the normal heart continues to pump out the same percentage of blood returned. This is called the ejection fraction. If more blood returns to the heart, the stretched heart pumps harder rather than allowing the blood to back up into the veins. The result is that more blood is pumped with each contraction, yet the ejection fraction remains unchanged (the amount of blood that is pumped out increases, but so does the amount of blood returned). This relationship maintains normal cardiac function when a person changes positions, coughs, breathes, and moves.

The Electrical Conduction System

Strands and clumps of specialized cardiac muscle contain only a few myofibrils, and are located throughout the heart. These areas initiate and distribute impulses through the myocardium, comprising the cardiac conduction system. The mechanical pumping action of the heart can only occur in response to an electrical stimulus. This impulse causes the heart to beat via a set of complex chemical changes within the myocardial cells. The brain partially controls the heart's rate and strength of contraction via the autonomic nervous system. Contractions of myocardial tissue, however, are initiated within the heart itself, in a group of complex electrical tissues that are part of the conduction system. The cardiac conduction system consists of six parts: the sinoatrial (SA) node, the atrioventricular (AV) node, the bundle of His, the right and left bundle branches, and the Purkinje fibers **Figure 6-9**.

The sinoatrial (SA) node is a small mass of specialized tissue just beneath the epicardium, in the right atrium. It is

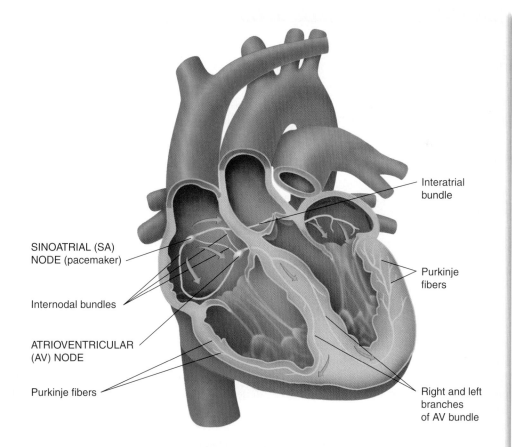

Interatrial bundle

SINOATRIAL (SA) NODE (pacemaker)

Internodal bundles

ATRIOVENTRICULAR (AV) NODE

Purkinje fibers

Purkinje fibers

Right and left branches of AV bundle

Figure 6-9 The cardiac conduction system. Specialized groups of cardiac muscle cells initiate an electrical impulse throughout the heart. The normal conduction pathway travels through the six parts of the cardiac conduction system. The impulse begins in the sinoatrial (SA) node and spreads through internodal bundles to the atrioventricular (AV) node. The AV node slows the impulse and initiates a signal that is conducted through the ventricles by way of the bundle of His, right and left bundle branches, and the Purkinje fibers.

located near the opening of the superior vena cava, with fibers continuous with those of the atrial syncytium (a mass of merging atrial cells that function as a unit). Because the SA node generates the heart's rhythmic contractions, it is often referred to as the pacemaker. Impulses originating in the SA node travel through the right and left atria, resulting in atrial contraction. The impulse then travels to the atrioventricular (AV) node, located in the right atrium adjacent to the septum, beneath the endocardium, where it transiently slows. Electrical stimulation of the heart muscle then continues toward the bundle of His, which is a continuation of the AV node. From here, it proceeds rapidly to the right and left bundle branches, stimulating the intraventricular septum. The impulse then spreads out, via the Purkinje fibers, to the left, then the right ventricular myocardium, resulting in ventricular contraction or systole.

The ability of cells to respond to electrical impulses is referred to as the property of excitability. The ability of the cells to conduct electrical impulses is referred to as the property of conductivity. Cardiac cells possess an ability to generate an impulse to contract even when there is no external nerve stimulus, a process called intrinsic automaticity.

Regulation of Heart Function

The brain, via the autonomic nervous system, the endocrine system, and the heart tissue, monitors and controls cardiac function. These functions include the heart's chronotropic effect (effect of the rate of contraction), dromotropic effect (effect of the rate of electrical conduction), and inotropic effect (effect of the strength of contraction). Homeostasis is maintained by the continuous monitoring of body functions by receptors in the brain, heart, blood vessels, and kidneys. Chemoreceptors sense changes in the chemical composition of the blood. Baroreceptors respond to changes in pressure, usually within the heart or the main arteries. If homeostasis is interrupted, receptors begin to fire and neurotransmitters or hormones are released. The transmission of nerve signals stops when conditions return to normal.

Often, stimulation of receptors causes activation of either the parasympathetic or sympathetic branches of the autonomic nervous system, affecting both the heart rate and the strength of heart muscle contraction (contractility). Parasympathetic stimulation slows the heart rate, primarily by affecting the AV node. Sympathetic stimulation has two potential effects, alpha effects or beta effects, depending on which nerve receptor is stimulated. An alpha effect occurs when alpha receptors are stimulated, resulting in vasoconstriction. A beta effect occurs when beta receptors are stimulated, resulting in increased inotropic, dromotropic, and chronotropic states.

Epinephrine and norepinephrine are naturally occurring hormones that also may be given as cardiac drugs. Epinephrine has a greater stimulatory effect on beta receptors, and norepinephrine has predominant stimulatory actions on alpha receptors.

Pathophysiology

If a patient is bleeding or severely dehydrated, baroreceptors sense abnormally low blood volume. Although several different body responses occur at once, a major response is the release of epinephrine and norepinephrine from the adrenal glands, causing sympathetic (adrenergic) stimulation, resulting in an increased pulse rate, as well as increased contractility.

Electrolytes (Ions)

Like all other cells in the body, myocardial cells are bathed in solutions of chemicals, or electrolytes (also called ions). Three positively charged ions, sodium (Na^+), potassium (K^+), and calcium (Ca^{2+}), are responsible for initiating and conducting electrical signals in the heart. In the resting cell, the concentration of potassium is greater inside the cell, whereas the concentration of sodium is greater outside the cell. To maintain this difference, sodium is pumped out of the cell by a special ion-transporting mechanism called the sodium-potassium pump, and potassium is moved in. This process requires the expenditure of energy.

The most important ions that influence heart action are potassium and calcium. Excess extracellular potassium ions (hyperkalemia) decrease contraction rates and forces, whereas deficient extracellular potassium ions (hypokalemia) may cause a potentially life-threatening abnormal heart rhythm (dysrhythmia). Excess extracellular calcium ions (hypercalcemia) can cause the heart to contract for an abnormally long time, whereas deficient extracellular calcium ions (hypocalcemia) depress heart action.

Clinical Tip

Sodium, potassium, and calcium move between cells through protein-lined passages known as ion channels. Cardiac drugs such as lidocaine, procainamide, and calcium-channel blockers affect the function of these channels. Numerous genetic abnormalities of the ion channel proteins have been described, some of which can predispose a patient to sudden death.

The Electrical Potential

The difference in sodium and potassium concentration across a cell membrane at any given instant produces an electrical charge difference referred to as an electrical potential. An electrical potential is measured in millivolts. In a resting cell, the area outside the cell is more positively charged than the inside of the cell. Hence, a negative electrical potential exists across the cell membrane. The resting cell normally has a net negative charge with respect to the outside of the cell. This is referred to as the polarized state.

Depolarization and Repolarization of Cardiac Cells

When a myocardial cell receives a stimulus from the conduction system, the permeability of the cell wall changes and sodium rushes into the cell. This causes the inside of the cell to become more positive. Calcium also enters the cell, although its passage occurs more slowly. The resulting exchange of ions generates an electrical current. The rapid influx of sodium and the slow influx of calcium continue, causing the inside of the cell to continue to become more positively charged, eventually achieving a slightly positive electrical potential. The process of electrical discharge and flow of electrical activity is called depolarization.

The flow of electrical current is passed from cell to cell along the conduction pathway in a wave-like motion throughout the heart. As the myocardial cells are depolarized, calcium is released and comes into close proximity with the actin and myosin filaments, as discussed in the Musculoskeletal System chapter. This process causes the filaments to slide together, resulting in muscle contraction. Contraction of heart muscle squeezes blood out of the chambers. The combination of electrical stimulation and the resultant muscle contraction sometimes is referred to as excitation-contraction coupling.

Once the cardiac cells depolarize, they begin to return to their resting or polarized state, a process called repolarization. At this time, the inside of the cell returns to its negative charge. Repolarization begins when the entry of sodium into the cells slows down and positively charged potassium ions begin to flow out of the cells. Following the efflux of potassium, sodium is actively pumped out of the cells, and

Case Study | PART 2

You discover that the patient has been experiencing these periods of chest "discomfort" over the past month, when he is actively doing physical labor. He says he figured he was having a bad case of heartburn and has been taking antacids. The rapid physical examination reveals a severely distressed overweight patient with mild dyspnea, some crackles (rales) in the bases of both lungs and normal heart sounds, no jugular vein distention, pale and moist skin, no scars on his chest or abdomen, and no peripheral edema. The patient says he feels weak and is nauseated.

Your SAMPLE history reveals a family history of cardiac events and he is taking medicine for his hypertension and high cholesterol. The ECG shows sinus tachycardia with occasional PVCs, and you apply the rest of the leads for a baseline 12-lead ECG.

Nitroglycerin spray did not relieve the patient's pain. Because his vital signs are the same as the initial set, you administer a second nitroglycerin spray. The paramedic has started an IV line, and the patient is being carefully transferred to a stair chair so he can be taken down the stairs to the stretcher waiting on the first floor and then out of the house to your ambulance.

Once in the ambulance, morphine is administered for the pain. The 12-lead ECG is transmitted to the hospital in your region that is a coronary catheterization center since the paramedic states that the patient meets the STEMI criteria.

Recording Time: 5 minutes	
Appearance	Significant distress
Level of consciousness	Alert (oriented to person, place, and day)
Airway	Open and clear
Breathing	Labored
Circulation	Pale, cool, and clammy

4. What blood vessels are most likely to be occluded if a 12-lead ECG is showing features of ischemia and infarction to the left ventricle of the heart?

5. What vessels supply the conduction system of the heart?

potassium is pumped back in. Calcium is returned to storage sites in the cells. As a result, the transmembrane potential returns to its baseline negative resting membrane potential and the cells regain both their polarized state and resting length.

In the early phase of repolarization, the cell contains such a large concentration of ions that it cannot be stimulated to depolarize. This period is known as the absolute refractory period. In the latter phase of repolarization, the cells are able to respond to a stronger-than-normal stimulus. This period is known as the relative refractory period.

The Electrocardiogram

An electrocardiogram (ECG) is used to record electrical changes in the myocardium during the cardiac cycle. Because body fluids conduct electrical currents, these electrical changes can be detected on the body's surface. The electrical currents generated during depolarization and repolarization of the heart can be visualized on an ECG. The standard ECG consists of 12 leads that record different "views" of the electrical activity of the heart. The shape of the normal ECG reading differs for each lead.

Several deflections, or waves, are noted on the ECG Figure 6-10. These represent the normal cardiac conduction pattern. The P wave occurs first and represents movement of the electrical impulse through the atria that results in atrial contraction. Following this is a flat line, or electrical pause, called the PR segment, representing the time delay that occurs within the AV node.

Next is a larger wave, the QRS complex, which represents depolarization of the ventricles. This complex corresponds to ventricular contraction, or systole. Another pause then occurs, known as the ST segment. During this period,

repolarization of the heart is beginning. The T wave follows, representing completion of repolarization.

A normal ECG cycle, representing a single heart beat in a normal sinus rhythm, consists of P waves that occur at regular intervals at a rate of 60 to 100 times per minute, a PR interval of normal duration (less than 0.2 seconds) followed by a QRS complex of normal contour and configuration, and a pause known as the ST segment, which is flat, followed by a T wave of normal contour and configuration.

■ Blood Vessels

There are five general classes of blood vessels in the cardiovascular system: the arteries, arterioles, capillaries, venules, and veins. Arteries are elastic vessels that are very strong, able to carry blood away from the heart under high pressure. They subdivide into thinner tubes that give rise to branched, finer arterioles. An artery's wall consists of three distinct layers. The innermost tunica interna is made up of a layer of simple squamous epithelium known as endothelium. It rests on a connective tissue membrane with many elastic, collagenous fibers. The endothelium helps prevent blood clotting and may also help in regulating blood flow. It releases nitric oxide to relax smooth muscle of the vessel. The middle tunica media makes up most of an arterial wall, including smooth muscle fibers and a thick elastic connective tissue layer. The outer tunica externa is thinner, made mostly of connective tissue with irregular fibers. It is attached to the surrounding tissues Figure 6-11.

Smooth artery and arteriole muscles are innervated by the sympathetic nervous system. Vasomotor fibers receive impulses to contract and reduce blood vessel diameter

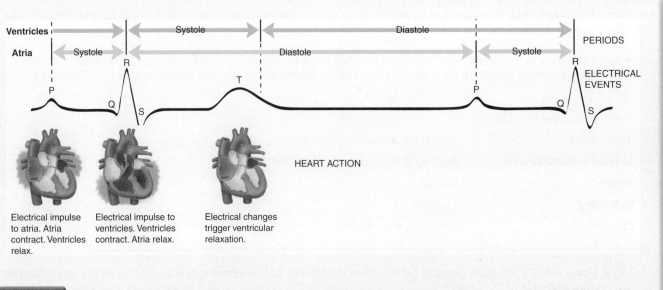

Figure 6-10 The normal deflections or waves of the electrocardiogram. The electrical impulse corresponds with muscle contraction and relaxation within the heart.

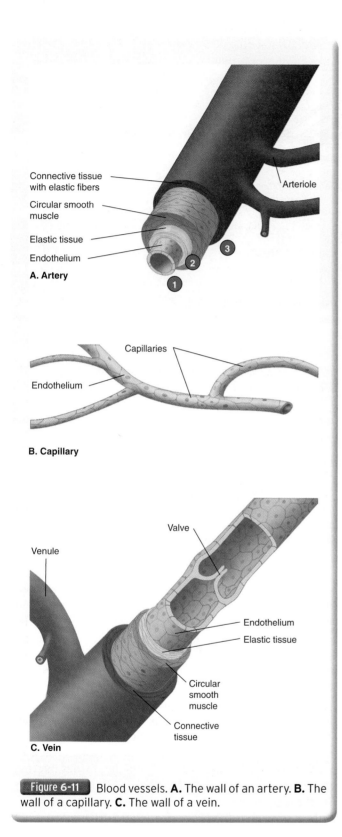

Connective tissue with elastic fibers

Circular smooth muscle

Elastic tissue

Endothelium

A. Artery

Arteriole

1 2 3

Capillaries

Endothelium

B. Capillary

Venule

Valve

Endothelium

Elastic tissue

Circular smooth muscle

Connective tissue

C. Vein

Figure 6-11 Blood vessels. **A.** The wall of an artery. **B.** The wall of a capillary. **C.** The wall of a vein.

Larger arterioles also have three layers in their walls, which get thinner as arterioles lead to capillaries. Very small arteriole walls only have an endothelial lining and some smooth muscle fibers, with a small amount of surrounding connective tissue.

The smallest-diameter blood vessels are <u>capillaries</u>, which connect the smallest arterioles to the smallest venules. The walls of capillaries are also composed of endothelium and form the semipermeable layer through which substances in blood are exchanged with substances in tissue fluids surrounding cells of the body Figure 6-12.

Capillary walls have thin slits where endothelial cells overlap. These slits have various sizes, affecting permeability. Capillaries of muscles have smaller openings than those of the glands, kidneys, and small intestine. Tissues with higher metabolic rates (such as muscles) have many more capillaries than those with slower metabolic rates (such as cartilage).

Some capillaries pass directly from arterioles to venules whereas others have highly branched networks Figure 6-13. Precapillary sphincters control blood distribution through capillaries. Based on the demands of cells, these sphincters constrict or relax so that blood can follow specific pathways to meet tissue cellular requirements.

Gases, metabolic by-products, and nutrients are exchanged between capillaries and the tissue fluid surrounding body cells. Capillary walls allow diffusion of blood with high levels of oxygen and nutrients. They also allow high levels of carbon dioxide and other wastes to move from the tissues into the capillaries. Plasma proteins usually cannot move through the capillary walls due to their large size, so they remain in the blood. Blood pressure generated when capillary walls contract provides force for filtration via hydrostatic pressure.

Blood pressure is strongest when blood leaves the heart, and weaker as the distance from the heart increases, because of friction (peripheral resistance) between the blood and the vessel walls. Therefore, blood pressure is highest in the arteries, less so in the arterioles, and lowest in the capillaries. Filtration occurs mostly at the arteriolar ends of capillaries because the pressure is higher than at the venular ends. Plasma proteins trapped in capillaries create an osmotic pressure that pulls water into the capillaries (colloid osmotic pressure).

Capillary blood pressure favors filtration whereas plasma colloid osmotic pressure favors reabsorption. At the venular ends of capillaries, blood pressure is decreased due to resistance, so reabsorption can occur.

More fluid usually leaves capillaries than returns into them. Lymphatic capillaries have closed ends and collect excess fluid to return it via lymphatic vessels to the venous circulation. Unusual events may cause excess fluid to enter spaces between tissue cells, often in response to chemicals such as histamine, a chemical found in <u>mast cells</u>. Histamine causes vasodilation of the arterioles near the capillaries, to increase capillary permeability. If enough fluid leaks out, the

(<u>vasoconstriction</u>). When inhibited, the muscle fibers relax, and the diameter of the vessel increases (<u>vasodilation</u>). Changes in artery and arteriole diameters greatly affect blood flow and pressure.

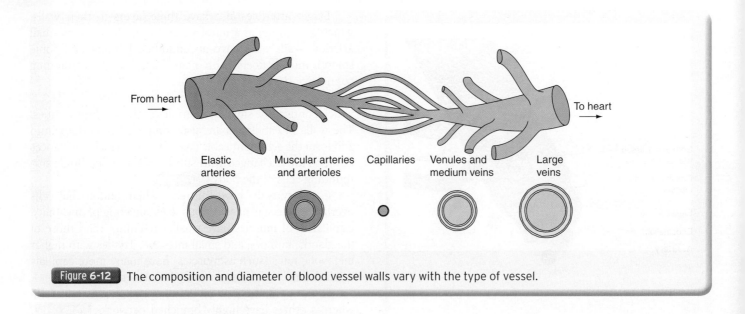

Figure 6-12 The composition and diameter of blood vessel walls vary with the type of vessel.

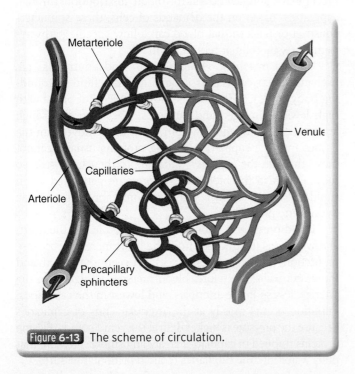

Figure 6-13 The scheme of circulation.

capillaries can be overwhelmed, causing lymphatic drainage and affected tissues to swell and become painful.

Venules are microscopic vessels that link capillaries to veins, which carry blood back to the atria. Vein walls are similar but not identical to arteries, but have poorly developed middle layers. Because they have thinner walls and are less elastic than arteries, their lumens have a greater diameter.

Many veins have flap-like valves projecting inward from their linings. These valves often have two structures that close if blood begins to back up in the vein. They aid in returning blood to the heart, opening if blood flow is toward the heart and closing if it reverses.

Veins also act as reservoirs for blood in certain conditions, such as during arterial hemorrhage. Resulting venous constrictions help to maintain blood pressure by returning more blood to the heart, ensuring an almost normal blood flow even when up to one quarter of the blood volume is lost.

Circulation to the Heart

The heart, like any other muscle, requires oxygen and nutrients. These are supplied via the coronary arteries, which arise from the aorta shortly after it leaves the left ventricle. The coronary circulation emanates from the left and right coronary arteries **Figure 6-14**.

The right coronary artery divides into nine important branches: the conus branch, sinus node branch, right ventricular branch, atrial branch, acute marginal branch, atrioventricular node branch, posterior descending branch, left ventricular branch, and left atrial branch. Not all branches are always present in all people. These branches supply blood to the walls of the right atrium and ventricle, a portion of the inferior part of the left ventricle, and portions of the conduction system (the sinus and AV nodes). When vessels to the conduction system fail to arise from the right coronary artery, they originate from the left side instead.

The left main coronary artery is the largest and shortest of the myocardial blood vessels. It rapidly divides into two branches, the left anterior descending (LAD) coronary artery and the circumflex coronary artery. These arteries subdivide further, supplying blood to most of the left ventricle, the intraventricular septum, and, at times, the AV node.

Arteriosclerosis is characterized by the deposition of calcium in the arterial walls. These deposits cause a loss of elasticity (thus, the term "hardening of the arteries") with a concomitant reduction in blood flow. Usually, atherosclerosis and arteriosclerosis are present together, and the resulting condition is referred to as coronary artery disease.

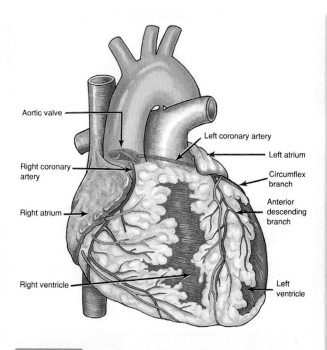

Figure 6-14　The coronary arteries supply oxygen and nutrients to the cardiac muscle cells.

Pulmonary Circulation

Pulmonary circulation carries blood from the right side of the heart to the lungs and back to the left side of the heart, and systemic circulation is responsible for blood flow in other areas of the body. Deoxygenated blood from the right ventricle is pumped through the pulmonic valve into the pulmonary artery Figure 6-16. This artery rapidly divides into the right and left pulmonary arteries. These arteries transport the blood to the right and left lungs. Inside the lungs, the arteries branch, becoming smaller and smaller. At the level of the capillary, waste products are exchanged and the blood is reoxygenated. The reoxygenated blood travels through venules into the pulmonary veins. The four pulmonary veins empty into the left atrium, two from each lung.

Systemic Arterial Circulation

Oxygenated blood leaves the heart through the aortic valve and passes into the aorta. From the aorta, blood is distributed to all parts of the body. All arteries of the body are derived from the aorta Figure 6-17. The aorta is divided into three portions: the ascending aorta, the aortic arch, and the descending aorta.

Pathophysiology

Various changes in the walls of coronary arteries can result in certain disease states. Atherosclerosis is a disorder characterized by the formation of plaques of material, mostly lipids and cholesterol, on the intima of the artery Figure 6-15. This process gradually narrows the lumen (opening or hollow part of the artery), resulting in a reduction in arterial blood flow.

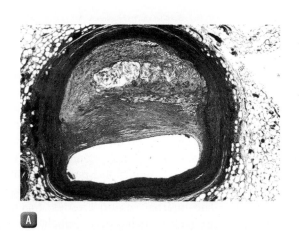

A

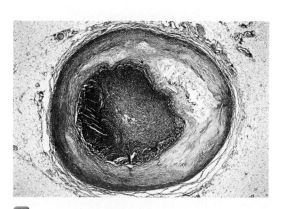

B

Figure 6-15　The formation of a plaque. **A.** The coronary artery exhibits severe atherosclerosis, and much of the passage of blood is blocked by buildup of cholesterol and other lipids on the intima of the artery, forming masses or plaques. **B.** The coronary artery is almost completely blocked. A blood clot blocks blood flow on the right side of the artery.

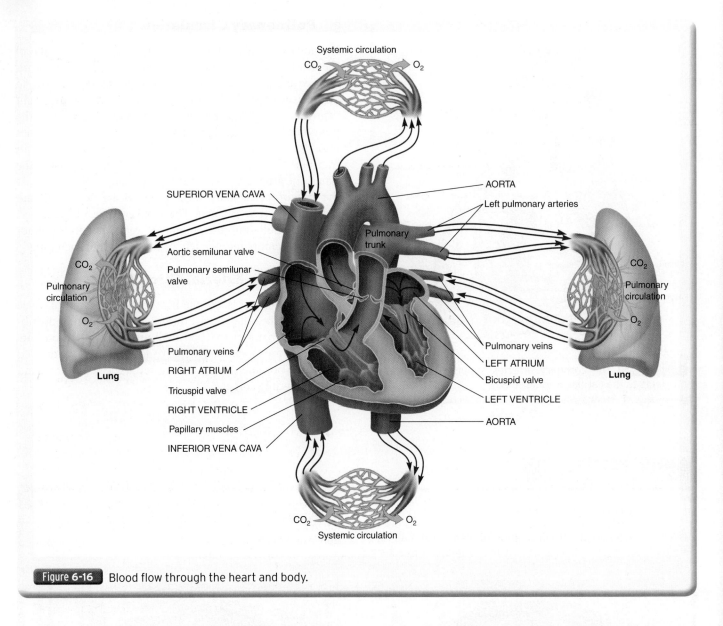

Figure 6-16 Blood flow through the heart and body.

The ascending aorta arises from the left ventricle and consists of only two branches, the right and left main coronary arteries. The aorta then arches posteriorly and to the left, forming the aortic arch. Three major arteries arise from the aortic arch: the brachiocephalic (innominate) artery, the left common carotid artery, and the left subclavian artery.

The descending aorta is the longest portion of the aorta and is subdivided into the thoracic aorta and the abdominal aorta. The descending aorta extends through the thorax and abdomen into the pelvis. In the pelvis, the descending aorta divides into the two common iliac arteries, which further divide into the internal and external iliac arteries. The thoracic aorta and the abdominal aorta will be discussed later in this chapter.

The Head and Neck

The brachiocephalic artery is the first vessel to branch from the aortic arch. It is relatively short and rapidly divides into the right common carotid artery and the right subclavian

artery. The carotid arteries transport blood to the head and neck, whereas the subclavian arteries transport blood to the upper extremities.

Each common carotid artery branches at the angle of the mandible into the internal and external carotid arteries. This point of division is called the carotid bifurcation. Here, a slight dilation, the carotid sinus, contains structures that are important in regulating blood pressure. Branches of the external carotid artery supply blood to the face, nose, and mouth. The internal carotid arteries, together with the vertebral arteries (branches of the subclavian arteries), supply blood to the brain **Figure 6-18** .

Circulation to the brain is provided through the vertebral arteries and the internal carotid arteries. The left and right vertebral arteries enter the cranial vault through the foramen magnum. They then unite to form the basilar artery. After branching to the pons (the mass of nerve fibers at the end of the medulla oblongata) and the cerebellum (the part

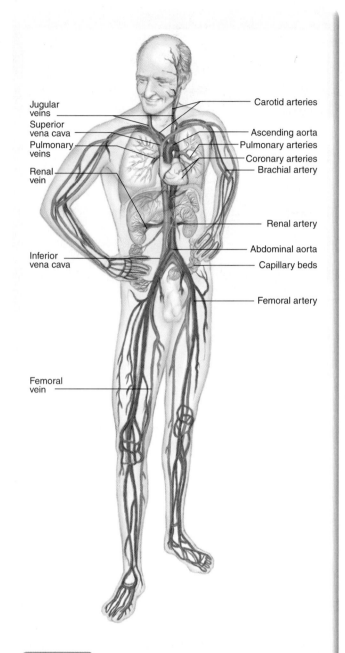

Figure 6-17 The cardiovascular system. The systemic arterial circulation is noted in red, and the systemic venous system is noted in blue.

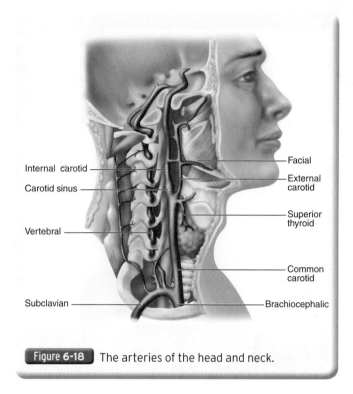

Figure 6-18 The arteries of the head and neck.

cerebral arteries interconnect via the anterior communicating artery. This interconnection of arteries forms a collateral network to deliver circulation to the brain, known as the circle of Willis **Figure 6-19** . This helps ensure that circulation to any portion of the brain is not interrupted if a single major artery leading to the brain becomes occluded.

Pathophysiology

Occlusion of one artery in the brain outside of the circle of Willis is a common cause of a stroke, damaging the brain from lack of oxygen.

The Upper Extremity

The subclavian artery supplies blood to the brain, neck, anterior chest wall, and shoulder. Shortly after its point of origin, each subclavian artery gives rise to a vertebral artery. The subclavian system then continues from the thorax into the upper extremity. At the shoulder joint, it becomes the axillary artery, then the brachial artery below the head of the humerus **Figure 6-20** . The transitions from subclavian to axillary to brachial are continuous and not due to branching. The brachial artery divides into the ulnar and radial arteries. These arteries form the two palmar arches of vessels within the hand: the superficial palmar arch and the deep palmar arch. Digital arteries extend from the superficial palmar arch to each digit.

of the brain that is dorsal to the pons and is responsible for coordination and balance), the basilar artery bifurcates into the posterior cerebral arteries. These arteries supply the posterior portion of the brain.

The carotid arteries enter the cranial vault through the carotid canals and soon give rise to the middle cerebral arteries, which supply blood to large portions of the brain cortex. The middle cerebral arteries give rise to several important branches. The posterior communicating arteries connect with the posterior cerebral arteries. The anterior

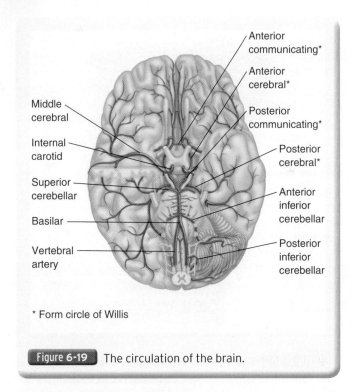

* Form circle of Willis

Figure 6-19 The circulation of the brain.

Pathophysiology

Raynaud phenomenon occurs when spasms in the digital arteries develop, particularly following emotional stress or exposure to cold. The fingertips become white and cool. Usually, the process reverses spontaneously within a few minutes.

Pathophysiology

The digital arteries are end arteries, meaning that they are the final source of blood to the fingers. Each finger has two digital arteries, and if both are damaged, tissue loss may occur. This fact becomes an important consideration during repair of finger lacerations. Inappropriate use of an anesthetic containing epinephrine can result in spasm in the digital arteries and possible necrosis of the fingertip.

The Thoracic Aorta

Two types of branches of arteries make up the thoracic aorta: the visceral arteries and the parietal arteries. Visceral arteries supply blood to the thoracic organs, and parietal arteries supply blood to the thoracic wall.

Intercostal arteries run along the ribs and provide circulation to the chest wall. Intercostal arteries branch into anterior and posterior intercostal arteries. The anterior

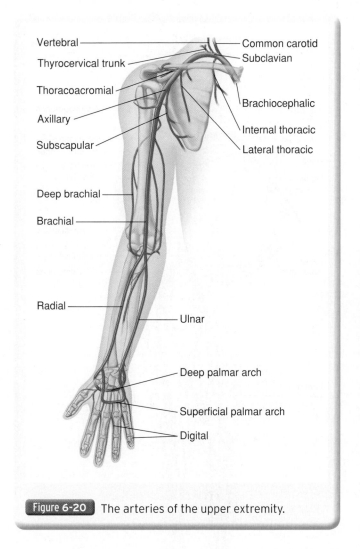

Figure 6-20 The arteries of the upper extremity.

intercostal arteries originate as branches of the subclavian system. The posterior intercostal arteries arise directly from the aorta. Visceral branches of the thoracic aorta supply the bronchial arteries in the lungs and the esophageal arteries (see Figure 6-4).

The Abdominal Aorta

Like their thoracic counterpart, branches of the abdominal aorta are divided into visceral and parietal portions. The visceral arteries are subdivided into paired and nonpaired arteries. The three major unpaired branches of the abdominal aorta's visceral arteries include the celiac trunk, the superior mesenteric, and the inferior mesenteric arteries **Figure 6-21**. The celiac trunk supplies blood to the esophagus, stomach, duodenum, spleen, liver, and pancreas. The superior mesenteric artery and its branches supply blood to the pancreas, small intestine, and colon. The inferior mesenteric artery and its branches supply blood to the descending colon and rectum **Figure 6-22**. Paired branches of the visceral abdominal aorta supply blood to the kidneys, adrenal gland, and gonads. The parietal branches supply blood to the diaphragm and abdominal wall.

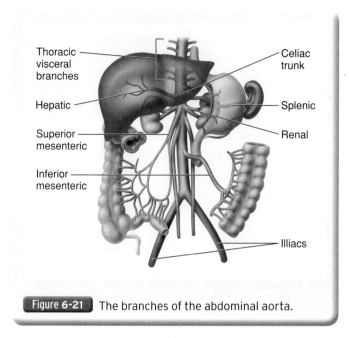

Figure 6-21 The branches of the abdominal aorta.

The Pelvis and Lower Extremity

At the level of the fourth lumbar vertebra, the aorta divides into the two common iliac arteries. These arteries further divide into the internal iliac arteries, which supply blood to the pelvis, and the external iliac arteries, which enter the lower extremity **Figure 6-23**. The internal iliac artery sends out visceral branches to the rectum, vagina, uterus, and ovary. Parietal branches supply blood to the sacrum, gluteal muscles of the buttocks region, the pubic region, rectum, external genitalia, and proximal thigh.

Like the upper extremity, the vessels of the lower extremity form a continuum. The external iliac arteries become the femoral arteries. Each femoral artery supplies blood to the thigh, external genitalia, anterior abdominal wall, and knee. The femoral artery becomes the popliteal artery in the lower thigh. Each popliteal artery then trifurcates, branching into anterior and posterior tibial and peroneal arteries. At the foot, the anterior tibial artery becomes the dorsalis pedis artery. Plantar arteries arise from the posterior tibial artery and subdivide into digital branches that supply blood to the toes **Figure 6-24**.

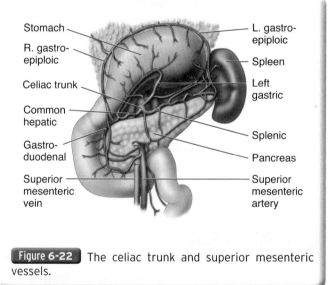

Figure 6-22 The celiac trunk and superior mesenteric vessels.

Pathophysiology

Atherosclerosis can affect the mesenteric arteries. When this occurs, patients experience cramping pain after eating because the narrowed artery is no longer able to supply adequate oxygen to the intestine for digestive processes to occur. The pain is called mesenteric angina. Complete blockage of a mesenteric artery can result in necrosis (death) of a portion of the bowel, a serious life-threatening condition known as mesenteric infarction.

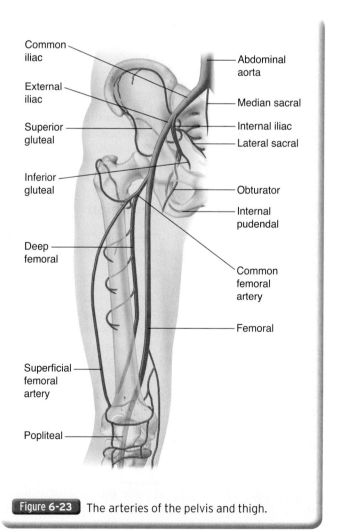

Figure 6-23 The arteries of the pelvis and thigh.

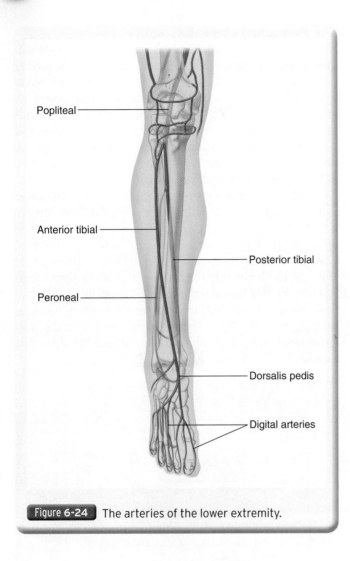

Figure 6-24 The arteries of the lower extremity.

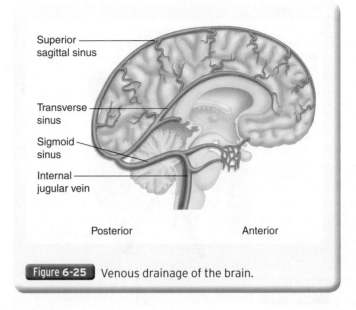

Figure 6-25 Venous drainage of the brain.

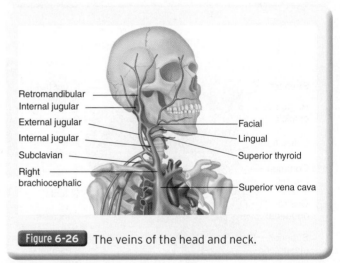

Figure 6-26 The veins of the head and neck.

Systemic Venous Circulation

As a rule, veins accompany the major arteries. Many veins have the same names as the arteries they accompany.

The Head and Neck

The two major veins that drain the head and neck are called the external and internal 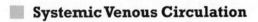. The external jugular vein is more superficial and often is visible immediately beneath the skin. The external jugular vein primarily drains the posterior head and neck. The internal jugular vein drains the cranial vault as well as the anterior portion of the head, face, and neck. Spaces between membranes surrounding the brain form venous sinuses. These sinuses are the primary means of venous drainage from the brain and feed into the internal jugular vein **Figure 6-25**.

The external jugular vein joins the internal jugular vein at the base of the neck **Figure 6-26**. The internal jugular veins join the subclavian veins (the proximal part of the main vein of the arm) to form the brachiocephalic veins, which drain into the superior vena cava.

Clinical Tip

The right subclavian or internal jugular veins are common sites for placement of percutaneous catheters, referred to as central lines, into the main or central circulation. Using the guide-wire or Seldinger technique, a needle is placed through the skin, into the deep vein. A guide wire that serves as a guide for placement of the catheter is placed through the needle.

The Upper Extremity

The veins of the upper extremity vary somewhat from person to person **Figure 6-27**. The names of the veins of the hands, wrists, and forearm follow the arteries of the same name. In the upper forearm, these veins combine to form the basilic vein and the cephalic vein, the major veins of the arm. The basilic and cephalic veins combine to form the axillary vein, which drains into the subclavian vein.

The Thorax

In the thorax, venous drainage begins at the anterior and posterior intercostal veins. The intercostal veins empty into the azygos vein on the right side of the thorax and the hemiazygos vein on the left side. These veins, along with the right and left brachiocephalic veins, provide the major source of flow into the superior vena cava.

The Abdomen and Pelvis

Ultimately, all venous drainage from the lower part of the body passes through the inferior vena cava. The inferior vena cava returns deoxygenated blood from the lower parts of the body to the right atrium for oxygenation. Within the abdominal and pelvic cavities, veins of the same name accompany the major arteries, providing venous drainage from structures including the kidney, adrenal glands, gonads, and diaphragm. The internal iliac veins drain the pelvis, and the external iliac veins drain the lower limbs. The internal and external iliac veins combine together in the pelvis, forming the common iliac veins, which combine to form the inferior vena cava.

The hepatic portal system is a specialized part of the venous system that drains blood from the liver, stomach, intestines, and spleen Figure 6-28 . Blood from the system flows first through the liver, where blood collects in the sinusoids. In the sinusoids, the liver extracts nutrients, filters the blood, and metabolizes various drugs. The blood then empties into the hepatic veins, which join the inferior vena cava.

The Lower Extremity

The longest vein in the body is the great saphenous vein. It drains the foot, leg, and thigh. The saphenous vein originates over the dorsal and medial side of the foot, ascends along the medial side of the leg and thigh, and empties into the femoral vein, which then drains into the external iliac vein. Laterally, the small saphenous vein helps drain the leg and lateral side of the foot. The veins of the feet also drain into the anterior and posterior tibial veins, which accompany their respective arteries, uniting at the knee to form the popliteal vein. The popliteal vein ascends through the thigh, becoming the femoral vein Figure 6-29 .

■ Blood Composition

Blood is made up of cells, fragments of cells, and dissolved biochemicals containing nutrients, oxygen, hormones, and wastes. Blood is the substance that is pumped by the heart through the arteries, veins, and capillaries Figure 6-30 . Blood helps to distribute body heat and maintain stable interstitial fluid. It is actually a connective tissue with its cells suspended in a liquid, extracellular matrix, and it is heavier and thicker than water. Blood contains red blood cells (RBCs), which transport gases, and white blood cells (WBCs), which fight disease. Platelets are cell fragments that aid in clotting. RBCs, WBCs, and platelets are collectively

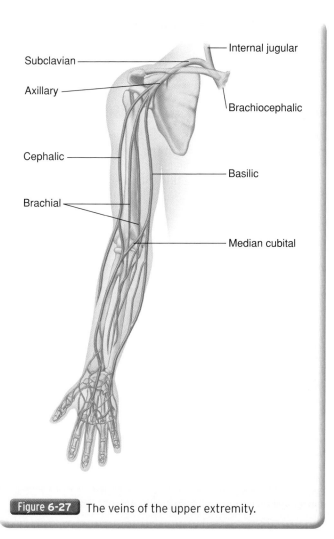

Figure 6-27   The veins of the upper extremity.

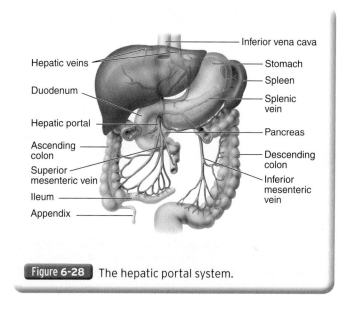

Figure 6-28   The hepatic portal system.

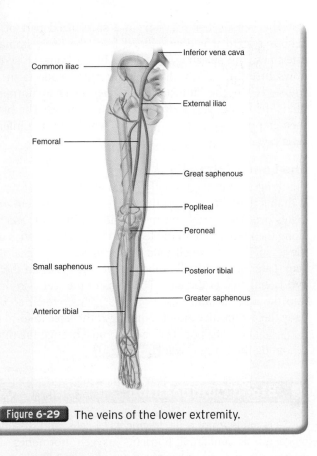

Figure 6-29 The veins of the lower extremity.

called formed elements **Figure 6-31** . The liquid portion of blood is called plasma.

Red blood cells make up about 45% of blood volume, which is known as the hematocrit. WBCs and platelets make up less than 1%. The remainder is plasma, which appears as a clear, straw-colored liquid. Plasma contains water, amino acids, carbohydrates, lipids, proteins, hormones, electrolytes, vitamins, and cellular wastes. The most abundant solutes in the plasma are plasma proteins. Albumins are the smallest of the plasma proteins and play an important role in the plasma's osmotic pressure, transporting molecules such as hormones and ions. An average adult male has approximately 5 to 6 liters of blood in his body, whereas an adult female has about 4 to 5 liters.

Red Blood Cells

Red blood cells are also known as erythrocytes and are disk-shaped cells that carry oxygen to the tissues. These are the most numerous of the formed elements. An average human has between 4.2 and 5.8 million erythrocytes per cubic millimeter of blood. RBCs are unable to move on their own; the flowing plasma passively propels them. RBCs contain a protein known as hemoglobin, which gives them their reddish color. Hemoglobin binds with oxygen that is absorbed in the lungs and transports

Case Study PART 3

After the patient has been moved to the ambulance and transport has begun, you perform a secondary assessment. The patient's symptoms have not improved, he is still feeling short of breath, the intensity of the chest pain has not lessened, he is sweaty, and the nausea is persisting. Vital signs have not changed from the last set obtained 5 minutes ago. Lungs have slight rales at the bases and the heart sounds are normal, oxygen saturation (Spo_2) is 98%, and the ECG is continuing to show irritability of the heart. You give the patient another nitroglycerin tablet since his BP has not dropped and call medical control.

Recording Time: 10 minutes	
Appearance	Still in severe distress
Level of consciousness	Alert (oriented to person, place, and day)
Airway	Open and clear
Breathing	Labored with rales at the bases
Circulation	Normal heart sounds, ECG shows persistent irritability
Pulse	110 beats/min, irregular, strong
Blood pressure	142/90 mm Hg
Respirations	24 breaths/min, labored
Spo_2	98%

6. "If this patient were not already en route to a STEMI center, would he be a candidate for fibrinolytic "clot-buster" therapy in a local hospital? Why or why not?"

7. Besides aspirin, oxygen, and the nitroglycerin, what other interventions could benefit this patient now?

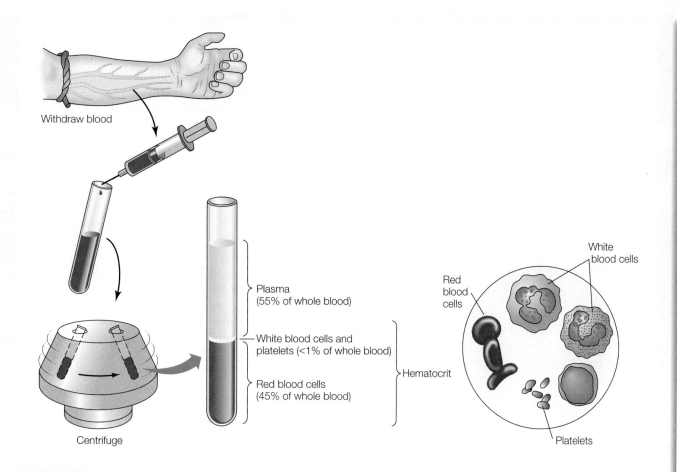

Withdraw blood

Centrifuge

Plasma
(55% of whole blood)

White blood cells and
platelets (<1% of whole blood)

Red blood cells
(45% of whole blood)

Hematocrit

Red
blood
cells

White
blood cells

Platelets

Figure 6-30 When blood is withdrawn from a vein and spun in a centrifuge, it separates into plasma and cellular layers. The cellular layer includes red cells, white cells, and platelets.

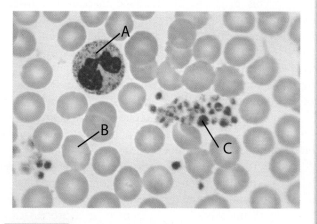

© Carolina Biological Supply, Co/Visuals Unlimited, Inc.

Figure 6-31 The microscopic appearance of blood cells. **A.** White blood cells. **B.** Red blood cells. **C.** Platelets.

it to the tissues where it is needed. Increased numbers of circulating RBCs increase the blood's oxygen-carrying capacity, which can affect health positively. RBC counts are taken to diagnose many diseases and evaluate their courses.

Erythropoiesis is the ongoing process by which RBCs are made. Production of red blood cells continues at a heightened rate until the amount of them in the blood circulation is enough to supply oxygen to the body tissues. Approximately 25 trillion erythrocytes are contained in the normal adult circulation; of these, 2.5 million erythrocytes are destroyed every second.

B-complex vitamins such as vitamin B_{12} and folic acid greatly influence RBC production as well as being necessary for DNA synthesis. Hematopoietic (blood-cell-forming) tissue is very vulnerable to deficiency of both of these vitamins. Iron is required for normal RBC production and for hemoglobin synthesis. Iron is slowly absorbed from the small intestine, and the body reuses much of the iron released by decomposition of hemoglobin from damaged RBCs. Only small amounts of iron must be taken in via the diet.

RBCs usually live for 120 days, with replacement cells created to maintain a relatively stable RBC count. Those cells that are destined for destruction decompose in the spleen and other tissues that are rich in cells known as macrophages. Macrophages protect the body against infection. The body "recycles" some components of hemoglobin, such as the protein, globin, and iron. The part of hemoglobin that is not recycled is converted to bilirubin, which is a waste product that undergoes further metabolism in the liver. Normally, a chemical derivative of bilirubin, urobilinogen, is excreted in the stool and in the urine.

RBCs contain antigens on their surface, which are proteins recognized by the immune system. Within the plasma are antibodies, which are proteins that react with antigens. Persons are classified as having one of four blood types based on the presence or absence of these specific antigens. This process of classification is referred to as blood typing, or determining the ABO blood group.

Type A blood contains erythrocytes with type A surface antigens and plasma containing type B antibodies; type B blood contains type B surface antigens and plasma containing type A antibodies. Type AB blood contains both types of antigens but the plasma contains no ABO antibodies. Type O contains neither A nor B antigens but contains both A and B plasma antibodies. A person's blood type determines which type of blood he or she may receive in a blood transfusion.

The Rh blood group got its name from the rhesus monkey, because it was in this type of monkey that it was first studied. There are several Rh antigens (factors) in humans, the most prevalent of which is antigen D. If present on the RBC membranes, the blood is called Rh-positive. If not, it is called Rh-negative. Only 15% of the US population is Rh-negative. The presence or absence of Rh antigen is inherited, but the antibodies that react with it, called anti-Rh antibodies, are not spontaneous. They form only in Rh-negative people because of specific stimulation. If a person with Rh-negative blood were to be exposed to Rh-positive blood, antibodies to the antigens could be produced.

Pathophysiology

Bilirubin may accumulate in the blood for a number of reasons, ranging from liver disease to bleeding. When blood concentrations of bilirubin are increased, jaundice occurs, in which the skin and sclera of the eyes often turn yellow.

White Blood Cells

White blood cells are also known as leukocytes. There are several different types of white blood cells and each has a different function. The primary function of all white blood cells is to fight infection. Antibodies to fight infection may be produced, or leukocytes may directly attack and kill bacterial invaders. Leukocytes are larger than erythrocytes. Most leukocytes are motile and leave the blood vessels by a process known as diapedesis to move toward the tissue where they are needed most.

Leukocytes are named according to their appearance in a stained preparation of blood. In general, granulocytes have large cytoplasmic granules that are easily seen with a simple light microscope; agranulocytes are leukocytes that lack these granules. There are three types of granulocytes (neutrophils, eosinophils, and basophils) and two types of agranulocytes (monocytes and lymphocytes).

Neutrophils are normally the most common type of granulocyte in the blood. Their nuclei are commonly multi-lobed, resembling a string of baseballs held together by a thin strand of thread. For this reason, these cells often are called polymorphonuclear cells or "polys." Neutrophils destroy bacteria, antigen-antibody complexes, and foreign matter. Eosinophils are granulocytes that contain granules that stain bright red with the acidic stain, eosin. Eosinophils function in the body's allergic response and are, thus, increased in people with allergies. Certain parasitic infections, such as trichinosis, also result in an increase in the number of eosinophils present. Basophils are the least common of all granulocytes and play a role in both allergic and inflammatory reactions. Basophils contain large amounts of histamine, a substance that increases tissue inflammation, and heparin, a substance that inhibits blood clotting.

Lymphocytes are the smallest of the agranulocytes. Lymphocytes originate in the bone marrow but migrate through the blood to the lymphatic tissues. Most lymphocytes are located in the lymph nodes, spleen, tonsils, lymph nodules, and thymus. Different types of lymphocytes will be described in the chapter, The Lymphatic and Immune System. B cells are lymphocytes that produce and secrete antibodies that bind and destroy foreign antigens. T cells are lymphocytes that interact directly with antigens, producing the cellular immune response; they also stimulate the B lymphocytes to produce antibodies.

Monocytes and macrophages are among the first lines of defense in the inflammatory process. Monocytes migrate out of the blood and into the tissues in response to an infection. They engulf microbes and digest them in a process called phagocytosis. Unlike their counterparts the neutrophils, which are short lived, once in the tissues monocytes mature into long-lived macrophages. **Figure 6-32** summarizes blood composition.

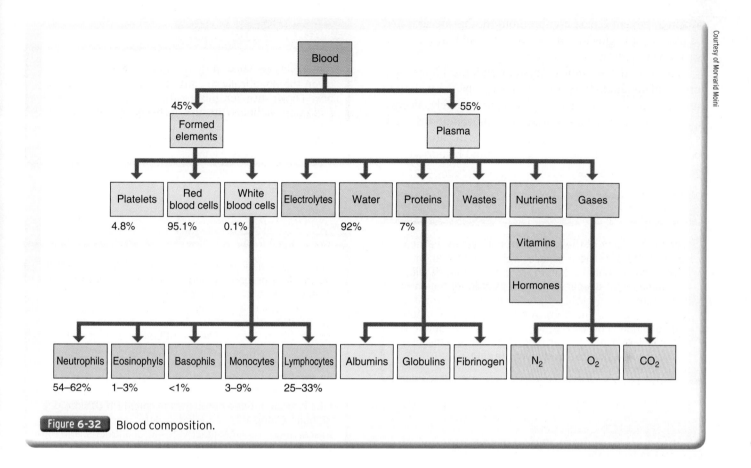

Figure 6-32 Blood composition.

Pathophysiology

All blood cells are produced in the bone marrow. This process is called hematopoiesis or hemopoiesis. Leukemia is a cancerous condition in which certain cell lines begin to grow abnormally fast. These cells function abnormally and invade other tissues, ultimately resulting in death if treatment fails.

■ Platelets and Blood Clotting

Platelets (also called thrombocytes) are small cells in the blood that are essential for clot formation. Clots are formed as a result of a series of chemical reactions. The blood clotting or coagulation process is a complex set of events involving platelets, clotting proteins in the plasma (clotting factors), other proteins, and calcium. During this process, platelets aggregate together in a clump and form much of the foundation of a blood clot. Clotting proteins produced by the liver solidify the remainder of the clot, which eventually includes red and white blood cells.

Following injury to a blood vessel wall, a predictable series of events takes place, resulting in hemostasis (cessation of bleeding) and formation of the final blood clot. Chemicals released from the vessel wall cause local vasoconstriction, as well as activation of the platelets. The combination of vessel contraction and loose platelet aggregation forms a temporary "plug." When a smaller blood vessel is cut or broken, smooth muscles in its walls contract (vasospasm), and loss of blood slows nearly immediately. A vasospasm has the potential to completely close the ends of a severed vessel. Other factors released by the tissues, known as tissue thromboplastin, activate a cascade of clotting proteins. Eventually, thrombin is formed from prothrombin, clotting protein made in the liver. This triggers the conversion of fibrinogen to fibrin, which binds to the platelet plug, forming the final mature clot.

The body also has two systems to counterbalance the clotting system. One, the fibrinolytic system, lyses or disrupts clots that have already formed. The main steps in the fibrinolytic system are the activation of tissue plasminogen activator, which then converts plasminogen to plasmin.

The other counterbalance to the clotting system consists of three naturally occurring blood thinners (anticoagulants), protein S, protein C, and antithrombin III, that are activated if a blood clot begins to form in an abnormal location, such as a coronary artery.

Together, the fibrinolytic system and the body's own anticoagulants attempt to provide a balance between clotting and bleeding; however, neither system is absolutely effective (for example, in patients with thrombotic conditions, such as myocardial infarction or stroke, as well as in patients with spontaneous bleeding, such as subarachnoid hemorrhage).

Pathophysiology

Venous anatomy of the lower extremity varies, particularly of the superficial, smaller veins. Inflammation of these veins, a condition known as phlebitis, may develop. Inflammation of deeper veins can result in formation of blood clots, or thrombi, which can break off and travel to other parts of the body. A potentially life-threatening condition known as pulmonary embolism develops when a piece of a clot, or an embolus, travels to the lung, blocking blood flow to a portion of the lung.

Pathophysiology

Any decrease in the number of red blood cells in the body is called anemia. Anemia may be caused by inadequate nutrition (such as iron deficiency), inadequate production of erythrocytes by bone marrow, increased destruction of red blood cells by the body (hemolysis), or bleeding.

Pathophysiology

Genetically engineered tissue plasminogen activator is given therapeutically to cause lysis of blood clots. The best known use for this treatment is for myocardial infarction, although its use is becoming increasingly more popular as a treatment of thrombotic stroke and pulmonary embolism.

Pathophysiology

During pregnancy, Rh grouping is very important. During late pregnancy and delivery, the mother often is exposed to a small amount of fetal blood. If the mother's blood is Rh negative and the fetus' blood is Rh positive, the mother's body will produce antibodies to Rh antigens. These antibodies may enter the fetal circulation and destroy the fetus' red blood cells. This condition, known as erythroblastosis fetalis, can be fatal to the child. Erythroblastosis fetalis usually is prevented if the mother is given an injection of a specific type of antibody preparation called Rh_o(D) immune globulin (RhoGAM) immediately after each delivery or miscarriage. RhoGAM inactivates fetal antigens, and the mother's body does not produce Rh-positive antibodies.

Case Study PART 4

While you are en route to the hospital, medical control advises that you give the patient morphine to help alleviate the pain as well as further dilate the coronary vessels. In this patient, morphine may be helpful because the 12-lead ECG shows indications of an acute myocardial infarction. You obtain serial vital signs every 5 minutes, and the patient seems to be breathing easier and calming down. You transmit a second 12-lead ECG and vital signs to the physician in the emergency department and discuss if you should bypass the emergency department and take the patient directly up to the cath lab for a percutaneous coronary intervention (PCI). As you engage in casual conversation with the patient, trying to keep him calm, he tells you that his father died suddenly while in his 40s and owns up to this pain having occurred for months now.

Prep Kit

Chapter Summary

- The human heart pumps blood through the arteries, which connect to smaller arterioles, and then even smaller capillaries.

- The heart (myocardium) is surrounded by a thick pericardial membrane, which contains visceral and parietal layers, separated by pericardial fluid. The upper chambers, or the atria, receive blood returning to the heart from other parts of the body. The lower chambers, the ventricles, pump blood out of the heart.

- The heart valves include the tricuspid, mitral, pulmonic, and aortic valves.

- Blood flow within the heart begins with the delivery of deoxygenated blood to the right atrium by the superior and inferior venae cavae.

- Strands and clumps of specialized cardiac muscle contain only a few myofibrils, and are located throughout the heart. These areas initiate and distribute impulses through the myocardium, comprising the cardiac conduction system that coordinates the cardiac cycle.

- The electrical activity of the heart is influenced by the brain and autonomic nervous system and the intrinsic conduction system of the heart including the sinoatrial node, atrioventricular node, bundle of His, bundle branches, and the Purkinje fibers.

- The regulation of heart function involves the control of the heart rate (chronotropic effect), conductivity (dromotropic effect), and strength of the contraction (inotropic effect). Receptors, such as baroreceptors and chemoreceptors, constantly monitor body functions.

- Three positively charged ions, sodium (Na^+), potassium (K^+), and calcium (Ca^{2+}) are responsible for initiating and conducting electrical charges in the heart.

- The process of electrical discharge and flow of electrical activity is called depolarization.

- Repolarization of cardiac cells occurs as they begin to return to their resting state. The two phases of repolarization are the early or absolute refractory period, in which depolarization cannot occur, and the latter or relative refractory period, in which cells can respond to a stronger-than-normal stimulus.

- An electrocardiogram (ECG) is a visualization of the electrical currents generated during depolarization and repolarization of the heart. The normal sinus rhythm ECG consists of P waves occurring at regular intervals, a PR segment of normal duration (less than 0.2 seconds), followed by a QRS complex (ventricular depolarization), an ST segment that is flat, and by a T wave (ventricular repolarization).

- The cardiac cycle is the repetitive pumping process that begins with the onset of cardiac muscle contraction and ends immediately prior to the start of the next contraction.

- Contraction of the ventricles is known as systole. A pressure also may be determined in the vessels during diastole, the relaxation phase of the heart cycle.

- The amount of blood pumped through the circulatory system in 1 minute is referred to as the cardiac output. The arteries are blood vessels that carry blood away from the heart. Veins are blood vessels that transport blood back to the heart. Arterioles are the smallest arteries and venules are the smallest veins. Capillaries are microscopic, thin-walled vessels through which oxygen and other nutrients and carbon dioxide and waste products are exchanged.

- The coronary arteries supply the heart with blood and arise from the aorta shortly after it leaves the left ventricle. The right coronary artery divides into several important branches and the left main coronary artery divides into two branches, the anterior descending and the circumflex coronary arteries.

- Pulmonary circulation carries blood from the right side of the heart to the lungs and back to the left side of the heart.

- Systemic arterial circulation carries oxygenated blood from the heart through the aortic valve, into the aorta, and out to the body.

- Circulation to the head and neck involves the brachiocephalic artery, the left common carotid artery, and the left subclavian artery.

- Circulation in the upper extremity involves the subclavian artery, vertebral artery, axillary artery, brachial artery, and ulnar and radial arteries.

- The thoracic aorta branches into the visceral arteries, supplying the thoracic organs, and the parietal arteries, supplying the thoracic wall.

- Intercostal arteries run along the ribs and provide circulation to the chest wall.

- The abdominal aorta divides into visceral arteries and parietal arteries. The major arteries are the celiac trunk, superior mesenteric, and inferior mesenteric arteries. Paired branches of the visceral abdominal aorta supply the kidneys, adrenal gland, and gonads. The parietal branches supply the diaphragm and abdominal wall.

- The circulation to the pelvis and lower extremities involves the aorta, the two common iliac arteries, the internal and external iliac arteries, the femoral arteries, popliteal arteries, tibial arteries, and dorsalis pedis arteries.

- The major veins of the head and neck include the external and internal jugular veins. The internal jugular veins join the subclavian veins to form the brachiocephalic veins, which drain into the superior vena cava.

- The venous circulation from the upper extremity involves the veins of the hands, wrists, and forearm and the basilic, cephalic, and axillary veins.

- The venous drainage from the thorax includes the anterior and posterior intercostal veins, the azygos vein, the hemiazygos vein, the brachiocephalic veins, and the superior vena cava.

- The venous drainage from the abdomen and pelvis empties into the inferior vena cava. Within the abdominal and pelvic cavities, veins of the same name accompany the major arteries, as well as the internal and external iliac veins.

- The hepatic portal system is a specialized part of the venous system that drains blood from the liver, stomach, intestines, and spleen.

- Venous circulation from the lower extremity involves the greater and lesser saphenous, femoral, anterior and posterior tibial, and popliteal veins.

- Blood is a combination of plasma and formed elements (cells) and serves to carry oxygen and nutrients to the tissues and waste products away. Adult men have approximately 70 mL/kg of blood, or 5 to 6 liters, and adult women have approximately 65 mL/kg, or 4 to 5 liters.

- The red blood cells (erythrocytes) carry oxygen to the tissues. Hemoglobin gives red blood cells their color and binds to oxygen that is absorbed in the lungs. Red blood cells have a lifespan of 120 days; they then decompose in the spleen and at other sites. The body "recycles" some components of hemoglobin and converts the remainder to bilirubin.

- Erythrocytes contain antigens on their surface; within the plasma are antibodies that react with these antigens. Blood typing is based on the presence or absence of these substances.

- The white blood cells (leukocytes) primarily fight infection by the production of antibodies or by directly attacking and killing bacterial invaders. The process by which clots are formed and bleeding stops is known as hemostasis.

- The platelets and blood clotting process can be very helpful or harmful to the circulation. The blood clotting or coagulation process is a complex set of events involving platelets, clotting proteins in the plasma, other proteins, and calcium. Other factors known as tissue thromboplastin activate a cascade of clotting proteins.

■ Vital Vocabulary

absolute refractory period The early phase of repolarization in which the cell contains such a large concentration of ions that it cannot be stimulated to depolarize.

afterload The pressure in the aorta against which the left ventricle must pump blood.

agranulocytes Leukocytes that lack granules.

albumins The smallest of plasma proteins; they make up about 60% of these proteins by weight.

alpha effect Stimulation of alpha receptors that results in vasoconstriction.

anemia A lower than normal hemoglobin or erythrocyte level.

anterior descending (LAD) coronary artery One of the two branches of the left main coronary artery.

antibodies Proteins secreted by certain immune cells that react against foreign antigens in the body by binding to the antigens, making them more visible to the immune system.

antigens Substances or molecules that, when taken into the body, stimulate immune system response and cause formation of specific protective proteins called antibodies.

aorta The principal artery leaving the left side of the heart and carrying freshly oxygenated blood to the body; the largest artery in the body.

aortic arch One of the three described portions of the aorta; the section of the aorta between the ascending and descending portions that gives rise to the right brachiocephalic (innominate), left common carotid, and left subclavian arteries.

aortic valve The semilunar valve that regulates blood flow from the left ventricle to the aorta.

arteries The muscular, thick-walled blood vessels that carry blood away from the heart.

arterioles Subdivisions of arteries that are thinner and have muscles in their walls that are innervated by the sympathetic nervous system.

arteriosclerosis A pathologic condition in which the arterial walls become thickened and inelastic.

ascending aorta The first of three portions of the aorta; originates from the left ventricle and gives rise to two branches, the right and left main coronary arteries.

atherosclerosis A disorder characterized by the formation of plaques of material, mostly lipids and cholesterol, on the inner arterial walls.

atria The upper chambers of the heart; they receive blood returning to the heart.

atrioventricular (AV) node A specialized structure located in the AV junction that slow conduction through the AV junction.

atrioventricular valves The mitral and tricuspid valves through which blood flows from the atria to the ventricles.

automaticity A state in which the cardiac cells are at rest, waiting for the generation of a spontaneous impulse from within.

axillary vein The vein that is formed from the combination of the basilic and cephalic veins; it drains into the subclavian vein.

B cells Lymphocytes that produce and secrete antibodies that bind and destroy foreign antigens.

baroreceptors Receptors in the blood vessels, kidneys, brain, and heart that respond to changes in pressure in the heart or main arteries to help maintain homeostasis.

basilar artery The artery that is formed when the left and right vertebral arteries unite after entering the brain through the foramen magnum.

basilic vein One of the two major veins of the arm; it combines with the cephalic vein to form the axillary vein.

basophils White blood cells that work to produce chemical mediators during an immune response; make up approximately 1% of leukocytes.

beta effect Stimulation of beta receptors that results in increased inotropic, dromotropic, and chronotropic states.

bilirubin A waste product of red blood cell destruction that undergoes further metabolism in the liver.

blood The fluid tissue that is pumped by the heart through the arteries, veins, and capillaries and consists of plasma and formed elements or cells, such as red blood cells, white blood cells, and platelets.

bruit An abnormal whooshing sound indicating turbulent blood flow within a narrowed blood vessel; usually heard in the carotid arteries.

bundle of His The portion of the electric conduction system in the interventricular septum that conducts the depolarizing impulse from the atrioventricular junction to the right and left bundle branches.

capillaries Thin-walled vessels that allow oxygen and nutrients to pass out into the cells and allow carbon dioxide and waste products to pass from the cells into the capillaries.

cardiac conduction system A group of complex electrical tissues within the heart that initiate and transmit stimuli that result in contractions of myocardial tissue.

cardiac cycle A heartbeat; each cardiac cycle consists of ventricular contraction (systole) and relaxation (diastole).

cardiac output The amount of blood pumped by the heart per minute, calculated by multiplying the stroke volume by the heart rate per minute.

cardiac tamponade Restriction of cardiac contraction, failing cardiac output, and shock, caused by the accumulation of fluid or blood in the pericardium.

cardiac veins Veins that branch out and drain blood from the myocardial capillaries to join the coronary sinus.

carotid bifurcation The point of division at which the common carotid artery branches at the angle of the mandible into the internal and external carotid arteries.

carotid canals An opening in the cranial vault through which the carotid arteries enter.

carotid sinus A slight dilation in the carotid bifurcation that contains structures that are important in the regulation of blood pressure.

cephalic vein One of the two major veins of the arm that combine to form the axillary vein.

cerebellum The part of the brain that is located dorsal to the pons and is responsible for coordination and balance.

cerebral arteries The arteries that supply blood to large portions of the cerebral cortex of the brain.

chemoreceptors Sense organs that monitor the levels of oxygen and carbon dioxide and the pH of the cerebrospinal fluid and blood and provide feedback to the respiratory centers to modify the rate and depth of breathing based on the body's needs at any given time.

chordae tendineae Thin bands of fibrous tissue that attach to the valves in the heart and prevent them from inverting.

chronotropic effect The effect on the rate of contraction of the heart.

circle of Willis An interconnection of the anterior, middle, and posterior cerebral arteries and the anterior communicating artery, which forms an important source of collateral circulation to the brain.

circulatory system The complex arrangement of tubes, including the arteries, arterioles, capillaries, venules, and veins, that moves blood, oxygen, nutrients, carbon dioxide, and cellular waste throughout the body.

circumflex coronary artery One of the two branches of the left main coronary artery.

coagulation The formation of a blood clot.

conductivity The ability of cardiac cells to conduct electrical impulses.

contractility The strength of heart muscle contraction.

coronary arteries Arteries that arise from the aorta shortly after it leaves the left ventricle and supply the heart with oxygen and nutrients.

coronary artery disease The condition that results when either atherosclerosis or arteriosclerosis is present in the arterial walls of the coronary arteries.

coronary sinus Veins that collect blood that is returning from the walls of the heart.

cusps The flaps that comprise the heart valves.

depolarization The rapid movement of electrolytes across a cell membrane that changes the cell's overall charge. This rapid shifting of electrolytes and cellular charges is the main catalyst for muscle contractions and neural transmissions.

descending aorta One of the three portions of the aorta; it is the longest portion and extends through the thorax and abdomen into the pelvis.

diapedesis A process whereby leukocytes leave blood vessels to move toward tissue where they are needed most.

dorsalis pedis artery A continuation of the anterior tibial artery at the foot.

dromotropic effect Related to the effect of the heart's conduction rate.

ejection fraction The percentage of blood that leaves the heart each time it contracts.

electrical potential An electrical charge difference that is created by the difference in sodium and potassium concentration across the cell membrane at any given instant.

electrocardiogram (ECG) A graphic recording of the electrical activity of the heart.

embolus A piece of clot that travels from one part of the body to another, potentially becoming an obstruction to blood flow.

endocarditis Infection of a heart valve.

eosinophils White blood cells with a major role in allergic reactions and bronchoconstriction during an asthma attack; make up approximately 1% to 3% of leukocytes.

epicardium The layer of the serous pericardium that lies closely against the heart; also called the visceral pericardium.

epinephrine A hormone produced by the adrenal medulla that has a vital role in the function of the sympathetic nervous system.

erythroblastosis fetalis A serious condition that results when a pregnant woman's blood type is incompatible with the fetus' blood type and antibodies from the mother enter the fetal circulation and destroy the fetus' red blood cells.

erythrocytes Disk-shaped cells that carry oxygen to the tissues; also known as red blood cells.

erythropoiesis The process by which red blood cells are made.

excitability A property of cardiac cells that provides the cells with the ability to respond to electrical impulses.

femoral arteries The principal arteries of the thigh, a continuation of the external iliac artery. They supply circulation to the thigh, external genitalia, anterior abdominal wall, and knee.

femoral vein A continuation of the saphenous vein that drains into the external iliac vein.

fibrin A white insoluble protein formed from fibrinogen in the clotting process.

fibrinogen A plasma protein that is important for blood coagulation.

foramen ovale An opening between the two atria that is present in the fetus but closes shortly after birth.

fossa ovalis A depression between the right and left atria that indicates where the foramen ovale had been located in the fetus.

granulocytes A type of leukocyte that has large cytoplasmic granules that are easily seen with a simple light microscope.

heart A hollow muscular organ that pumps blood throughout the body.

hematocrit The percentage of blood volume made up by red blood cells.

hematopoiesis The process of blood cell production in the bone marrow; also called hemopoiesis.

hemoglobin An iron-containing protein within red blood cells that has the ability to bind to oxygen.

hemostasis Control of bleeding by formation of a blood clot.

heparin A substance found in large amounts in basophils that inhibits blood clotting.

hepatic portal system A specialized part of the venous system that drains blood from the liver, stomach, intestines, and spleen.

hepatic veins The veins to which blood empties after liver cells in the sinusoids of the liver extract nutrients, filter the blood, and metabolize various drugs.

histamine A chemical found in mast cells that, when released, causes vasodilation, capillary leaking, and bronchiole constriction.

inferior vena cava One of the two largest veins in the body; carries blood from the lower extremities and the pelvic and the abdominal organs to the heart.

inotropic effect The effect on the contractility of muscle tissue, especially cardiac muscle.

ischemia Insufficient oxygen at a particular tissue site often associated with obstruction of arterial blood flow to the site.

jaundice A yellowing of the skin and sclera of the eyes because of excessive concentrations of bilirubin in the blood.

jugular veins The two main veins that drain the head and neck.

leukemia A cancerous condition in which certain white blood cell lines begin to grow abnormally fast and invade other tissues.

leukocytes White blood cells that are responsible for fighting infection.

lumen The inside of an artery, vein, or other hollow structure.

lymphocytes The white blood cells responsible for a large part of the body's immune protection.

macrophages Cells that develop from the monocytes that provide some of the body's first line of defense in the inflammatory process.

mast cells Cells to which antibodies attach, formed in response to allergens. When allergens attach to antigens on the mast cell surface, the cells release potent inflammatory mediators resulting in allergic symptoms or potentially anaphylaxis.

mediastinum The space between the lungs, in the center of the chest, that contains the heart, trachea, mainstem bronchi, part of the esophagus, and large blood vessels.

mesenteric angina Pain caused by partial occlusion of the mesenteric artery from atherosclerosis.

mesenteric infarction Blockage of a mesenteric artery, resulting in necrosis of a portion of the bowel.

mitral valve The valve in the heart that separates the left atrium from the left ventricle.

monocytes Granulocytes that migrate out of the blood and into the tissues in response to an infection.

murmur An abnormal heart sound, heard as "whooshing," indicating turbulent blood flow within the heart.

myocardial infarction Blockage of one or more of the arteries that supply oxygen to the heart, resulting in death to a portion of the myocardium.

myocardium The heart muscle.

neutrophils White blood cells that are one of the three types of granulocytes; they have multi-lobed nuclei that resemble a string of baseballs held together by a thin strand of thread; they destroy bacteria, antigen-antibody complexes, and foreign matter.

norepinephrine A naturally occurring hormone with a greater stimulatory effect on alpha receptors that also may be given as a cardiac drug.

P wave The first wave in the ECG complex, representing depolarization of the ventricles.

palmar arches The two arches formed from the radial and ulnar vessels within the hand, creating the superficial and deep palmar arches.

papillary muscles Specialized muscles that attach the ventricles to the cusps of the valves by muscular strands called chordae tendineae.

parietal layer One of two layers of the serous pericardium; it is separated from the visceral pericardium by a small amount of pericardial fluid.

pericardial effusion A condition, often caused by trauma, in which the pericardial sac fills with too much fluid, impairing the heart's ability to expand and contract properly.

pericardial fluid A serous fluid that fills the space between the visceral pericardium and the parietal pericardium and helps to reduce friction.

pericardial sac A thick, fibrous membrane that surrounds the heart; also called the pericardium.

pericardiocentesis A life-saving procedure to correct cardiac tamponade, in which a needle is inserted into the pericardial sac to remove excess fluid that is restricting the heart from expanding and contracting properly.

pericarditis Infection or inflammation of the pericardial membranes, resulting in severe chest pain.

pericardium A thick, fibrous membrane that surrounds the heart; also called the pericardial sac.

phlebitis Inflammation of the wall of the vein, sometimes caused by an IV line, manifested by tenderness, redness, and slight edema along part of the length of the vein.

plasma A sticky yellow fluid that carries the blood cells and nutrients and transports cellular waste material to the organs of excretion; makes up 55% of the total blood volume.

plasma proteins The most abundant solutes (dissolved substances) in the plasma.

plasmin A naturally occurring clot-dissolving enzyme, usually present in the body in its inactive form, plasminogen.

platelets Tiny, disk-shaped cell fragments that are much smaller than the red or white blood cells; they are essential in the initial formation of a blood clot, the mechanism that stops bleeding.

polarized state The state of the resting cell, which normally has a net negative charge with respect to the outside of the cell.

pons The mass of nerve fibers at the end of the medulla oblongata.

popliteal artery A continuation of the femoral artery at the knee.

popliteal vein The vein that forms when the anterior and posterior tibial veins unite at the knee.

PR segment The period between the beginning of the P wave (atrial depolarization) and the onset of the QRS complex (ventricular depolarization), signifying the time required for atrial depolarization and passage of the excitation impulse through the atrioventricular junction.

prothrombin An alpha globulin made in the liver that is converted to thrombin.

pulmonary circuit The venules and veins, which send deoxygenated blood to the lungs to receive oxygen and unload carbon dioxide.

pulmonary embolism A blood clot or foreign matter trapped within the pulmonary circulation.

pulmonary valve The semilunar valve that regulates blood flow between the right ventricle and the pulmonary artery.

QRS complex Deflections of the ECG produced by ventricular depolarization.

Raynaud phenomenon Spasms that develop in the digital arteries, particularly following emotional stress or cold exposure, resulting in white and cool fingertips.

red blood cells Cells that transport gases, including oxygen; also called erythrocytes.

relative refractory period The latter phase of repolarization in which the cells are able to respond to a stronger-than-normal stimulus.

repolarization The process by which ions are moved across the cell wall to return to a polarized state.

rheumatic fever An inflammatory disease caused by streptococcal bacterial infection that can cause a stenosis of the mitral valve or aortic valve.

saphenous vein The longest vein in the body, it drains the leg, thigh, and dorsum of the foot.

semilunar valves The two valves, the aortic and pulmonic valves, that divide the heart from the aorta and pulmonary artery.

septum A solid, wall-like structure that separates the left atrium and ventricle from the right atrium and ventricle.

serous pericardium The inner membrane of the pericardium, which contains two layers called the visceral pericardium and the parietal pericardium.

sinoatrial (SA) node The dominant pacemaker of the heart, located at the junction of the superior vena cava and the right atrium.

sinusoids A part of the hepatic portal system in which blood collects within the liver and the liver cells extract nutrients from the blood, filter the blood, and metabolize various drugs.

sodium-potassium pump A molecular (ion-transporting) mechanism whereby sodium is actively moved out of a cell and potassium moved in.

ST segment The interval between the end of the QRS complex and the beginning of the T wave; often elevated or depressed with respect to the isoelectric line when there is significant myocardial ischemia.

stroke volume The volume of blood pumped forward with each ventricular contraction.

subclavian artery The proximal part of the main artery of the arm, which supplies the brain, neck, anterior chest wall, and shoulder.

subclavian vein The proximal part of the main vein of the arm, which unites with the internal jugular vein and terminates at the superior vena cava.

superior vena cava One of the two largest veins in the body; carries blood from the upper extremities, head, neck, and chest into the heart.

systemic circuit The arteries and arterioles, which send oxygenated blood and nutrients to the body cells while removing wastes.

systole The period of time when the atria or ventricles are contracting; also called atrial or ventricular systole.

T cells Lymphocytes that interact directly with antigens, producing the cellular immune response; they also stimulate the B lymphocytes to produce antibodies.

T wave The upright, flat, or inverted wave following the QRS complex of the ECG, representing ventricular repolarization.

thrombi Blood clots.

thrombin An enzyme that causes the conversion of fibrinogen to fibrin, which binds to the platelet plug, forming the final mature clot.

thrombocytes Incomplete cells important in blood clotting; also called platelets.

tibial veins A continuation of the veins of the feet that unite at the knee to form the popliteal vein, which then drains into the femoral vein.

tissue plasminogen activator An important element of the fibrinolytic system; causes clots that have already formed to lyse or be disrupted; works by converting plasminogen to plasmin.

tricuspid valve The heart valve that separates the right atrium from the right ventricle.

tunica media The middle and thickest layer of tissue of a blood vessel wall, composed of elastic tissue and smooth muscle cells that allow the vessel to expand or contract in response to changes in blood pressure and tissue demand.

vasoconstriction The contraction of blood vessels, which decreases their diameter.

vasodilation The relaxation of blood vessels, which increases their diameter.

vasospasm The action of a muscle contraction in a small blood vessel that occurs after it is cut or broken; this action can completely close the ends of a severed vessel.

veins The blood vessels that bring blood back to the heart.

venous sinuses Spaces between the membranes surrounding the brain that are the primary means of venous drainage from the brain.

ventricles The two lower chambers of the heart that pump blood out of the heart.

venules Microscopic vessels that link capillaries to veins.

visceral layer The layer of the serous pericardium that lies closely against the heart; also called the epicardium.

white blood cells Cells that protect the body against disease, particularly infectious disease; also called leukocytes.

■ Case Study Answers

1. What is cardiac output?

   Answer: Cardiac output is the amount of blood pumped through the circulatory system in 1 minute. It is expressed in liters per minute (L/min). The cardiac output equals the heart rate multiplied by the stroke volume or amount of blood (volume) pumped with each heartbeat: Cardiac Output = Stroke Volume × Heart Rate.

2. How does a heart attack affect the patient's cardiac output?

   Answer: Factors that influence the heart rate, the stroke volume, or both will affect cardiac output. A heart attack can cause ischemia or infarction to the electrical conduction system, the myocardium, or both, resulting in decreased cardiac output. The less functioning the cardiac muscle mass, the more likely an effect on the cardiac output. This can have a cumulative effect such as in the case of a patient who experienced a previous AMI and is now experiencing another one.

3. Which blood vessels supply oxygen and nutrients to the myocardium and are the location for partial or full occlusion(s) that can result in a heart attack?

   Answer: The right and left coronary arteries arise from the aorta shortly after it leaves the left ventricle and divide into several important branches that supply the heart with oxygen and nutrients.

4. What blood vessels are most likely to be occluded if a 12-lead ECG is showing features of ischemia and infarction to the left ventricle of the heart?

   Answer: Most blood vessels supplying the left ventricle rise from the left main coronary artery. This vessel is the largest and shortest of the myocardial blood vessels. It divides into two branches, the anterior descending and the circumflex coronary arteries. These arteries subdivide further, supplying most of the left ventricle, the intraventricular septum, and, at times, the atrioventricular node. The occlusion may be partial or full and could be in the left main coronary artery or any of its branches.

5. What vessels supply the conduction system of the heart?

   Answer: The right coronary artery and its branches supply portions of the conduction system (ie, the primary pacemakers of the heart); however, when vessels to the conduction system do not arise from the right coronary artery, they originate from the left side instead.

6. If this patient were not already en route to a STEMI center, would he be a candidate for fibrinolytic "clot-buster" therapy in a local hospital? Why or why not?

   Answer: At this point, most EMS systems in the United States would have protocols in place to transfer the STEMI patient directly to a hospital with a coronary catheterization lab because the effectiveness of this intervention is better than the fibrinolytic drugs that were used primarily in the 1980s to 2005. Check with your Medical Director to review the specific protocols and procedures for transport of a suspected STEMI patient in your system.

7. Besides aspirin, oxygen, and the nitroglycerin, what other interventions could benefit this patient now?

Answer: The morphine should be helpful to vaso-dilate the coronary vessels and as an analgesic, provided his blood pressure stays stable. A beta-blocker may be of value for a patient with these signs and symptoms. In the regulation of heart function, beta effects result in an increased heart rate, cardiac conduction, and contractility, all of which are stressing the patient's myocardium and increasing oxygen demand. A beta-blocker helps to block the stimulation of beta receptors and reduce the stress and oxygen demand on the heart.

The Lymphatic and Immune System

Learning Objectives

1. Describe the functions of the lymphatic system. (p 148)
2. Describe the system of lymph vessels and explain how lymph is returned to the blood. (p 148-151)
3. State how lymph is formed. (p 149)
4. State the location and function of the lymph nodes, the thymus, and the spleen. (p 152-155)
5. Explain the role of the thymus in immunity. (p 153)
6. Define immunity. (p 154-155)
7. Explain the differences between humoral response and cellular immune response. (p 157)
8. Compare and contrast the development and function of B cells and T cells. (p 157-158)
9. Describe the differences between active and passive immunity. (p 158-159)
10. List the five types of immunoglobulins and explain which type is important in the activation of B cells. (p 158)
11. Differentiate between primary and secondary immune responses. (p 158)
12. Explain how vaccines work. (p 158)
13. Define infectious disease. (p 159-160)
14. Name some important infectious diseases found in prehospital care. (p 159-160)
15. Explain how microorganisms are named and classified. (p 160)
16. Describe the distribution of and the benefits of normal flora. (p 160)
17. List different methods by which infectious diseases are spread. (p 160)

■ Introduction

Similar to the cardiovascular system, the lymphatic system transports fluids through a network of vessels. The primary function of the lymphatic system is the production, maintenance, and distribution of lymphocytes Figure 7-1. Another major function is to transport excess fluid out of interstitial spaces in tissues and return it to the bloodstream. Without the lymphatic system, fluid would accumulate in tissue spaces. Lacteals are special lymphatic capillaries located in the small intestine's lining that absorb digested fats and carry them to the venous circulation.

The biochemicals and cells of the lymphatic system attack foreign particles in the body, allowing the destruction of infectious microorganisms and viruses, as well as toxins and cancer cells. Many organs and body systems work together to maintain life and proper health. The lymphatic system is vital in this capacity because it is responsible for defending the body against environmental hazards (such as various pathogens) and internal threats (such as cancer cells). Lymphocytes are vital for the body's ability to resist or overcome diseases and infections.

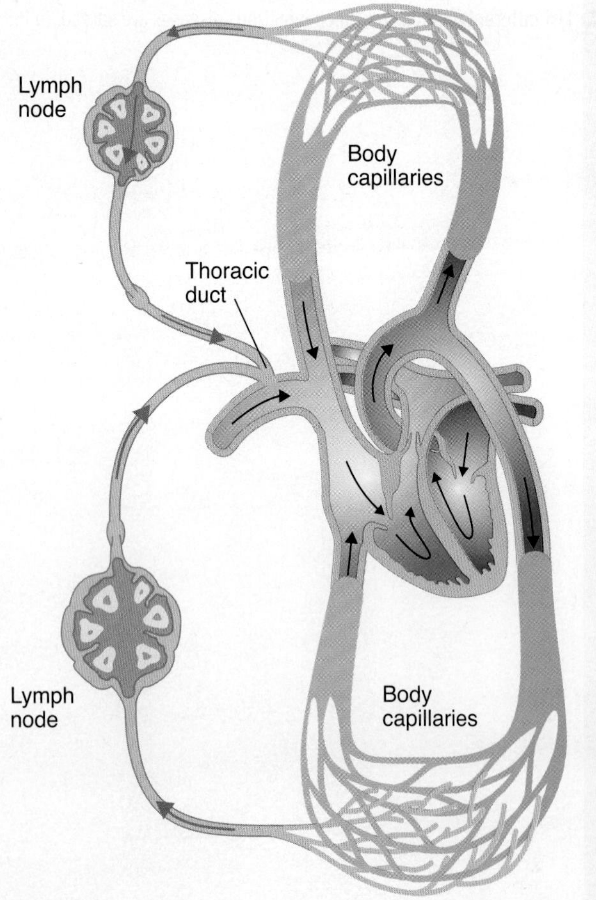

■ Lymphatic Vessels

Lymphatic vessels only carry fluid away from the tissues. Lymphatic capillaries form tiny tubes called lymphatic pathways, which merge to form larger vessels, eventually uniting with veins in the thorax. Microscopic lymphatic capillaries extend into interstitial spaces in complex networks Figure 7-2. Their walls consist of a single layer of squamous epithelium that allows tissue fluid to enter. The fluid inside these capillaries is called lymph.

Similar to veins, but with thinner walls, lymphatic vessels have valves preventing backflow of lymph. Larger vessels lead to specialized organs known as lymph nodes, and then continue on to form larger lymphatic trunks.

Lymphatic trunks drain lymph from lymphatic vessels and join one of two collecting ducts (the thoracic duct or the right lymphatic duct). Figure 7-3 shows the right lymphatic duct and lymph drainage of the right breast. Of the two collecting ducts, the thoracic duct is larger and longer, receiving lymph from the lower limbs, abdominal regions, left upper limb, and left side of the head, neck, and thorax. It empties into the left subclavian vein near the left jugular vein. The right lymphatic duct receives lymph from the right side of the head and neck, right upper limb, and right thorax. It empties into the right subclavian vein near the right jugular vein.

Lymph then moves from the two collecting ducts into the venous system, becoming part of the plasma. This occurs just before the blood is returned to the right atrium.

Figure 7-1   The lymphatic system transports fluids through a network of vessels.

Pathophysiology

The lay term for lymph nodes is "glands." The term swollen glands refers to inflammation and enlargement of the cervical lymph nodes, a common occurrence in response to various types of upper respiratory and throat infections. Lymph nodes in the axilla or groin may swell in response to infections of the arm or leg, respectively. Inflammation of lymph nodes caused by infection is called lymphadenitis.

Any swelling of the lymph nodes, whether painful or not, is called lymphadenopathy. This condition may indicate the presence of a malignancy or an infectious disease, such as strep throat. Many forms of cancer, especially of the breasts and colon, tend to spread or metastasize to the lymph nodes.

Tissue Fluid and Lymph Formation

Lymph is a thin, plasma-like fluid formed from interstitial or extracellular fluid. Lymph is basically the same as tissue fluid. It is referred to as lymph once it has entered a lymphatic capillary. Tissue fluid is made up of water and dissolved substances from the blood capillaries. It is very similar to blood plasma, containing gases, hormones, and nutrients. However, it lacks plasma proteins because their size does not permit them to leave the blood capillaries. Plasma colloid osmotic pressure helps to draw fluid back into the capillaries using the process of osmosis.

Lymph forms because filtration from blood plasma occurs at a higher rate than does reabsorption. The hydrostatic pressure of tissue fluid is increased, inducing tissue fluid movement into the lymphatic capillaries. Most of the small proteins that the blood capillaries filtered earlier are returned to the bloodstream via the lymph. Lymph also carries foreign particles (including bacteria and viruses) to the lymph nodes.

Movement of Lymph

The movement of lymph is influenced by muscular activity. Lymph itself is under low hydrostatic pressure. Without contraction of skeletal muscles, smooth muscle contraction in the larger lymphatic trunks, and breathing-related pressure changes, lymph may not flow easily. Skeletal muscles, for example, compress lymphatic vessels to move the lymph inside, with valves preventing any backflow. Breathing creates a relatively low thoracic cavity pressure during inhalation, aiding lymph circulation. The diaphragm increases abdominal cavity pressure, squeezing lymph out of abdominal vessels and into thoracic vessels.

Case Study | PART 1

At 3:00 PM, your unit arrives at a trailhead to await a mountain rescue team that will be carrying out an injured hiker. According to the latest radio report, at approximately 1:00 AM, the patient was bitten in the right leg by a rattlesnake. When the rescue team arrives, they introduce you to a 22-year-old man who is accompanied by two friends. Your general impression is an average-size young man with very pale and clammy skin, who is in apparent pain. The patient has an open airway with shallow breathing, no serious external bleeding, and you are able to detect a pulse. A bandage has been applied to his right lower leg. You immediately apply oxygen with a nonrebreathing mask as your partner obtains vital signs. One of the patient's friends tells you that the wound bled initially, but once they were safely back on the trail, he made a pressure bandage from a piece of a shirt while the other friend ran for help. The bleeding has since stopped. After a quick set of baseline vitals, you decide to transport the patient immediately.

Recording Time: 0 Minutes

Appearance	Pale and diaphoretic young man adult in pain
Level of consciousness	Alert (oriented to person, place, and day)
Airway	Appears patent
Breathing	Shallow respirations
Circulation	A weak pulse is detected
Pulse	Weak and rapid radial pulse
Blood pressure	98 mm Hg by palpation
Respirations	22 breaths/min, regular
Spo_2	97%

1. What are the body's first routes of defense against a sting, bite, or local infection?

2. What can be done immediately to minimize the spread of a foreign substance through the lymphatic system?

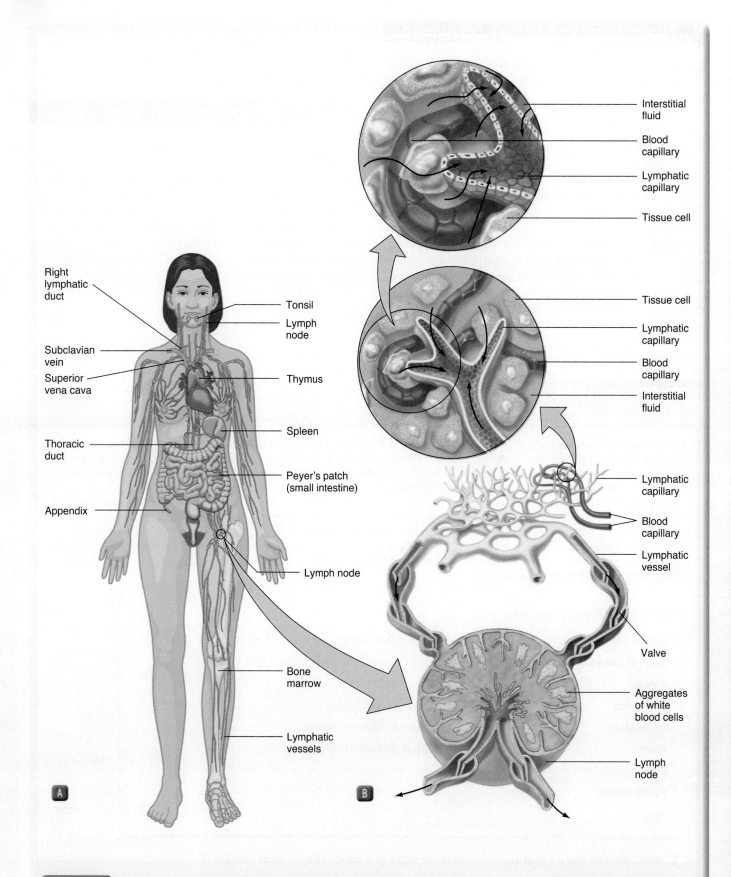

Figure 7-2 The lymphatic system. **A.** The lymphatic system consists of vessels that transport lymph back to the circulatory system. **B.** Lymph nodes interspersed along the vessels filter the lymph.

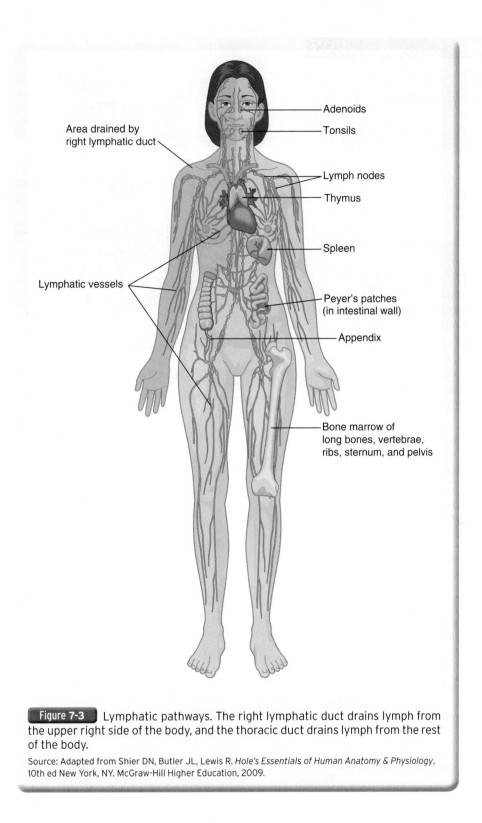

Area drained by
right lymphatic duct

Adenoids

Tonsils

Lymph nodes

Thymus

Spleen

Lymphatic vessels

Peyer's patches
(in intestinal wall)

Appendix

Bone marrow of
long bones, vertebrae,
ribs, sternum, and pelvis

Figure 7-3 Lymphatic pathways. The right lymphatic duct drains lymph from the upper right side of the body, and the thoracic duct drains lymph from the rest of the body.

Source: Adapted from Shier DN, Butler JL, Lewis R. *Hole's Essentials of Human Anatomy & Physiology,* 10th ed New York, NY. McGraw-Hill Higher Education, 2009.

The continuous movement of lymph stabilizes fluid volume in the body's interstitial spaces. When tissue fluid accumulates in the interstitial spaces (edema), it is due to an interference with lymph movement. To prevent the tissues from becoming edematous, the lymphatic vessel must absorb this excess fluid and return it to the central venous circulation. After surgery involving the lymph nodes in the axilla or groin some patients can develop a severely swollen extremity, which can be painful and disabling.

Lymph Nodes

Lymph nodes are actually lymph glands. They are found along the lymphatic pathways and contain many lymphocytes and macrophages that fight invading microorganisms. Although they vary in size and shape, lymph nodes are generally bean shaped and less than 2.5 centimeters long Figure 7-4. An indented region of each node, called the hilum, is where blood vessels and nerves are attached. Lymphatic vessels leading to a node are called afferent vessels, and enter separately at various points on its surface. Lymphatic vessels that leave the node's hilum are called efferent vessels.

Each lymph node is enclosed and subdivided by a capsule. The functional units of a lymph node are the lymph nodules (follicles), which are denser arrangements of lymphoid tissue that are found in the loose connective tissue of the digestive, respiratory, and urinary systems. Lymph nodules occur either alone or in groups. Major collections of lymph nodes are located in the axilla (axillary nodes), neck (cervical nodes), and groin (inguinal nodes).

Three sets of lymphatic organs comprise the tonsils: the palatine tonsils, the pharyngeal tonsils (adenoids), and the lingual tonsils. The tonsils are located in the back of the throat and nasopharynx and protect the body from bacteria introduced through the nose and mouth Figure 7-5. In most adults, the tonsils have decreased in size since childhood; in some adults the tonsils have actually disappeared.

The palatine tonsils are located in the back of the throat, on each side of the posterior opening of the oral cavity. The pharyngeal tonsils (or adenoids) are located near the internal opening of the nasal cavity. The lingual tonsils are located on the posterior margin of the tongue.

Groups of nodules called Peyer's patches are found in the lining of the small intestine. Lymph sinuses are spaces inside a node that comprise complex channels through which lymph moves. There are more macrophages in the lymph sinuses than in any other parts of a node.

Lymph nodes are grouped along larger lymphatic vessels, but do not exist in the central nervous system Figure 7-6. Lymph nodes have two main functions. They filter potentially harmful particles from the lymph before it is returned to the bloodstream, and they also monitor body fluids. Immune surveillance occurs via the action of the lymphocytes and macrophages. Lymphocytes are produced in the lymph nodes as well as in the red bone marrow. They attack viruses, bacteria, and parasitic cells. Macrophages engulf and destroy cellular debris, damaged cells, and foreign substances.

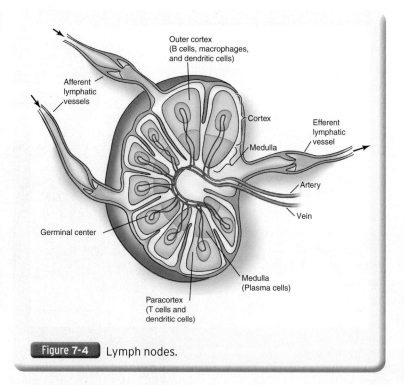

Figure 7-4   Lymph nodes.

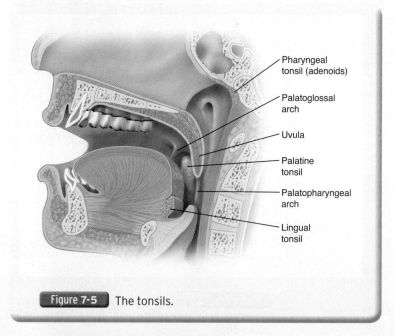

Figure 7-5   The tonsils.

Pathophysiology

Years ago, the palatine tonsils and adenoids were commonly removed surgically in an attempt to reduce the frequency of colds and sore throats, particularly those that were caused by the *Streptococcus* organism. Today, the procedure usually is performed only if a patient has an abscess of the tonsils, severe and frequent infections, or an intermittent airway obstruction problem such as sleep apnea.

The Thymus

The thymus is located in the thorax, anterior to the aorta and posterior to the upper sternum. It is soft and consists of two lobes that are enclosed in a connective tissue capsule Figure 7-7 . Although relatively large in infancy and early childhood, the thymus shrinks after puberty, becoming much smaller in adults. Its lymphatic tissue is replaced during the later years of life by adipose and connective tissues. The thymus produces lymphocytes, which move to other lymph tissues to help fight infection. The thymus plays a major role in immunity, especially in early life.

The thymus is divided into lobules by inward-extending connective tissues. The lobules contain large amounts of lymphocytes, including primarily inactive thymocytes. Some thymocytes mature into T lymphocytes, which leave the thymus after 3 weeks and provide immunity in the body.

Thymosins are secreted by the epithelial cells of the thymus. This hormone causes T lymphocytes to mature.

The Spleen

The spleen is located in the upper left abdominal cavity, inferior to the diaphragm and posterior and lateral to the stomach. It is the body's largest lymphatic organ, resembling a large, subdivided lymph node. The spleen contains the largest amount of lymphatic tissue in an adult's body. It differs from lymph nodes in that its venous sinuses are filled with blood, not lymph. There are two types of tissues inside the splenic lobules. White pulp is located throughout the spleen in small "islands," made up of splenic nodules containing many lymphocytes. The remainder of the lobules is filled by red pulp, which contains many red blood cells, lymphocytes, and macrophages Figure 7-8 .

Case Study | PART 2

The patient is placed on the ambulance stretcher, and you apply a splint to the injured extremity to immobilize it, carefully keeping it below the level of the heart. You attach the ECG monitor; two large-bore IV lines of saline will be started en route. Because of the local injury and the systemic effect it is having on this patient, he is quickly loaded into the ambulance and you start out for the regional trauma center, which is about 25 minutes away. As soon as the ambulance begins moving, you call the hospital to prepare the staff for the arrival of this patient.

You learn that the patient is a 22-year-old man who weighs 90 kg. The patient has pale, clammy skin and swelling around the injured area. The patient has no known medication allergies and uses an Albuterol inhaler for his asthma, as needed. The patient's only medical history is exercise-induced asthma. The last food intake was snack bars and water for lunch around 1 PM. Prior to the onset of symptoms, the patient and his friends were hiking off the trail when they confronted a rattlesnake.

Recording Time: 5 Minutes	
Appearance	He has a look of "impending doom"
Level of consciousness	Alert (oriented to person, place, and day)
Airway	Open and clear
Breathing	Becoming rapid and shallow
Circulation	Skin is pale, diaphoretic
Pulse	110 beats/min, weak and thready
Blood pressure	100/70 mm Hg
Respirations	24 breaths/min, shallow
Spo$_2$	97%
Pupils	Equal and reactive

3. What potential problem is of most concern for a patient who has been bitten or stung?

4. What type of cells help fight infection in the body and are the most important component of the immune system?

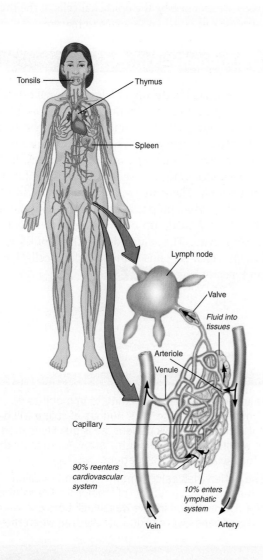

Figure 7-6 The lymphatic vessel. The enlarged diagram of a lymph node and vessels shows the path of the excess fluid that leaves the capillary, enters the adjacent tissue spaces, and is absorbed by lymphatic capillaries.

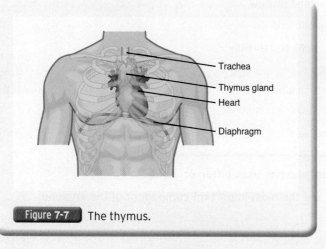

Figure 7-7 The thymus.

Pathophysiology

Trapping of bacteria by the lymphatic system is one of the body's first routes of defense against a local infection, such as that around a splinter in the finger. Often, this process occurs at the site of the wound, resulting in localized redness, pain, and swelling. Sometimes, the infection spreads beyond the local area into the lymphatic vessel. This condition, known as lymphangitis, causes red streaks to run from the wound toward the central part of the body. The associated lymph nodes may become swollen and painful as well.

The blood capillaries of the red pulp are extremely permeable, and red blood cells easily squeeze through the capillary walls to enter the venous sinuses. Older red blood cells may be damaged during this process, so they are engulfed by macrophages inside the splenic sinuses. Virtually all of the blood in the body transverses the splenic tissue, where it is filtered and worn out blood cells, foreign substances, and bacteria are removed.

Pathophysiology

The spleen is a highly vascular organ. Persons with injuries to this organ may easily bleed to death. In the past, the routine treatment of splenic injury was a splenectomy, or removal of the spleen, to stop the bleeding. Today, common practice is to preserve the spleen, if at all possible, because the spleen performs an important infection-fighting function. It filters out certain types of bacteria from the blood. Persons who have undergone a splenectomy are susceptible to overwhelming and occasionally life-threatening infections from these bacteria. At a motor vehicle crash, suspect the spleen when your unrestrained driver has lower left rib pain.

■ Body Defenses and Fighting Infection

The immune system is integrally related to the lymphatic system and is the body system that is responsible for providing immunity, the ability to resist damage from foreign substances or harmful chemicals. The human body has multiple defense mechanisms that work together to provide resistance. An infection may be caused by the presence and multiplication of a disease-causing agent (pathogen), which can be a virus, bacterium, fungus, or protozoan. Body defenses can be divided into two general categories: innate (nonspecific) and adaptive (specific) defenses. Innate

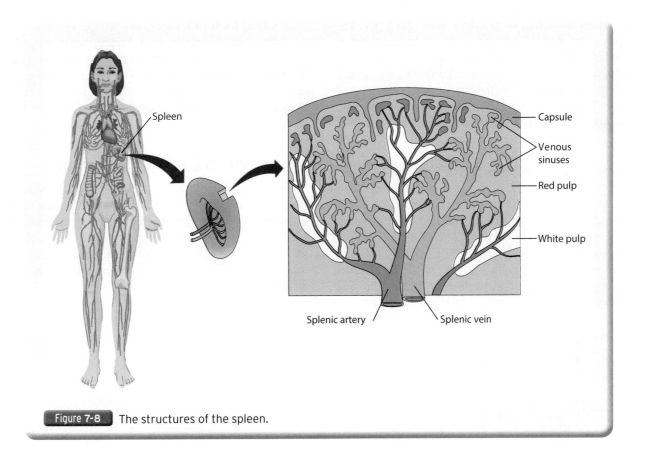

Figure 7-8   The structures of the spleen.

(nonspecific) defense defends against many different types of pathogens. This type of defense, which is present at birth, is an immune response that is predictable each time the body is exposed to a particular challenge. Specific defenses are more precise and target specific pathogens to provide adaptive (specific) defense or immunity. In this type of defense, specialized lymphocytes recognize foreign molecules and act against them. The response to a given substance is faster and stronger after each subsequent exposure.

Innate (Nonspecific) Defenses

Nonspecific defenses prevent or limit microorganisms and other environmental hazards from approaching, entering, or spreading. Nonspecific defenses are classified as follows, with mechanical barriers being the first line of defense and the others being second lines of defense:

- **Mechanical barriers.** Also known as physical barriers, they include the skin and the mucous membranes that line the respiratory, digestive, urinary (basement membranes), and reproductive passageways. They protect against certain infectious agents. The body's hair, sweat, and mucus also act as mechanical barriers.
- **Chemical barriers.** Provided by enzymes and other chemical substances in body fluids; these include pepsin and hydrochloric acid in the stomach, tears, lysozyme (present in tears, saliva, breast milk, and mucus), salt

(exists in perspiration), interferons (hormone-like peptides) that bind to uninfected cells and stimulate them to make protective proteins, and complement (a group of proteins in plasma and other body fluids that interact to cause inflammation and phagocytic activities). Plasma contains 11 special complement (C) proteins that comprise the complement system. The term complement refers to the way that this system "complements" the action of antibodies. The complement proteins interact in chain reactions (cascades) that are similar to those of the clotting system.

- **Fever.** Elevation of body temperature that reduces iron in the blood, which inhibits bacterial and fungal reproduction; fever also causes increased phagocytosis (macrophages).
- **Inflammation.** A tissue response to injury or infection that may include redness, swelling, heat, and pain; infected cells attract white blood cells, which engulf them. Many chemicals involved in the immune system promote inflammation. This inflammatory response results in the influx of cells and other chemicals that fight the foreign challenge. The most common chemicals are histamine, kinins, complement, prostaglandins, leukotrienes, pyrogens, and interferon. All of these substances are produced in response to different types of infection, as well as to the presence of foreign matter. Masses of leukocytes, bacterial cells, and

damaged tissue may form a thick fluid called pus. The body may react to inflammation by forming a network of fibrin threads where the infection is centered. This closes off the infected area to inhibit the spread of pathogens. An inflammatory response is triggered when mast cells release histamine, serotonin, and heparin. The inflammatory response is a tissue-level reaction, and is therefore related to the tissues and integumentary system.

- **Immunologic surveillance.** The constant monitoring, recognition, and destruction of abnormal cells by natural killer (NK) cells in peripheral tissues. NK cells defend the body against cancer cells and various viruses.
- **Phagocytosis.** Injured tissues attract neutrophils and monocytes, which engulf and digest particles (pathogens and cell debris); monocytes influence the development of macrophages that attach to blood and lymphatic vessels. Together, these various phagocytic cells make up the mononuclear phagocytic system to remove foreign particles from the lymph and also the blood.

A final form of innate (nonspecific) defense is species resistance. In this example, a human being may be resistant to certain diseases that affect other species of animals. A pathogen effective against a dog, for example, may be unable to survive in a human. In reverse, humans can be infected with measles, gonorrhea, mumps, and syphilis, none of which affect other animal species.

Immunity (Specific Defenses)

Immunity is also known as the third line of defense. It is defined as resistance to specific pathogens or their toxins and metabolic by-products. Specific immunity basically implies that the body is able to recognize, respond to, and remember a particular substance. Adaptive immune responses are carried out by lymphocytes and macrophages that recognize and remember certain foreign substances known as antigens (or allergens).

A small molecule that cannot stimulate an immune response by itself is known as a hapten. The molecule is found in certain drugs such as penicillin, in dust particles,

Case Study | PART 3

While en route to the hospital, the patient rests but is still reporting pain. Because infusion of the IV fluids has stabilized his blood pressure, you contact medical control to discuss an order for morphine or fentanyl. The medical control physician agrees that pain relief is appropriate and also asks the patient to describe what the snake looked like. The patient said he was so scared he did not get a good look at the snake but his friend did and identified the snake as a rattlesnake.

Recording Time: 10 Minutes	
Appearance	Starting to calm down and in less distress, but still in pain
Level of consciousness	Alert (oriented to person, place, and day)
Airway	Open and clear
Breathing	Regular
Circulation	Skin is pale, warm, and less sweating
Pulse	100 beats/min, strong and regular
Blood pressure	116/70 mm Hg
Respirations	24 breaths/min, improved effort from baseline
Spo$_2$	98%
Pupils	Equal and reactive

5. Could a vaccination have prevented the patient's reaction to the snakebite?

6. How are foreign substances removed from the body?

Pathophysiology

Tests for AIDS are used to diagnose the presence of the human immunodeficiency virus 1 (HIV-1) and 2 (HIV-2) in the blood. The presence of HIV-1 occurs more commonly in the United States, and HIV-2 occurs more commonly in West Africa. The mere presence of the virus does not necessarily indicate that a person has AIDS. A diagnosis of AIDS requires confirmatory clinical and laboratory findings, as well as a positive test result for HIV. While HIV is the virus that causes AIDS, with proper treatment today, most patients infected with HIV will never develop AIDS.

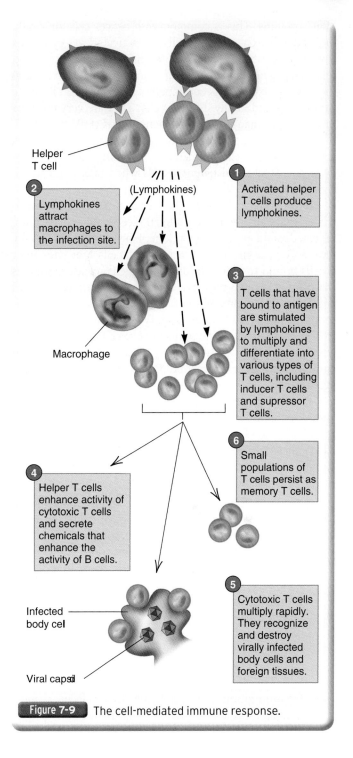

1 Activated helper T cells produce lymphokines.

2 Lymphokines attract macrophages to the infection site.

3 T cells that have bound to antigen are stimulated by lymphokines to multiply and differentiate into various types of T cells, including inducer T cells and supressor T cells.

4 Helper T cells enhance activity of cytotoxic T cells and secrete chemicals that enhance the activity of B cells.

5 Cytotoxic T cells multiply rapidly. They recognize and destroy virally infected body cells and foreign tissues.

6 Small populations of T cells persist as memory T cells.

Figure 7-9 The cell-mediated immune response.

in animal dander, and in various chemicals. Haptens usually combine with larger, more complex molecules to elicit an immune response.

Before birth, red bone marrow releases lymphocyte precursors, about half of which reach the thymus. They specialize into T lymphocytes (T cells), which later make up between 70% and 80% of circulated blood lymphocytes. Other T cells exist in lymphatic organs, particularly in lymph nodes, the white pulp of the spleen, and the thoracic duct. Others remain in the red bone marrow, eventually differentiating into B lymphocytes (B cells). They are distributed by the blood, and make up between 20% and 30% of the circulating lymphocytes. B cells are abundant in the lymph nodes, bone marrow, intestinal lining, and spleen.

T cells attach to foreign, antigen-bearing cells such as bacterial cells, and interact with direct cell-to-cell contact. This is known as cellular immune response, or cell-mediated immunity **Figure 7-9**. T cells, along with some macrophages, also synthesize polypeptides called cytokines, or, more specifically, lymphokines, that enhance responses to antigens. Interleukin-1 and interleukin-2 stimulate synthesis of cytokines from other T cells. Other cytokines called colony-stimulating factors (CSFs) stimulate leukocyte production in red bone marrow, activate macrophages, and cause B cells to grow.

B cells divide and differentiate into plasma cells, producing antibodies (immunoglobulins) that react to destroy antigens or antigen-containing particles. This is called the humoral immune response. There are millions of different types of T and B cells. Each variety originates from a single early cell to form a clone of cells (identical to the original cell). Each variety has a certain antigen receptor responding to only a specific antigen.

Before a lymphocyte can respond to an antigen, it must be activated. T cells are activated by the presence of processed antigen fragments attached to the surface of an antigen-presenting cell (accessory cell), which may be macrophages, B cells, or other types of cells. When a macrophage phagocytizes a bacterium and digests it in its lysosomes, T cell activation begins. Some bacterial antigens then move to the surface of the macrophage. They are displayed near certain protein molecules that make up the major histocompatibility complex (MHC). MHC antigens help T cells recognize foreign antigens. Helper T cells contact displayed foreign antigens. If the antigen combines with the helper T cell's antigen receptors, it becomes activated and stimulates a B cell to produce antibodies specific for the displayed antigen.

A cytotoxic T cell recognizes and combines with foreign antigens displayed on cell surfaces near certain

MHC proteins. This is common with cancer cells or virally infected cells. Cytotoxic T cells are activated via cytokines from helper T cells. They bind to antigen-bearing cells and release a protein that cuts openings into these cells to destroy them. Cytotoxic T cells continually recognize and eliminate tumor cells and virally infected cells. They are very effective in fighting human immunodeficiency virus (HIV) infection, but are often killed by the viruses they combat. Some T cells act as memory cells, immediately dividing to yield more cytotoxic T cells and helper T cells when reexposed to the same antigen.

B cells may activate when encountering an antigen whose shape fits the B cell's antigen receptor shape, dividing repeatedly and expanding its clone. However, B cells usually require T cells in order to activate. T cells that encounter B cells bound to identical foreign antigens release cytokines that stimulate the B cells. The cytokines attract macrophages and leukocytes. Some of the B cell's clones differentiate into more memory cells. These memory B cells respond quickly to reexposure to specific antigens. Other B cell clones differentiate into antibody-secreting plasma cells, which can combine with their corresponding foreign antigens and react against them.

B cells can produce between 10 million and 1 billion varieties of antibodies, each specific to an antigen. Antibody response therefore defends against many pathogens. Antibodies are round, soluble proteins making up the gamma globulin part of the plasma proteins. There are five major types of antibodies:

- **Immunoglobulin G (IgG).** A single molecule in plasma and tissue fluids; very effective against bacteria, viruses, and toxins. It activates complement.
- **Immunoglobulin A (IgA).** In exocrine gland secretions, breast milk, tears, nasal fluid, gastric juice, intestinal juice, bile, and urine.
- **Immunoglobulin M (IgM).** Composed of five single molecules found together; it is the first antibody to be produced in response to infection. IgM in plasma responds to certain antigens in foods or bacteria. The antibodies known as anti-A and anti-B are examples of IgM. This antibody also activates complement.
- **Immunoglobulin D (IgD).** On the surfaces of most B cells, especially in infants; important in the activation of B cells. It may play a role in regulation of the humoral immune response.
- **Immunoglobulin E (IgE).** Attaches to mast cells, basophils, and eosinophils and is involved in allergic reactions.

Antibodies commonly attack antigens directly, activate complement, or stimulate inflammation. They combine with antigens, causing clumping (agglutination) or forming insoluble substances (precipitation). Phagocytosis then can occur more easily. Sometimes antibodies neutralize the toxic effects of antigens. Complement activation is generally more important in protecting against infection than direct antibody attack, however.

When some IgM or IgG antibodies combine with antigens, they trigger many reactions that lead to the activation of the complement proteins. Effects include coating the antigen–antibody complexes (opsonization), attracting macrophages and neutrophils (chemotaxis), making the complexes more susceptible to phagocytosis, clumping antigen-bearing cells, rupturing foreign cell membranes (lysis), and altering viral molecular structures to make them harmless.

A primary immune response is constituted by activation of B cells or T cells after they first encounter the antigens for which they are specialized to react. Plasma cells release IgM into the lymph, followed by IgG. The antibodies are transported to the blood and throughout the body to help destroy antigen-bearing agents. This continues for several weeks.

Some of the B cells then remain as memory cells so that if the identical antigen is reencountered, clones of these memory cells enlarge and send IgG to the antigen. These memory B cells, along with memory T cells, produce a secondary immune response. After a primary immune response, detectable concentrations of antibodies appear in the blood plasma, usually 5 to 10 days after exposure to antigens, and a secondary immune response can then occur within 1 to 2 days. Memory cells live much longer than newly formed antibodies (which live between a few months and a few years). Secondary immune responses may last a long time.

Adaptive (acquired) immunity can be caused by natural events or by administration (oral or injected) of suspensions of killed or weakened pathogens or their molecules. This type of immunity may be active or passive. Active immunity is long-lasting, and occurs when a person produces an immune response to an antigen. Passive immunity occurs when antibodies produced by another person are received by a patient; it has only short-term effects. Naturally acquired active immunity occurs when a disease develops from exposure to a pathogen. Resistance then occurs as a result of the primary immune response.

A preparation known as a vaccine produces another type of active immunity. A vaccine may consist of killed or weakened bacteria or viruses, or pathogenic molecules. It cannot cause serious infections or diseases. Vaccines can also be made of a toxoid, with a toxin from an infectious organism chemically altered so that it is not dangerous. Vaccines cause artificially acquired active immunity to develop.

If a person has been exposed to a disease-causing microorganism, but there is not enough time to develop active immunity, an injection of antiserum may be given. Antiserum consists of ready-made antibodies that can be obtained from gamma globulin acquired from people who are already immune to the same disease. Injection of such gamma globulin provides artificially acquired passive immunity.

IgG antibodies pass from maternal blood to the fetus during pregnancy, giving the fetus limited immunity against the pathogens to which the mother is immune. The fetus therefore has naturally acquired passive immunity, which lasts from 6 months to 1 year after birth.

When an immune response occurs because of a non-harmful substance, it is called an allergic response. This is similar to an immune response. Both responses sensitize the lymphocytes, and the antibodies produced may combine with antigens. Allergic reactions can damage tissues, however, whereas normal immune responses cannot. Allergens are a type of antigen that triggers allergic responses. Allergens are classified as:

- **Delayed-reaction allergy.** Results from repeated exposure of the skin to certain chemicals; it usually takes about 48 hours to occur
- **Immediate-reaction allergy.** Affects people with inherited tendencies to overproduce IgE antibodies because of certain antigens; it takes only a few minutes to occur, and subsequent reexposure continues to trigger allergic reactions

Another type of reaction concerns transplantation and tissue rejection. When a body part is transplanted from one person to another, the receiving patient's immune system may recognize the transplanted part as foreign and attempt to destroy its tissues, causing a tissue rejection reaction. The greater the difference between the antigens on cell surface molecules of the donor and recipient, the greater and more rapid the rejection reaction. Therefore, donor and recipient tissues must be matched to minimize these reactions. Immunosuppressive drugs are used to reduce tissue rejection. Although they reduce the immune response by suppressing antibody and T cell formation and therefore decreasing the likelihood of rejection of the transplanted organ, they weaken the recipient's immune system. Occasionally, transplant patients survive the transplant but die of a secondary infection caused by a weakened immune system.

When the immune system fails to distinguish self from nonself, it may produce autoantibodies as well as cytotoxic T cells that attack and damage the body's tissues and organs. This "attack against self" is called autoimmunity. About 5% of all people have an autoimmune disorder. It is believed that this type of condition occurs in one of three ways:

- When a replicating virus "borrows" proteins from a host cell, incorporating them onto its own surface, the immune system "learns" the surface of the virus to destroy it, and also begins to attack the original cells bearing the same proteins.
- T cells may not learn to distinguish self from nonself.
- A nonself antigen happens to resemble a self antigen, such as when a *Streptococcus* bacterial infection triggers inflammation of the heart valves.

Pathophysiology

Often, when a person is exposed to an antigen for the first time, no problems are clinically apparent. The body responds by forming an IgE antibody to that particular substance. This antibody remains in the plasma. If the person is exposed to the same antigen again, the antigen and the antibody may react, causing the release of various substances from the mast cells. These substances can cause severe allergic shock, or anaphylaxis. Wheezing, edema or swelling caused by leaking from the blood vessels, and, ultimately, shock may occur. Known allergens such as shellfish, bees, or chocolate should be avoided, and if anaphylaxis occurs, the drug adrenaline (epinephrine) should be administered. Adrenaline is a naturally occurring hormone that also may be given as a cardiac drug and has alpha and beta effects.

Pathophysiology

Vaccines prevent infection by exposing the recipient to attenuated (weakened) or dead bacteria or viruses, or their protein coats. This exposure does not cause disease, but usually it is sufficient to stimulate the person's own immune system to produce antibodies, disease-specific T cells, or both. Any subsequent exposure will be "nipped in the bud" before causing any significant problems.

Pathophysiology

Acquired immune deficiency syndrome (AIDS) is a disease process that occurs following infection with the human immunodeficiency virus (HIV). The virus adversely affects a protein on T helper cells, the CD4 antigen, causing it to appear as an antigen to healthy cells. As a result, T helper cells are destroyed and the body becomes unable to fight many different types of infections and tumors.

■ Practical Applications—Infectious Diseases

An infectious disease is one that may be transmitted from one person to another via some type of specific microscopic organism, such as a bacterium. The most frequent infectious diseases seen in prehospital care are serious infections such as pneumonia and hepatitis.

Hepatitis is among the most serious infectious diseases in the United States and infects nearly 70,000 people annually. This infectious disease causes inflammation of the liver, which interferes with liver function. There are seven types of hepatitis labeled A-G, but only the first four are common in the United States.

Tuberculosis (TB) is an infectious disease that is spread through droplets from coughing and sneezing. Once the leading cause of death in the United States, today it is a major health problem throughout the world. It is not a serious threat in the United States with the exception of some outbreaks in certain metropolitan areas. TB is prevalent in nursing homes, homeless shelters, hospitals, prisons, migrant farm camps, and among IV drug users and people who are HIV-positive. It is making a comeback because of the development of more resistant strains.

Common means of disease transmission from person to person include airborne, body substance, injection, and oral transmission. Airborne transmission is a common form of disease transmission and occurs when microorganisms become aerosolized by coughing or sneezing. Virtually any body fluid, including tears, blood, saliva, urine, stool, semen, and vaginal secretions, can potentially transmit microorganisms to a susceptible recipient, causing disease. Drug addicts may pass HIV or hepatitis infection from one to another by sharing needles. A needle, a foreign body such as a splinter, or an insect bite or sting can cause transmission by injection. Bites and stings are an unusual initial cause of infection. More commonly, a wound becomes infected from frequent scratching or other response to the irritation. However, an important exception to this rule is human bites that often become seriously infected because of direct contamination from the oral bacteria. Oral transmission occurs from inhalation of airborne secretions, oral absorption of splattered body fluids, or ingestion of infected substances.

Literally thousands of different types of microorganisms cause disease. The common denominator is that these organisms are not visible to the naked eye. Several known infectious agents include bacteria, viruses, fungi, protozoans, nematodes, and prions. Bacteria are small, one-cell organisms that are capable of independent existence. They often are classified based on their shape: rod-shaped (bacilli), spherical (cocci), comma-shaped (vibrio), or spiral (spirochete). Bacteria cause most serious human infections, including tuberculosis, urinary tract infection, pneumonia, and plague.

Conversely, viruses are small particles that are incapable of living independently. Viruses contain genetic material (either RNA or DNA) and typically live and reproduce within another living cell. Viruses cause most "common colds."

Fungi are small, plant-like organisms, such as yeast. Fungi cause many common conditions such as athlete's foot and jock itch. Other less common fungal infections such as blastomycosis may be fatal. Protozoans are single-cell animal-like microorganisms such as amoeba and plasmodium. Exposure to plasmodium can cause malaria.

Nematodes are unsegmented worms that are tapered at both ends and include roundworms, pinworms, and hookworms. Exposure to nematodes is a known cause of intestinal or skin disease. Prions are abnormal proteins, previously believed to be incapable of a free-living existence, that somehow survive independently and transmit disease from person to person.

Certain body sites are normally colonized by various bacteria, called the normal flora, that help maintain homeostasis. The best known of these bacteria, *Escherichia coli*, are located in the gastrointestinal tract. Although certain types of *E coli* may cause serious diseases, the presence of this bacteria in the normal flora in the intestines is essential. In addition to aiding in digestion and absorption of food, the flora are important in the metabolism of waste products (eg, protein and bilirubin). Normal flora also colonizes the skin, oral, vaginal and nasal cavities.

Clinical Tip

The use of gloves and other personal protective equipment clearly helps to reduce a rescuer's risk of exposure to HIV and other communicable diseases. However, changing gloves and paying attention to properly cleaning and disinfecting equipment between patients is critical to minimize the risk of exposure from one patient to another. Many patients have a depressed immune system because of their current illness or disease process. These patients require only minimal exposure to infection to become sicker.

Case Study | PART 4

The SAMPLE history was unremarkable and did not add any pertinent information regarding the patient other than the fact that he is very thirsty. The hikers packed only one water bottle, and half of that was used to clean out the wound before applying the bandage. The patient may be dehydrated in addition to his snakebite injury. En route to the hospital the patient remains alert, and you and the patient have an interesting conversation about how the rest of his summer has been. Because his serial vital signs are improving, infusion of IV fluid is slowed somewhat.

Prep Kit

Chapter Summary

- The lymphatic system is related very closely to the cardiovascular system. It transports excess tissue fluid to the bloodstream.

- The lymphatic system also absorbs fats and helps to defend against disease-causing agents.

- Lymphatic vessels only carry fluid away from the tissues. Lymphatic capillaries are in all tissues except the central nervous system, bone marrow, cartilage, epidermis, and cornea.

- To prevent tissues from becoming edematous, the lymphatic vessels absorb excess fluid and return it to the central venous circulation.

- Lymph capillaries join to form larger lymph vessels and tend to follow the course of an associated artery and vein. Valves prevent backflow through these vessels when they are squeezed. The lymphatic vessels empty into the subclavian vein by the lymphatic or thoracic ducts.

- The thymus and spleen are the predominant organs of the lymphatic system, along with structures known as lymph nodes.

- Lymphatic vessels pass through lymph nodes where lymph is filtered and foreign material is removed by lymphocytes.

- Denser arrangements of lymphoid tissue are called lymph nodules.

- Major collections of lymph nodes are located in the axilla, neck, and groin.

- Three sets of lymphatic organs comprise the tonsils: the palatine, pharyngeal, and lingual tonsils.

- Lymph nodes are round or bean-shaped structures distributed along the course of the lymph vessels, which filter the lymph and serve as a source of lymphocytes.

- The spleen is located in the left upper quadrant of the abdomen and consists of two types of lymph tissue: red pulp and white pulp.

- The thymus, located below the sternum in the superior mediastinum, is quite large in the infant and decreases in size with age.

- The thymus produces lymphocytes, a type of white blood cell that helps fight infection and aids immunity.

- The immune system, which controls the body's ability to resist damage from foreign substances, is integrally related to the lymphatic system and provides specific and nonspecific immune defenses.

- T and B cells reside in lymphatic tissues and organs and are vital for the body's self-protection.

- Numerous chemicals, which promote inflammation, are involved in the immune system. The most common chemicals are histamines, kinins, complement, prostaglandins, leukotrienes, pyrogens, and interferon.

- Leukocytes released into the blood will move toward areas of bacterial invasion or foreign bodies through a process called chemotaxis.

- Neutrophils usually are the first cells to enter infected tissues and will ingest bacteria through a process called phagocytosis. Larger cells called macrophages leave the bloodstream and enter diseased tissues to "clean up" the dead bacteria.

- Two types of specific immunity exist in the body: cellular immune response and humoral immune response.

- Cellular immune response is achieved by the actions of T lymphocytes, or T cells.

- Antibodies are gamma globulin proteins called immunoglobulins and include five major types: IgM, IgA, IgE, IgD, and IgG.

- Active immunity lasts much longer than passive immunity.

- The presence of allergens in the body can produce various types of allergies that the body may respond to either immediately or in a delayed manner.

- An infectious disease is one that may be transmitted from one person to another via some type of specific microscopic organism.

- Diseases are commonly transmitted from person to person by airborne, body substance, injection, or oral transmission.

- Thousands of types of microorganisms can cause disease; not all are visible to the naked eye. Several infectious agents include bacteria, viruses, fungi, protozoans, nematodes, and prions.

- The body normally contains numerous bacteria in its normal flora, which help maintain homeostasis. Normal flora colonizes areas including the skin, gastrointestinal tract and the oral and nasal cavities.

Vital Vocabulary

acquired immune deficiency syndrome (AIDS) The disease process that occurs following infection with the human immunodeficiency virus (HIV).

adaptive (specific) defense Immunity; it targets specific pathogens and acts more slowly than innate defenses.

adrenaline A naturally occurring hormone that also may be given as a cardiac drug and has alpha and beta effects; also called epinephrine.

allergens Antigens; chemicals that stimulate B cells to produce antibodies or allergies.

anaphylaxis An extreme systemic form of an allergic reaction involving two or more body systems.

antibodies Immunoglobulins; proteins secreted by certain immune cells that react against foreign antigens in the body by binding to the antigens, making them more visible to the immune system.

antigen-presenting cell An accessory cell, which may be a macrophage, B cell, or other type of cell that has processed antigen fragments on its surface.

antigens Substances foreign to the body.

autoantibodies Antibodies produced by the body in reaction to any of its own cells or cell products.

autoimmunity An abnormal immune response in which the body attacks its own tissues.

axillary nodes A large collection of lymph nodes located in the axilla (armpit).

B lymphocytes (B cells) Lymphocytes that exist in the blood and are abundant in the lymph nodes, bone marrow, intestinal lining, and spleen.

basophils White blood cells that work to produce chemical mediators during an immune response; they make up approximately 1% of leukocytes.

CD4 antigen A protein found on the surface of helper T cells that is adversely affected by exposure to HIV.

cell-mediated immunity The immune process by which T cell lymphocytes and macrophages attack and destroy pathogens or foreign substances; the process involves recognizing antigens, then secreting cytokines (specifically lymphokines) that attract other cells or stimulate the production of cytotoxic cells that kill the infected cells.

cellular immune response Cell-mediated immunity; it occurs when T cells attach to foreign, antigen-bearing cells such as bacterial cells, and interact with direct cell-to-cell contact.

cervical nodes A large collection of lymph nodes located in the neck.

chemotaxis The movement of additional white blood cells to an area of inflammation in response to the release of chemical mediators.

collecting ducts The thoracic duct and right lymphatic duct.

eosinophils White blood cells with a major role in allergic reactions and bronchoconstriction during an asthma attack; make up approximately 1% to 3% of leukocytes.

hapten A substance that normally does not stimulate an immune response but can be combined with an antigen and at a later point initiate an antibody response; found in certain drugs, dust particles, animal dander, and various chemicals.

helper T cells Cells that aid other white blood cells in carrying out cell-mediated immune functions, including maturation of B cells into plasma cells and memory B cells, and activation of cytotoxic T cells and macrophages.

hilum An indented region of a lymph node where blood vessels and nerves are attached.

human immunodeficiency virus (HIV) A virus that may lead to acquired immunodeficiency syndrome (AIDS); cells in the immune system are killed or damaged so that the body is unable to fight infections and certain cancers.

humoral immune response When antibodies react to destroy antigens or antigen-containing particles.

immune system The body system that includes all of the structures and processes designed to mount a defense against foreign substances and disease-causing agents.

immunity Physiologically, refers to the body's ability to protect itself from infectious disease.

immunoglobulins See antibodies.

infection The invasion of a host or tissue by pathogenic organisms such as bacteria, viruses, or parasites that produces illness that may or may not have clinical manifestations.

infectious disease A disease that is caused by infection or one that is capable of being transmitted to another person with or without direct contact.

inflammatory response A reaction by tissues of the body to irritation or injury, characterized by pain, swelling, redness, and heat.

inguinal nodes A large collection of lymph nodes located in the groin.

innate (nonspecific) defense An immune response that is predictable each time the body is exposed to a particular challenge. One that protects the body from pathogens involving mechanical barriers, chemical barriers, natural killer cells, inflammation, phagocytosis, fever, or species resistance.

lingual tonsils One of three sets of lymphatic organs that comprise the tonsils, they are located on the posterior margin of the tongue and help protect the body from bacteria introduced into the mouth and nose.

lymph A thin plasma-like liquid formed from interstitial or extracellular fluid that bathes the tissues of the body.

lymph nodes Round or bean-shaped structures interspersed along the course of the lymph vessels, which filter the lymph and serve as a source of lymphocytes.

lymph nodules Tissue that is denser than diffuse lymphatic tissue, found in the loose connective tissue of the digestive, respiratory, and urinary systems.

lymph sinuses Spaces inside lymph nodes that comprise complex channels through which lymph moves.

lymphadenitis Inflammation of a lymph node caused by infection.

lymphadenopathy Any swelling of the lymph nodes, with or without pain.

lymphangitis An infection that spreads beyond the local area into a lymphatic vessel causing red streaks to run from the infected area proximally.

lymphatic capillaries Vessels of the lymphatic system that carry fluid away from the tissues and toward one of the great lymph vessels.

lymphatic duct One of two great lymph vessels; it empties into the subclavian vein.

lymphatic pathways Tiny tubes formed from lymphatic capillaries that merge to form larger vessels.

lymphatic system A passive circulatory system that transports a plasma-like liquid called lymph, a thin fluid that bathes the tissues of the body.

lymphatic trunks Structures that drain lymph from lymphatic vessels and join either the thoracic duct or the right lymphatic duct.

lymphatic vessels Thin-walled vessels through which lymph circulates in the body, they travel close to the major arteries and veins.

lymphocytes The white blood cells responsible for a large part of the body's immune protection.

lymphokines Cytokines produced by T cells that recruits mast cells and other nonspecific inflammatory mediators to aid in destruction of antigens.

lysis The process of disintegration or breakdown of cells that occurs when excess water enters the cell through osmosis.

macrophages Cells that develop from the monocytes that provide the body's first line of defense in the inflammatory process.

mast cells The cells that resemble basophils but do not circulate in the blood; have a role in allergic reaction, immunity, and wound healing.

memory T cells The form into which T cells differentiate when activated by an antigen; memory T cells remain within the body, ready to respond to a second challenge.

metastasize The spreading of a disease from one part of the body to another, especially with many forms of cancer.

microorganisms Organisms of microscopic size.

mononuclear phagocytic system Phagocytic cells that remove foreign particles from the lymph and blood.

neutrophils Usually the first cells to enter infected tissues, they ingest bacteria through phagocytosis.

normal flora Bacteria found in certain sites in the body, such as the gastrointestinal tract, vagina, skin, and oral and nasal cavities, that help maintain homeostasis.

palatine tonsils One of three sets of lymphatic organs that comprise the tonsils. They are located in the back of the throat, on each side of the posterior opening of the oral cavity, and help protect the body from bacteria introduced into the mouth and nose.

pathogen A disease-causing agent, which may be a virus, bacterium, fungus, or protozoan.

phagocytosis The process of ingesting and destroying foreign matter by certain types of leukocytes.

pharyngeal tonsils One of three sets of lymphatic organs that comprise the tonsils, they are located near the internal opening of the nasal cavity and help protect the body from bacteria introduced into the mouth and nose. Also called adenoids.

plasma cells Cells that produce antibodies (immunoglobulins) to destroy antigens or antigen-containing particles; plasma cells are formed from divided and differentiated B cells.

primary immune response The activation of B or T cells after they first encounter the antigens for which they are specialized to react; the process continues for several weeks.

right lymphatic duct The smaller of the two collecting ducts; it receives lymph from the right side of the head and neck, right upper limb, and right thorax.

secondary immune response The appearance of concentrations of antibodies in the blood plasma, usually 5 to 10 days after exposure to antigens.

species resistance An innate (nonspecific) defense wherein one species is resistant to certain diseases that may affect other species.

spleen The largest lymphatic organ; filters the blood via the actions of lymphocytes and macrophages.

splenectomy Surgical removal of the spleen.

T lymphocytes (T cells) Specialized lymphocyte precursors that make up the majority of circulated blood lymphocytes.

thoracic duct One of two great lymph vessels; it empties into the superior vena cava.

thymus A gland that is larger in children but shrinks with age; it secretes thymosins, which are important in early immunity by affecting production and differentiation of lymphocytes.

tonsils Three sets of lymphatic organs—the palatine tonsils, pharyngeal tonsils, and lingual tonsils—that are located in the back of the throat and nasopharynx and protect the body from bacteria introduced into the mouth and nose.

vaccine A substance that includes antigens that stimulate an immune response against a particular pathogen.

Prep Kit, continued

Case Study Answers

1. What are the body's first routes of defense against a sting, bite, or local infection?

   Answer: The skin is the first route of defense against venoms. In this situation, the skin has been breached. Whenever a sting, bite, or local infection occurs, the body activates the lymphatic system to trap the foreign bacteria. This process often causes localized pain, swelling, and redness at the site.

2. What can be done immediately to minimize the spread of a foreign substance through the lymphatic system?

   Answer: The heart does not pump lymph fluid through the body. Compression of lymph vessels occurs by muscle movements, as well as by changes in the intrathoracic pressure during breathing. To minimize the movement of lymph from the injured extremity, the extremity should be immobilized to prevent muscle movement.

3. What potential problem is of most concern for a patient who has been bitten or stung?

   Answer: The most common problem associated with bites and stings is the potential for an allergic reaction or anaphylaxis (severe allergic shock). In the case of envenomation, the signs and symptoms begin with swelling (edema), bruising, bleeding, and pain. Progressive signs and symptoms may vary and can include difficulty breathing, swallowing, weakness, diaphoresis (sweating), hypotension, dysrhythmias, muscle twitching, and seizures.

4. What type of cells help fight infection in the body and are the most important component of the immune system?

   Answer: The most important component of the immune system is the leukocytes (white blood cells). Various types of leukocytes perform specific tasks, and when released into the blood, they move toward areas of bacterial invasion or foreign bodies and ingest and destroy the invaders.

5. Could a vaccination have prevented the patient's reaction to the snakebite?

   Answer: Vaccinations prevent infection by exposing the recipient to attenuated or dead bacteria, viruses, or their protein coats. For patients who have sustained serious snakebites, specific antivenin treatment may occasionally be helpful; therefore, early communication with the hospital regarding access to antivenin should be included in the prehospital care.

6. How are foreign substances removed from the body?

   Answer: Through the process of chemotaxis, leukocytes attack invading bacteria or foreign bodies, then, through the process of phagocytosis, neutrophils ingest and destroy the bacteria, and finally, macrophages enter diseased tissues to clean up the dead bacteria.

The Nervous System

Learning Objectives

1. Name the anatomic and functional divisions of the nervous system. (p 166)
2. Name the parts of a neuron and the function of each. (p 166-168)
3. Describe the types of neurons, nerves, and nerve tracts. (p 166-169)
4. Explain the importance of Schwann cells in the peripheral nervous system and neuroglia in the central nervous system. (p 166-168)
5. Describe the electrical nerve impulse and impulse transmission at the synapse. (p 166-169)
6. State the functions of the parts of the brain and locate each part on a diagram. (p 168-174)
7. Explain the importance of stretch reflexes, flexor reflexes, and a reflex arc. (p 170)
8. Name the meninges and point out their locations on a diagram. (p 172-174)
9. State the functions of cerebrospinal fluid. (p 173-174)
10. Name the cranial nerves. (p 181-182)
11. Distinguish between the sympathetic and parasympathetic divisions of the autonomic nervous system. (p 182-184)

Introduction

The nervous system is a complex array of structures that help control body function. It is composed of two major structures, the brain and the spinal cord, and thousands of nerves that allow every part of the body to communicate. This system is responsible for fundamental functions such as controlling breathing, pulse rate, and blood pressure. However, what makes the nervous system so special is that it allows the performance of higher lever activity, such as memory, understanding, and thought.

The nervous system is divided into two main portions: the central nervous system (CNS) and the peripheral nervous system **Figure 8-1**. The somatic nervous system is the part of the peripheral nervous system that regulates activities over which there is voluntary control, such as walking. The autonomic nervous system (ANS) controls the many body functions that occur without voluntary control, such as digestion. Together, as a whole, the nervous system can be divided anatomically into the central and peripheral nervous systems and functionally into somatic (voluntary) and autonomic (involuntary) components **Figure 8-2**.

The Nervous System

The nervous system is composed of specialized tissue that conducts electrical impulses between the brain and the rest of the body. Neural tissue contains two basic types of cells: nerve cells, which are known as neurons and contain projections called axons and dendrites that make connections between adjacent cells **Figure 8-3**, and neuroglia, which are supporting cells that have five basic functions. Neuroglia provide a supporting skeleton for neural tissue, isolate and protect the cell membranes of neurons, regulate the composition of interstitial fluid, defend neural tissue from pathogens, and aid in the repair of injury.

Axons may or may not be surrounded by a membrane sheath. In unsheathed or unmyelinated axons, action potential electrical signals in the nerves propagate along the entire axon membrane. Myelinated nerves are surrounded by a myelin sheath manufactured by a form of nervous tissue called Schwann cells **Figure 8-4**.

Nodes of Ranvier, which are narrow gaps between the Schwann cells, are located between the cells at intervals of

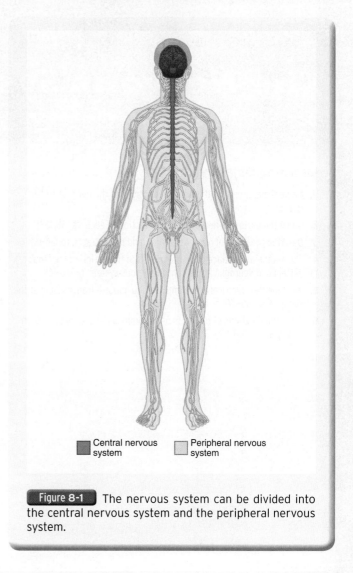

Central nervous system   Peripheral nervous system

Figure 8-1 The nervous system can be divided into the central nervous system and the peripheral nervous system.

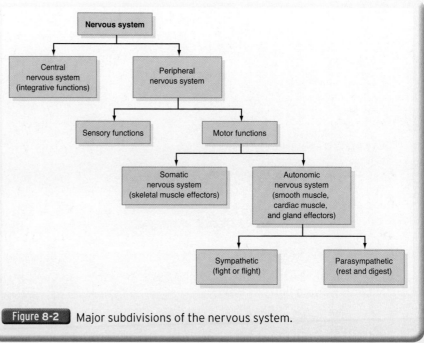

Figure 8-2 Major subdivisions of the nervous system.

approximately 1 to 1.5 mm (see Figure 8-5). In myelinated nerves, the action potential jumps between these regions, resulting in increased speed of transmission of the impulse. Bundles of myelinated nerves are referred to as white matter.

Between the nerve cells lies a gap called the synapse, which consists of a terminal bouton or other type of axon terminal, the synaptic cleft, and the membrane of the post-synaptic cell. The presynaptic terminal is at one end of a nerve. The synaptic cleft is the space between neurons. Opposite of the presynaptic terminal, across the synaptic cleft, is the postsynaptic terminal. Electrical impulses travel down the nerve and trigger the release of chemicals known as neurotransmitters from the presynaptic terminal. These neurotransmitters cross the synaptic cleft to stimulate an electrical reaction in adjacent neurons. Neurotransmitters are contained within synaptic vesicles

and are released into the synaptic cleft at the presynaptic terminal. This electrical reaction passes through the neuron to the next synapse, and the process is repeated Figure 8-5 .

Groups of nerve cells are bundled together to form nerve fibers. Groups of nerve fibers are bundled together to form a nerve, which is tissue that connects the nervous system with body parts or organs. As described earlier, the nervous system is divided into the central nervous system (CNS), the peripheral nervous system (PNS), and the autonomic nervous system (ANS). The CNS is composed of the brain and spinal cord. The CNS includes the second cranial or optic nerve which is actually a tract of the central nervous system as opposed to an independent nerve. The remaining 11 pairs of cranial nerves that branch directly from the brain as well as the 31 pairs of spinal nerves that exit the spinal cord via the vertebral column

Case Study PART 1

At 7:00 PM on a summer evening, you respond to a call at a high bridge at the riverfront. The regional swift water team has pulled a 50-year-old man from the river after he jumped 70 feet into the river from the bridge railing.

Your general impression is a conscious, thin, middle-aged man. He has already been immobilized on a long backboard. You are told that the patient initially was very confused and disoriented. At this time, he is able to answer questions although he is not willing to talk about how he ended up in the river.

The patient's airway is open, and he is having difficulty breathing. His pulse is weak and rapid with a regular rate and he is cold from the river water. He tells you that he has no feeling in his legs. You administer oxygen using a nonrebreathing mask.

Recording Time: 0 minutes	
Appearance	Pale, and struggling to breathe
Level of consciousness	Alert (oriented to person, place, and day)
Airway	Appears patent
Breathing	Struggling to breathe
Circulation	Cold skin, weak distal pulse, no external bleeding
Pulse	100 beats/min, regular and weak
Blood pressure	100 mm Hg by palpation
Respirations	24 breaths/min, labored
Spo$_2$	92%

1. What part of the nervous system contains the nerves and sensors that are responsible for motor and sensory function of the body?

2. How can the knowledge of dermatomes help you to anticipate the level of treatment that may be required for a patient with a traumatic injury?

are part of the PNS. The ANS controls smooth muscle, cardiac muscle, and glands and is responsible for the "fight-or-flight" response. Autonomic functions are not under conscious control and include such activities as maintaining the pulse rate and blood pressure, intestinal motility, and pupillary response.

The Central Nervous System

The central nervous system consists of the brain and the spinal cord, both of which are encased in and protected

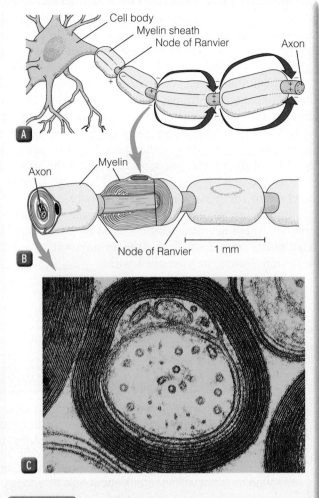

© Visuals Unlimited, Inc.

Figure 8-4 A myelinated nerve. **A.** The myelin sheath allows impulses to "jump" from node to node, greatly accelerating the rate of transmission. **B.** The node of Ranvier. **C.** A transmission electron micrograph of an axon in a cross section, showing a myelin sheath.

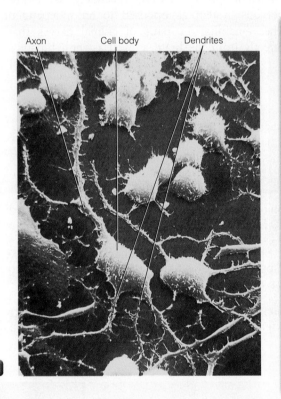

© David M. Phillips/Visuals Unlimited

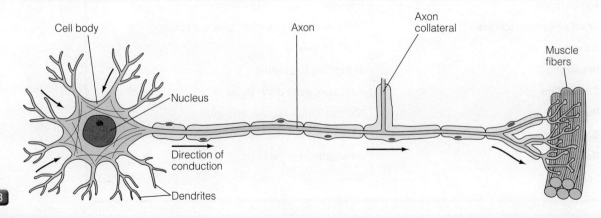

Figure 8-3 A neuron. **A.** A scanning electron micrograph of the cell body (the nucleus-containing central part of a neuron exclusive of its axons and dendrites) and dendrites. **B.** Collateral branches may occur along the length of the axon. In motor neurons, when the axon terminates, it branches many times, ending on individual muscle fibers.

by bone. The <u>brain</u> is located within the cranial cavity and contains billions of neurons that serve a variety of vital functions. It is the controlling organ of the body. It is the center of consciousness. It is responsible for all of your voluntary body activities, your perception of your surroundings, and the control of your reactions to the environment.

The brain is subdivided into several areas, all of which have specific functions. The major subdivisions of the brain are the cerebrum, diencephalon (thalamus and hypothalamus), cerebellum, and the brainstem. Collectively, the midbrain, pons, and medulla are referred to as the <u>brainstem</u> **Figure 8-7**. The largest part of the brain is the

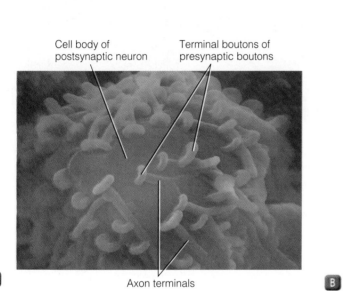

A · Cell body of postsynaptic neuron · Terminal boutons of presynaptic boutons · Axon terminals

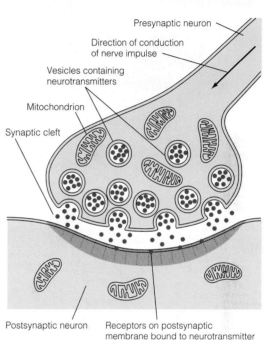

B · Presynaptic neuron · Direction of conduction of nerve impulse · Vesicles containing neurotransmitters · Mitochondrion · Synaptic cleft · Postsynaptic neuron · Receptors on postsynaptic membrane bound to neurotransmitter

© Science VU/E.R. Lewis/Visuals Unlimited

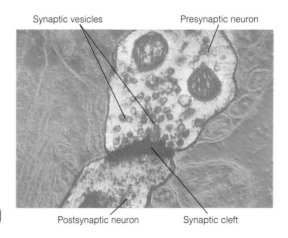

C · Synaptic vesicles · Presynaptic neuron · Postsynaptic neuron · Synaptic cleft

© Science VU/Lewis-Everhart-Zeevi/Visuals Unlimited

Figure 8-5 The function of neurotransmitters in the synaptic cleft. **A.** A scanning electron micrograph showing the terminal boutons of an axon ending on the cell body of another neuron. **B.** The arrival of the impulse stimulates the release of neurotransmitters held in synaptic vesicles in the axon terminals. Neurotransmitter diffuses across the synaptic cleft and binds to the postsynaptic membrane, where it elicits another action potential that travels down the dendrite to the cell body. **C.** A transmission electron micrograph showing the details of the synapse.

Pathophysiology

Spinal reflex arcs are automatic reactions to stimuli that occur without conscious thought Figure 8-6 . For example, the tendon stretch reflex occurs when the patella is tapped gently with a reflex hammer. The lower leg first moves sharply forward, then backward (extends and flexes). The flexor reflex is a withdrawal reflex, which affects the muscles of a limb, as when someone touches a very hot object or other unpleasant stimulus, the hand rapidly withdraws without any conscious action. These reactions are mediated locally within the spinal cord, although impulses from higher centers in the CNS normally regulate reflex activity.

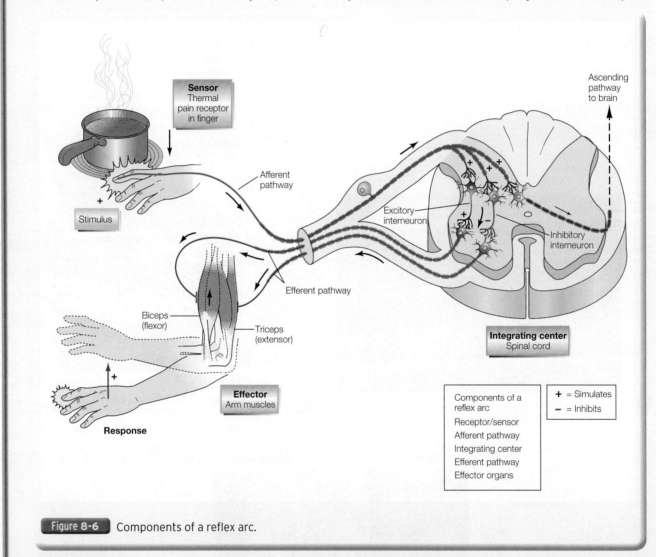

Figure 8-6   Components of a reflex arc.

Pathophysiology

A lesion of the substantia nigra, a layer of gray matter in the midbrain that helps produce dopamine, is believed to be responsible for Parkinson disease, a disorder resulting in tremor and decreased coordination.

Pathophysiology

In the brainstem, most nerves cross from one side to the other. Motor and sensory nerves on the left side of the brain, for example, serve the right side of the body. This is why a person who has had a stroke or trauma in one hemisphere has nerve deficits on the opposite side of the body. Because the cranial nerves are above this crossover point, their function will be affected on the same side of the body as the injury or stroke.

cerebrum, which makes up three fourths of the volume of the brain Figure 8-8 .

The Cerebrum

The cerebrum controls the higher thought processes. The cerebrum is divided into right and left hemispheres, or halves, by a longitudinal fissure. Numerous folds, called gyri, greatly increase the surface area of the cortex. Between the gyri are grooves called sulci.

Within each hemisphere are subdivisions known as lobes. Each lobe has the same name as that of the bone of the skull that overlies it. The frontal lobe is important in voluntary motor action as well as personality traits. The parietal lobe is the site for reception and evaluation of some sensory information, such as skin sensation, but excludes smell, hearing, and vision, and is separated from the frontal lobe by the central sulcus. Posteriorly, the occipital lobe is responsible for the processing of visual information. The temporal lobe plays an important role in hearing and memory and is separated from the rest of the cerebrum by a lateral fissure. Taste and smell receptors are located deeper within the cerebrum.

The cerebral cortex is a thin layer of gray matter comprising the outer portion of the cerebrum. It contains about 75% of all the neuron cell bodies of the nervous system. Beneath the cerebral cortex is white matter comprising most of the cerebrum. It contains myelinated axon bundles, some of which pass from one cerebral hemisphere to the other. Others carry impulses from the cortex to nerve centers of the brain and spinal cord.

The Diencephalon

The diencephalon is the part of the brain between the brainstem and the cerebrum and includes the thalamus, subthalamus, hypothalamus, and epithalamus Figure 8-9 . The thalamus processes most sensory input and influences mood and general body movements, especially those associated with fear or rage. The subthalamus is involved in controlling motor functions. The functions of the epithalamus,

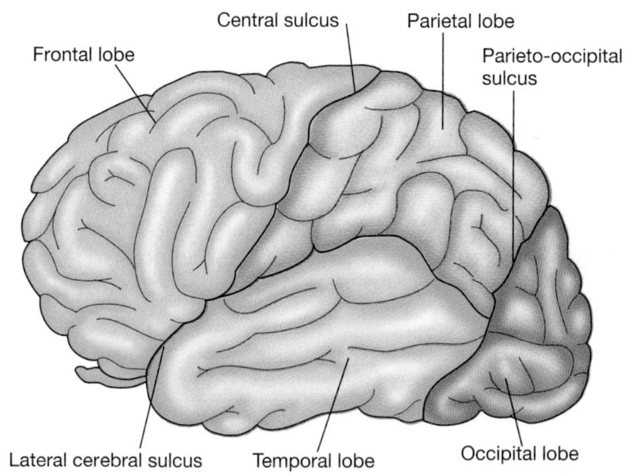

Pathophysiology

Several structures associated with the ascending reticular activating system are located throughout the brainstem. This region is responsible for maintenance of consciousness. This is why a sharp blow to the back of the neck, as with a karate chop, results in unconsciousness.

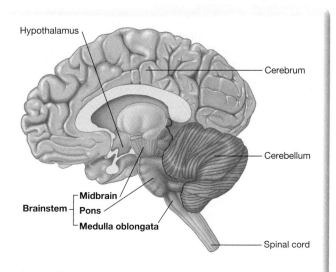

Figure 8-7 The brainstem consists of the medulla oblongata, pons, and midbrain.

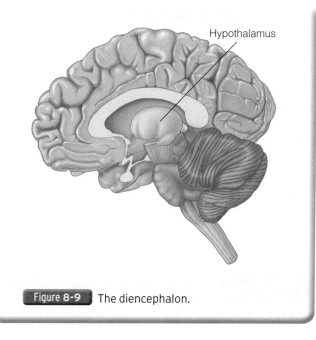

Figure 8-8 The lobes of the cerebrum.

Figure 8-9 The diencephalon.

especially the pineal body, involve control of emotions, circadian rhythms (our biological clock), and connecting the limbic system with the rest of the brain. The most inferior portion of the diencephalon is the hypothalamus. This organ is vital in the control of many body functions, including pulse rate, digestion, sexual development, temperature regulation, emotion, hunger, thirst, and regulation of the sleep cycle.

The Brainstem

The brainstem consists of the medulla, pons, and midbrain and connects the spinal cord to the remainder of the brain. The brainstem is vital for many very basic body functions. Damage to portions of the brainstem can easily result in death. All but two of the twelve cranial nerves exit from the brainstem. The midbrain lies immediately below the diencephalon and is the smallest region of the brainstem.

Deep within the cerebrum, diencephalon, and midbrain is a set of important structures known as the basal ganglia. The basal ganglia (or basal nuclei) play an important role in coordination of motor movements and posture. Portions of the cerebrum and diencephalon are referred to as the limbic system, which includes several structures that influence emotions, motivation, mood, and sensations of pain and pleasure Figure 8-10 .

The pons lies below the midbrain and above the medulla Figure 8-11 . It contains numerous important nerve fibers, including those for sleep, respiration, and the medullary respiratory center.

The inferior portion of the midbrain, the medulla, is continuous inferiorly with the spinal cord (see Figure 8-7).

The medulla serves as a conduction pathway for both ascending and descending nerve tracts. It also coordinates the pulse rate, blood vessel diameter, breathing, swallowing, vomiting, coughing, and sneezing. The pons and medullary respiratory centers are responsible for all respiratory movements.

The Cerebellum

The cerebellum communicates with the other regions of the CNS through the cerebellar peduncles, a set of three bands of nerve fibers. The cerebellum is essential in coordinating muscle movements of the body. Normal cerebellar function is necessary for proper balance and movement.

Pathophysiology

Stroke is a serious medical condition in which blood supply to areas of the brain is interrupted, causing brain damage and abnormal neurologic findings. Stroke in 85% of patients is caused by occlusion of the arteries to the brain. Most of the time, an artery is blocked by atherosclerotic plaques, similar to those that block arteries of the heart in coronary artery disease. Sometimes, small clots or emboli that are formed elsewhere flow to and block the lumen of an artery. Stroke also can result from bleeding within the brain or surrounding membranes.

The major risk factors for stroke are cigarette smoking and alcohol abuse. Embolic stroke often is a result of a blood clot that arises in the heart because of a cardiac rhythm disorder. The most common underlying condition resulting in embolic stroke is atrial fibrillation. Hemorrhagic stroke (bleeding) may be caused by trauma, or it may occur as a result of high blood pressure, cocaine use, or several systemic illnesses. Patients may have a severe headache, seizure, or loss of consciousness. Typically, blood pressure is elevated because the normal response of the body is to try to maintain blood flow to the compromised area.

Computed tomographic (CT) scans often are obtained for patients with a suspected stroke, and patients are immediately referred to a neurosurgeon if bleeding is seen on the scan. In some areas, physicians are using thrombolytic therapy or "clot busters" for acute treatment of embolic stroke.

A transient ischemic attack (TIA) is an episode of neurologic impairment that lasts less than 24 hours. However, TIA is a serious warning sign of impending stroke, particularly within the first 2 weeks following the attack.

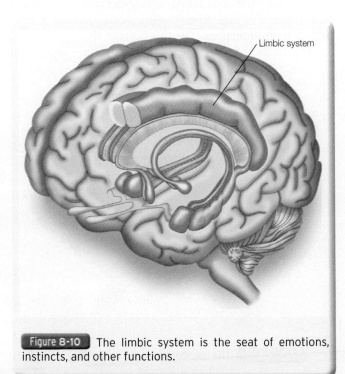

Limbic system

Figure 8-10 The limbic system is the seat of emotions, instincts, and other functions.

The Meninges

The entire CNS is enclosed by a set of three tough membranes known as the meninges Figure 8-12 . The outer membrane is the dura mater and is the toughest membrane. The dura mater is made up of fibrous, tough,

Cerebral cortex

- Receives sensory information from skin, muscles, glands, and organs
- Sends messages to move skeletal muscles
- Integrates incoming and outgoing nerve impulses
- Performs associative activities such as thinking, learning, and remembering

Basal nuclei

- Plays a role in the coordination of slow, sustained movements
- Suppresses useless patterns of movement

Thalamus

- Relays most sensory information from the spinal cord and certain parts of the brain to the cerebral cortex
- Interprets certain sensory messages such as those of pain, temperature, and pressure

Hypothalamus

- Controls various homeostatic functions such as body temperature, respiration, and heartbeat
- Directs hormone secretions of the pituitary

Cerebellum

- Coordinates subconscious movements of skeletal muscles
- Contributes to muscle tone, posture, balance, and equilibrium

Brainstem

- Origin of many cranial nerves
- Reflex center for movements of eyeballs, head, and trunk
- Regulates heartbeat and breathing
- Plays a role in consciousness
- Transmits impulses between brain and spinal cord

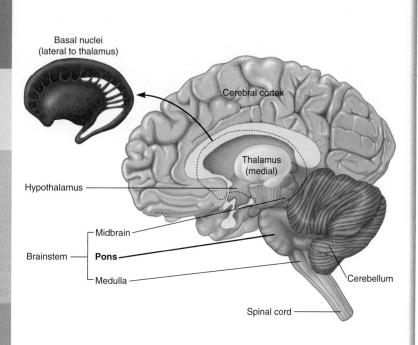

Figure 8-11   The relative position of the brainstem and pons in the brain.

white connective tissue. It has many blood vessels and nerves, and attaches to the inside of the cranial cavity; it also extends inward between the brain lobes to form protective partitions. It continues into the vertebral canal to surround the spinal cord, ending in a sac at its end. The second layer, the thin, weblike arachnoid, lies between the dura and pia maters. The innermost layer, resting directly on the brain or spinal cord, is the pia mater. The thin pia mater has many blood vessels and nerves that nourish the brain and spinal cord. The pia mater is closely aligned with the surfaces of these organs. When a hematoma develops, it can be classified according to its location in respect to the meninges (an epidural or a subdural hematoma). The meninges float in watery, clear cerebrospinal fluid (CSF),

Pathophysiology

Meningitis is an inflammation of the meninges and CSF, usually caused by infection. Acute bacterial meningitis can be life threatening. Early suspicion and antibiotic therapy are essential. Diagnosis is made by a physician withdrawing a specimen of CSF using a needle inserted into the vertebral canal in a procedure known as a lumbar puncture or spinal tap.

Pathophysiology

Bleeding can occur between the meninges and the brain, usually as a result of trauma. The most common type of bleeding occurs with a subarachnoid hemorrhage, in which the blood lies between the arachnoid and the pia mater.

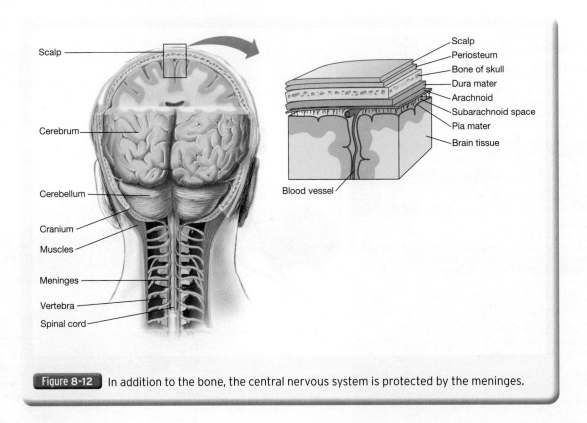

Scalp
Cerebrum
Cerebellum
Cranium
Muscles
Meninges
Vertebra
Spinal cord

Scalp
Periosteum
Bone of skull
Dura mater
Arachnoid
Subarachnoid space
Pia mater
Brain tissue
Blood vessel

Figure 8-12   In addition to the bone, the central nervous system is protected by the meninges.

Pathophysiology

Obstruction to the flow of CSF results in increased pressure within the brain tissue, dilation of the ventricles, and compression of the brain, a condition known as hydrocephalus **Figure 8-13**.

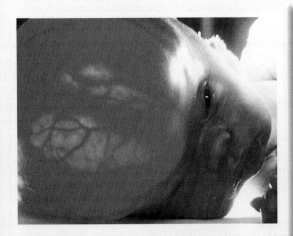

© Stu/Visuals Unlimited

Figure 8-13   Hydrocephalus. The birth defect results from a blockage in the ventricles that causes CSF to build up, thinning the cortex and causing severe brain damage.

Pathophysiology

In patients with a fracture at the base of the skull, CSF can leak into the eustachian tubes, past the eardrums, and out through the ears. Because CSF does not mix well with blood, it sometimes appears as a halo of clear fluid around drops of blood when it leaks onto a gauze pad. CSF that leaks into the back of a patient's throat because the patient is in a seated position, often is described as having a "salty taste." Ironically, CSF is of the same chemical consistency as seawater, thus accounting for its salty taste.

which is manufactured in the ventricles of the brain and flows in the subarachnoid space. The subarachnoid space is located between the pia mater and the arachnoid.

CSF is manufactured by specialized cells within the choroid plexus in the ventricles, specialized hollow areas in the brain. These areas normally are interconnected, and CSF flows freely between them. CSF is similar in composition to plasma. The meninges and CSF form a fluid-filled sac that cushions and protects the brain and spinal cord.

The Spinal Cord

At the base of the brain, the spinal cord, a thin column of nerves leading from the brain to the vertebral canal, represents the continuation of the central nervous system

Case Study | **PART 2**

Because of the significance of the mechanism of injury (MOI), you decide to limit time at the scene. You begin the rapid trauma exam and obtain serial vital signs, as your paramedic partner starts two large-bore IV lines of normal saline. The physical examination shows the following:

- Head: Unremarkable
- Neck: Unremarkable
- Chest: Tenderness of the right lower ribs
- Abdomen and pelvis: Contusions to the RUQ and LLQ
- Back and buttocks: Line of demarcation for loss of sensation noted at approximately T12, L1 (the lower abdomen and buttocks)
- Upper extremities: A possible closed fracture to the right humerus, contusions, and swelling
- Lower extremities: No sensation or motor function to either leg

Because the patient is alert and able to speak, you obtain a SAMPLE history during transit to the regional trauma center. His vital signs are monitored every 5 minutes during transport. The SAMPLE history shows the following:

- **S**igns and symptoms: Nausea, dizziness, thirst, and chills
- **A**llergies to medications: Codeine and penicillin
- **M**edications taken: Paxil, Valium, and Librium
- **P**ast pertinent medical history: Depression and stress-related syndrome
- **L**ast food/oral intake: Breakfast this morning
- **E**vents prior to onset: Patient felt depressed and had not taken his medications because they make him sleepy. He states that he jumped off the bridge in an attempt to kill himself.

Recording Time: 5 minutes

Level of consciousness	Alert (oriented to person, place, and day)
Airway	Appears open and patent
Breathing	Labored and shallow
Circulation	Pale and clammy, no external bleeding
Pulse	94 beats/min, weak
Blood pressure	100/70 mm Hg
Respirations	24 breaths/min and labored
Spo$_2$	92%
Electrocardiogram	Normal sinus rhythm with no ectopy

3. What part of the nervous system is responsible for the "fight-or-flight" response associated with stress or shock?

4. Is the response to shock normal in this patient? Explain.

5. How is an impulse transmitted from nerve to nerve?

Clinical Tip

Cerebrospinal fluid (CSF) is a clear body fluid that can carry the same infectious diseases as blood. The risk of exposure to infectious agents from CSF can be even greater than from blood, because its presence is not as obvious as blood is at first sight. To avoid exposure to infectious agents, you should always wear gloves when making patient contact.

Figure 8-14. The spinal cord is composed of bundles of nerve fibers and leaves the skull through a large opening at the base called the <u>foramen magnum</u>. The principal

function of the spinal cord is to transmit messages between the brain and the body. These messages are passed along the nerve fibers as electrical impulses, just as messages are passed along a telephone cable. The nerve fibers are arranged in specific bundles within the spinal cord to carry the messages from one specific area of the body to the brain and back.

The spinal cord has spinal nerves that arise from each of its 31 segments. In the neck, the spinal cord thickens to form the cervical enlargement, which supplies nerves to the upper limbs. The lumbar enlargement in the lower back supplies nerves to the lower limbs. The spinal cord is divided into right and left halves by a deep anterior median fissure and a shallow posterior median fissure **Figure 8-15**.

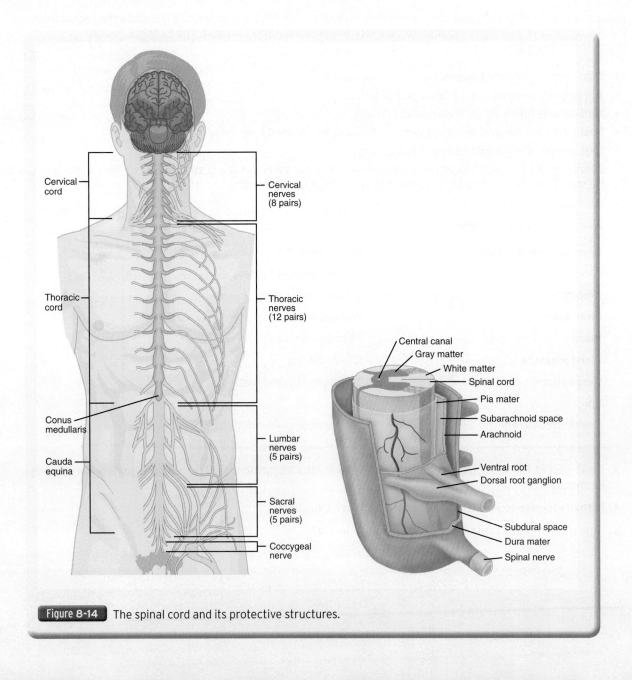

Figure 8-14   The spinal cord and its protective structures.

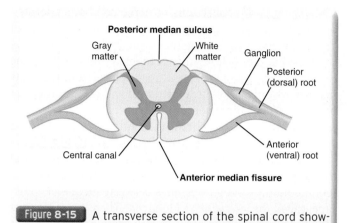

Figure 8-15 A transverse section of the spinal cord showing spinal nerve roots.

to the level at which they exit the spinal canal. Within the spinal cord are numerous tracts, or pathways, that contain nerve fibers **Figure 8-16**.

Pathophysiology

Various lesions of the spinal cord result in typical sensory deficits or losses. The physician uses the known patterns of nerve distribution, dermatomes, to aid in localizing the anatomic position of the lesion.

Pathophysiology

Injuries to the intervertebral disks of the lumbar spine can result in irritation of the spinal nerve roots. Muscle weakness and pain may then travel from the back, down the buttocks, along the entire leg and into the foot. This pain often is called sciatica.

The spinal cord extends to approximately the level of the space between the first and second lumbar vertebrae. At this point, it gives rise to numerous individual nerve roots, called the cauda equina. Throughout its length, the spinal cord is encased in the bony vertebral canal formed by the individual vertebrae. Nerves branch off at regular intervals between vertebrae and are numbered according

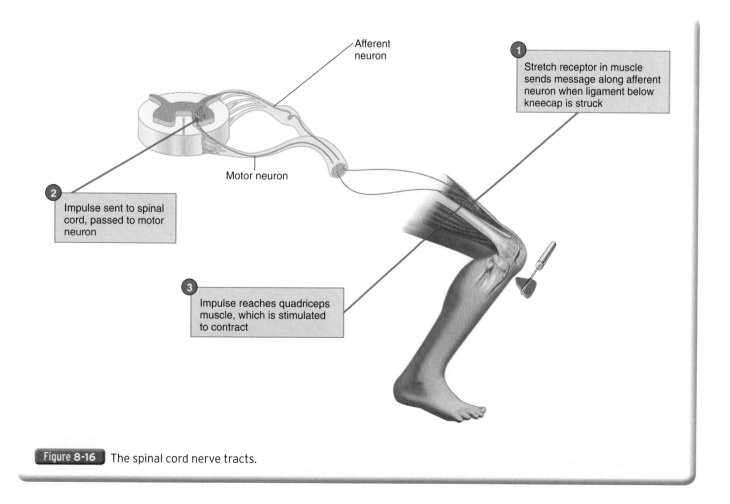

Figure 8-16 The spinal cord nerve tracts.

Two-way communication flows between the brain and other body parts because of the spinal cord. Ascending tracts carry sensory information in the form of action potentials, from the periphery back to the brain. Descending tracts carry motor impulses, also in the form of action potentials, from the brain to the fibers of the peripheral nervous system.

Major ascending tracts include the spinothalamic tract and the spinocerebellar tract. The anterior spinothalamic tracts carry light touch, pressure, and tickling and itching sensations. The lateral spinothalamic tracts carry pain and temperature information. The spinocerebellar tracts carry information regarding body position (proprioception) to the cerebellum. In addition, the posterior columns carry positional and vibration signals to the brain. Descending tracts, including the corticospinal tracts, coordinate voluntary movements, especially of the limbs. The vestibulospinal and reticulospinal tracts control involuntary body movements.

The Peripheral Nervous System

The peripheral nervous system consists of nerves that extend from the CNS to peripheral structures outside the CNS. Ganglia are collections of nerve cell bodies located outside the CNS. Spinal nerves arise from numerous small nerves called rootlets along the dorsal and ventral surfaces of the spinal cord. Roughly six to eight rootlets combine to form a ventral root; a dorsal root is formed in the same manner by other rootlets. One dorsal and one ventral root unite to form a spinal nerve, which eventually divides into several parts. The dorsal root is identified by an enlarged structure known as the dorsal root ganglion Figure 8-17.

With the exception of the first pair of spinal nerves and those in the sacrum, the remaining spinal nerves exit the vertebral column through openings between successive vertebrae, called the intervertebral foramen. There are eight pairs of spinal nerves in the cervical region, twelve in the thoracic region, five in the lumbar region, five in the sacral region, and one in the coccygeal region. Each of these pairs is numbered based on the vertebral level at which it exits the spinal canal (C1, T12).

The peripheral nervous system is made up of two types of nerves: sensory and motor nerves. Sensory nerves, or afferent nerves, carry impulses from the body to the brain and provide input to the brain about sensations that are felt, such as touch, pain, pressure, and temperature. When sensory nerve endings in the extremities

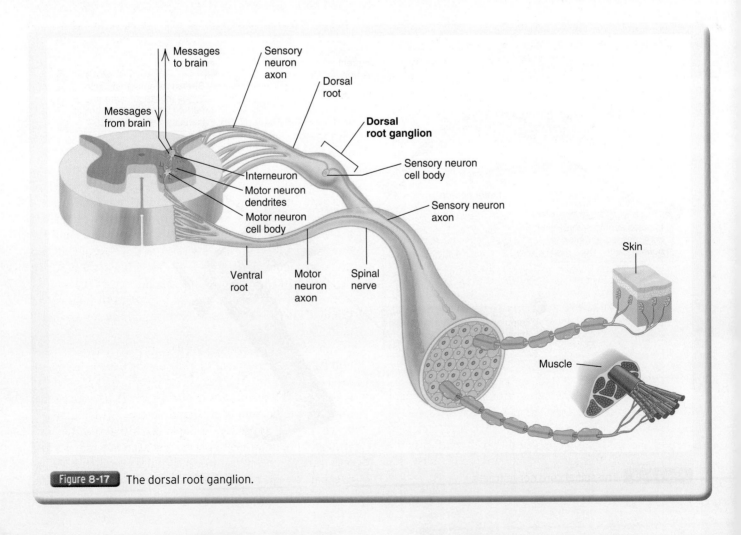

Figure 8-17 The dorsal root ganglion.

are stimulated, the impulses are transmitted along a peripheral nerve to the spinal cord. The cell body of the peripheral nerve lies in the spinal cord. The impulse is then transmitted from that cell body to another nerve ending in the spinal cord and from there up the spinal cord to the sensory area in the parietal lobe of the brain, where the sensory information can be interpreted and acted on by the brain. A dermatome is the area of skin supplied by a given pair of spinal sensory nerves. Except for C1, each spinal nerve has a specific sensory distribution on the surface of the body.

Motor nerves, or efferent nerves, carry commands from the brain to the receptor on the muscle for nerve impulses (neuromuscular junction), resulting in muscle contraction and motion. Each muscle in the body has its own motor nerve. The cell body for each motor nerve lies in the spinal cord, and a fiber from the cell body extends as part of the peripheral nerve to its specific muscle. Electrical impulses that are produced by the cell body in the spinal cord are transmitted along the motor nerve to the muscle and cause it to contract. The cell body in the spinal cord is stimulated by an impulse produced in the motor strip of the cerebral cortex. This impulse is transmitted along the spinal cord to the cell body of the motor nerve. Most nerves are mixed nerves, consisting of both sensory and motor nerves.

The main portions of the spinal nerves combine (except in the thoracic region) to form complex networks called plexuses. There are four plexuses in the body: the cervical plexus consists of spinal nerves C1 to C4; the brachial plexus, C5 to T1; the lumbar plexus, L1 to L4; and the sacral plexus, L4 to S4. The plexuses give rise to the peripheral nerves, which branch and eventually supply motor function and sensation to many areas of the body.

Clinical Tip

The agent curare prevents transmission of neural impulses across the neuromuscular junction. Large doses result in complete paralysis that is reversible with certain drugs. Various derivatives of curare, called neuromuscular blockers, are used in anesthesia to induce muscle relaxation. In the field, the most commonly used neuromuscular blocker is succinylcholine.

The Cervical Plexus

The cervical plexus provides innervation to the neck and posterior portion of the head. Fibers from the third, fourth, and fifth cervical nerves are combined into the right and left phrenic nerves **Figure 8-18**. These nerves conduct motor impulses to the diaphragm, causing the contraction that occurs during breathing.

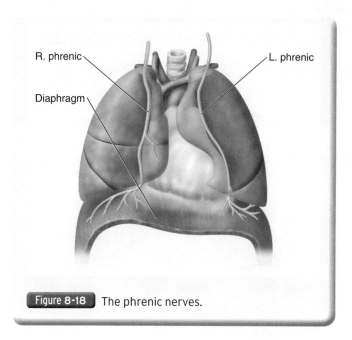

R. phrenic   L. phrenic

Diaphragm

Figure 8-18   The phrenic nerves.

The Brachial Plexus

The brachial plexus is divided into rami, trunks, divisions, cords, and branches. Together, the nerves in these divisions innervate the shoulder and upper extremity. The major nerves emanating from the brachial plexus are the axillary, radial, musculocutaneous, ulnar, and median nerves.

The axillary nerve supplies the deltoid and teres minor muscles, enabling arm abduction and lateral rotation. The radial nerve supplies the muscles that extend the elbow (brachioradialis and triceps brachii), supinate the forearm (supinator), and extend the wrist (extensor carpi muscles), fingers (extensor digitorum), and thumb muscles.

The musculocutaneous nerve innervates muscles that flex the shoulder and elbow (coracobrachialis, biceps brachii, and brachialis). The median nerve supplies the pronator muscles of the forearm, as well as those that flex the wrist (flexor carpi muscles and palmaris longus), the fingers (flexor digitorum muscles), and the thumb (flexor pollicis longus). The ulnar nerve innervates muscles that flex the wrist (flexor carpi ulnaris) and fingers (flexor digitorum muscles) and abduct and adduct the fingers and thumb (interossei, adductor pollicis, and the abductor pollicis).

In terms of sensory distribution, the axillary nerve innervates a small patch of skin on the lateral border of the proximal arm. The radial nerve provides sensation to the posterior arm and forearm as well as to the lateral two thirds of the dorsum of the hand. The musculocutaneous nerve provides sensation to the lateral surface of the forearm, and the ulnar nerve provides sensation to the medial one third of the hand, the little finger, and the medial one half of the ring finger. The median nerve provides sensation to the lateral two thirds of the palm of the hand, including the lateral half of the ring finger **Figure 8-19**.

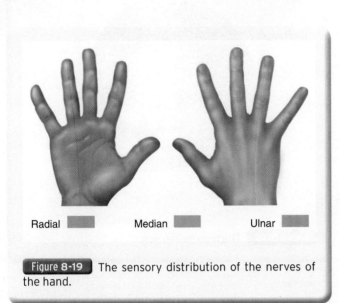

Radial   Median   Ulnar

Figure 8-19   The sensory distribution of the nerves of the hand.

Pathophysiology

The median nerve enters the wrist through the carpal tunnel, a narrow area between the carpal bones and the flexor retinaculum on the anterior surface of the wrist. Inflammation, overuse, and various disease states can result in carpal tunnel syndrome. In this condition, edema compresses the nerve, causing pain and difficulty in using the hand and wrist. Carpal tunnel syndrome often is claimed as a cause of occupational disability, especially in persons whose job involves the use of his or her hands for repetitive motion.

Pathophysiology

Damage to the radial nerve results in unopposed action of the muscles that flex the wrist and forearm, and the characteristic "wrist drop" develops.
Injury to the ulnar nerve results in unopposed extension of the thumb and first two fingers. This is called a "clawhand" deformity.

Case Study | PART 3

En route to the hospital, the patient tells you that this is not the first time he has tried to harm himself. You can see scars on his wrists from previous attempts at suicide. The patient's mental status remains alert and vital signs relatively unchanged from the baseline set. Your estimated time to arrival at the trauma center is only 6 minutes. You continue to keep the patient warm and reassess physical findings. The patient still has no sensation or motor function in either leg. When you assess for neurologic function, you find that the line of demarcation for loss of sensation noted at approximately T12, L1 (the lower abdomen and buttocks) is unchanged.

Recording Time: 10 minutes	
Level of consciousness	Alert (oriented to person, place, and day)
Airway	Open and patent
Breathing	Still labored but visible chest rise
Circulation	Pale, cool, and shivering
Pulse	90 beats/min, weak and regular
Blood pressure	106/70 mm Hg
Respirations	20 breaths/min, improved effort from baseline
Pupils	Equal and reactive
Spo$_2$	98%
Electrocardiogram	Normal sinus rhythm with no ectopy

6. If the patient's spinal cord has actually been severed, what nerves will most likely be dysfunctional?

7. Is the spinal cord injury in this patient currently a life-threatening condition?

The Lumbosacral Plexus

Four major nerves exit the lumbosacral plexus and supply the lower extremity: the obturator, femoral, tibial, and common peroneal nerves. Other nerves supply the lower back, hip, and lower abdomen.

The obturator nerve innervates muscles that adduct the thigh (adductor muscles and the gracilis) and rotate it laterally (obturator externus). The femoral nerve innervates the muscles that flex the hip (psoas major and sartorius) and extend the knee (rectus femoris and the vastus muscles). The tibial nerve innervates muscles that extend the hip and flex the knee (biceps femoris, semitendinosus, semimembranosus, and popliteus), plantar flex the ankle (gastrocnemius, soleus, plantaris, and tibialis posterior), and flex the toes (flexor muscles).

The common peroneal branch of the sciatic nerve innervates the short head of the biceps femoris muscle, causing extension of the hip and flexion of the knee. Along with the tibial nerve, the common peroneal nerve travels within a connective tissue sheath for the length of the thigh. Combined, these two nerves are called the sciatic nerve. The sciatic nerve is the largest peripheral nerve in the body **Figure 8-20**.

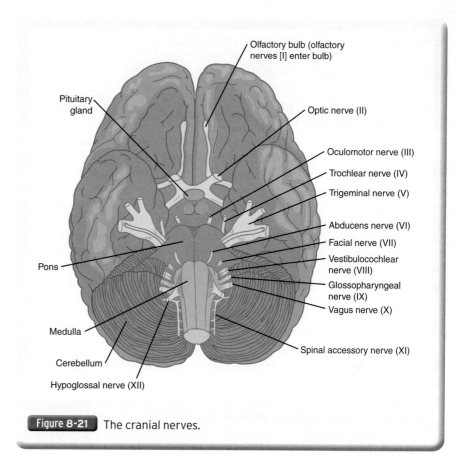

Figure 8-21   The cranial nerves.

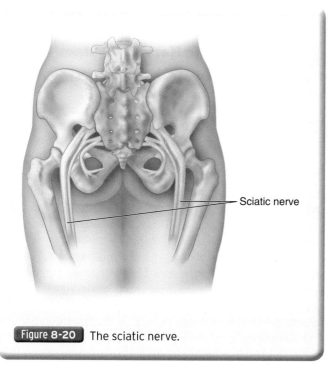

Figure 8-20   The sciatic nerve.

After wrapping around the neck of the fibula below the knee joint, the common peroneal nerve branches into the deep peroneal nerve and the superficial peroneal nerve. The deep branch innervates muscles that dorsiflex the ankle (tibialis anterior) and extend the toes (extensor hallucis longus and extensor digitorum longus). The superficial branch stimulates the muscles of plantar foot eversion (peroneus muscles).

The obturator nerve provides sensation to the upper medial side of the thigh. Sensory branches of the femoral nerve supply the thigh, medial leg, and medial aspect of the ankle. The tibial nerve provides sensation to the sole of the foot as well as to the posterior leg. The common peroneal nerve and its branches provide sensation over the lateral surface of the knee, the skin over the great and second toes, the dorsum of the foot, and the distal anterior one third of the leg.

The Cranial Nerves

Twelve pairs of cranial nerves arise from the base of the brain. All but two pairs, the olfactory nerves and the optic nerves, exit from the brainstem **Figure 8-21**.

Some of the cranial nerves carry only sensory fibers (I, II, and VIII), and others carry only motor fibers (III, IV, VI, XI, and XII). Many are mixed nerves, carrying a combination of sensory fibers and motor fibers (V, VII, IX, and X). Some cranial nerves also carry nerves of the parasympathetic nervous system in combination with motor, sensory, or both types of nerves (III, VII, IX, and X). Each nerve passes from the brain through a foramen in the skull to reach its endpoint.

The olfactory nerve (I) provides the sense of smell. The nerve arises at the base of the brain as the olfactory tract. The tract forms the olfactory bulb, which lies on the cribriform plate of the ethmoid bone. Nerve fibers penetrate the cribriform plate providing sensations of smell to the nose.

The optic nerve (II) provides the sense of vision. The optic tracts arise at the base of the brain, forming the optic chiasm, anterior to the pituitary gland. The optic nerves extend from the optic chiasm to each eyeball, passing through the optic foramina **Figure 8-22**.

The oculomotor nerve (III) innervates the muscles that cause motion of the eyeballs and upper lid. The oculomotor nerve also carries parasympathetic nerve fibers that cause constriction of the pupil (sphincter muscle), and accommodation of the lens (ciliary muscle).

The trochlear nerve (IV) innervates the superior oblique muscle of the eyeball, which allows a downward gaze. The trigeminal nerve (V) supplies sensation to the scalp, forehead, face, and lower jaw via three branches: the ophthalmic, maxillary, and mandibular divisions. The trigeminal nerve also provides motor innervation to the muscles of mastication, the throat, and the inner ear.

The abducens nerve (VI) supplies the lateral rectus muscle of the eyeball (lateral movement). The facial nerve (VII) supplies motor activity to all muscles of facial expression, the sense of taste to the anterior two thirds of the tongue, and cutaneous sensation to the external ear, tongue, and palate. The facial nerve also carries parasympathetic stimulation to the salivary glands, lacrimal gland, and the glands of the nasal cavity and palate.

The vestibulocochlear nerve (VIII) passes through the internal auditory meatus and provides the senses of hearing and balance. The glossopharyngeal nerve (IX) supplies motor fibers to the pharyngeal muscles. It provides taste sensation to the posterior portion of the tongue and carries parasympathetic fibers to the salivary glands (parotid glands) located on each side of the face.

The vagus nerve (X) provides motor functions to the soft palate, pharynx, and larynx (voice). The vagus nerve carries sensory fibers from the inferior pharynx, larynx, thoracic, and abdominal organs, taste bud fibers from the posterior tongue, and parasympathetic fibers to thoracic and abdominal organs.

The spinal accessory nerve (XI) (also referred to as the spinal accessory nerve) provides motor innervation to the muscles of the soft palate and the pharynx and to the sternocleidomastoid and trapezius muscles. The spinal accessory nerve controls swallowing, speech, head, and shoulder movements. The hypoglossal nerve (XII) provides motor function to the muscles of the tongue and throat and contains fibers from C1 to C3 of the upper spinal cord.

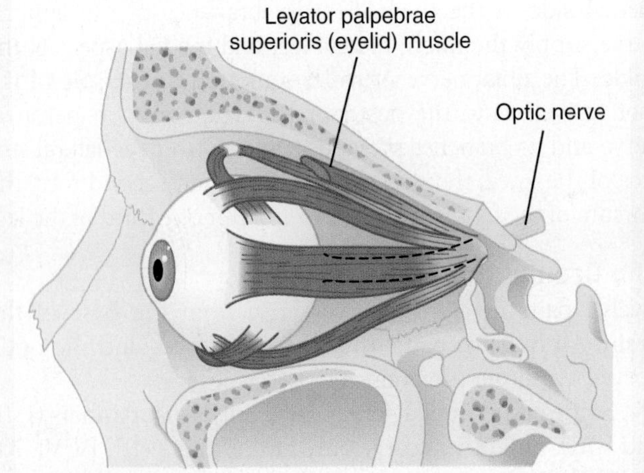

Pathophysiology

Unilateral paralysis of the facial nerve (Bells palsy) is relatively common. Although most causes of Bells palsy are idiopathic, physicians believe that viral infection may result in inflammation of the nerve leading to paralysis of muscles innervated by it. Alternatively, direct face, head, or brain injury can cause the condition in some persons. Sometimes, Bells palsy may accompany other signs of a stroke. In those cases, stroke must be ruled out by CT scan or MRI prior to initiating treatment. Patients with idiopathic paralysis have a relatively good prognosis, especially when they are treated early with corticosteroids to fight inflammation in the nerve.

The Autonomic Nervous System

The autonomic nervous system is part of the peripheral nervous system. Efferent neurons in the peripheral nervous system are separated into somatic and autonomic divisions **Figure 8-23**. The somatic division comprises the nerves of the peripheral nervous system that innervate functions under conscious control. The autonomic division, the autonomic nervous system (ANS), operates without conscious control and regulates the function of the internal organs, glands, and smooth muscle. The two divisions of the autonomic nervous system are the parasympathetic division and the sympathetic division.

The sympathetic pathway is responsible for the body's response to shock and stress. This response is associated with the release of adrenaline from the adrenal glands. Sympathetic responses include shunting of blood from the extremities to the vital core organs, increasing the pulse rate and respirations, increasing blood pressure, dilation of the pupils, and reduction of digestive system activity.

Figure 8-22 The optic nerve.

Levator palpebrae superioris (eyelid) muscle

Optic nerve

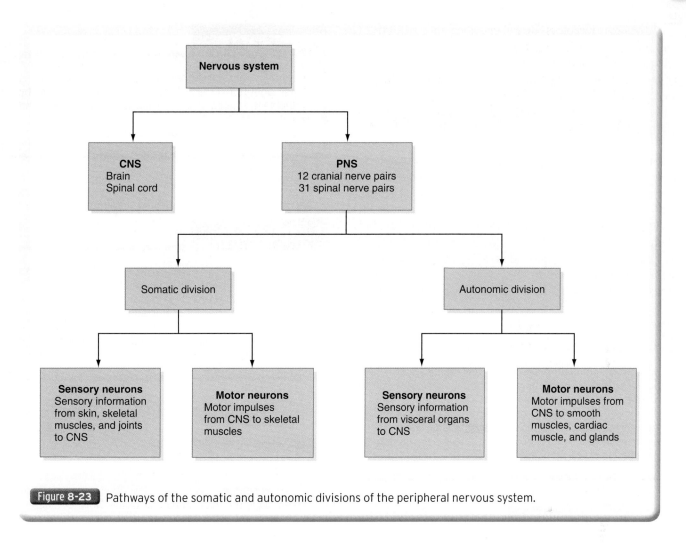

Figure 8-23 Pathways of the somatic and autonomic divisions of the peripheral nervous system.

The parasympathetic nervous system relaxes the body. The parasympathetic responses include slowing the pulse and respiratory rates, lowering the blood pressure, constricting the pupils, and increasing digestive system activity.

Preganglionic and Postganglionic Neurons

Although somatomotor nerves (sensory and motor nerves of the peripheral nervous system) extend directly from the CNS to skeletal muscle, nerves of the ANS contain two neurons in a series located between the CNS and the organs that are innervated. The first nerve, or preganglionic neuron, is separated from the second, the postganglionic neuron, by a ganglionic synapse. The preganglionic cell bodies are located within the central gray matter of the brainstem (the parasympathetic nervous system) and the spinal cord (the parasympathetic and sympathetic nervous systems). The cell bodies of the postganglionic neurons are located in autonomic ganglia and send their axons through nerves to various organs, where they synapse with the neuroeffector cells (target tissues).

Neurotransmitters and Receptors

The sympathetic and parasympathetic divisions secrete one of two neurotransmitters. A neuron that secretes acetylcholine is a cholinergic fiber. A neuron that secretes norepinephrine is an adrenergic fiber.

Both sympathetic and parasympathetic nerves release acetylcholine molecules from preganglionic fibers into the synaptic cleft. These molecules diffuse across to nicotinic receptors in the postganglionic neuron. These receptors are so named because they can be stimulated in the laboratory by the alkaloid nicotine. The impulse travels down the postganglionic neuron to reach the synapse at the target tissue with the neuroeffector cell. Acetylcholine is normally then rapidly destroyed by an enzyme, acetylcholinesterase.

At the target tissue, parasympathetic nerves release acetylcholine, which stimulates muscarinic receptors. Muscarinic receptors can be stimulated in the laboratory by the compound extracted from muscarine mushrooms. Sympathetic fibers release either norepinephrine, stimulating adrenergic receptors, or acetylcholine, stimulating muscarinic receptors.

All preganglionic neurons of the sympathetic and parasympathetic divisions and all postganglionic neurons of the parasympathetic division are cholinergic. Most postganglionic neurons of the sympathetic division are adrenergic, but a few, such as the postganglionic neurons that innervate sweat glands and a few blood vessels, are cholinergic.

Adrenergic receptors are subclassified into two structural and functional categories: alpha receptors and beta receptors. Norepinephrine binds to both but has somewhat greater affinity for alpha receptors. The substance epinephrine (adrenaline) is secreted by the adrenal gland and has nearly equal affinity for both receptor types. Alpha and beta receptors are further subdivided into alpha-1, alpha-2, beta-1, and beta-2 receptors.

Stimulation of various alpha and beta receptors can have either excitatory or inhibitory effects, depending on the location and type of the receptor. The primary type of stimulation in the heart involves beta-1 fibers. Such stimulation results in enhancement of myocardial cell contractility and an increased pulse rate. Beta-2 stimulation primarily affects the lungs, causing bronchodilation. Most alpha effects occur in the peripheral blood vessels, causing vasoconstrictions (alpha-1), and in the brain, having variable effects (alpha-2).

Pathophysiology

Muscarinic stimulation results in increased sweating, increased secretion of glands in the digestive system, decreased pulse rate, constriction of the pupils, and contraction of respiratory, digestive, and urinary system smooth muscles. Poisoning with agents such as nerve gas or pesticides inhibits acetylcholinesterase, resulting in excessive acetylcholine stimulation.

Pathophysiology

The symptoms of pathologic parasympathetic over-stimulation that would be seen in nerve gas poisoning are remembered by the mnemonic SLUDGE syndrome, which stands for: **s**alivation, **l**acrimation, **u**rination, **d**efecation, **g**astrointestinal cramping, and **e**mesis (vomiting).

Clinical Tip

A common class of cardiac drugs is the beta-blockers. These agents decrease the workload on the heart by reducing the speed of contraction, as well as by reducing the blood pressure. Because they also slow the patient's heart rate, they can possibly cause bradycardia.

Clinical Tip

The parasympathetic-blocking drug atropine blocks acetylcholine at the synapse with the neuroeffector cell, but it has no effect on transmission at autonomic ganglia. Administration of this agent results in a reduction of parasympathetic nervous system activity and is important in the treatment of patients with certain cardiac problems.

Pathophysiology

Beta-3 receptors have been described recently. They are found in the heart and in fat tissue. Normally, beta-3 receptors are minimally expressed; they only play a significant role, based on current knowledge, in heart failure when they come to the cell surface and bind to epinephrine and norepinephrine. Current thought is that their purpose may be to counteract the adverse effects of beta-1 and beta-2 overactivation. Beta-3 stimulation therefore has the opposite effect on the heart's contractility of beta-1 stimulation.

Case Study PART 4

On arrival at the hospital, you transfer patient care to the emergency department staff and give them an oral report. The patient has remained conscious and his vital signs have been maintained despite the progressing shock from his spinal injury. He has received approximately a liter of fluid at this point. Unfortunately, the patient's sensory and motor function below the umbilicus has not returned.

Prep Kit

Chapter Summary

- The nervous system is composed of neurons, which conduct electrical impulses and contain projections called axons and dendrites.

- The nervous system is divided into two main portions: the central nervous system and the peripheral nervous system.

- The somatic nervous system is the part of the peripheral nervous system that regulates activities over which there is voluntary control, such as walking.

- The autonomic nervous system controls the many body functions that occur without voluntary control, such as digestion.

- Axons that are sheathed by a membrane are called myelinated nerves, and when they are bundled together, they are referred to as white matter.

- The transmission across the synaptic cleft, between two neurons, is done by way of chemicals called neurotransmitters.

- The major regions of the adult's brain are the cerebrum (the largest portion), diencephalon, cerebellum, and brainstem.

- Each lobe of the cerebrum shares the name of the bone of the skull that overlies it.

- Portions of the cerebrum and diencephalon are referred to as the limbic system, which influences emotions, motivation, mood, and sensations of pain and pleasure.

- The cerebellum is essential in coordinating muscle movements and balance of the body.

- The brain and spinal cord are enclosed by three membranes called the meninges (the dura mater, arachnoid, and pia mater).

- The spinal cord extends from the base of the brain to the level of the second lumbar vertebra and then gives rise to the cauda equina.

- Within the spinal cord are numerous tracts or pathways containing axons, such as the afferent, or ascending, tracts and the efferent, or descending, tracts.

- The peripheral nervous system consists of nerves that extend from the CNS to peripheral structures outside the CNS.

- The two types of nerves in the peripheral nervous system are sensory and motor nerves. Sensory, or afferent, nerves carry impulses from the body to the brain, and motor, or efferent, nerves carry commands from the brain to the muscle.

- Several nerves come together to form a plexus, which then gives rise to peripheral nerves that supply motor function and sensation to many areas of the body.

- Twelve pairs of cranial nerves arise from the base of the brain. Each nerve passes from the brain through an opening in the skull to reach its endpoint.

- The parasympathetic and the sympathetic divisions comprise the autonomic nervous system.

- The parasympathetic nervous system functions as part of the rest-and-digest response, decreasing the pulse rate and the breathing rate.

- The sympathetic nervous system prepares the body for stressful or emergency situations and is part of the fight-or-flight response, increasing the pulse rate and the breathing rate.

- The sensory and motor nerves of the autonomic nervous system contain two neurons in a series, called the preganglionic neuron and the postganglionic neuron, that are located between the CNS and the organs that are innervated.

- The sympathetic and parasympathetic divisions secrete one of two neurotransmitters. A neuron that secretes acetylcholine is cholinergic and one that secretes norepinephrine is adrenergic.

- Both sympathetic and parasympathetic nerves release acetylcholine molecules from preganglionic fibers into the synaptic cleft. Adrenergic receptors are classified into two structural and functional categories: alpha receptors and beta receptors. Stimulation of these receptors can have either excitatory or inhibitory effects, depending on the location and type of the receptor.

Vital Vocabulary

abducens nerve The cranial nerve (VI) that supplies the lateral rectus muscle of the eyeball (lateral movement).

accessory nerve (also referred to as the spinal accessory nerve) The cranial nerve (XI) that provides motor innervation to the muscles of the soft palate and the pharynx and to the sternocleidomastoid and trapezius muscles.

acetylcholine A chemical neurotransmitter that serves as a mediator in both the sympathetic and parasympathetic nervous system.

acetylcholinesterase An enzyme that causes muscle relaxation by helping to break down acetylcholine.

action potentials An electrochemical event associated with cell membrane depolarization where stimulation of a nearby cell could cause excitation of another cell.

adrenal glands Endocrine glands located on top of the kidneys that release epinephrine and norepinephrine when stimulated by the sympathetic nervous system.

adrenergic Description of a neuron that secretes the neurotransmitter norepinephrine.

adrenergic receptors A type of receptor that is associated with the sympathetic nerves and is stimulated by epinephrine and norepinephrine.

afferent nerves Nerves that send information to the brain; also called sensory nerves.

alpha receptors One of two adrenergic receptors classified into two structural and functional categories; alpha receptors are further subdivided into alpha-1 and alpha-2 receptors.

anterior spinothalamic tracts Ascending fiber tracts that carry information to the brain about light touch, pressure, and tickling and itching sensations.

arachnoid The middle membrane of the three meninges that enclose the brain and spinal cord.

ascending tracts Fibers that carry sensory information from the periphery to the brain; also called afferent tracts.

ascending reticular activating system Several structures located throughout the brainstem that are responsible for maintenance of consciousness.

autonomic nervous system A subdivision of the nervous system that operates without conscious control and regulates the function of the internal organs, glands, and smooth muscle; comprised of the sympathetic and parasympathetic nervous systems.

axillary nerve One of the major nerves emanating from the brachial plexus; it supplies the deltoid and teres minor muscles, enabling arm abduction and lateral rotation.

axons Long, slender filaments projecting from a nerve cell that conduct impulses to adjacent cells.

basal ganglia (basal nuclei) Structures located deep within the cerebrum, diencephalon, and midbrain that play an important role in coordination of motor movements and posture.

beta-blockers A common class of cardiac drugs that blocks beta effects, causing a decrease in the workload of the heart by reducing the speed of contraction, as well as reducing blood pressure.

beta receptors One of two adrenergic receptors classified into two structural and functional categories; beta receptors are further subdivided into beta-1, beta-2, and beta-3 receptors.

brachial plexus The plexus of spinal nerves that consists of nerves C5 to T1 and innervates the shoulder and upper extremity.

brain The controlling organ of the body and center of consciousness; functions include perception, control of reactions to the environment, emotional responses, and judgment.

brainstem The area of the brain between the spinal cord and cerebrum, surrounded by the cerebellum; controls functions that are necessary for life, such as respiration.

cauda equina Numerous individual nerve roots that extend from the spinal cord at the level of the second lumbar vertebra.

central nervous system The brain and spinal cord.

cerebellar peduncles One of three bands of nerve fibers through which the cerebellum communicates with other regions of the central nervous system.

cerebellum The region of the brain essential in coordinating muscle movements of the body.

cerebral cortex The largest portion of the brain, it controls the higher thought processes; also called the cerebrum.

cerebrospinal fluid (CSF) Fluid produced in the ventricles of the brain that flows in the subarachnoid space and bathes the meninges.

cerebrum The largest portion of the brain that controls the higher thought processes, including control of movement, hearing, balance, speech, visual perception, emotions, and personality; also called the cerebral cortex.

cholinergic A term used to describe the fibers in the parasympathetic nervous system that release a chemical called acetylcholine.

choroid plexus Specialized cells within hollow areas in the ventricles of the brain that produce cerebrospinal fluid.

common peroneal nerve A major nerve of the leg, providing sensation to the lateral leg and dorsum of the foot and motor activity to hip extensors, knee flexors, ankle dorsiflexors, and toe extensors.

corticospinal tracts Descending tracts that coordinate movements, especially of the hands.

cranial nerves The 12 pairs of nerves that arise from the base of the brain.

curare An agent that blocks transmission of neural motor impulses at the neuromuscular junction.

deep peroneal nerve A component and branch of the common peroneal nerve that innervates the muscles that dorsiflex the ankle and extend the toes.

dendrites The parts of the neuron that receive impulses from the axon and contain vesicles for release of neurotransmitters.

dermatome An area of skin that corresponds to the sensory distribution of a specific cranial or spinal nerve.

descending tracts Fibers that carry motor impulses from the brain to the fibers of the peripheral nervous system; also called efferent tracts.

diencephalon The part of the brain between the brainstem and the cerebrum that includes the thalamus and hypothalamus.

dorsal root One of two roots of a spinal nerve that passes posteriorly into the spinal cord and contains the dorsal root ganglion.

dorsal root ganglion A ganglion on the dorsal root of each spinal nerve.

dura mater The outermost of the three meninges that enclose the brain and spinal cord; it is the toughest membrane.

efferent nerves Nerves that carry commands from the brain to peripheral muscles; also called motor nerves.

epithalamus Part of the diencephalon with functions related to emotions, circadian rhythms, and connecting the limbic system with other parts of the brain.

facial nerve The cranial nerve (VII) that supplies motor activity to all muscles of facial expression, the sense of taste to the anterior two thirds of the tongue, and cutaneous sensation to the external ear, tongue, and palate.

femoral nerve The branch of the lumbosacral plexus that innervates the muscles that flex the hip and extend the knee.

flexor reflex A withdrawal reflex in the flexor muscles of the limbs that contract in response to an unpleasant stimulus.

foramen magnum A large opening at the base of the skull through which the spinal cord exits the brain.

frontal lobe The portion of the brain that is important in voluntary motor actions and personality traits.

ganglia Collections of nerve cell bodies located outside the central nervous system.

ganglionic synapse The separation between two nerves (preganglionic and postganglionic neurons), that serves to connect the central nervous system and the organs innervated.

glossopharyngeal nerve The cranial nerve (IX) that supplies motor fibers to the pharyngeal muscle, provides taste sensation to the posterior portion of the tongue, and carries parasympathetic fibers to the parotid gland.

gyri The numerous folds in the cerebrum, which greatly increase the surface area of the cortex.

hypoglossal nerve The cranial nerve (XII) that provides motor function to the muscles of the tongue and throat.

hypothalamus The most inferior portion of the diencephalon; it is responsible for control of many body functions, including pulse rate, digestion, sexual development, temperature regulation, emotion, hunger, thirst, and regulation of the sleep cycle.

internal auditory meatus A short canal through which auditory and facial nerves pass.

intervertebral foramen Openings between successive vertebrae through which nerves exit the vertebral column.

lateral spinothalamic tracts Ascending tracts that carry information to the brain about pain and temperature.

limbic system Structures within the cerebrum and diencephalon that influence emotions, motivation, mood, and sensations of pain and pleasure.

lobes Subdivisions within each hemisphere of the cerebrum; each lobe shares the name of the bone of the skull that overlies it.

longitudinal fissure The crevasse that separates the right and left hemispheres of the cerebrum.

lumbar puncture A needle insertion through the vertebral canal into the subarachnoid space to obtain a specimen of cerebrospinal fluid.

lumbosacral plexus A combination of the lumbar plexus, the sacral plexus, and the coccygeal root.

median nerve The nerve in the brachial plexus that innervates the pronator muscles of the forearm, as well as those that flex the wrist, fingers, and thumb.

medulla The inferior portion of the midbrain, which serves as a conduction pathway for both ascending and descending nerve tracts.

meninges A set of three tough membranes, the dura mater, arachnoid, and pia mater, that encloses the entire brain and spinal cord.

meningitis An inflammation of the meninges and cerebrospinal fluid, usually caused by infection.

motor nerves Nerves that carry commands from the brain to the muscle; also called efferent nerves.

muscarinic receptors Receptors at the target tissue that are stimulated by acetylcholine and can also be stimulated in the laboratory by the compound extracted from muscarine mushrooms.

musculocutaneous nerve A nerve in the upper extremity that innervates muscles that flex the shoulder and elbow.

myelin sheath A membrane formed by Schwann cells, which cover the axons of certain neurons.

myelinated nerves An axon surrounded by a membrane sheath produced by Schwann cells.

nerve Nervous tissue that connects the nervous system with body parts or organs.

nerve fibers Groups of nerve cells that are bundled together.

nervous system The system that controls virtually all activities of the body, both voluntary and involuntary.

neuroeffector cells The target tissues of the autonomic nervous system.

neuroglia One of two basic types of neural tissue, neuroglia support, protect, defend, and aid in the repair of injury of neural tissue, and regulate composition of nervous system interstitial fluid.

neuromuscular blockers A group of drugs derived from curare that are used in anesthesia to induce muscle relaxation.

neuromuscular junction The receptor on the muscle for nerve impulses.

neurons The basic nerve cells of the nervous system, containing a nucleus within a cell body and extending one or more processes; they exist in masses to form nervous tissue.

neurotransmitters Chemicals produced by neurons that stimulate electrical reactions in adjacent cells.

nicotinic receptors Receptors in the postganglionic neuron that can be stimulated in the laboratory by the alkaloid nicotine.

nodes of Ranvier Regions between individual Schwann cells in myelinated neurons, between which action potentials jump.

norepinephrine A neurotransmitter secreted by the autonomic nervous system.

obturator nerve A nerve emanating from the lumbosacral plexus that innervates muscles that adduct the thigh and rotate it medially.

occipital lobe The portion of the brain that is responsible for the processing of visual information.

oculomotor nerve The cranial nerve (III) that innervates the muscles that cause motion of the eyeballs and upper lid.

olfactory bulb The portion of the olfactory nerve formed by the olfactory tract that lies on the cribriform plate of the ethmoid bone and is penetrated by nerve fibers that provide information about smell from the nose.

olfactory nerve The cranial nerve (I) that transmits information about the sense of smell.

olfactory tract The part of the olfactory nerve that arises at the base of the brain.

optic chiasm Location where approximately half of the nerve fibers from each eye cross over to the opposite side of the brain.

optic foramina The openings through which the optic nerves pass to reach each eyeball.

optic nerve The cranial nerve (II) that transmits visual information to the brain. This is the only of the cranial nerves considered to be part of the central nervous system.

optic tracts The parts of the optic nerve that arise at the base of the brain, forming the optic chiasm.

parasympathetic nervous system The part of the autonomic nervous system that relaxes the body.

parasympathetic-blocking drug A drug that blocks acetylcholine at the neuroeffector synapse.

parietal lobe The portion of the brain that is the site for reception and evaluation of most sensory information, except smell, hearing, and vision.

peripheral nerves Nerves that arise from the different plexuses to branch and supply motor function to and convey sensory information from many areas of the body.

peripheral nervous system The portion of the nervous system that consists of 31 pairs of spinal nerves and 11 of the 12 pairs of cranial nerves; these nerves may be sensory, motor, or connecting nerves.

pia mater The innermost of the three meninges that enclose the brain and spinal cord; it rests directly on the brain and spinal cord.

pineal body Part of the epithalamus in the diencephalon.

plexuses Complex networks made up by the combination of the main portions of the spinal nerves.

pons The portion of the brainstem that lies below the midbrain and contains nerve fibers that affect sleep and respiration.

postganglionic neuron The second of two nerves, separated by a ganglionic synapse, in a series between the central nervous system and the organs that are innervated.

postsynaptic terminal The end of a nerve where electrical impulses are received from the synaptic cleft.

preganglionic neuron The first of two nerves, separated by a ganglionic synapse, in a series between the central nervous system and the organs that are innervated.

presynaptic terminal The end of a nerve where neurotransmitters are released into the synaptic cleft.

proprioception Information about the body's position and of its parts in relation to itself, to one another, and to the pull of gravity.

radial nerve One of the major nerves in the upper extremity, it supplies muscles that extend the elbow, supinate the forearm, and extend the wrist, fingers, and thumb.

reticulospinal tracts Descending tracts that are involved in involuntary body movements.

rootlets Small nerves.

Schwann cells Nervous tissue that helps form the myelin sheath around certain neurons.

sciatic nerve The longest peripheral nerve in the body, formed by the combination of the common peroneal nerve and the tibial nerve.

sciatica Pain and muscle weakness that travels from the back, into the buttocks, and along the leg into the foot as a result of irritation of the sciatic nerve or a lumbar spinal nerve root.

sensory nerves Nerves that carry sensations of touch, taste, heat, cold, pain, and other modalities from the body to the central nervous system.

somatic nervous system The part of the nervous system that regulates activities over which there is voluntary control.

spinal cord An extension of the brain, composed of virtually all the nerves carrying messages between the brain and the rest of the body; it lies inside of and is protected by the spinal canal.

spinal nerves Thirty one pairs of nerves each responsible for sending and receiving sensory and motor messages to and from the central nervous system from a portion of the body.

spinal reflex arcs Automatic reactions to stimuli mediated by neuronal pathways within the spinal cord that occur without conscious thought.

spinal tap A needle insertion through the vertebral canal to the subarachnoid space to obtain a specimen of cerebrospinal fluid.

spinocerebellar tracts Ascending tracts that carry information regarding body position (proprioception) to the cerebellum.

stroke Brain damage typically resulting from a disruption of the circulation to the brain, causing abnormal neurologic findings.

subarachnoid hemorrhage A hemorrhage into the brain tissue beneath the arachnoid membrane.

subarachnoid space The space located between the pia mater and the arachnoid in which the cerebrospinal fluid is contained.

substantia nigra A layer of gray matter located in the midbrain.

subthalamus The part of the diencephalon that is involved in controlling motor functions.

sulci Grooves located between the gyri in the cerebrum.

superficial peroneal nerve The nerve in the leg that innervates the muscles of foot eversion.

superior oblique muscle The muscle that controls the downward gaze of the eyeball.

sympathetic pathway The part of the autonomic nervous system that is responsible for the body's response to shock and stress.

synapse The junction between nerve cells across which nervous stimuli are transmitted. Includes the synaptic cleft, presynaptic cell membrane with synaptic vesicles and axon terminal and postsynaptic cell membrane.

synaptic cleft The space between neurons where electrical impulses trigger the release of neurotransmitters, which in turn stimulate an electrical reaction in adjacent neurons.

synaptic vesicles Vesicles that contain neurotransmitters.

temporal lobe The portion of the brain that plays an important role in hearing and memory.

thalamus The part of the diencephalon that processes most sensory input and influences mood and general body movements, especially those associated with fear or rage.

tibial nerve The nerve in the leg that innervates the muscles that extend the hip, flex the knee, plantar flex the ankle, and flex the toes.

tracts Pathways within the spinal cord that contain nerves.

transient ischemic attack An episode of neurologic impairment that lasts less than 24 hours and represents a warning sign of an impending stroke.

trigeminal nerve The cranial nerve (V) that supplies sensation to the scalp, forehead, face, and lower jaw and innervates the muscles of mastication, the throat, and the inner ear.

trochlear nerve The cranial nerve (IV) that innervates the superior oblique muscle of the eyeball, which controls a downward gaze.

ulnar nerve The nerve in the arm that innervates muscles that flex the wrist and fingers and abduct and adduct the fingers and thumb.

unmyelinated axons Neurons with no myelin sheath or white matter.

vagus nerve The cranial nerve (X) that provides motor functions to the soft palate, pharynx, and larynx and carries taste bud fibers from the posterior tongue, sensory fibers from the inferior pharynx, larynx, thoracic, and abdominal organs, and parasympathetic fibers to thoracic and abdominal organs.

ventral root One of two roots of a spinal nerve that is formed from six to eight rootlets.

ventricles Specialized fluid-filled areas in the brain.

vertebral canal The bony canal formed by vertebrae that houses and protects the spinal cord.

vestibulocochlear nerve The cranial nerve (VIII) that passes through the internal auditory meatus and transmits information important to the senses of hearing and balance.

vestibulospinal tracts Descending tracts that are involved in involuntary body movements.

white matter Bundles of myelinated nerves.

Case Study Answers

1. What part of the nervous system contains the nerves and sensors that are responsible for motor and sensory function of the body?

Answer: The peripheral nervous system consists of nerves that extend from the central nervous system to peripheral structures outside the CNS. One division of the PNS, the somatic system, controls voluntary functions, while the other division, the autonomic nervous system, controls the involuntary functions.

2. How can the knowledge of dermatomes help you to anticipate the level of treatment that may be required for a patient with a traumatic injury?

Answer: A dermatome is a particular area where a spinal nerve provides sensation. A dermatome can be mapped out by the level of the spinal nerve and can be a useful tool to determine the specific level of a spinal cord injury.

3. What part of the nervous system is responsible for the "fight-or-flight" response associated with stress or shock?

Answer: The autonomic nervous system consists of two divisions: the sympathetic and parasympathetic divisions. The sympathetic pathway is responsible for increasing the body's response to stress and shock.

4. Is the response to shock normal in this patient? Explain.

Answer: The normal response to shock is a release of adrenaline from the adrenal glands, which in turn causes the body to shunt blood to the vital organs (the heart, brain, and lungs), increase the respiratory rate and the pulse rate, and constrict the pupils. In this patient, a spinal cord injury may be preventing the message to release adrenaline from getting to the adrenal glands.

5. How is an impulse transmitted from nerve to nerve?

Answer: Nerve cells communicate with each other primarily through synapses. The message may be propagated from cell to cell by either more synapses (synaptic transmission) or by the movement of ions (electrical transmission).

6. If the patient's spinal cord has actually been severed, what nerves will most likely be dysfunctional?

Answer: If there is a complete transection of the spinal cord, the peripheral nerves below the level of injury will be damaged. If there is associated swelling or bleeding at the injury site, higher levels in the spinal cord may be affected temporarily or permanently.

7. Is the spinal cord injury in this patient currently a life-threatening condition?

Answer: The mechanism of injury was severe and the patient has sustained injuries that could quickly become unstable or critical. Close evaluation of the patient's mental status and the ABCs are paramount. The spinal cord injury most likely is not life threatening; however, the other internal injuries he may also have sustained, such as bleeding, are potentially life threatening. The presence of the spinal cord injury should be a sign that the mechanism of injury was significant and that associated internal abdominal or intrathoracic injury is a significant possibility.

The Integumentary System

Learning Objectives

1. State the three functions of the integumentary system. (p 192)
2. Name the two layers of skin. (p 193)
3. Name the tissues that make up the subcutaneous layer and describe their functions. (p 193)
4. Name the five layers of the epidermis. (p 193)
5. State the function of the stratum corneum and the stratum germinativum. (p 193-195)
6. Describe the function of melanin and melanocytes. (p 195-196)

7. Describe how the blood vessels in the dermis respond to heat, cold, and stress. (p 196-197)
8. Describe the function of hair and how hairs grow out of the skin. (p 197-198)
9. Explain how sweat glands play a major role in regulating body temperature. (p 198)
10. Distinguish between eccrine and apocrine glands. (p 198)
11. Describe the structure of nails. (p 198)

Introduction

The skin is the largest organ of the human body and serves as the interface between the body and the outside world. The integumentary system includes the skin, nails, hair, and sweat and oil glands, and accounts for 15% of the total body weight of an adult. The integumentary system is responsible for temperature regulation and maintaining tissue water balance. In addition, the integumentary system is the body's first line of defense against disease-causing organisms. The layers of the skin contain nerve receptors for temperature, touch, pain, and pressure. The skin is continually bombarded by many environmental components including microorganisms, sunlight, and chemicals. Injury to the skin can result in an abrasion, a laceration, a penetrating wound, or an amputation.

Clinical Tip

The term hypodermic refers to "below the skin" and is commonly applied to injections or shots. A health care provider uses a hypodermic syringe to give a hypodermic injection.

The Integumentary System

The external surface of the body is covered by the integumentary system, which includes the skin and sweat glands. The integumentary system has three functions: temperature regulation, maintenance of water balance, and defense against external elements Table 9-1.

Case Study PART 1

At 5:00 PM, your unit is dispatched to a local park for a person who has been burned. As you arrive at the picnic area, you see that the park police and the fire department are on the scene, as well as what seems to be a group of families having a barbecue. You determine that the scene is safe, and you approach a 20-year-old man who was burned about 15 minutes earlier. The fire department had hosed him down to cool him off. The patient had been having difficulty starting a fire, so he tried to pour a pint of gasoline onto the wood to help start the fire. Sparks that were already present lit the fumes, sending flames onto his face and hair. He and his friends had been drinking beer since about 1:00 PM.

You begin your primary assessment and determine that the patient is alert and has an open airway. He is breathing rapidly, yet adequately. The patient's pulse is strong, rapid, and regular, and there is no life-threatening external bleeding. You apply a nonrebreathing mask and explain to the patient that your partner will be removing the patient's soaked and burned clothing. After the patient's outer clothes have been removed, you ask him to sit on the burn sheet that has been spread out on the stretcher. Next, your partner obtains a set of baseline vital signs.

Recording Time: 0 minutes	
Appearance	Severely distressed
Level of consciousness	Alert (oriented to person, place, and day) and in severe pain
Airway	Appears patent
Breathing	Rapid but adequate
Circulation	Strong, rapid, regular pulse
Pulse	100 beats/min, regular and strong
Blood pressure	120/70 mm Hg
Respirations	22 breaths/min, adequate
Spo$_2$	97%

1. How is the skin attached to the underlying bones or muscles?

2. What gives the skin its strength and permeability and where does it come from?

Table 9-1	**Major Functions of the Integumentary System**
Temperature regulation	
First-line of defense against infection	
Fluid balance regulation	

The Layers of the Skin

The skin protects the body and helps to maintain homeostasis. It also aids in the regulation of body temperature, slows water loss from deep tissues, synthesizes biochemicals, excretes certain wastes, and contains sensory receptors for touch, pressure, pain, and temperature stimuli. The skin also helps to produce vitamin D when dehydrocholesterol in the diet reaches the skin via the blood and becomes exposed to the sun's ultraviolet light. Vitamin D is essential for normal bone and tooth development. It also stores lipids in adipocytes (in the dermis) and in adipose tissue (in the subcutaneous layer). Keratinocytes are special skin cells that produce hormone-like substances that stimulate the development of white blood cells known as T lymphocytes, which are important in defending against infection.

There are two main layers of skin **Figure 9-1**. The epidermis is the outer layer, and is made up of stratified squamous epithelium. The dermis is the inner layer, and is much thicker than the epidermis. The dermis consists of papillary and reticular regions. The papillary region contains fine elastic fibers and dermal papillae. The reticular region is composed of connective tissue containing collagen, elastic fibers, fat tissue, hair follicles, nerves, sebaceous (oil) glands, and the ducts of sweat glands. The epidermis is connected to the dermis by a basement membrane. Loose connective tissue below the dermis binds the skin to the organs underneath. This tissue, which is predominantly adipose (fatty), forms the subcutaneous layer, also known as the hypodermis. It is deep below the dermis, and not actually part of the skin. This adipose tissue insulates the body, conserving inner heat and helping to keep excessive heat from outside the body from entering. The major blood vessels that supply the skin and adipose tissue are contained within the subcutaneous layer.

The Epidermis

The epidermis is the outermost layer of the skin. It is composed of stratified squamous epithelia. The epidermis does not contain blood vessels, although its deepest layer, the stratum basale, receives blood via the dermal blood vessels. Cells in this layer of the epidermis divide and grow, moving toward the skin surface, away from the

dermis below. As they move upwards, they receive less nutrients, and eventually die. Older cells are called keratinocytes, which harden with age in the process known as keratinization. Keratin protein fills the cytoplasm of these skin cells, which collectively form a layer called the stratum corneum. Dead skin cells in this layer are eventually shed from the body.

The five layers of the epidermis include the following:

- Stratum germinativum
- Stratum spinosum
- Stratum granulosum
- Stratum lucidum
- Stratum corneum

The stratum germinativum is the innermost epidermal layer, and is also known as the stratum basale. It is interlocked with the underlying dermis. This layer forms the epidermal ridges, extending into the dermis, which are adjacent to dermal projections (dermal papillae). These structures are important because the strength of the attachment of the layer is proportional to the surface area of the basal lamina. The stratum germinativum forms the epidermal ridges. Ridge shapes are genetically determined, and the pattern of epidermal ridges does not change during the entire lifespan of a person. The ridge patterns on the tip of each finger are instrumental in the forming of fingerprints. Each person's fingerprints are unique, including those of identical twins. As a result, fingerprints are commonly used in criminal cases to identify people. Large basal (germinative) cells dominate the stratum germinativum. They are stem cells with divisions that replace superficial keratinocytes that are lost or shed on the epithelial surface.

When a stem cell divides into daughter cells, they are pushed from the stratum germinativum upward into the next layer, the stratum spinosum. This layer is made up of 8 to 10 layers of keratinocytes that are bound together by desmosomes. This "spiny layer" contains cells that look like tiny pincushions because of exposure to chemicals that caused them to shrink slightly. This layer also contains Langerhans cells, which stimulate immune defenses against microorganisms and superficial skin cancers.

The next region is called the stratum granulosum ("grainy layer") and consists of three to five layers of keratinocytes. Cells in this layer have mostly stopped dividing and are now making the proteins keratin and keratohyalin. Keratin is tough and fibrous, making up hairs and nails. Keratohyalin forms cytoplasmic granules that dehydrate cells and aggregate and cross-link keratin fibers. The cells die as the nuclei and other organelles disintegrate.

The fourth region is the stratum lucidum, which is thicker on the palms of the hands and soles of the feet, with a glassy or clear appearance. In this layer, the cells are flattened, densely packed, and contain eleidin, which is eventually transformed to keratin.

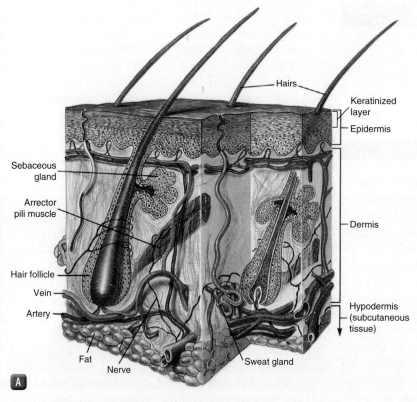

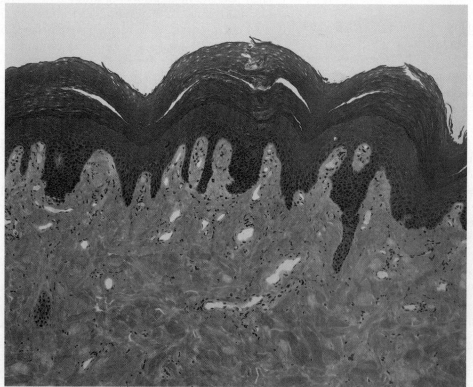

Figure 9-1   Anatomy of the skin. **A.** The structural anatomy. **B.** The microscopic appearance of the two main layers of the skin.

The surface of the skin is made up of the stratum corneum, and contains 15 to 30 layers of keratinized cells that are protective and filled with keratin. The dead cells of the stratum corneum are tightly interconnected by desmosomes. Keratinized cells of this layer are shed in large sheets rather than individually. Cells move from the stratum germinativum to the stratum corneum in 15 to 30 days, remaining in the stratum corneum for about 2 weeks. The dryness of the stratum corneum reduces the amount of potential microbial growth, and this layer is coated with lipid secretions from the sebaceous glands. This layer is water resistant but not waterproof. About 500 mL of water is lost from this layer via evaporation every day (a process known as insensible perspiration). **Figure 9-2** shows the relative thickness of the epidermal layers. Healthy skin balances the production of epidermal cells with the loss of dead cells on an ongoing basis.

The epidermis protects the underlying tissues against the effects of harmful chemicals, excess water loss, mechanical injury, and pathogenic microorganisms. Layers of pigment in the epidermis help protect both epidermal and dermal tissues. Melanin is a brown, yellow-brown, or black pigment produced by melanocytes located in the stratum germinativum, either between or deeply rooted in the epithelial cells **Figure 9-3**. Melanin absorbs ultraviolet (UV) radiation from sunlight, protecting the epidermis and dermis from its harmful effects. Sunlight contains significant amounts of UV radiation. Small amounts of UV radiation are beneficial because they stimulate the epidermal production of a compound required for calcium ion homeostasis (the production of vitamin D). However, larger amounts of UV radiation damage DNA, causing mutations and promoting the development of cancer. UV radiation can also produce burns. When severe, they can damage the epidermis and the dermis.

Differences in skin color are based on the amount of melanin produced and how it is distributed throughout the skin. Skin color is based on a person's genetics, which regulates the amount of melanin that will be produced by the melanocytes. Other factors that affect skin color include sunlight, ultraviolet light, and x-rays. Dermal vessel blood also affects the color of the skin. Well-oxygenated blood makes light-skinned people appear more pink, whereas poorly oxygenated blood makes them appear more blue, as in the condition known as cyanosis. Diet also affects skin color, as do biochemical imbalances. For example, the buildup of the substance known as bilirubin

---

Clinical Tip

The skin provides an excellent protective barrier to infection, especially if good handwashing techniques and disposable vinyl or nitrile gloves are used. Some EMS providers have dry, flaky skin, small cuts, or cracked cuticles. Although frequent handwashing is very necessary, it can contribute to dry skin. Infection of these areas of the skin can be avoided by keeping the skin clean and covering any cuts or cracks in the skin with a bandage and disposable gloves. A moisturizing cream also should be considered.

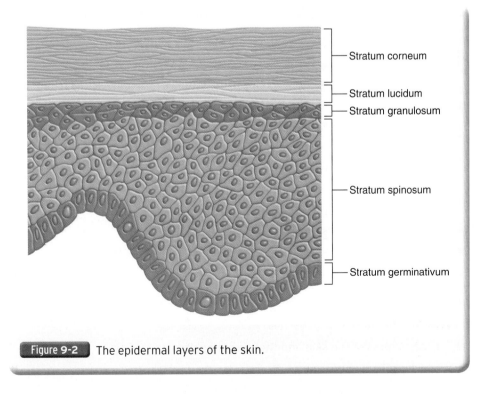

— Stratum corneum

— Stratum lucidum
— Stratum granulosum

— Stratum spinosum

— Stratum germinativum

Figure 9-2 The epidermal layers of the skin.

makes the skin appear yellowish, as in the condition called jaundice. Albinism is a condition resulting from the skin's inability to synthesize melanin and is characterized by milky or translucent skin, pale or colorless hair, and pink or blue irises.

The Dermis

The dermis lies between the epidermis and the subcutaneous layer, immediately above the hypodermis, and contains dense and irregular connective tissue, with very little fat tissue. It has two major components: (1) a superficial papillary layer and (2) a deeper reticular layer. The papillary layer consists of areolar tissue and contains capillaries, lymphatics, and sensory neurons. The papillary layer is named for the dermal papillae that project between the epidermal ridges. The reticular layer is made up of a meshwork of connective tissue containing collagen and elastic fibers. The boundary between both layers is not distinct. The dermis also contains all the cells of connective tissue proper. Epidermal accessory organs extend into the dermis, and both the papillary and reticular layers of the dermis contain blood vessels, lymph vessels, and nerve fibers.

The collagenous and elastic fibers of the dermis make it both tough and elastic. Processes from nerve cells are located throughout the dermis. Motor processes carry impulses to the dermal glands and muscles, while sensory

Case Study PART 2

It is clear that this patient should be transported to the regional burn center, and a helicopter has been called to the scene. Fortunately, there does not seem to be a respiratory burn because his nasal hairs are not burned and he has no breathing difficulty. With the patient seated on the burn sheet, you begin a rapid trauma exam as a part of your secondary assessment while your partner obtains the patient's vital signs.

You perform a rapid trauma examination and find:

- Head: Superficial burns to the chin
- Neck: Superficial burns
- Chest: Partial- and full-thickness burns
- Abdomen: Partial-thickness burns
- Pelvis: Superficial burns
- Extremities: Partial- and full-thickness burns on right arm
- Back and buttocks: No injury

Recording Time: 5 minutes

Appearance	Burns of varying degrees ranging from superficial to full thickness
Level of consciousness	Alert (oriented to person, place, and day)
Airway	Open and patent
Breathing	Rapid but adequate
Circulation	Pale in the areas that do not involve the burn
Pulse	110 beats/min, strong and regular
Blood pressure	120/78 mm Hg
Respirations	24 breaths/min, regular
Pupils	Equal and reactive
Spo$_2$	97%

3. Describe the five layers that compose the epidermis.

4. What are the accessory structures of the skin and their functions?

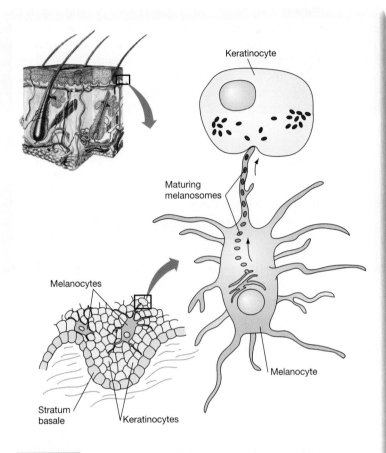

Figure 9-3 Melanocytes produce melanin, the pigment of skin, package it in melanosomes, and transfer it to keratinocytes.

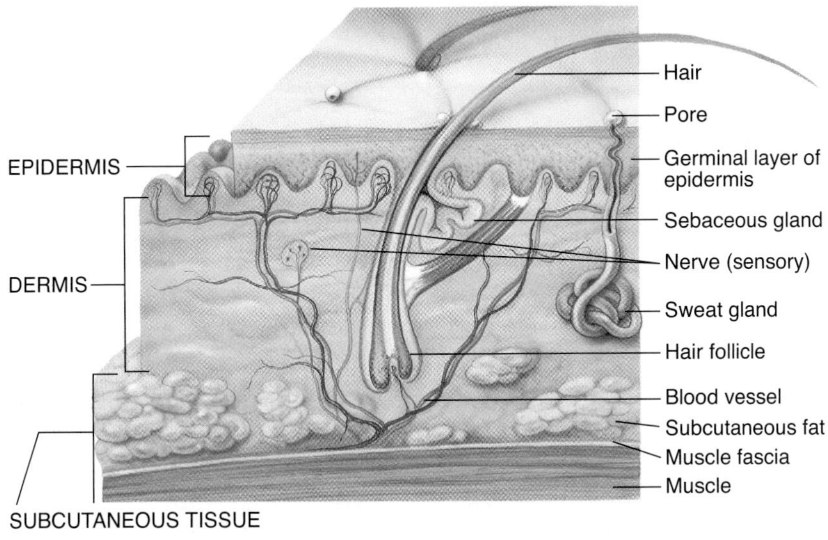

processes carry impulses back to the brain and spinal cord. The blood vessels of the dermis play an important role in the body's response to touch, hot, cold, and pain by vasoconstricting or vasodilating in response to stimulation from the autonomic nervous system.

Accessory Skin Structures

Hair

Hair is a threadlike, keratin-containing appendage of the outer layer of the skin Figure 9-4 . Hairs project above the skin surface over most of the body, except for the sides and soles of the feet, the palms of the hands, the sides of the fingers and toes, the lips, and parts of the external genitalia. There are about 2.5 million hairs on the human body. Over 75% of body hair is on the general body surface, and not the head. Hairs are dead structures produced in organs called hair follicles Figure 9-5 . Hair follicles extend from the skin surface into the dermis, containing hair roots that are nourished with dermal blood. Each hair follicle is attached to an arrector pili muscle, which helps the hair shaft to stand on end when it contracts. This occurs during emotional upset and cold temperatures. Hairs are pushed upward as epidermal hair cells divide and grow, becoming keratinized and then dying. Hair shafts are actually composed of dead epidermal cells.

Hair color is reflected by genetics, and variations in the pigment produced by melanocytes at the hair papilla. Darker hair has more eumelanin (which is brownish-black), whereas lighter hair has more pheomelanin (which is reddish-yellow). The different forms of melanin give hair a wide variety of shades, ranging from dark brown to yellow brown, to red. Albinos have white hair because their hair shafts completely lack melanin. Hormonal and environmental factors also influence the hair's condition. As pigment production decreases with age, hair color lightens. White hair results from a lack of pigment along with the presence of air bubbles in the medulla of the hair shaft. As the proportion of white hairs increases, the overall hair color is described as gray.

EPIDERMIS

DERMIS

SUBCUTANEOUS TISSUE

Hair
Pore
Germinal layer of epidermis
Sebaceous gland
Nerve (sensory)
Sweat gland
Hair follicle
Blood vessel
Subcutaneous fat
Muscle fascia
Muscle

Figure 9-4 Hair and its associated structures.

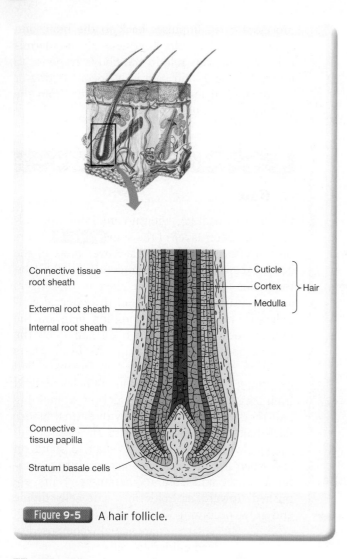

Figure 9-5   A hair follicle.

Connective tissue root sheath
External root sheath
Internal root sheath
Connective tissue papilla
Stratum basale cells
Cuticle
Cortex
Medulla
Hair

Glands

Sebaceous glands and sweat glands are the two types of exocrine glands in the skin. Sebaceous glands (oil glands) are made up of specialized epidermal cells and are primarily located near hair follicles. They are actually holocrine glands, secreting sebum, which is an oily mixture of fatty material and debris from cells. Sebaceous glands are especially abundant on the scalp, face, nose, mouth, and ears. Generally, sebum is secreted into hair follicles, but in some places (such as the labia minora and the lips), it is secreted onto the surface of the skin. Sebum oils the hair and skin and helps to retain body heat and prevent evaporation of sweat.

Sweat glands consist of a small tube originating as a coil in the deep dermis or superficial subcutaneous layers. The coiled portion is lined with sweat-secreting epithelial cells. Sweat glands are divided into two types: merocrine and apocrine glands. Merocrine (eccrine) glands produce a solution containing salt and urea that is secreted directly onto the surface of the skin through sweat pores. Merocrine glands are distributed over the body and promote cooling

of the body. Apocrine glands are coiled tubular glands that usually open into hair follicles of the axillae and genitalia, as well as around the anus. They are similar to odiferous glands in mammals. Their secretion is thicker than sweat and is metabolized by skin bacteria, resulting in body odors. Ceruminous glands are modified sweat glands in the ear that produce cerumen, which is a component of earwax.

Nails

The nail is a flattened structure that protects the ends of each finger and toe. It is made of keratin from the epidermis. In humans, nails do little except provide additional protection over the skin of the nail bed Figure 9-6. Each nail contains a root, a body, and a free edge. The root fits into a groove in the skin (the eponychium or cuticle at the base and the paronychium along the edges) and is closely molded to the skin of the finger or toe, with the nail fold overlying the root. The body of the nail lies over the nail bed. The part of the nail plate that grows most actively is covered by a whitish, half-moon-shaped lunula, where epithelial cells divide and become keratinized. As the stratum germinativum of the root proliferates, nails grow longer. The nail of the middle finger grows fastest whereas the nail of the thumb grows slowest.

Pathophysiology

The skin's most important function is to serve as a physical barrier to invasion of the body by germs. Persons with widespread burns lose this protection. Thus, infection is a frequent complication in patients with burns. In fact, severe infections are the most common cause of death in patients with burns to a large portion of the body.

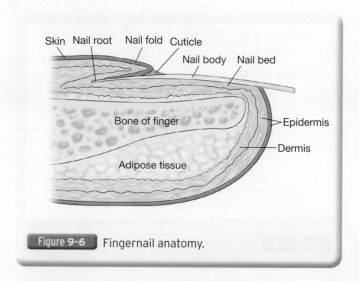

Skin   Nail root   Nail fold   Cuticle
Nail body   Nail bed
Bone of finger
Epidermis
Dermis
Adipose tissue

Figure 9-6   Fingernail anatomy.

While you are waiting the 8 minutes it takes for the helicopter to arrive, your paramedic partner starts a large-bore IV line in the patient's uninjured arm and removes the rings from his fingers because they are already beginning to swell. Using the rule of nines, your partner determines that the patient has burns to approximately 25% of the body surface area. You obtain a patient history and also note that the patient's vital signs remain stable. Your partner calls medical control for an order to administer analgesics for the patient's pain. As he does this, you quickly prepare some notes on your assessment card to give to the flight medics because there will be no room for you on the helicopter.

The patient history reveals a 20-year-old man who weighs 75 kg. The SAMPLE history shows:

- **A**ge, gender, weight: 20-year-old man, 75 kg
- **S**igns and symptoms: Severe pain at the site of the burns, blisters forming on the chest and abdomen, and swelling in the right upper extremity
- **A**llergies to medications: No known drug allergies
- **M**edications taken: Taking an antibiotic for an inner ear infection
- **P**ast pertinent medical history: A recent flare up of swimmer's ear
- **L**ast food/fluid intake: Several beers, chicken, salad, and chips over the past few hours
- **E**vents prior to onset: Carelessness with fire and fuel

The OPQRST history shows:

- **O**nset of symptoms: Immediate with the time of the burns
- **P**rovoking factors: Alcohol consumption
- **Q**uality of discomfort: Severe burns
- **R**adiating/related signs/symptoms/relief:
    - Head – Superficial burns to the chin
    - Neck – Superficial burns to the neck
    - Chest – Partial- and full-thickness burns
    - Abdomen – Partial-thickness burns
    - Pelvis – Superficial burns
    - Extremities – Partial- and full-thickness burns to right arm
    - Back and buttocks – No injury
- **S**everity of complaint: Excruciating pain
- **T**ime: 30 minutes ago

Recording Time: 15 minutes

Appearance	Still in significant pain
Level of consciousness	Alert (oriented to person, place, and day)
Airway	Still open and patent
Breathing	Breathing rate is increasing but adequate volume
Circulation	Pulse is still fast and regular
Pulse	120 beats/min, regular
Blood pressure	110/70 mm Hg
Respirations	26 breaths/min, adequate
Spo$_2$	97%

5. What is the most important function of the skin?

6. How devastating can burn injuries be to the body?

■ Injuries and Wounds to the Skin

The skin responds to injuries and wounds with inflammation, which causes redness, increased warmth, and painful swelling. The blood vessels of the wounded area dilate and allow fluids to leak into the damaged tissues. This provides more nutrients and oxygen to the tissues, aiding in healing. Shallow breaks in the skin cause epithelial cells to divide more rapidly, with the new cells filling the break.

An abrasion is an injury in which the involved body part has lost its outer layer of skin or mucous membrane because it has been rubbed or scratched off. A laceration is a wound with a smooth or jagged edge, resulting from a tearing or scraping action. This type of wound can be caused by a sharp object, broken glass, a jagged piece of metal, or a severe blow or impact. A penetrating wound is made by a sharp instrument that passes through the skin, affecting all tissues in its path. An incision is a smooth cut, usually made by a sharp object. Incisions may be quite deep, involving muscle, blood vessels, tendons, and nerves. Bleeding may or may not be severe. Nails, splinters, or knives can cause penetrating wounds. In an avulsion, flaps of skin and tissue are torn loose or pulled off completely **Figure 9-7** . An amputation involves the cutting or tearing off of a body part. Most commonly this refers to an extremity or a part of an extremity, such as a finger, toe, arm, or leg.

A cut that extends into the dermis or subcutaneous layers usually involves blood vessels. The escaping blood then forms a clot in the wound, eventually forming a scab as it dries. The scab protects the underlying tissues. Cells called fibroblasts move to the injury to form new collagenous fibers that bind the edges of the wound together.

Large skin breaks may require suturing or other methods of closing in order to promote healing with minimal scar tissue and without infection. This actually helps to speed up the action of the fibroblasts in healing.

Wound healing proceeds as blood vessels extend into the area below the scab, allowing phagocytic cells to remove dead cells and debris. As tissue is replaced, the scab eventually falls off. Extensive wounds may cause the newly formed tissue to appear on the skin surface as a scar. Large open wounds may develop small round masses of granulation tissue, which consist of new blood vessel branches and clusters of fibroblasts. Once the fibroblasts eventually move away, the resultant scar is mostly composed of collagenous fibers.

If a wound is large or occurs in an area where the skin is thin, epithelial cells cannot cover the surface until dermal repairs are already under way. Circulation to the area is enhanced so that blood clotting, fibroblasts, and an extensive capillary network can combine to combat the injury. (Together, these components are known as granulation tissue.) Repairs do not restore the dermis to its original condition, and collagen fibers dominate with relatively few new blood vessels. Scar tissue is relatively inflexible and noncellular. Thickened, raised scar tissue forms in some people who are genetically predisposed and is referred to as a keloid, featuring a shiny and smooth surface. Keloids are harmless but unsightly.

Pathophysiology

Burns result from heat or other thermal injury to the skin and are classified based on the levels of skin involved. Burns involving only the epidermis are called superficial burns, or first-degree burns. Burns that involve the epidermis and a portion of the dermis are classified as partial-thickness burns, or second-degree burns. Full-thickness burns, or third-degree burns, involve the hypodermis and may extend to bone, muscle, and internal organs. Some EMS agencies recognize a category of burn called the "fourth-degree" burn. This is a burn involving charring down to the bone.

Case Study   PART 4

As you place the patient into the helicopter, he says "What an idiot you must think I am." You think first before you speak, then you look at him and say, "You are very lucky that you did not burn your face. Now it is important for you to concentrate on getting through this injury." You know that it is neither the first nor last time that you will see the results of alcohol-related trauma.

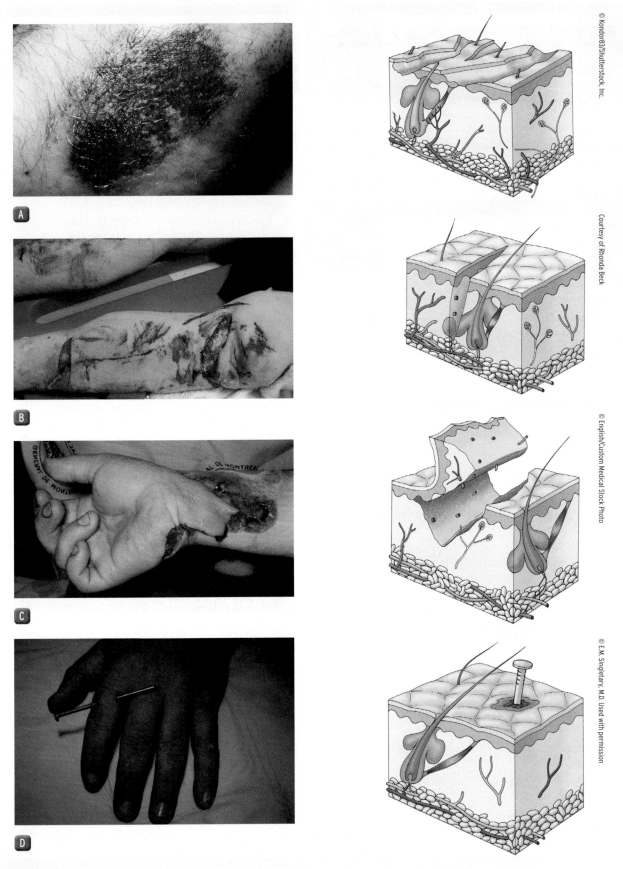

© Kondor83/Shutterstock, Inc.

Courtesy of Rhonda Beck

© English/Custom Medical Stock Photo

© E.M. Singletary, M.D. Used with permission

Figure 9-7 Types of wounds. **A.** Abrasion. **B.** Laceration. **C.** Avulsion. **D.** Penetrating wound.

Prep Kit

Chapter Summary

- The external surface of the body is covered by the integumentary system. As the body's largest organ system, this system is responsible for temperature regulation, tissue water balance, and defense against disease-causing organisms.

- The layers of the skin contain nerve receptors for temperature, touch, pain, and pressure.

- The epidermis is the outer skin layer, made up of stratified squamous epithelium.

- The epidermis contains numerous nerve vessels but no nerve endings.

- The epidermis is composed of five layers: the stratum corneum, stratum lucidum, stratum granulosum, stratum spinosum, and the stratum germinativum.

- The dermis is the inner layer, and is much thicker than the epidermis.

- The dermis is located immediately above the hypodermis and contains dense and irregular connective tissue and very little fat tissue.

- The blood vessels of the dermis vasoconstrict or vasodilate in response to stimulation from the autonomic nervous system. The hypodermis is the layer of tissue immediately below the skin that attaches the skin to the underlying bone or muscle and stores the body's fat. It also is rich in blood vessels and nerves.

- Melanocytes contribute to skin color by producing a dark pigment called melanin that protects the skin from the sun's ultraviolet rays.

- Differences in skin color are based on the amount of melanin produced and how it is distributed throughout the skin.

- Hair is a threadlike, keratin-containing appendage of the outer layer of the skin that is present on the body surface, except for the palms, soles, lips, and a few areas of the external genitalia.

- Each hair follicle is attached to an arrector pili muscle, which helps the hair shaft to stand on end.

- Hair aids in thermal regulation, as well as in sensation.

- Skin glands include sebaceous glands and sweat glands.

- Sebaceous glands are primarily located near hair follicles, and secrete sebum, an oily mixture of fatty material and cellular debris.

- Together with sweat, sebum moisturizes and protects the skin. Sebum oils the hair and skin and helps to retain body heat and prevent evaporation of sweat.

- Sweat glands originate in the deep dermis or superficial subcutaneous layers, and secrete sweat.

- Sweat glands are divided into two types: merocrine (eccrine) and apocrine glands.

- Merocrine glands produce a solution containing salt and urea that is secreted directly onto the surface of the skin through sweat pores.

- Apocrine glands are coiled tubular glands that usually open into hair follicles of the axillae and genitalia, as well as around the anus.

- The sweat glands help to regulate body temperature by releasing sweat to the skin surface, which evaporates to cool the skin.

- The nail is a flattened structure at the end of each finger and toe made of keratin from the epidermis.

- The part of the nail that grows most actively is covered by a whitish, half-moon shaped lunula, where epithelial cells divide and become keratinized.

- The nail cells push forward over the nail bed, causing the nail to continually grow outward.

- A laceration is a wound with a smooth or jagged edge caused by a sharp object.

- A penetrating wound is made by a sharp instrument that passes through the skin.

- An avulsion occurs when flaps of skin and tissue are torn loose or pulled off completely.

- An amputation involves the cutting or tearing off of a body part.

Vital Vocabulary

abrasion An injury in which the involved body part has lost its outer layer of skin or mucous membrane because it has been rubbed or scratched off.

albinism A condition of the skin resulting from the inability to synthesize melanin.

amputation Completely cutting or tearing off of a body part.

apocrine glands Coiled tubular glands that usually open into hair follicles of the axillae and genitalia, as well as around the anus.

arrector pili muscle Muscle attached at the base of the hair that pulls the hair perpendicular to the surface of the skin in cold or threatening situations.

avulsion A wound in which flaps of skin and tissue are torn loose or pulled off completely.

basal lamina A thin, noncellular layer of ground substance lying under epithelial surfaces that separates the epidermis from the areolar tissue of the adjacent dermis.

burns The result of heat or other thermal injury to the skin.

dermis The inner layer of the skin, containing hair follicles, sweat glands, nerve endings, and blood vessels; located immediately above the hypodermis.

desmosomes Cell structures specialized for cell-to-cell adhesion.

eleidin Granules within the stratum lucidum that are formed from keratohyaline and are eventually transformed to keratin.

epidermis The superficial, outer layer of the skin that contains numerous nerve vessels, but no nerve endings; acts as the body's first line of defense.

first-degree burns Burns involving only the epidermis; also called superficial burns.

full-thickness burns Burns that involve the hypodermis and possibly bone, muscle, or internal organs; also called third-degree burns.

hair Threadlike, keratin-containing appendage of the outer layer of the skin.

hair follicles Tubelike structures in which hairs develop; they extend from the skin surface into the dermis.

hair shafts The portions of hair that extend above the skin.

holocrine glands Glands that secrete sebum; also called sebaceous glands.

hypodermic Referring to below the skin.

hypodermis The layer of tissue immediately below the dermis; also called the subcutaneous layer.

incision A smooth cut, usually made by a sharp object such as a scalpel.

integumentary system The body's external surface, including the skin, nails, hair, and sweat and oil glands.

keratin A protein in the skin that is responsible for the strength and permeability of the epidermis.

keratinocytes The cells in the epidermis that produce a protein called keratin.

keratohyalin A precursor of keratin that is located in the stratum granulosum of the epidermis.

laceration A wound with a smooth or jagged edge, resulting from a tearing, scraping, or sharp cutting action.

lunula A whitish, crescent-shaped structure at the base of the nail body.

melanin The dark pigment in skin that protects the skin from the sun's ultraviolet rays.

melanocytes Epidermal cells that contribute to skin color by producing a dark pigment called melanin.

merocrine (eccrine) glands Sweat glands that produce a solution containing salt and urea that is secreted directly onto the surface of the skin through sweat pores.

nail A flattened structure at the end of each finger and toe made of keratin from the epidermis.

nail bed The portion of the nail over which the nail body lies.

partial-thickness burns Burns that involve the epidermis and a portion of the dermis; also called second-degree burns.

penetrating wound Wound made by a sharp instrument that passes through the skin, affecting all tissues in its path.

sebaceous glands Glands that produce sebum and are located in the dermis of the entire body, except for the palms and soles.

sebum Material produced by sebaceous glands that contains a combination of fatty material and cellular debris.

second-degree burns Burns that involve the epidermis and a portion of the dermis; also called partial-thickness burns.

squamous epithelia The flat sheets of cells that make up the epidermis.

stratum corneum The outer layer of the epidermis, which contains about 25 layers of dead cells that continuously shed as new cells push upward.

stratum germinativum The innermost layer of epidermis.

stratum granulosum The layer of epidermis between the stratum lucidum and the stratum spinosum that is composed of flattened cells that contain granules of keratohyalin.

stratum lucidum The first inner layer of the epidermis, it is readily visible only in the thick epithelium of the palms of the hands and the soles of the feet.

stratum spinosum The layer of epidermis between the stratum granulosum and the stratum germinativum that contains cells known as keratinocytes, which synthesize the keratohyaline, a precursor of keratin.

subcutaneous layer The layer of soft tissue immediately below the dermis; also called the hypodermis.

superficial burns Burns involving only the epidermis; also called first-degree burns.

sweat pores Pores in the skin through which sweat is secreted.

third-degree burns Burns that involve the hypodermis and possibly bone, muscle, or internal organs; also called full-thickness burns.

wounds Breaks in the integrity of the integumentary system.

Case Study Answers

1. How is the skin attached to the underlying bones or muscles?

   Answer: The subcutaneous tissue attaches the skin to underlying structures such as bone or muscle. The subcutaneous tissue also contains many blood vessels, nerves, and body fat stores.

2. What gives the skin its strength and permeability and where does it come from?

   Answer: Fibrous proteins called keratin, which are produced by keratinocytes, give the skin its strength and permeability. However, each of the five layers of the epidermis contributes to synthesis of keratin.

3. Describe the five layers that compose the epidermis.

   Answer:

   1. Stratum corneum—the outer layer of the epidermis, which forms the main superficial skin barrier.

   2. Stratum lucidum—the first inner layer, which is easily visible only in the thick epithelium of the palms of the hands and the soles of the feet.

   3. Stratum granulosum—the next layer, which is composed of flattened cells that contain granules of keratohyalin, the precursor of eleidin.

   4. Stratum spinosum—the layer below the stratum granulosum that contains keratinocytes, which synthesize the protein keratin.

   5. Stratum germinativum—the inner-most layer of epidermis is a single layer of cells in which cell division occurs frequently.

4. What are the accessory structures of the skin and their functions?

   Answer: Hair, glands, and nails are the accessory structures of skin. Hair, present on most body surfaces, aids in thermal regulation as well as in sensation. There are two types of glands: sebaceous and sweat glands. These glands protect the skin, moisturize, and produce wax and sweat. Nails are made of keratin from the epidermis, and provide protection over the skin of the nail bed of each finger and toe.

5. What is the most important function of the skin?

   Answer: The skin serves as a physical barrier to invasion of the body by germs. When the integumentary system is breached, the body is at increased risk for infection. The larger the injury; the more susceptibility there is for infection.

6. How devastating can burn injuries be to the body?

   Answer: The severity of a burn injury, the amount of body surface area (BSA) involved, as well as the depth of the burn, can be a good predictor of how physically destructive a burn can be. Depending on the location of the burn, there can be permanent loss of mobility or function when an extremity is involved. The psychological effects cannot be predicted, but they can be devastating, especially when the face is involved.

The Gastrointestinal System

Learning Objectives

1. Identify the organs of the digestive system. (p 206)
2. Describe the wall of the alimentary canal. (p 206-207)
3. Identify the accessory organs of digestion. (p 206)
4. Describe the structure and function of the teeth and tongue in digestion. (p 207)
5. Explain the processes by which materials move through the digestive tract. (p 207-208)
6. Explain the difference between mechanical and chemical digestion. (p 207-208)
7. Define peristalsis. (p 208)
8. Explain the function of saliva. (p 210)
9. Describe the location and function of the pharynx and esophagus. (p 211)
10. Define chyme. (p 211)
11. Describe the anatomy of the stomach. (p 211-212)
12. Describe the difference in absorption between the large and small intestine. (p 212-216)
13. Describe the function of the normal flora in the colon. (p 215)
14. Describe the functions of the liver. (p 217)
15. Describe the importance of the mesenteries. (p 217)

Introduction

Life is sustained by obtaining nutrients from the environment. Nutrients are the raw materials needed to synthesize essential compounds in the body. They may also be decomposed to provide energy required by the cells to continue functioning. The mechanical and chemical breakdown of foods and the absorption of resulting nutrients by the body's cells are known as digestion. The organs of the digestive system, also known as the gastrointestinal (GI) system, carry out the processes of mechanical digestion and chemical digestion Figure 10-1. Mechanical digestion is the process of breaking large pieces of food into smaller ones without altering their chemical makeup. Chemical digestion uses chemicals, such as the action of saliva on starches, to break food into simpler chemicals. Both of these processes begin to occur in the pharynx and are sometimes referred to as oral digestion.

The alimentary canal, through which food passes, extends from the mouth to the anus. It includes the mouth, pharynx, esophagus, stomach, small intestine, large intestine, rectum, and anus. Its accessory organs include the teeth, tongue, salivary glands, liver, gallbladder, and the pancreas. The secretions from these accessory organs empty via ducts into the digestive tract. Glandular organ secretions are made up of water, enzymes, buffers, and other components. These secretions assist in preparing organic and inorganic nutrients for absorption across the epithelium of the digestive tract. The digestive system is basically a tube that is open at both ends that supplies nutrients for body cells. The surface area of the small intestine alone in an adult is approximately 250 square meters.

The Alimentary Canal

The alimentary canal is an 8-meter-long muscular tube passing through the thoracic and abdominopelvic cavities

Case Study PART 1

At 9:00 PM, your unit is dispatched to a fifth-floor apartment in the city. The patient's wife quickly leads you to the bathroom where her 49-year-old husband is sitting in a chair near the toilet. Your general impression is a thin man who appears diaphoretic and very pale.

As you begin your primary assessment, you note that the patient clearly is alert, has an open airway, and has been vomiting coffee-ground-colored material into a basin. You quickly apply a nonrebreathing mask and then assess the patient's pulse.

The patient's wife tells you that her husband has been having pain in the left upper quadrant of his abdomen all evening and has had dark-colored, tarry diarrhea with a very distinctive odor. She also tells you that the patient has a history of stomach problems caused by eating spicy foods. Several years ago, he had an endoscopic procedure that revealed a peptic ulcer. You assist the patient into a supine position on your stretcher and complete your primary assessment and take some baseline vital signs.

Recording Time: 0 minutes	
Appearance	Pale, diaphoretic skin
Level of consciousness	Alert (oriented to person, place, and day)
Airway	Appears patent
Breathing	Regular, nonlabored
Circulation	Pale, diaphoretic skin; regular, thready pulse
Pulse	100 beats/min and shallow
Blood pressure	110/70 mm Hg
Respirations	20 breaths/min and regular
SpO_2	98%

1. Why is the patient vomiting dark-colored material?

2. Describe the components of the upper gastrointestinal tract and their functions.

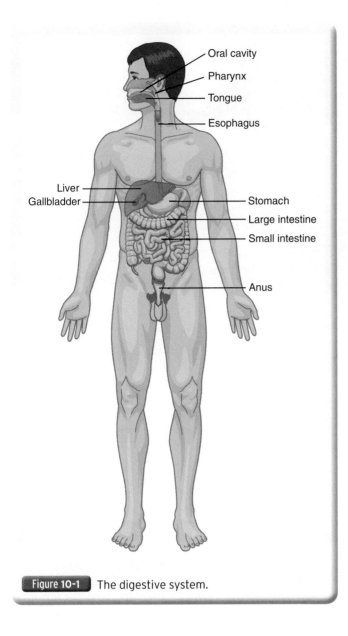

Figure 10-1 The digestive system.

Figure 10-2. Its wall consists of four layers, specialized in certain regions for particular functions, as follows:

- Mucosa (mucous membrane). Surface epithelium, underlying connective tissue, and a small amount of smooth muscle; it is folded in some regions, with projections extending into the lumen that increase its absorptive surface. The mucosa carries out secretion and absorption.
- Submucosa Loose connective tissue with glands, blood vessels, lymphatic vessels, and nerves; it nourishes surrounding tissues and carries away absorbed materials.
- Adventitia (muscular layer). Produces movements of the tube and is made of two smooth muscle tissue coats: circular fibers of the inner coat encircle the tube, causing contraction, and longitudinal fibers run lengthwise, causing shortening of the tube.
- Serosa (serous layer). Composed of a visceral peritoneum on the outside and connective tissue beneath; it protects underlying tissues and secretes serous fluid so that abdominal organs slide freely against each other.

Figure 10-3 shows the layers of the alimentary canal.

Functions of the Digestive System

The functions of the digestive system consist of a series of steps that include the following:

- Ingestion. Materials enter the digestive tract via the mouth.
- Mechanical processing. Materials are crushed and broken into smaller fragments by the teeth (mastication), making them easier to move through the digestive tract. This is also referred to as mechanical digestion, as the teeth and tongue are used to tear and mash food; additional mechanical processing is provided by the mixing motions of the stomach and intestines.

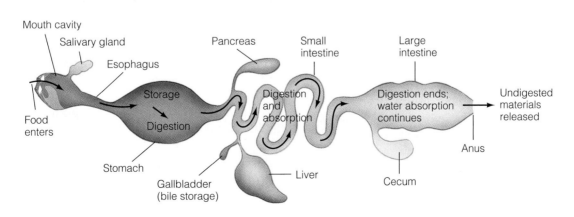

Figure 10-2   The alimentary canal.

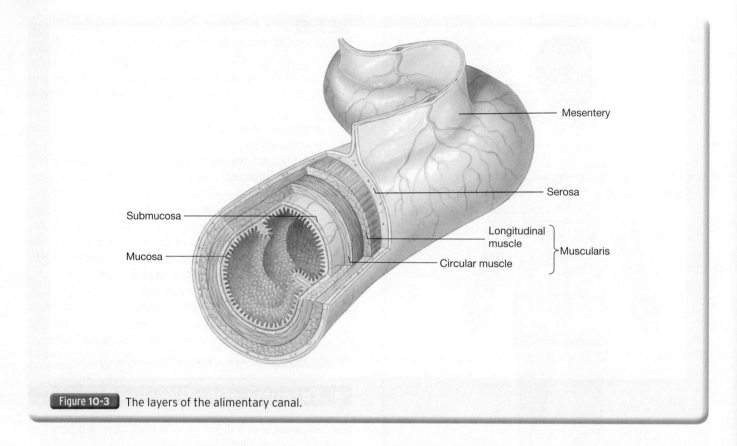

Figure 10-3   The layers of the alimentary canal.

- Digestion. The chemical breakdown of food into particles that are small enough to be absorbed by the digestive epithelium, which is a process called chemical digestion. Simple molecules such as glucose are absorbed intact while others (polysaccharides, proteins, triglycerides) must first be broken down before they can be absorbed. This begins in the mouth with enzymes in the saliva attacking the particles of food during chewing. This is also referred to as oral digestion.
- Secretion. Release of water, acids, buffers, enzymes, and salts by the epithelium and glandular organs of the digestive tract.
- Absorption. The movement of organic substrates (molecules acted on by enzymes), electrolytes, vitamins, and water across the epithelium of the digestive tract into the interstitial fluid.
- Excretion. The removal of waste products from body fluids via secretions from the digestive tract and glandular organs. After mixing with residue that cannot be digested, the waste products become feces, which are eliminated during the process of defecation.

The digestive system's lining protects surrounding tissues against digestive acids and enzymes that may corrode them, abrasion and other mechanical stress, and bacteria that may be consumed with food or that normally live inside the digestive tract. Should bacteria reach areas of areolar tissue such as the lamina propria, immune cells such as macrophages will attack them. The lamina propria lies beneath the epithelium and constitutes the mucosa (mucous membranes) of the digestive tract.

Movement of Digestive Materials

There are two basic types of motor functions in the alimentary canal: mixing movements and propelling movements. When smooth muscles contract rhythmically, mixing occurs. Waves of contractions mix food with digestive juices. In the small intestine, mixing movements are aided by segmentation, involving alternating contraction and relaxation of smooth muscle in nonadjacent segments. Materials are not propelled along the tract in one direction because segmentation follows no set pattern. Peristalsis consists of the propelling, wavelike movements of the tube. Contraction appears in the wall of the tube in a "ring," while the muscular wall immediately ahead of the ring relaxes. The peristaltic wave moves along, pushing contents of the tube toward the anus.

Abdominal Quadrants

For prehospital providers, the training curricula have traditionally used the quadrant system. The abdomen is divided into four quadrants in order to reference the location of abdominal organs. If two intersecting perpendicular lines are drawn through the umbilicus, four quadrants are formed

Figure 10-4. The diaphragm forms the top of the abdominal cavity. The pelvis forms the bottom of the abdominal cavity.

The four quadrants are: the right upper quadrant (RUQ), left upper quadrant (LUQ), right lower quadrant (RLQ), and left lower quadrant (LLQ). The major organs in the RUQ include

Case Study | PART 2

Your partner obtains a set of baseline vital signs, and you continue with your assessment that includes a history and a physical examination. The patient history reveals a 49-year-old man who weighs 90 kg. The SAMPLE history shows:

- **A**ge, gender, weight: 49-year-old man, 90 kg
- **S**igns and symptoms: Dizziness, nausea, and GI distress
- **A**llergies to medications: Codeine and sulfa-based drugs
- **M**edications taken: Tagamet, Maalox, and vitamins
- **P**ast pertinent medical history: Peptic ulcer disease
- **L**ast food/fluid intake: Dinner at 5:00 PM, which consisted of bland food and a glass of white wine
- **E**vents prior to onset: Excessive stress at work over a period of time

The OPQRST history shows:

- **O**nset of symptoms: Pain had been present earlier in the day, subsided for a few hours, and returned about 2 hours ago
- **P**rovoking factors: The patient is the CEO of a large company that is going through bankruptcy, and he has been experiencing tremendous stress recently.
- **Q**uality of discomfort: Sharp and cramping pain
- **R**adiating/related signs/symptoms: The pain is located in the left upper quadrant of the abdomen. The patient experienced temporary relief earlier in the day from antacids and a glass of milk.
- **S**everity of complaint: On a scale of 1 to 10, with 10 being the worst pain he has ever experienced, the patient says the pain is a 7.
- **T**ime: The latest flare-up of pain occurred about 2.5 hours ago.

You place the patient on the stretcher in the Trendelenburg position and the paramedic starts a large-bore saline IV line. As the patient is loaded into the ambulance, he once again vomits coffee-ground colored material into a plastic bag.

Recording Time: 5 minutes

Appearance	Pale, diaphoretic skin
Level of consciousness	Alert (oriented to person, place, and day)
Airway	Appears patent
Breathing	Regular, nonlabored
Circulation	Pale, diaphoretic skin; regular, thready pulse
Pulse	120 beats/min, thready
Blood pressure	96/70 mm Hg
Respirations	24 breaths/min, regular
Spo$_2$	96%
Pupils	Equal and reactive
Electrocardiogram	Sinus tachycardia with no ectopy

3. The patient has a past medical history of peptic ulcer disease. What is the impact of this condition on the stomach?

4. Which hormones are responsible for increasing and decreasing gastric motility?

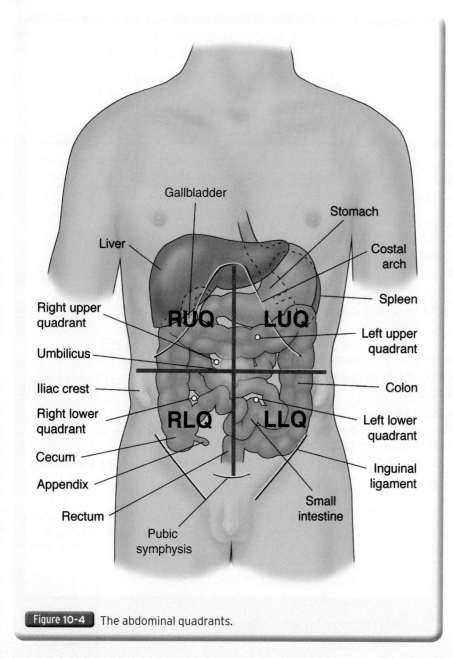

Figure 10-4 The abdominal quadrants.

the liver, gallbladder, part of the large intestine, and the right kidney; in the LUQ, they are the stomach, spleen, pancreas, part of the large intestine, and the left kidney. The RLQ contains the appendix, part of the large intestine, the right ovary,

Pathophysiology

Inflammation of the appendix, or appendicitis, is a common malady. If the condition goes untreated or unrecognized, the appendix may burst, resulting in the release of pus into the abdominal cavity. Peritonitis, a life-threatening infection of the abdominal cavity, may result. Persons with appendicitis often experience tenderness over an area of the right lower quadrant known as McBurney point.

right ureter, and part of the uterus and urinary bladder, and the LLQ contains part of the large intestine, the left ovary, left ureter, and part of the uterus and urinary bladder.

■ Gastrointestinal Tract Organs

■ The Mouth

Digestion begins in the mouth with mastication, or the chewing of food by the teeth. Mastication prepares the food for further breakdown in the stomach and intestines. During mastication, food is mixed with secretions from the salivary glands Figure 10-5.

The tongue, a muscular process in the floor of the mouth, manipulates materials in the mouth to assist in chewing by mechanical process and preparing the material for swallowing. The tongue provides sensory analysis by touch, temperature, and taste receptors.

Saliva is secreted by the salivary glands. It moistens food and begins the chemical digestion of carbohydrates. Saliva is also a solvent that dissolves foods so they can be tasted, and it helps to cleanse the mouth and teeth of bacteria. Each salivary gland has secretory serous cells and mucous cells, in varying proportions. Serous cells produce a watery fluid containing the digestive enzyme salivary amylase, which breaks starches and other polysaccharides into simple sugars.

Mucous cells secrete mucus, a thick liquid that binds food particles and lubricates them during swallowing. Parasympathetic nerve impulses cause saliva secretion when appealing food is seen, smelled, tasted, or even thought about. Unappealing food actually inhibits parasympathetic activity, producing less saliva, and making swallowing difficult.

The three pairs of major salivary glands are as follows:

- Parotid glands. The largest glands; they lie anterior and slightly inferior to each ear, between the cheek and masseter muscle, producing a clear and watery fluid rich in amylase.
- Submandibular glands. Located in the floor of the mouth on the inside lower jaw surface; they secrete a more viscous fluid than the parotid glands.
- Sublingual glands. The smallest; they lie on the floor of the mouth inferior to the tongue, and produce thick and stringy secretions.

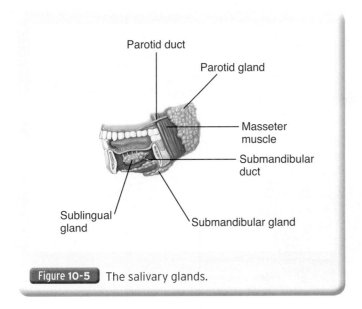

Parotid duct

Parotid gland

Masseter
muscle

Submandibular
duct

Sublingual
gland

Submandibular gland

Figure 10-5 The salivary glands.

The Hollow Abdominal Organs

Abdominal organs are either hollow (such as the intestines) or solid (such as the liver). The hollow organs are tubular structures through which food or secretions move—the esophagus, stomach, intestines, and gallbladder.

Pathophysiology

Injury to a hollow organ may puncture or rupture it. In either case, the internal contents will be dumped into the abdominal cavity, resulting in irritation and possibly infection.

The Esophagus

The esophagus is a hollow muscular tube, about 25 centimeters (10 inches) in length, with a diameter of about 2 centimeters. It is basically a straight but collapsible tube. The main function of the esophagus is to pass solid food and liquids to the stomach. Food passes through the esophagus from the pharynx to the stomach, beginning at the base of the pharynx and descending posterior to the trachea. The esophagus passes through the mediastinum, penetrating the diaphragm through the esophageal hiatus, and is continuous with the stomach on the abdominal side of the diaphragm.

Throughout the submucosa of the esophagus there are many mucous glands that moisten and lubricate the inner lining of the tube. Above the area where the esophagus joins the stomach, circular smooth muscle fibers thicken to form the lower esophageal sphincter (cardiac sphincter). Two muscular rings, the upper and lower esophageal sphincters, regulate the movement of material into and out of the esophagus.

Pathophysiology

At times, a weakness in the esophageal hiatus develops so that the stomach and esophagus move above the diaphragm. This hiatal hernia may result in backflow of stomach acid into the esophagus and the production of heartburn or reflux esophagitis.

The Stomach

The stomach is a pouch-like organ shaped like a J. It hangs inferior to the diaphragm in the upper left abdominal cavity. Its capacity is approximately 1 liter, and its inner lining consists of thick folds of mucosal and submucosal layers. When the stomach is distended, these folds (rugae) disappear. The stomach mixes food from the esophagus with gastric juice, begins protein digestion and limited absorption, and moves food into the small intestine **Figure 10-6**. It is divided into the cardiac, fundic, body, and pyloric regions, as follows:

- Cardiac region. A small area near the esophageal opening. This portion of the stomach that attaches to the esophagus is called the cardia.
- Fundic region. The fundus is the portion of the stomach that balloons superior to the cardiac portion and acts as a temporary storage area.
- Body region. The dilated, main portion of the stomach.
- Pyloric region. Narrower than the rest of the stomach, this region becomes the pyloric antrum connecting the body of the stomach to the pyloric canal as it nears the small intestine. At its end, the muscular wall thickens to form a powerful, circular pyloric sphincter, which acts as a valve controlling gastric emptying into the duodenum of the intestine.

In the stomach, the food is churned and mixed with digestive juices, forming a semiliquid mass called chyme. The stomach's volume increases during eating, and decreases as chyme leaves the stomach to enter the small intestine. The chyme is pushed via peristalsis toward the pyloric region of the stomach, causing the pyloric sphincter to relax. Stomach contractions slowly push the chyme into the small intestine. Liquids pass through more quickly than solids. Carbohydrates pass most quickly, then proteins, and finally fatty foods (which may remain in the stomach for up to 6 hours). Secretions from the pancreas, liver, and gallbladder are added in the duodenum of the small intestine.

The mucosa includes many gastric pits, or invaginations, that contain openings for glands of the stomach. The glands consist of three types of cells: the parietal, chief, and endocrine cells.

Parietal cells produce hydrochloric acid, used to digest food, and intrinsic factor, which is important in the absorption of vitamin B_{12}. Chief cells produce pepsinogen, an important enzyme in the digestion of food. Pepsinogen is inactive until

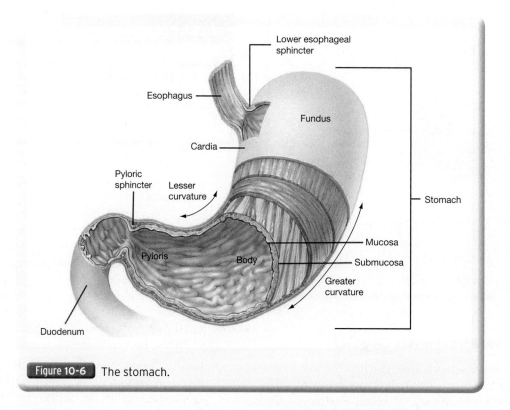

Figure 10-6   The stomach.

it is exposed to hydrochloric acid, at which time it is rapidly converted to its activated form, pepsin. Pepsin breaks down proteins. Endocrine cells produce regulatory hormones.

Hormones produced by the endocrine cells of the stomach and intestine have significant effects on the motility (motion) of substances through the stomach. Gastrin increases stomach secretions as well as the rate of gastric emptying. Secretin, which is produced by the duodenum, inhibits gastric secretion and stimulates the production of alkaline pancreatic secretions. Secretin inhibits gastric motility.

Cholecystokinin is a hormone produced in the intestine that stimulates the production of pancreatic secretions, stimulates gallbladder contractions, and inhibits gastric motility. Gastric inhibitory peptide inhibits both gastric secretion and motility.

Pathophysiology

Surgical removal of large portions of the stomach will result in the body's inability to make intrinsic factor. This substance is necessary for the proper intestinal absorption of vitamin B$_{12}$. If vitamin B$_{12}$ levels decrease enough, a condition known as pernicious anemia will develop.

Pathophysiology

Gastritis is one type of stomach irritation often caused by overproduction of stomach acid by the parietal cells. Peptic ulcer disease, in which parts of the stomach and duodenal lining actually erode, is another cause of stomach irritation Figure 10-7.

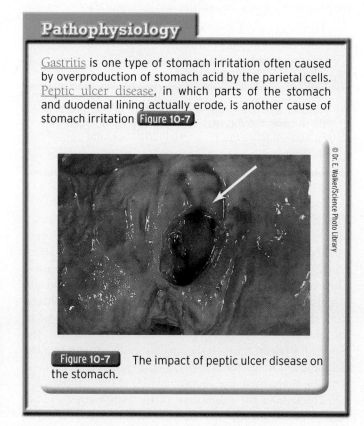

© Dr. E. Walker/Science Photo Library

Figure 10-7   The impact of peptic ulcer disease on the stomach.

The Small Intestine

The small intestine is the longest part of the digestive tract and the major site of food digestion and absorption of nutrients. Secretions from the pancreas and liver lubricate and protect the intestinal wall from the acidic chyme and the action of digestive enzymes. The release of secretin and cholecystokinin stimulate the production of liver and pancreatic digestive enzymes. The small intestine contains three portions: the duodenum, jejunum, and ileum. The entire small intestine is approximately 7 meters long in an adult. The first portion, or duodenum, forms a 180° arch within the abdomen. It is located posterior to the parietal peritoneum, following a C-shaped path by passing anterior to the right kidney and upper three lumbar vertebrae. It is broken into four sections, two of which are retroperitoneal and then reenter the peritoneal cavity at the duodenojejunal flexure or the ligament of Treitz. The pancreas is located within this C-shaped loop. This portion of the small intestine functions as a mixing area, receiving chyme from the stomach and digestive secretions from the pancreas and liver. The remainder of the small intestine is more mobile, lying free inside the peritoneal cavity. The duodenum takes a sharp bend and, at the duodenojejunal flexure, continues into the jejunum. The jejunum has thicker walls and more folds than the other portions of the small intestine. The jejunum is the proximal two fifths of the small intestine, and is about 2.5 meters in length. Most chemical digestion and nutrient absorption occur in the jejunum. The ileum is the last portion of the small intestine and continues on to become the large intestine. The ileum is not distinctly

Case Study PART 3

After administration of the first liter of saline, you note the patient's blood pressure while lying down has risen slightly to 110 mm Hg by palpation, and his pulse rate is now 110 beats/min. You now begin the physical examination. You keep the patient supine and warm your hands before touching his belly.

The results of the physical examination are:

- Head: Pale skin
- Neck: Flat neck veins
- Chest: No scars, patches, or medical identification chains or bracelets
- Lung sounds: Clear in all fields
- Abdomen: Soft with no masses, diffusely tender, no bruising or discoloration
- Pelvis: Unremarkable
- Upper extremities: Unremarkable
- Lower extremities: Unremarkable

The patient states that the dizziness has subsided while lying supine, but he still feels nauseated. You give him an emesis bag and keep alert for more vomiting while your partner prepares to administer medication for the nausea.

Recording Time: 15 minutes	
Appearance	Pale and clammy
Level of consciousness	Alert (oriented to person, place, and day)
Airway	Open and clear
Breathing	Rapid with no distress
Circulation	Pale, clammy skin and rapid pulse
Pulse	120 beats/min, fast and weak
Blood pressure	110/70 mm Hg
Respirations	22 breaths/min and normal
Spo$_2$	97%
Pupils	Equal and reactive to light
Electrocardiogram	Sinus tachycardia with no ectopy

5. Describe the landmarks of the left upper quadrant of the abdomen and the internal organs within that area.
6. Which part of the GI system is the major site for digestion of food and absorption of nutrients?

separate from the jejunum, but has a smaller diameter, with a thinner, less vascular, and less active wall. It is the longest portion of the small intestine, totaling about 3.5 meters in length. Also differentiating the ileum from the jejunum are the Peyer patches, which are defined as organized lymphoid tissue that are similar in appearance to lymph nodes. They function to protect the ileum from invasive pathogenic microorganisms.

Plicae circulares are circular folds that run perpendicular to the long axis of the digestive tract. These folds greatly increase the surface area available for absorption, allowing for much more efficient digestion. Each fold contains numerous fingerlike projections, or villi, that are 0.5 to 1.5 mm long. Each villus contains a capillary and lymph capillary called a lacteal. Absorptive cells produce digestive enzymes and absorb digested food **Figure 10-8**. Disaccharidases break down sugars, and peptidases break down proteins. Goblet cells produce a protective mucous lining, and endocrine cells produce regulatory hormones.

The common bile duct and the hepatic duct drain into the opening, or lumen, of the duodenum at the ampulla of Vater **Figure 10-9**.

The diameter of the small intestine gradually decreases from the duodenum distally so that the jejunum and ileum are smaller structures than the duodenum. The jejunum and ileum are the primary sites for absorption of nutrients. The ileum also contains numerous intermittent lymph nodules, called Peyer patches. The ileocecal junction is located between the ileum and the large intestine. The ileocecal valve prevents backflow of intestinal contents.

The small intestine is the most important absorbing organ of the alimentary canal. Very little absorbable material

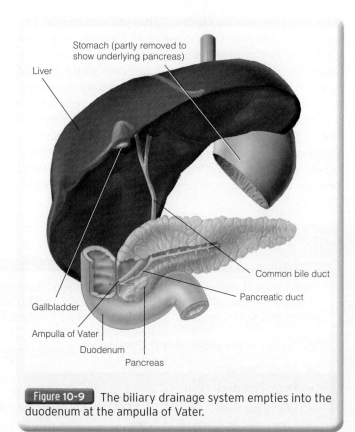

Stomach (partly removed to show underlying pancreas)

Liver

Common bile duct

Pancreatic duct

Gallbladder

Ampulla of Vater

Duodenum

Pancreas

Figure 10-9 The biliary drainage system empties into the duodenum at the ampulla of Vater.

reaches its distal end. The digestion of carbohydrates begins in the mouth and is completed by enzymes from the intestinal mucosa and pancreas. Monosaccharides that result from this process are absorbed by the villi, and simple sugars are absorbed by active transport or facilitated diffusion.

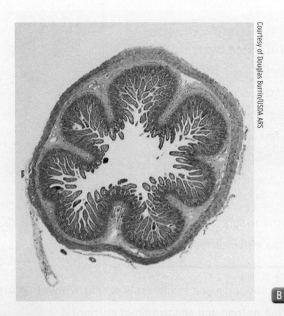

Courtesy of Douglas Burrin/USDA ARS

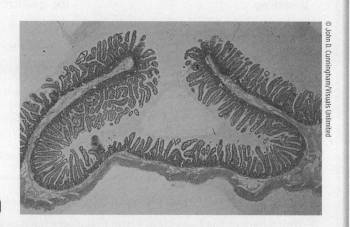

© John D. Cunningham/Visuals Unlimited

A

B

Figure 10-8 The small intestine mucosa is folded into villi. **A.** Villi in the small intestine. **B.** Close-up of villi.

Overdistention or irritation of the small intestine results in a peristaltic rush, which moves the small intestine's contents into the large intestine quickly. Normal absorption of nutrients, water, and electrolytes therefore does not occur in this situation. Peristaltic rush results in diarrhea, and prolonged diarrhea results in water and electrolyte imbalances.

The small intestine connects to the large intestine via the ileocecal sphincter, or junction. This sphincter is usually constricted to keep the contents of each intestine separate. After eating, peristalsis in the ileum relaxes the sphincter to force some small intestine contents into the cecum of the large intestine.

Pathophysiology

Gastrointestinal bleeding, whether it is upper or lower, can be a source of significant hemorrhage. Often, the patient has nausea, vomiting, and diarrhea that may contain bright red or partially digested blood. Vomiting can occur rapidly and forcefully, and if you are not prepared you could be exposed to the patient's blood. The stool and emesis associated with this type of hemorrhage can be identified by the distinct odor that accompanies it. It is overwhelming and unforgettable. Gloves should always be worn with every patient encounter, but they are especially necessary in this situation. You should be prepared for vomitus and fecal material to be present on the patient and in the surrounding areas.

The Large Intestine

The large intestine begins at the cecum **Figure 10-10**. Typically, the ileum enters the cecum at the ileocecal valve, forming a blind sac, attached to the end of which is the vermiform appendix. The appendix contains large numbers of lymph nodules.

The large intestine has little or no digestive function. It contains many tubular glands composed almost entirely of goblet cells. Mucus is the only important secretion of the large intestine. It protects the intestinal wall against abrasion and binds particles of fecal matter. The mucus is alkaline, helping to control pH of the large intestine.

The colon consists of four portions: the ascending colon, transverse colon, descending colon, and sigmoid colon. The ascending colon extends upward from the cecum. It ends at the hepatic flexure, where the colon takes a sharp left turn near the inferior border of the liver. The transverse colon, the longest, most movable part, continues across the abdomen to the splenic flexure, where it turns sharply and becomes the descending colon. The sigmoid colon forms an S-shaped tube that extends into the pelvis and ends at the rectum which is the exit of the intestine.

The colon lacks the folds and villi of the small intestine. Rather, it contains numerous straight tubular glands called crypts. These glands contain many mucus-producing goblet cells. A portion of the longitudinal muscle layer of the wall of the large intestine, the teniae coli, encircles the colon. Contractions of the teniae coli produce haustra, recesses that give the colon a puckered appearance.

The mixing actions of the large intestine are usually slower than those of the small intestine. The peristaltic waves of the large intestine happen only between twice and three times per day. The intestinal walls constrict vigorously (mass movements) to force contents toward the rectum. These movements usually follow a meal, but may also be caused by irritations of the intestinal mucosa. Conditions such as colitis (inflamed colon) may also cause frequent mass movements.

The rectum is a straight, muscular tube that ends at the anus. Its function is to store stool. Stretching of the rectum by stool results in the urge to defecate. The anal canal is very short (1 inch to 2 inches). It contains two circular sphincters, the internal sphincter and the external sphincter, which help regulate the passage of stool. The external muscle is under voluntary control.

Pathophysiology

The colon normally contains many bacteria that are helpful in breaking down food. Without these bacteria, called normal flora, severe diarrhea develops. The normal flora produces gases called flatus. The amount of colonic gas present depends partly on the number of bacteria present and partly on the foods consumed. Beans and cauliflower, for example, are well known for their flatogenic effect.

Pathophysiology

Weakness in the walls of the colon can develop, resulting in outpouchings, or diverticuli. Diverticuli can become inflamed, causing diverticulitis, or they may bleed. Most persons with diverticuli, however, remain asymptomatic.

Pathophysiology

Cancer of the colon is very common, especially in the sigmoid and descending region. A fiberoptic scope, the colonoscope, allows the physician to view the lining of this portion of the colon and biopsy suspicious lesions. Early symptoms include a change in bowel movements and blood in the stool. Most physicians recommend regular stool examination for this disease in persons older than age 40 years. Persons at high risk (those with a family history of colon cancer) as well as persons older than age 50 years should undergo regular colonoscopic examination.

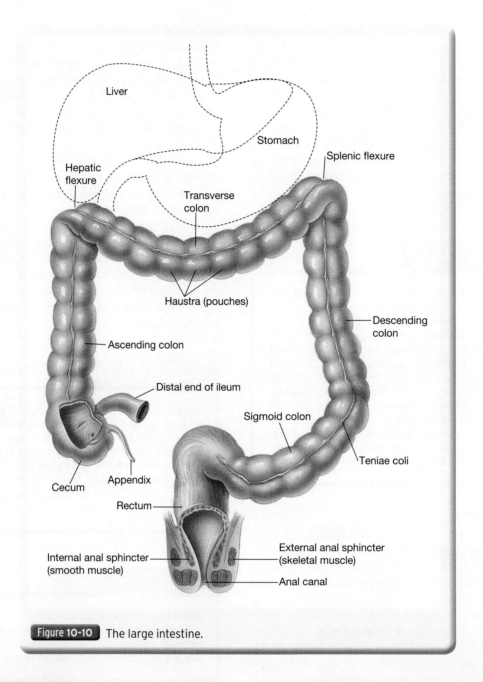

Figure 10-10 The large intestine.

Pathophysiology

Large veins line the inside of the anal canal. These vessels constitute the hemorrhoidal plexus. Medications that are given rectally are quickly absorbed into these veins and into the remainder of the body. Abnormal dilations of these veins result in the formation of hemorrhoids.

The Gallbladder

The gallbladder is a pear-shaped sac located on the lower surface of the liver (see Figure 10-9). It is connected to the cystic duct, which joins the common hepatic duct.

The gallbladder has an epithelial lining and strong muscles in its wall. It stores bile—one of the digestive enzymes produced by the liver—reabsorbs water, and contracts to release bile into the small intestine.

The common bile duct is formed by the joining of the common hepatic and cystic ducts. It leads to the duodenum, where the hepatopancreatic sphincter is normally contracted. As bile collects in the common bile duct, it backs up into the cystic duct and flows into the gallbladder for storage.

Bile usually enters the duodenum once cholecystokinin stimulates gallbladder contraction. The hepatopancreatic sphincter is contracted until a peristaltic wave in the duodenal wall influences its relaxation, resulting in the passage of bile into the small intestine.

Pathophysiology

Digestive enzymes contained within the gallbladder can, at times, form stones called gallstones. If gallstones occlude the cystic duct, the gallbladder becomes swollen, with resultant pain, nausea, and vomiting. The presence of gallstones is termed cholelithiasis. Cholecystitis, or a "gallbladder attack," occurs with the presence of symptoms from cholelithiasis.

The Solid Abdominal Organs

The major solid abdominal organs are the liver, spleen, and pancreas. When crushed or penetrated, these organs bleed profusely.

Pathophysiology

Injury to a solid organ may result in significant bleeding into the abdominal cavity.

The Liver

The liver is located in the right upper quadrant of the abdominal cavity, inferior to the diaphragm, and is the largest internal organ of the body, normally weighing about 3 pounds. It is reddish-brown, well-supplied with blood vessels, and extends from the level of the fifth intercostal space to the lower margin of the ribs. The liver is enclosed in a fibrous capsule and is divided into lobes by connective tissue. Its right lobe is larger than its left lobe. The liver's many functions include storage of glucose, protein synthesis, and filtering body wastes from the blood.

A specialized portion of the circulatory system, the hepatoportal system, directs blood from the intestines through the liver for processing.

The Spleen and Pancreas

The spleen is in the left upper quadrant lateral and posterior to the stomach. It is vascular and vital in fighting infection as well as in the removal of red blood cells from circulation. Like the spleen, the pancreas is mostly located posterior to behind the stomach within the lesser omental space, extending laterally from the duodenum toward the spleen. It is an elongated organ, about 15 centimeters long, and weighing about 3 ounces. The pancreas makes insulin, glucagons, and digestive enzymes and secretes insulin and glucagons into the bloodstream.

Digestive enzymes travel via the main pancreatic duct into the common hepatic duct and empty into the duodenum at the ampulla of Vater. Pancreatic enzymes that digest proteins include trypsin, chymotrypsin, and carboxypeptidase. Other enzymes, collectively referred to as lipases, break down fats.

The Peritoneum and Mesenteries

The digestive organs are surrounded by the peritoneum, a two-layer, smooth membrane of connective tissue. The parietal peritoneum lines the abdominal cavity; the visceral peritoneum is in close contact with the organs. The kidneys, pancreas, duodenum, and major blood vessels of the abdominal cavity are located in an area behind the parietal peritoneum known as the retroperitoneal space. These are sometimes referred to as retroperitoneal organs.

Mesenteries are parts of the peritoneum that hold the abdominal organs in place and provide a passageway for blood vessels and nerves to the organs. The omenta are folds of the peritoneum from the stomach to adjacent organs. The lesser omentum is the portion of mesentery that connects the lesser curvature of the stomach to the liver and diaphragm. The greater omentum connects the greater curvature of the stomach to the transverse colon and posterior body wall. This long, double fold of mesentery extends inferiorly from the stomach to create a cavity called the omental bursa.

Case Study PART 4

While en route to the hospital, you conduct a reassessment that includes repeating the primary assessment, obtaining serial vital signs every 5 minutes, and reassessing interventions such as administering oxygen and monitoring IV fluids. The patient is still very pale, but he is not cyanotic. He denies shortness of breath. The patient vomits once again, and you collect the vomitus in a disposable plastic suction canister to deliver to the emergency department physician.

Prep Kit

Chapter Summary

- All portions of the alimentary canal contain four similar layers: the mucosa, submucosa, adventitia (muscle layer), and serosa (or outer lining of the bowel).

- Digestion begins in the mouth; food then travels via the esophagus to the stomach, where it is further digested before moving to the small intestine.

- The abdomen is divided into quadrants with the umbilicus as the central reference point.

- The right upper quadrant contains the liver, gallbladder, part of the large intestine, and the right kidney.

- The left upper quadrant contains the stomach, spleen, pancreas, part of the large intestine, and the left kidney.

- The right lower quadrant contains the appendix, part of the large intestine, the right ovary, right ureter, and part of the uterus and urinary bladder.

- The left lower quadrant contains part of the large intestine, the left ovary, left ureter, and part of the uterus and urinary bladder.

- The esophagus is a hollow tube with a thick muscular wall that transports food and liquid from the mouth to the stomach.

- The stomach is an expandable organ where food is churned and mixed with digestive juices, forming a semiliquid mass called chyme.

- The stomach begins protein digestion and limited absorption and moves food into the small intestine.

- Thick folds of the stomach wall are called rugae, which allow the stomach lining to stretch when the stomach is full.

- The lining of the inner stomach mucosa has many gastric pits, which contain the parietal, chief, and endocrine cells.

- The small intestine is the longest part of the digestive tract, approximately 7 meters in the adult, and is the major site of food digestion and absorption of nutrients.

- The small intestine contains three portions: the duodenum, jejunum, and ileum.

- The large intestine (or colon) begins at the cecum. The appendix is located at the end of the cecum and contains large numbers of lymph nodes.

- The large intestine has little or no digestive function.

- The colon consists of four portions: the ascending colon, transverse colon, descending colon, and sigmoid colon.

- The rectum is a straight, muscular tube that ends at the anal canal. Stretching of the rectum by stool results in the urge to defecate.

- The gallbladder is a pear-shaped sac located on the lower surface of the liver that acts as a reservoir for bile, one of the digestive enzymes.

- The liver is the largest internal organ of the body and has many functions, including storage of glucose, protein synthesis, and filtering body wastes from the blood.

- The spleen is a highly vascular organ that aids in the removal of old blood cells from circulation as well as in fighting infection.

- The pancreas is an elongated organ that has several functions, including the manufacture of digestive enzymes and the hormones insulin and glucagon.

- The digestive organs are surrounded by the peritoneum, a two-layer smooth membrane of connective tissue. The parietal peritoneum lines the abdominal cavity; the visceral peritoneum is in close contact with the organs.

- The kidneys, pancreas, duodenum, and major blood vessels of the abdominal cavity are located in an area behind the parietal peritoneum known as the retroperitoneal space.

- Mesenteries are parts of the peritoneum that hold the abdominal organs in place and provide a passageway for blood vessels and nerves to the organs.

Vital Vocabulary

absorptive cells Cells that produce digestive enzymes and absorb digested food.

adventitia The muscular layer of the wall of the alimentary canal.

alimentary canal The mouth, pharynx, esophagus, stomach, small intestine, large intestine, rectum, and anus.

ampulla of Vater Opening in the duodenum into which the common bile duct and the pancreatic duct drain.

anal canal The short tube at the end of the rectum that contains two circular sphincters (internal and external), which help regulate the passage of stool.

anus The distal orifice of the alimentary canal, where stool passes from the body.

appendicitis Inflammation of the appendix.

ascending colon One of four portions of the colon; it extends upward from the cecum.

bile A digestive enzyme produced in the liver and stored in the gallbladder.

carboxypeptidase A pancreatic enzyme that digests proteins.

cecum The first part of the large intestine, into which the ileum opens.

chemical digestion Digestion of food by enzymes in the stomach and small bowel.

chief cells Cells in the stomach mucosa that produce pepsinogen, an important enzyme in the digestion of food.

cholecystitis Symptoms from cholelithiasis; also called a gallbladder attack.

cholecystokinin A hormone produced in the intestine that stimulates the production of pancreatic secretions and gallbladder contractions and inhibits gastric motility.

cholelithiasis The presence of gallstones.

chyme The name given to the substance that leaves the stomach once food is digested; it is a combination of all of the eaten foods with added stomach acids.

chymotrypsin A pancreatic enzyme that digests proteins.

colon A portion of the gastrointestinal system extending from the small intestine to the rectum that maintains water balance by absorbing and excreting water; also called the large intestine.

colonoscope A fiberoptic scope used in the visual examination of the colon.

crypts Tubular glands located in the colon, which contain many mucus-producing goblet cells.

cystic duct The route through which the gallbladder releases bile.

descending colon One of four portions of the colon; it extends from the splenic flexure to the sigmoid colon.

diaphragm Large dome-shaped muscle used for respiration that represents the boundary between the abdominal and thoracic cavities.

digestion The mechanical and chemical breakdown of foods and the absorption of resulting nutrients by the body's cells.

digestive system The body system that carries out the processes of mechanical and chemical digestion; also called the gastrointestinal system.

disaccharidases Enzymes that break down sugars.

diverticuli Weakened areas (outpouchings) in the walls of the colon.

diverticulitis Inflammation of the diverticuli.

duodenojejunal flexure The sharp bend in the small intestine between the duodenum and the jejunum.

duodenum The first of three sections of the small intestine; it extends posteriorly from the stomach and forms a 180° arch within the retroperitoneal portion of the abdomen.

endocrine cells Cells in the stomach mucosa that produce regulatory hormones.

esophageal hiatus An opening in the diaphragm through which the esophagus passes.

esophageal sphincters Two muscular rings (upper and lower) that regulate the movement of material into and out of the esophagus.

esophagus A collapsible tube that extends from the pharynx to the stomach; contractions of the muscle in the wall of the esophagus propel food and liquids through it to the stomach.

flatus Gas within the colon.

fundus The bottom of a hollow organ. In the stomach, it is the portion that balloons superior to the cardiac portion to act as a temporary storage area.

gallbladder A saclike organ located on the lower surface of the liver that acts as a reservoir for bile.

gallstones Rigid stones formed by digestive enzymes within the gallbladder.

gastric inhibitory peptide A hormone that inhibits both gastric secretion and motility.

gastric pits Numerous pits in the stomach mucosa; also called invaginations.

gastrin A hormone produced by the endocrine cells of the stomach that increases stomach secretions as well as the rate of gastric emptying.

gastritis Irritation of the stomach often caused by overproduction of stomach acid by the parietal cells.

gastrointestinal (GI) system System composed of structures and organs involved in the consumption, digestion, and elimination of food; also called the digestive system or gastrointestinal tract.

goblet cells Cells that produce a protective mucous lining.

haustra Recesses in the colon caused by contractions of the teniae coli.

heartburn Sensation often caused by the back flow of stomach acid into the esophagus; also called reflux esophagitis.

hemorrhoidal plexus Large veins that line the inside of the anal canal.

hemorrhoids Abnormal dilation of veins in the hemorrhoidal plexus.

hepatic flexure The first turn (sharp left turn near the inferior border of the liver) in the large intestine at the end of the ascending colon and beginning of the transverse colon.

hepatoportal system A specialized portion of the circulatory system that directs blood from the stomach and intestine through the liver for processing.

hiatal hernia A weakening in the esophageal hiatus that allows the stomach to move above the diaphragm and may result in acid reflux, causing heartburn.

hydrochloric acid An acid produced by parietal cells in the stomach that aids in digestion.

ileocecal junction The junction between the ileum and large intestine.

ileum The last portion of the small intestine, which extends from the jejunum to the ileocecal valve at the beginning of the large intestine.

intrinsic factor The chemical substance produced by parietal cells in the stomach that is important in the absorption of vitamin B$_{12}$.

invaginations Numerous pits in the stomach mucosa; also called gastric pits.

jejunum The middle portion of the small intestine; it has thicker walls and more folds than the other portions of the small intestine.

lacteal A capillary and lymph channel contained in each villus.

large intestine A portion of the gastrointestinal system that extends from the small intestine to the rectum and maintains water balance by absorbing and excreting water; also called the colon.

lipases Pancreatic enzymes that break down fat.

liver A large abdominal organ that lies in the right upper quadrant immediately below the diaphragm; it produces bile, stores glucose for immediate use by the body, and produces many substances that help regulate immune responses.

lumen The opening of a vessel.

mastication Chewing.

McBurney point An anatomic landmark in the right lower quadrant of the abdomen that typically represents the location of pain associated with appendicitis.

mechanical digestion Chewing of food.

mesenteries Parts of the peritoneum that hold the abdominal organs in place and provide a passageway for blood vessels and nerves to the organs.

motility The motion that results in the passage of substances through the digestive tract.

mucosa The innermost lining of the lumen of each portion of the alimentary canal; rich in glands, lymphatic tissue, and blood vessels.

mucus Related to digestion, it is a thick liquid that binds food particles and lubricates them during swallowing.

normal flora Bacteria that are located in the colon and help in the digestion of food.

omental bursa A cavity created by a double fold of mesentery, which extends inferiorly from the stomach.

pancreas A flat, solid organ that lies below the liver and the stomach, and which is a digestive gland that secretes digestive enzymes into the duodenum through the pancreatic duct; considered both an endocrine gland and an exocrine gland.

pancreatic duct The duct through which digestive enzymes pass on their way through the common hepatic duct to the duodenum at the ampulla of Vater.

parietal cells Cells in the gastric mucosa that produce hydrochloric acid.

parietal peritoneum A smooth membrane of connective tissue that lines the abdominal cavity.

parotid glands One pair of the three sets of salivary glands.

pepsin The enzyme formed from the exposure of pepsinogen to hydrochloric acid in the stomach that is important in the initial breakdown of proteins.

pepsinogen An enzyme produced by the chief cells in the stomach that is converted to pepsin by hydrochloric acid

peptic ulcer disease A condition in which parts of the stomach and duodenal lining are eroded by stomach acid.

peptidases Enzymes that break down proteins.

peristalsis The process of contraction of the smooth muscle in the wall of the alimentary tract that serves to propel food through the system.

peritoneum A two-layer smooth membrane of connective tissue that surrounds a group of digestive organs within the abdomen.

peritonitis A potentially life-threatening inflammation of the lining of the abdominal cavity.

Peyer patches Intermittent patches of lymph nodes located in the ileum.

plicae circulares Circular folds that run perpendicular to the long axis of the digestive tract and increase the surface area available for absorption.

rectum The distal portion of the large intestine, ending at the anal canal.

reflux esophagitis The back flow of stomach acid into the esophagus; also called heartburn.

retroperitoneal space An area behind the parietal peritoneum that contains the kidneys, pancreas, duodenum, and major blood vessels of the abdominal cavity.

rugae Thick folds of the stomach wall.

saliva The fluid produced by the salivary glands that helps break down starches and other polysaccharides into simple sugars, washes the oral cavity, and helps weaken bacteria.

salivary amylase The primary enzyme in saliva.

salivary glands The glands that produce saliva to keep the mouth and pharynx moist; includes the parotid, sublingual, and submandibular glands.

secretin A hormone produced by the duodenum that inhibits gastric secretion and stimulates the production of alkaline pancreatic secretions.

segmentation Alternating contraction and relaxation of smooth muscle in nonadjacent segments of the small intestine.

serosa The outer lining of the bowel.

sigmoid colon One of four portions of the colon; it extends from the descending colon and forms an S-shaped tube that extends into the pelvis and ends as the rectum.

small intestine The portion of the gastrointestinal system that consists of the duodenum, jejunum, and ileum and is the major site of food digestion and nutrient absorption.

sphincters Rings of muscle that surround an opening, allowing for contraction or closing.

spleen The largest lymphatic organ; filters the blood via the actions of lymphocytes and macrophages.

splenic flexure The second sharp turn in the large intestine, connecting the transverse colon to the descending colon.

stomach An expandable organ that is located in the left upper quadrant, below the diaphragm.

sublingual glands One pair of the three sets of salivary glands.

submandibular glands One pair of the three sets of salivary glands.

submucosa The lining next to the mucosa in the gastrointestinal system that contains blood vessels and lymphatic channels.

teniae coli A portion of the longitudinal muscle layer of the wall of the large intestine that encircles the colon.

transverse colon One of four portions of the colon; it extends from the hepatic flexure across the abdomen to the splenic flexure.

trypsin A pancreatic enzyme that aids in the digestion of proteins.

umbilicus The navel, which serves as the central reference point in determining the location of organs in the abdominal quadrants.

vermiform appendix An appendage attached to the end of the cecum that contains large numbers of lymph nodules.

villi Fingerlike projections in the plicae circulares.

visceral peritoneum A smooth membrane of connective tissue that lies in immediate contact with the organs within the peritoneal cavity.

■ Case Study Answers

1. Why is the patient vomiting dark-colored material?

   Answer: He has bleeding somewhere in his upper gastrointestinal (GI) tract, and the blood has accumulated in his stomach. Blood is irritating to the stomach and causes sudden and unexpected nausea and vomiting. The dark or coffee-ground color indicates that the blood has been partially digested.

2. Describe the components of the upper gastrointestinal tract and their functions.

   Answer: The mouth, esophagus, and stomach make up the upper GI tract. Digestion begins in the mouth with chewing and the secretion of saliva, which breaks down starches and other polysaccharides into sugars. The esophagus transports food and liquid to the stomach where digestive juices are churned with the food, forming a semiliquid mass called chyme.

3. The patient has a past medical history of peptic ulcer disease. What is the impact of this condition on the stomach?

   Answer: Peptic ulcer disease can arise from overproduction of stomach acid, which causes parts of the stomach and duodenal lining to erode. GI bleeding can occur in the affected areas. Patients are prescribed medications that help inhibit the excessive release of stomach acid, giving the lining a chance to heal.

4. Which hormones are responsible for increasing and decreasing gastric motility?

   Answer: Gastrin, released by the gastric mucosa, increases the release of stomach secretions as well as the rate of gastric emptying. Secretin, produced by the duodenum, inhibits gastric secretion and motility. Cholecystokinin inhibits motility, and gastric inhibitory peptide inhibits both gastric secretion and motility.

5. Describe the landmarks of the left upper quadrant of the abdomen and the internal organs within that area.

   Answer: The top border of the abdomen is the diaphragm. The umbilicus is the center and two perpendicular imaginary lines mark the four quadrants. The left upper quadrant contains the stomach, spleen, pancreas, part of the large intestine, and the left kidney in the posterior.

6. Which part of the GI system is the major site for digestion of food and absorption of nutrients?

   Answer: The small intestine is the longest part of the digestive tract and contains three distinct portions: the duodenum, jejunum, and ileum. The small intestine is the major site of food digestion and absorption of nutrients.

The Endocrine System

Learning Objectives

1. Define endocrine glands, exocrine glands, hormones, and prostaglandin. (p 224)

2. Explain what prostaglandins are made of and state some of their functions. (p 224)

3. Discuss the relevance of understanding the function and structure of the endocrine system to conditions commonly found in the field. (p 224-235)

4. Explain how protein hormones and steroid hormones are believed to exert their effects. (p 225)

5. Identify the primary endocrine glands and list the major hormones secreted by each. (p 225-230)

6. Explain the roles of positive and negative feedback mechanisms in hormone secretions. (p 225)

7. List the hormones released from the anterior pituitary and posterior pituitary. (p 226)

8. Describe the location of the thyroid gland and identify the hormones produced by this gland. (p 229-230)

9. Describe the relationship between parathyroid hormone and calcitonin. (p 229-230)

10. Describe the relationship between insulin and glucagon. (p 231-232)

11. Describe the location, structure, and general functions of the adrenal glands. (p 233-234)

Introduction

The endocrine system works along with the nervous system to regulate the functions of the human body to maintain homeostasis. The endocrine system and its glands secrete hormones that diffuse from the interstitial fluid into the bloodstream. The hormones act on target cells. Paracrine secretions are those that affect only neighboring cells. Autocrine secretions are those that affect the secreting cell only. Exocrine glands are those that secrete outside the body through ducts, and include the sweat glands and tear ducts.

The Endocrine System

The brain controls the body through both the nervous system and the endocrine system. The endocrine system is a complex message and control system that integrates many body functions. Through endocrine glands, the endocrine system releases hormones such as insulin into the bloodstream. Each endocrine gland produces one or more hormones. Each hormone has a specific effect on some organ, tissue, or process.

The major endocrine glands include the pituitary gland, thyroid gland, parathyroid glands, adrenal glands, pancreas, pineal gland, thymus gland, and reproductive glands Figure 11-1 .

Prostaglandins are a group of hormone-like fatty acids that are produced in body tissues such as the uterus, brain, and kidneys. Semen also contains prostaglandins. Prostaglandins act on target organs to produce wide-ranging effects such as uterine contraction, regulation of blood pressure, smooth muscle contraction, and pain and inflammation. Aspirin and nonsteroidal anti-inflammatory drugs are believed to act by interfering with the synthesis of certain prostaglandins.

Case Study | PART 1

At 12:00 PM, your unit is dispatched to a local shopping mall parking lot for a minor, low-speed crash. The police are already on the scene, and they want you to check out a driver who is acting strange. A police officer tells you that a witness saw the patient leave the mall and stumble to her car before she backed her car into two parked vehicles.

You determine that the scene is safe and begin to assess the patient. You note that the patient has an open airway with no breathing problems, but she is obviously distressed. She knows her name but is a little confused about the day and exactly where she is. She has a weak, rapid distal pulse and no external bleeding. Your general impression is a patient in her 40s who is confused and very diaphoretic. Although the patient is cooperative, she acts like she is intoxicated; however, you do not smell alcohol. You apply oxygen via a nonrebreathing mask and note that the patient does not appear to have sustained any trauma, despite the dent in the rear of her car. You have your partner get a set of baseline vital signs.

Recording Time: 0 minutes	
Appearance	Pale, diaphoretic skin
Level of consciousness	Verbal (knows her name, but confused as to where she is and what day it is)
Airway	Appears patent
Breathing	Regular
Circulation	Thready distal pulse; no obvious external hemorrhaging
Pulse	100 beats/min and regular
Blood pressure	120 /70 mm Hg
Respirations	20 breaths/min and regular
Spo$_2$	98%

1. What is the hormone that is influencing the sympathetic nervous system during this time of stress?

2. What is the name of the organ known as the "master gland," and why is it called that?

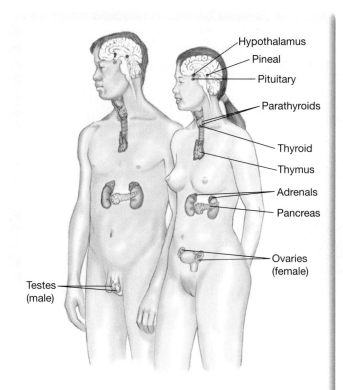

Figure 11-1 The organs of the endocrine system: the endocrine glands.

Labels: Hypothalamus, Pineal, Pituitary, Parathyroids, Thyroid, Thymus, Adrenals, Pancreas, Ovaries (female), Testes (male)

Hormones, regardless of their source, act by binding to receptors. Steroids and thyroid hormones bind to receptors located within cells. All other hormones, as a rule, bind to receptors located on the surface of cells. Hormones stimulate the production of intracellular proteins and other substances that carry out the next task in whatever body process the particular hormone is involved **Figure 11-2**.

In the absence of disease, hormones interact with each other to maintain homeostasis, or balance, in the body. Typically, this interaction involves positive feedback and negative feedback, or feedback inhibition. Negative feedback implies that when a hormone has exerted its desired effect, the result inhibits further production of the hormone until it is needed again (ie, cessation of insulin production because of low blood glucose concentration). Most feedback mechanisms in the human body are negative.

A few hormones, such as progressive labor and blood clotting hormones, work with positive feedback, in which the desired effect increases production of the hormone.

Pathophysiology

Several diseases of the central nervous system result in decreased production of antidiuretic hormone. As a result, a condition known as diabetes insipidus, the production of large volumes of dilute urine, develops.

Pathophysiology

Persons with hyperthyroidism, or an overactive thyroid gland, have increased metabolic rates with weight loss, rapid pulse rate, elevated blood pressure, diarrhea, and at times, abnormal protrusion of the eyes known as exophthalmos. Hypothyroidism, on the other hand, results in decreased metabolic rate with weight gain, dry skin, low pulse rate and blood pressure, constipation, and apathy. Either disease state may result in the presence of an enlarged thyroid gland, or goiter.

Pathophysiology

Excess secretion of parathyroid hormones results in hyperparathyroidism, or loss of calcium from the bones and increases in serum calcium levels. Loss of parathyroid function, such as results from surgical removal of the thyroid, may result in life-threatening hypocalcemia, which is a low blood calcium level. Painful muscle spasms, called tetany, may result from this condition.

Pathophysiology

Cushing syndrome is a disorder caused by excessive production of cortisol by the adrenal glands. Patients have a typical facial appearance, known as cushingoid facies, the so-called "moonface," as well as obesity, abnormal hair growth, high blood pressure, and emotional disturbances. The prolonged administration of synthetic corticosteroids also can result in this syndrome.

The Pituitary Gland and Hypothalamus

The pituitary gland, or hypophysis, is known as the master gland. The pituitary gland is located at the base of the brain in the cranial cavity, and it secretes hormones that regulate the function of many other glands in the body. The hypothalamus, the basal portion of the diencephalon, regulates the function of the pituitary gland. Compounds called releasing factors or inhibiting factors travel from the hypothalamus to the pituitary gland in a specialized set of blood vessels, the hypothalamohypophyseal portal system. The interactions of the hypothalamus and the pituitary gland often are referred to as the hypothalamic-pituitary axis.

The pituitary gland is located below the hypothalamus and is connected to it by a stalk, or infundibulum. The pituitary gland consists of two portions, the anterior pituitary (lobe), or adenohypophysis, and the posterior pituitary (lobe), or neurohypophysis **Figure 11-3**.

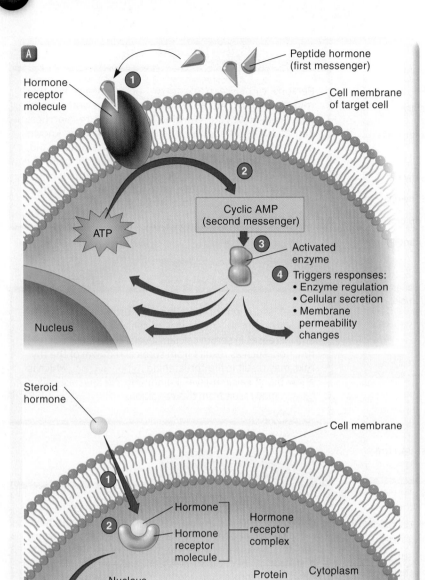

A.

Peptide hormone (first messenger)

Hormone receptor molecule

1

Cell membrane of target cell

2

Cyclic AMP (second messenger)

ATP

3   Activated enzyme

4   Triggers responses:
• Enzyme regulation
• Cellular secretion
• Membrane permeability changes

Nucleus

Steroid hormone

Cell membrane

1

2

Hormone

Hormone receptor molecule

Hormone receptor complex

Protein   Cytoplasm

Nucleus

Activated DNA (genes)

3

4

mRNA on ribosomes directs protein synthesis

B.

Figure 11-2 The mechanism of action of hormones. **A.** Peptide hormones. **B.** Steroid hormones.

The posterior pituitary differs from the anterior pituitary in that it is made up of mostly nerve fibers and neuroglial cells.

The Posterior Pituitary

The posterior portion of the pituitary gland is directly connected to and continuous with the brain. Because this area of the pituitary gland is an extension of the central nervous system, hormones produced by this region are called neurohormones. The two major hormones stored and

secreted by the neurohypophysis are antidiuretic hormone and oxytocin. Each of these hormones is secreted by different cells of the hypothalamus; however, both hormones are stored in and released by the posterior pituitary.

Antidiuretic hormone (ADH) is also called vasopressin. In high concentrations, ADH constricts blood vessels and raises the blood pressure. Its primary target tissue is the kidney, where it promotes retention of water and reduction in urine volume. The secretion of ADH changes in response to signals given to the brain by specialized neurons, called osmoreceptors, as well as by blood pressure receptors in the blood vessels.

Oxytocin causes the smooth muscles of the pregnant uterus to contract and milk to be released from the breasts of lactating women. Preparations of oxytocin sometimes are used to induce or augment labor or to contract uterine musculature after childbirth to reduce or prevent bleeding.

The Anterior Pituitary

Because the anterior portion of the pituitary gland is not considered part of the central nervous system, the hormones it produces are not neurohormones. The hypothalamus releases substances that are carried directly to the anterior pituitary via the blood. Releasing actions of the anterior pituitary are mostly stimulatory, although some have inhibitory effects.

The anterior pituitary consists of dense, collagenous connective tissue. It has five types of secretory cells, four of which—growth hormone (GH), prolactin (PRL), thyroid-stimulating hormone (TSH), and adrenocorticotropic hormone (ACTH)—secrete a single hormone. The fifth type secretes both follicle-stimulating hormone (FSH) and luteinizing hormone (LH).

Growth Hormone

Growth hormone (GH), or somatotropin, stimulates growth in most tissues, especially in long bones of the extremities. GH also increases protein synthesis and the use of fats for energy. GH stimulates the production of proteins called somatomedins by the liver, skeletal muscle, and other tissues. Somatomedins circulate in the blood and affect target tissues primarily by mediating the effects of somatotropin. Both somatomedins and somatotropin appear to be necessary for optimal growth.

Growth hormone–releasing hormone, produced by the hypothalamus, stimulates secretion of GH. Growth hormone

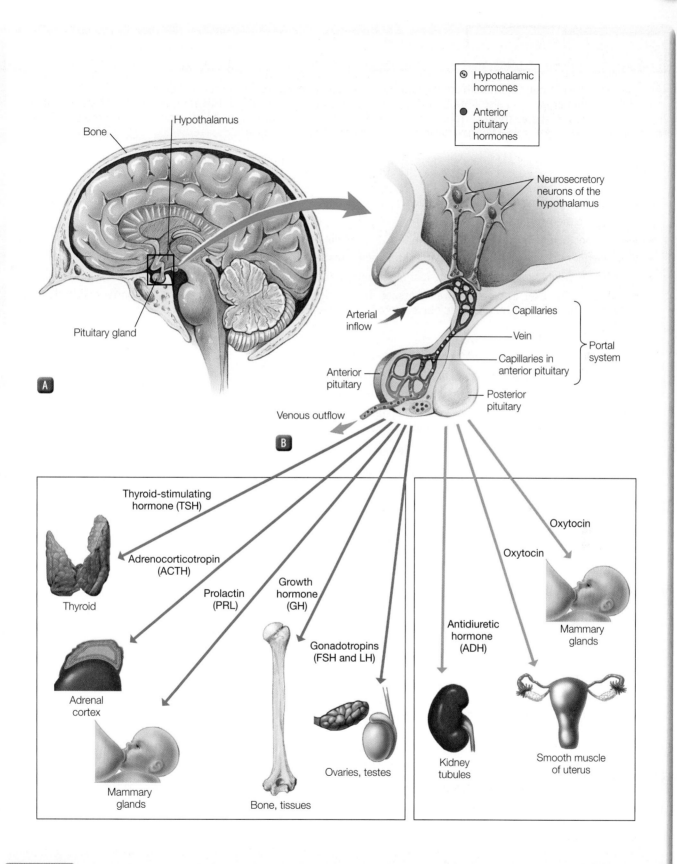

Figure 11-3 The pituitary gland. **A.** The location of the pituitary gland. **B.** Major structures of the pituitary and the hormones produced.

Case Study | PART 2

As you assist the patient onto the stretcher, you notice that a couple of pieces of partially unwrapped hard candy have fallen from her lap. You also note that the patient is wearing a medical identification bracelet that states she has insulin-dependent diabetes (type 1). Your partner obtains the patient's vital signs as you continue with the secondary assessment including history taking and the physical examination.

The patient history reveals a 44-year-old woman who weighs 75 kg. The SAMPLE history shows:

- **A**ge, gender, weight: 44-year-old woman, 75 kg
- **S**igns and symptoms: Nausea, slurred speech, light-headedness
- **A**llergies to medications: None are known
- **M**edications taken: The patient thinks she took her insulin this morning.
- **P**ast pertinent medical history: The patient has type 1 diabetes.
- **L**ast food/fluid intake: The patient ate last night before bed but skipped breakfast this morning.
- **E**vents prior to onset: The patient was shopping and suddenly started feeling confused. The patient stumbled from the mall to her car, and then backed her car into two parked cars.

The OPQRST history shows:

- **O**nset of symptoms: Rather suddenly, within the past 30 minutes
- **P**rovoking factors: Patient skipped breakfast this morning
- **Q**uality of discomfort: Patient is unable to relate her discomfort
- **R**adiating/related signs/symptoms/relief: No pain or specific local complaint
- **S**everity of complaint: Compared with the last time this happened, the patient became confused rather quickly.
- **T**ime: The confusion began about 30 minutes ago, and the patient thought she should get right home.

Because the patient's vital signs are stable and she has a gag reflex, you decide to follow your protocol and give her 25 grams of oral glucose on a tongue blade.

Recording Time: 5 minutes	
Appearance	Pale, diaphoretic skin
Level of consciousness	Verbal (confused about the place and day of the week)
Airway	Open and clear
Breathing	Rapid but not labored
Circulation	Pale and very clammy, no life-threatening external bleeding
Pulse	100 beats/min, thready and regular
Blood pressure	118/78 mm Hg
Respirations	24 breaths/min, regular
Pupils	Equal and reactive
Spo$_2$	98%
Electrocardiogram	Sinus tachycardia with no ectopy

3. What two primary hormones are vital for controlling the body's metabolism and blood glucose level, and where are they produced?

4. What is diabetes mellitus?

release–inhibiting hormone, or somatostatin, inhibits its release. Body stresses such as shock or low blood glucose levels increase the secretion of GH, whereas high blood glucose levels decrease it.

Pathophysiology

Excessive production of growth hormone results in an overly large size, or gigantism, which also is called acromegaly. A deficiency of growth hormone results in stunted growth, or dwarfism.

Thyroid-Stimulating Hormone

Thyroid-stimulating hormone (TSH), or thyrotropin, controls the release of thyroid hormone from the thyroid gland into the bloodstream. TSH is influenced by thyrotropin-releasing factor from the hypothalamus.

Adrenocorticotropic Hormone

Adrenocorticotropic hormone (ACTH) is one of several molecules derived from a common precursor, pro-opiomelanocortin. ACTH is essential for development of the cortex of the adrenal gland and its secretion of corticosteroids. ACTH secretion is stimulated by stress, trauma, major surgery, fever, and other conditions. Beta-endorphins are proteins that have the same effects as opiate drugs such as morphine and also are derived from pro-opiomelanocortin. They are found in the hypothalamus and anterior pituitary and have analgesic potency that is 80 times greater than that of morphine.

Pathophysiology

Stress causes increased production of pro-opiomelanocortin, resulting in higher levels of both adrenocorticotropic hormone and beta-endorphins. Some researchers believe that the production of opiates by the brain causes low blood pressure, compounding the already severe stress of shock states. Experimentally, some researchers have administered the narcotic antagonist agent, naloxone, to reverse the effects of the beta-endorphins. Animal studies looked very promising, but human data do not yet support the use of naloxone in the treatment of shock.

Clinical Tip

Synthetic corticosteroids are commonly administered to patients for medicinal purposes. Anti-inflammatory agents are the most commonly administered synthetic corticosteroids and aid in the treatment of conditions such as asthma and arthritis.

Pathophysiology

Persons who have been treated for longer than 2 to 3 weeks with large doses of corticosteroids lose the normal response patterns of their hypothalamic-pituitary-adrenal axis, resulting in their body's inability to manufacture cortisol appropriately in times of stress. During times of infection, surgery, and other stresses, these patients require supplemental corticosteroids in addition to those that their body already produces. Failure to appropriately administer supplemental corticosteroids may result in a life-threatening condition known as addisonian crisis.

Clinical Tip

One of the serious side effects of taking anabolic steroids is the potential for the person to become quickly agitated, aggressive, and physically violent. Affected persons can pose a physical threat to those around them, including EMS personnel.

Reproduction-Regulating Hormones

Luteinizing hormone (LH) and follicle-stimulating hormone (FSH) regulate the production of both eggs and sperm, as well as production of reproductive hormones (estrogen and progesterone in women, and testosterone in men). Gonadotropin-releasing hormone produced by the hypothalamus influences the release of both LH and FSH. Prolactin plays an important role in milk production in women; in men, it may also help to maintain sperm production. Elevated levels of prolactin can interrupt sexual function in both men and women. Prolactin-releasing hormones and prolactin-inhibiting hormones are released by the hypothalamus and influence the release or inhibition of prolactin.

The Thyroid Gland

The thyroid gland is located just below the larynx, on either side and in front of the trachea **Figure 11-4**. It consists of two large lobes that are connected by a band of tissue called an isthmus and is covered by a capsule of connective tissue with secretory parts called follicles. The thyroid is filled with a clear substance called colloid, which stores hormones produced by the follicles. The thyroid gland manufactures and secretes hormones that influence growth, development, and metabolism.

Microscopically, the thyroid gland contains numerous small cavity glands called follicles that are filled with thyroglobulin, a protein to which thyroid hormones are bound. Between the follicles are parafollicular cells that produce the hormone <u>calcitonin</u>, which is important in regulating calcium levels in the body. Calcitonin decreases the breakdown of bone by osteoclasts, resulting in a decrease in blood calcium and phosphate levels.

The two major hormones that the thyroid gland produces are <u>triiodothyronine (T_3)</u> and <u>tetraiodothyronine (T_4)</u>. These hormones are produced in response to stimulation from the anterior pituitary by TSH. In the blood, both T_3 and T_4 bind to a protein synthesized in the liver, <u>thyroxine-binding globulin</u>. T_3 interacts mostly with target tissues. Approximately 40% of T_4 is converted to T_3 in the body tissues. Both hormones are essential for normal growth and development in children. They also play an important role in the regulation of body metabolism.

The Parathyroid Glands

The <u>parathyroid glands</u> are located on the posterior surface of the thyroid gland. There are usually four parathyroid glands—one superior and one inferior gland on each lobe of the thyroid. They are covered in thin connective tissue capsules and appear yellowish-brown. They produce and secrete <u>parathyroid hormone</u>, which maintains normal levels of calcium in the blood and normal neuromuscular function **Figure 11-5**. Parathyroid hormone effects are opposite to those of calcitonin.

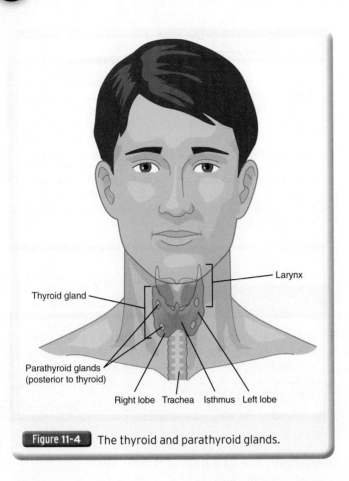

Larynx

Thyroid gland

Parathyroid glands (posterior to thyroid)

Right lobe   Trachea   Isthmus   Left lobe

Figure 11-4 The thyroid and parathyroid glands.

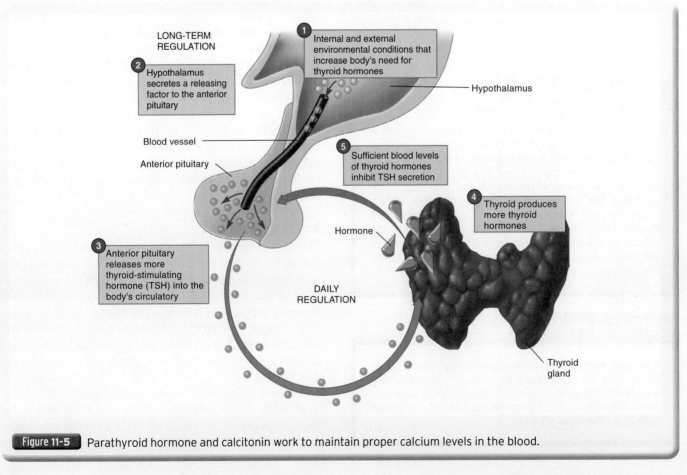

LONG-TERM REGULATION

2 Hypothalamus secretes a releasing factor to the anterior pituitary

1 Internal and external environmental conditions that increase body's need for thyroid hormones

Hypothalamus

Blood vessel

Anterior pituitary

5 Sufficient blood levels of thyroid hormones inhibit TSH secretion

4 Thyroid produces more thyroid hormones

Hormone

3 Anterior pituitary releases more thyroid-stimulating hormone (TSH) into the body's circulatory

DAILY REGULATION

Thyroid gland

Figure 11-5 Parathyroid hormone and calcitonin work to maintain proper calcium levels in the blood.

The Pancreas

The pancreas functions as an exocrine gland secreting digestive juice and an endocrine gland releasing hormones. The pancreas lies between the greater curvature of the stomach and the duodenum in the retroperitoneum, or space behind the peritoneum Figure 11-6 . The head of the pancreas rests near the duodenum; the body and tail of the pancreas project toward the spleen. It is joined to the duodenum of the small intestine, transporting digestive juice into the intestine.

In addition to digestive enzymes, the pancreas produces the hormones insulin and glucagon. Both of these hormones are vital in control of the body's metabolism and blood glucose level. Insulin and glucagon are produced in specialized groups of cells known as the islets of Langerhans (see Figure 11-7, parts B and C). Within each islet are alpha cells that secrete glucagon and beta cells that secrete insulin.

Glucagon stimulates the liver and kidneys to break down glycogen and convert certain noncarbohydrates (including amino acids) into glucose in a process known as gluconeogenesis. This raises the blood glucose concentration much more effectively than epinephrine is able to do. Glucagon secretion is regulated by negative feedback and prevents hypoglycemia from occurring when the glucose concentration is relatively low. In addition, glucagon activates an enzyme, hormone-sensitive lipase, that breaks triglycerides down into free fatty acids and glycerol.

Case Study PART 3

Shortly after you administer the oral glucose, the patient begins to look better and is no longer confused. She tells you that her glucose level was in a normal range this morning when she checked it and she is not sure why this episode occurred. The patient remembers starting to feel funny while in the store, so she began to eat some hard candies, which usually helps until she can eat something solid. The patient tells you that she has had a stomach virus for the past 24 hours and has had vomiting, diarrhea, and loss of appetite.

The results of the physical examination are:

- Skin signs: Pale and moist
- Head: Face is pale with drying beads of sweat on the forehead
- Neck: Flat neck veins
- Chest: No scars or patches
- Lung sounds: Clear in all fields
- Upper extremities: Strong and regular distal pulses
- Lower extremities: Unremarkable

Recording Time: 15 minutes	
Appearance	Pale, diaphoretic skin
Level of consciousness	Verbal yet progressively becoming alert
Airway	Open and clear
Breathing	Rapid but normal
Circulation	Pale and clammy with no external bleeding
Pulse	78 beats/min, regular
Blood pressure	124/80 mm Hg
Respirations	20 breaths/min, regular
Spo$_2$	98%

5. Why is oral glucose helpful for this patient?

6. Why is it so urgent that the patient's condition is managed?

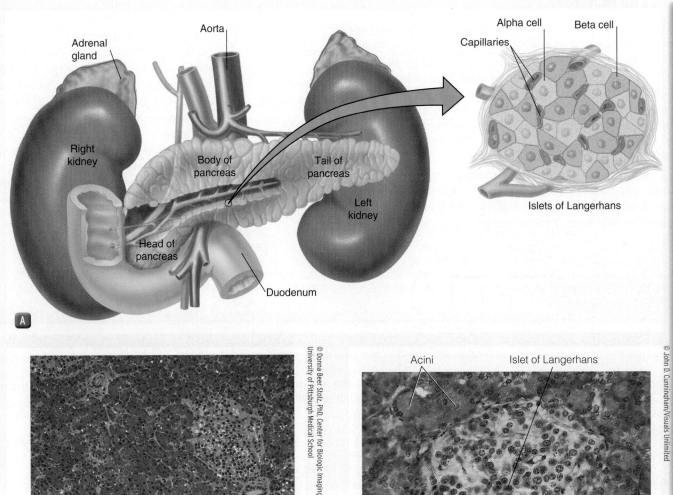

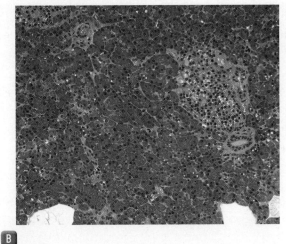

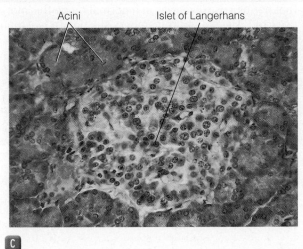

Figure 11-6   The pancreas. **A.** The pancreas produces two hormones, insulin and glucagon, as well as digestive enzymes. **B.** The islets of Langerhans are located among the acini, very small groups of digestive-enzyme-producing cells of the pancreas. **C.** Hormones are produced by specialized cells within the islets of Langerhans.

Insulin works in a manner opposite of glucagon, by stimulating the liver to form glycogen from glucose and inhibiting conversion of noncarbohydrates into glucose. Insulin causes foodstuffs (sugar, fatty acids, and amino acids) to be taken up and metabolized by cells. Fatty acids are converted into triglycerides and stored as fat. Amino acids are metabolized into proteins or glucose to be used for energy.

Insulin and glucagon function together to maintain a stable blood glucose concentration, even though the amount of carbohydrates ingested by a person may vary widely. Nerve cells are partially sensitive to blood glucose concentration changes. Such changes can alter brain function.

Clinical Tip

Vasopressin is sometimes administered to patients who are bleeding from the gastrointestinal tract. Vasopressin causes blood vessels to constrict, resulting in a decrease in the rate of bleeding. A potential side effect is unwanted constriction of the coronary arteries, resulting in myocardial ischemia. Vasopressin also is used in the treatment of cardiac arrest for patients with ventricular fibrillation. The drug is administered in a one-time dose of 40 units and given instead of the first or second dose of epinephrine.

Pathophysiology

Diabetes mellitus is a disease with life long implications on the health of the patient. There are three forms of the disease that affect the body's ability to balance the carbohydrate needs of the cells with the endocrine hormone insulin. Insulin is manufactured in the pancreas and is responsible for helping carbohydrates in the form of glucose enter the cells. It works like the key to your car. Your car may be sitting in the driveway, but without the key, you cannot turn it on. Without a sufficient amount of available functional insulin, the glucose in a patient's bloodstream will not enter the cells. Therefore, insulin works to keep blood glucose levels at a relatively stable and low level. By promoting carbohydrate metabolism, insulin also blocks fat metabolism, thereby preventing the breakdown of fat tissue in the body. Glucagon and epinephrine, so-called "stress hormones," have the opposite effects, resulting in increased circulating blood glucose. Glucagon, a protein hormone produced in the pancreas, stimulates an increase in blood glucose by stimulating the breakdown of glycogen to glucose.

There are three "types" of diabetes mellitus: type 1 (commonly referred to as juvenile-onset diabetes), type 2 (commonly referred to as adult-onset diabetes), and gestational diabetes. A patient with type 1 diabetes (insulin-dependent diabetes mellitus) has a pancreas that cannot produce insulin. These patients have to monitor their blood glucose levels very closely throughout the day and inject themselves with insulin.

A patient with type 2 diabetes (non-insulin-dependent diabetes mellitus) has a pancreas that produces insulin but that is relatively non-functional, resulting in a state of so-called insulin resistance. Also, over time, cell surface insulin receptors develop resistance to the body's own insulin, resulting in the progression of non-insulin-dependence. The net effect is the same as in the case of a patient with type 1 diabetes. Most of the time, a patient with type 2 diabetes can control the glucose/insulin balance through a combination of oral anti-diabetic medications and an appropriate diet. Many times insulin resistance is a function of advancing age and/or obesity.

The patient with gestational diabetes mellitus (GDM) is a pregnant woman who develops all the symptoms of diabetes during the pregnancy. In most cases, this resolves itself shortly after the pregnancy. GDM is the inability to process carbohydrates during pregnancy. This produces a high-risk pregnancy for both the mother and the fetus, and is also considered a risk factor for the development of type 2 diabetes later in life. Diabetic emergencies occur when the blood glucose levels becomes too low or too high, and insulin supply is imbalanced relative to carbohydrate demand. A normal blood glucose reading is approximately 70 to 120 mg/dL. The conditions associated with abnormal blood glucose levels include: hypoglycemia, hyperglycemia, diabetic ketoacidosis (DKA), and hyperosmolar hyperglycemic nonketotic coma (HHNC), or hyperosmolar nonketotic coma (HONK). Frequently, mild to moderate hyperglycemia is seen in association with states of physiologic stress such as acute illness or injury.

Hypoglycemia is a state of low blood glucose levels (less than 45 mg/dL) with associated clinical symptoms, and is a very common side effect of the treatment for diabetes. It happens when too much insulin is administered, too little food is taken in, or a combination of both. Patients with diabetes can also become hypoglycemic when they do not take in enough carbohydrates for exercise or unplanned activities. When the blood glucose level falls significantly, the brain becomes hypoperfused of glucose and altered states of consciousness may occur. Some patients may also become violent. When hypoglycemia is prolonged, a loss of consciousness results and may lead to permanent brain cell damage or insulin shock.

Hyperglycemia is a state of elevated blood glucose levels above the normal range (80-120 mg/dL) and occurs with or without symptoms. If left untreated, hyperglycemia can progress to diabetic ketoacidosis. Diabetic ketoacidosis is caused by a combination of insulin deficit and excessive glucagons. The result is an elevated blood glucose level with excessive fat breakdown with ketoacidosis. Dehydration and electrolyte disturbances are common.

When diabetic ketoacidosis is not treated adequately, diabetic coma may result. Diabetic coma is a state of unconsciousness, resulting from several problems, including ketoacidosis, dehydration due to excessive urination, and hyperglycemia. Blood glucose levels are greater than 800 mg/dL when a diabetic coma occurs.

HHNC or HONK involves very marked hyperglycemia (often greater than 1,000 mg/dL), dehydration, and usually coma, and occurs with insulin deficiency but without ketones and acidosis. This occurs principally in patients with type 2 diabetes.

The Adrenal Glands

The adrenal glands, sometimes called the suprarenal glands, sit on top of each kidney like caps. The adrenal gland manufactures and secretes certain sex hormones, as well as other hormones that are vital in maintaining the body's water and salt balance. In times of stress, the adrenal glands produce adrenaline (also called epinephrine), which mediates the "fight-or-flight" response of the sympathetic nervous system.

The adrenal glands have a central adrenal medulla and an outer adrenal cortex, each secreting different hormones.

The inner portion, or medulla, of the adrenal glands produces epinephrine and norepinephrine. These hormones are vital in the function of the sympathetic nervous system. The remainder of adrenal tissue, known as the adrenal cortex, consists of layers of cells, or zones: the zona glomerulosa, zona fasciculata, and zona reticularis Figure 11-7 .

The zona glomerulosa produces mineralocorticoids. These hormones are important in regulating the water and salt balance of the body. The most important mineralocorticoid is aldosterone. This compound increases the absorption of sodium by the kidneys. In addition,

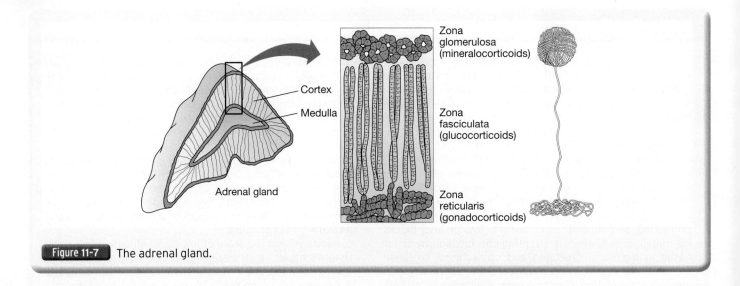

Figure 11-7   The adrenal gland.

aldosterone increases the rate at which water is reabsorbed. The result is an increase in both the blood volume and the concentration of sodium within the plasma. Secretion of aldosterone also increases the excretion of potassium by the kidneys.

The zona fasciculata secretes glucocorticoids, which are also known as corticosteroids. The most important of these compounds is cortisol. Cortisol has a myriad of roles in the body, including regulation of blood glucose, metabolism of fat tissue, and inhibition of inflammation. Secretion of corticosteroids is regulated by the hypothalamic-pituitary-adrenal axis, a complex set of interactions involving chemical signals delivered through the bloodstream from the brain to the adrenal glands.

The zona reticularis secretes a few relatively weak male sex hormones, or androgens. Androgens are produced in both women and men, but in different quantities. The most common androgen is androstenedione. Adrenal androgens stimulate growth of pubic and axillary hair, as well as sexual drive in women. In men, their effects are insignificant compared to the sex hormones produced by the gonads.

Clinical Tip

Some bodybuilders use synthetic androgens, sometimes called anabolic steroids, to increase muscle mass. These substances have numerous dangerous side effects, including cancer, and are outlawed by most athletic organizations.

The Reproductive Glands and Hormones

The gonads are the reproductive glands and consist of the ovaries in women and the testes in men. Testosterone is the major androgen manufactured by the testes. Testosterone also is produced in small amounts in the adrenal glands and in the ovaries. Testosterone is responsible for the development of male secondary sex characteristics, such as a deep voice and facial hair.

The three major female hormones are estrogen, progesterone, and human chorionic gonadotropin (hCG). The developing embryo in the uterus manufactures hCG if conception takes place to keep the lining of the uterus (endometrium) thick and able to sustain the pregnancy. The ovaries produce estrogen and progesterone. Estrogen functions in the menstrual cycle and in the development of secondary sex characteristics, such as breast development in adolescence. Progesterone, which is produced by the corpus luteum of the ovary, prepares the uterus for implantation of a fertilized egg. In men, small amounts of estrogen and progesterone also are produced in the testes and adrenal glands.

Pathophysiology

A condition known as Conn syndrome (also called primary hyperaldosteronism) results in excess secretion of aldosterone. Disturbances in salt and water balance develop, with symptoms of weakness, convulsions, muscular cramps and twitching, and itching or burning of the skin. The most common cause of Conn syndrome is a benign tumor.

Other Glands

The pineal gland is located deep in the cerebral hemispheres and is attached to the thalamus near the upper part of the third ventricle Figure 11-8 . It secretes the hormone melatonin in response to light conditions in the external environment. When it is dark, nerve impulses from the eyes decrease, and the secretion of melatonin increases.

Melatonin functions as a biologic clock and can help to regulate the circadian rhythms, which are associated with environmental day and night cycles. The circadian rhythms help the body to distinguish day from night. Melatonin is not fully understood, but appears to inhibit gonadotropin secretion, help regulate the female reproductive cycle, and control the onset of puberty.

The thymus, inside the mediastinum posterior to the sternum (between the lungs), is larger in children than in adults. It shrinks with age, and is important in early immunity. The thymus secretes hormones called thymosins, affecting production and differentiation of lymphocytes.

The digestive glands that secrete hormones are found in the linings of the stomach and small intestine. The heart secretes atrial natriuretic peptide, which stimulates urinary sodium excretion. The kidneys secrete erythropoietin, which is a red blood cell growth hormone.

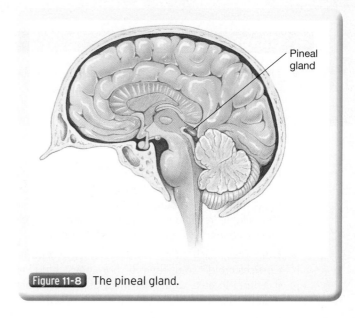

Pineal gland

Figure 11-8   The pineal gland.

Case Study PART 4

As your partner obtains a complete set of vital signs, you suggest that the patient be transported to the hospital for evaluation. The reassessment is completed while you are en route to the hospital.

Prep Kit

Chapter Summary

- The endocrine system works along with the nervous system to regulate the functions of the human body to maintain homeostasis.

- The endocrine system and its glands secrete hormones that diffuse from the interstitial fluid into the bloodstream to their target cells.

- Prostaglandins are a group of hormone-like fatty acids produced in many body tissues that act on target organs to produce effects such as uterine contraction, regulation of blood pressure, smooth muscle contraction, and pain and inflammation.

- Hormones act by binding to receptors. Corticosteroids and thyroid hormones bind to receptors located within cells. All other hormones bind to receptors located on the surface of cells.

- Hormones interact with each other to maintain homeostasis in an interaction that includes negative feedback, or feedback inhibition. A few hormones interact with positive feedback.

- The pituitary gland is known as the master gland and is located at the base of the brain. The pituitary gland secretes hormones that regulate the function of many other glands in the body.

- The hypothalamus regulates the function of the pituitary gland.

- The posterior portion of the pituitary gland is directly connected to and continuous with the brain and is called the neurohypophysis. Hormones produced by this region of the pituitary gland are called neurohormones.

- The two major hormones stored and secreted by the neurohypophysis are antidiuretic hormone and oxytocin.

- In high concentrations, antidiuretic hormone constricts blood vessels and raises the blood pressure. Its primary target tissue is the kidney, where it promotes retention of water and reduction in urine volume.

- Oxytocin causes the smooth muscles of the pregnant uterus to contract and milk to be released from the breasts of lactating women.

- Hormones produced by the anterior pituitary or the adenohypophysis are not neurohormones because this portion of the gland is not considered part of the central nervous system.

- Growth hormone, or somatotropin, stimulates growth in most tissues, especially of long bones in the extremities, increases protein synthesis and the use of fats for energy, and stimulates the production of proteins by the liver and skeletal muscle.

- The hypothalamus produces growth hormone–releasing hormone, which stimulates secretion of growth hormone. Growth hormone release–inhibiting hormone inhibits the release of growth hormone.

- Thyroid-stimulating hormone, or thyrotropin, controls the release of thyroid hormone from the thyroid gland.

- Adrenocorticotropic hormone (ACTH) is essential for development of the cortex of the adrenal gland and its secretion of corticosteroids. ACTH secretion is stimulated by stress, trauma, major surgery, fever, and other conditions.

- Luteinizing hormone and follicle-stimulating hormone regulate the production of both eggs and sperm, as well as production of reproductive hormones. Both are under the influence of gonadotropin-releasing hormone.

- Prolactin plays an important role in milk production in women.

- The thyroid gland is a large gland situated at the base of the neck consisting of two lobes that are connected by a band of tissue, the isthmus.

- The thyroid gland manufactures and secretes hormones that influence growth, development, and metabolism.

- Microscopically, the thyroid gland contains numerous follicles, each filled with thyroglobulin, a protein to which thyroid hormones are bound. Between the follicles are parafollicular cells that produce the hormone calcitonin, which is important in regulating calcium levels in the body.

- The thyroid gland produces two major hormones, triiodothyronine (T_3) and tetraiodothyronine (T_4). The hormones are produced in response to stimulation from the anterior pituitary gland by thyroid-stimulating hormone.

- The parathyroid glands are located on the posterior thyroid gland surface. They produce parathyroid hormone, which maintains normal levels of calcium in the blood and normal neuromuscular function.

- The pancreas functions as an exocrine gland secreting digestive juice and an endocrine gland releasing hormones. In addition to producing digestive enzymes, the pancreas manufactures the hormones insulin and glucagon, both of which are vital in control of the body's metabolism and blood glucose level.

- Insulin works in a manner opposite of glucagon, by stimulating the liver to form glycogen from glucose and inhibiting conversion of noncarbohydrates into glucose.

- Insulin causes sugar, fatty acids, and amino acids to be taken up and metabolized by cells.

- Glucagon stimulates the breakdown of glycogen to glucose. In addition, glucagon stimulates both the liver and the kidneys to produce glucose from noncarbohydrate sources in a process known as gluconeogenesis.

- The adrenal glands are located on top of each kidney. They manufacture and secrete sex hormones as well as hormones vital in maintaining the body's water and salt balance.

- The adrenal glands produce adrenaline, which mediates the "fight-or-flight" response of the sympathetic nervous system. The adrenal glands also secrete corticosteroids.

- The reproductive glands, or gonads, are the ovaries in women and the testes in men.

- Testosterone is the major androgen manufactured by the testes and is responsible for the development of male secondary sex characteristics.

- The three major female hormones are estrogen, progesterone, and human chorionic gonadotropin.

- The ovaries produce estrogen and progesterone. In women, estrogen functions in the menstrual cycle and in the development of secondary sex characteristics.

- The pineal gland is located deep in the cerebral hemispheres and secretes the hormone melatonin in response to light conditions in the external environment. When it is dark, nerve impulses from the eyes decrease, and the secretion of melatonin increases.

◼ Vital Vocabulary

acromegaly A disorder caused by chronic overproduction of growth hormone by the pituitary gland that is characterized by a gradual and permanent enlargement of the flat bones (the lower jaw) and of the hands and feet, abdominal organs, nose, lips, and tongue; also called gigantism.

addisonian crisis Acute adrenocortical insufficiency.

adenohypophysis One of the two portions of the pituitary gland, it produces hormones that are not neurohormones; also called the anterior pituitary.

adrenal cortex The outer layer of the adrenal gland, it produces hormones that are important in regulating the water and salt balance of the body.

adrenal glands Glands located on top of each kidney that produce and secrete certain sex hormones, as well as other hormones that are vital to maintaining the body's water and salt balance; also called suprarenal glands.

adrenaline Hormone with alpha and beta sympathomimetic properties, produced by the adrenal glands that mediates the "fight-or-flight" response of the sympathetic nervous system; also called epinephrine.

adrenocorticotropic hormone (ACTH) Hormone that targets the adrenal cortex to secrete cortisol.

aldosterone One of the two main hormones responsible for adjustments to the final composition of urine; increases the rate of active reabsorption of sodium and chloride ions into the blood and decreases reabsorption of potassium.

alpha cells Cells located in the islets of Langerhans that secrete glucagon.

anabolic steroids Synthetic androgens used to increase muscle mass.

androgens Male sex hormones.

androstenedione A steroid sex hormone secreted by the adrenal cortex, testes, and ovaries.

anterior pituitary (lobe) One of the two portions of the pituitary gland; it produces hormones that are not neurohormones; also called the adenohypophysis.

antidiuretic hormone (ADH) A hormone secreted by the posterior pituitary lobe of the pituitary gland; it constricts blood vessels and raises the blood pressure; also called vasopressin.

autocrine Denoting self-stimulation through cellular production of a factor and a specific receptor for it.

beta cells Cells located in the islets of Langerhans that secrete insulin.

beta-endorphins Proteins produced in the hypothalamus and anterior pituitary that have the same effects as opiate drugs such as morphine but are 80 times more potent.

calcitonin A hormone produced by the parafollicular cells of the thyroid gland that is important in the regulation of calcium levels in the body.

circadian rhythms Associated with environmental day and night cycles; these rhythms help the body to distinguish day from night.

Conn syndrome A condition that results in excess secretion of aldosterone, most commonly caused by a benign tumor.

corticosteroids Any of several steroids secreted by the adrenal gland.

cortisol The most important corticosteroid secreted by the zona fasciculata of the adrenal cortex, it has many effects on the body.

Cushing syndrome A condition caused by excessive production of cortisol by the adrenal glands resulting in obesity, abnormal hair growth, high blood pressure, emotional disturbances, and cushingoid facies or the so-called "moonface."

diabetes insipidus A disorder of the pituitary gland that results in production of very large volumes of dilute urine.

diabetes mellitus A condition that results from impaired production of insulin by the pancreas.

dwarfism Stunted growth caused by a deficiency of growth hormone.

endocrine glands Glands that produce and secrete hormones into the bloodstream.

endocrine system The complex message and control system that integrates many body functions, including the release of hormones.

epinephrine Hormone produced by the adrenal medulla that has a vital role in the function of the sympathetic nervous system; also called adrenaline.

estrogen A hormone released from the ovaries that stimulates the uterine lining during the menstrual cycle; it is one of three major female hormones.

exocrine glands Glands that secrete chemicals for elimination.

exophthalmos Protrusion of the eyes from the normal position within the socket.

feedback inhibition Negative feedback resulting in the decrease of an action in the body.

follicles Small cavity glands within the thyroid gland that contain thyroglobulin.

follicle-stimulating hormone (FSH) The hormone that regulates the production of both eggs and sperm, as well as production of reproductive hormones.

gigantism A disorder caused by chronic overproduction of growth hormone by the pituitary gland that is characterized by a gradual and permanent enlargement of the flat bones (the lower jaw) and of the hands and feet, abdominal organs, nose, lips, and tongue; also called acromegaly.

glands A cell, group of cells, or an organ that selectively removes, concentrates, or alters materials in the blood and secretes them back into the body.

glucagon Hormone produced by the pancreas that is vital to the control of the body's metabolism and blood glucose level; glucagon stimulates the breakdown of glycogen to glucose.

glucocorticoids Hormones secreted by the zona fasciculata of the adrenal glands that play an important role in metabolism and inhibit inflammation.

gluconeogenesis A process that stimulates both the liver and the kidneys to produce glucose from noncarbohydrate molecules.

glycogen A long polymer from which glucose is converted in the liver (animal starch).

goiter Enlarged visible mass in the anterior part of the neck caused by enlargement of the thyroid gland.

gonadotropin-releasing hormone A hormone released by the hypothalamus that influences the release of luteinizing hormone and follicle-stimulating hormone.

gonads The reproductive glands.

growth hormone (GH) A hormone that stimulates growth in most tissues, especially of long bones in the extremities; also called somatotropin.

growth hormone release–inhibiting hormone A hormone released by the hypothalamus that inhibits the secretion of growth hormone; also called somatostatin.

growth hormone–releasing hormone A hormone released by the hypothalamus that stimulates the secretion of growth hormone.

hormone-sensitive lipase An enzyme that is activated by glucagon; it breaks triglycerides down into free fatty acids and glycerol.

hormones Substances formed in specialized organs or glands and carried to another organ or group of cells in the same organism; regulate many body functions, including metabolism, growth, and body temperature.

human chorionic gonadotropin (hCG) One of three major female hormones; it is produced by a developing embryo after conception.

hyperparathyroidism A condition that results in a loss of calcium from the bones, as well as increases in serum calcium levels, caused by excess secretion of parathyroid hormones.

hyperthyroidism Overactivity of the thyroid gland, which results in increased metabolic rates, weight loss, rapid pulse rate, elevated blood pressure, diarrhea, and at times, abnormal protrusion of the eyes.

hypocalcemia Potentially life-threatening low blood calcium levels resulting from loss of parathyroid function.

hypophysis The gland that secretes hormones that regulate the function of many other glands in the body; also called the pituitary gland.

hypothalamic-pituitary axis The part of the neuroendocrine system that involves interactions of the hypothalamus and the pituitary gland.

hypothalamic-pituitary-adrenal axis A major part of the neuroendocrine system that controls reactions to stress; regulates the secretion of corticosteroids.

hypothalamohypophyseal portal system A specialized set of blood vessels that carry releasing factors from the hypothalamus to the anterior pituitary.

hypothalamus The basal part of the diencephalon; it regulates the function of the pituitary gland.

infundibulum The stalk that connects the hypothalamus to the pituitary gland.

inhibiting factors Compounds that travel from the hypothalamus to the pituitary gland in a specialized set of blood vessels; also called releasing factors.

insulin Hormone produced by the pancreas that is vital in the control of the body's metabolism and blood glucose level.

islets of Langerhans A specialized group of cells in the pancreas where insulin and glucagon are produced.

isthmus A band of tissue that connects the two lobes of the thyroid gland.

luteinizing hormone (LH) Hormone that regulates the production of both eggs and sperm, as well as production of reproductive hormones.

medulla The inner portion of the adrenal glands, which produces epinephrine and norepinephrine.

melatonin A hormone secreted by the pineal gland that functions as a biologic clock, helping to regulate the circadian rhythms.

mineralocorticoids Hormones produced in the zona glomerulosa of the adrenal cortex that are important in the regulation of water and salt balance in the body.

negative feedback The concept that once the desired effect of a hormone has been achieved, further production of the hormone is inhibited until it is needed again; also called feedback inhibition.

neurohormones Hormones secreted by the posterior pituitary.

neurohypophysis One of the two portions of the pituitary gland; it is an extension of the central nervous system and secretes hormones called neurohormones; also called the posterior pituitary.

norepinephrine A hormone produced by the adrenal glands that is vital in the function of the sympathetic nervous system.

osmoreceptors Specialized neurons in the brain that regulate the secretion of antidiuretic hormone.

ovaries The female reproductive glands.

oxytocin A hormone that causes the smooth muscles of the pregnant uterus to contract and milk to be released from the breasts of lactating women.

pancreas A flat, solid organ that lies below and behind the liver and the stomach, and which is a digestive gland that secretes digestive enzymes into the duodenum through the pancreatic duct; considered both an endocrine gland and an exocrine gland.

paracrine Relating to a kind of hormone function in which the effects of the hormone are restricted to the local environment.

parafollicular cells Cells located between the follicles in the thyroid gland that produce the hormone calcitonin.

parathyroid glands Four glands that are embedded in the posterior portion of the thyroid, they produce and secrete parathyroid hormone.

parathyroid hormone Hormone produced and secreted by the parathyroid glands; it maintains normal levels of calcium in the blood and normal neuromuscular function.

pineal gland Secretes the hormone melatonin in response to changes in light conditions.

pituitary gland An endocrine gland that secretes hormones that regulate the function of many other glands in the body; also called the hypophysis.

positive feedback The concept that once the desired effect of a hormone begins, further production of the hormone is stimulated.

posterior pituitary (lobe) One of the two portions of the pituitary gland; it is an extension of the central nervous system and produces hormones called neurohormones; also called the neurohypophysis.

progesterone A hormone released by the ovaries that stimulates the uterine lining during the menstrual cycle; it is one of three major female hormones.

prolactin A hormone that plays an important role in milk production in women.

prolactin-inhibiting hormones Hormones released by the hypothalamus that influence the inhibition of prolactin.

prolactin-releasing hormones Hormones released by the hypothalamus that influence the release of prolactin.

prostaglandins A group of hormone-like fatty acids that are produced in many body tissues, including the uterus, brain, and kidneys.

releasing factors Compounds that travel from the hypothalamus to the pituitary gland in a specialized set of blood vessels; also called inhibiting factors.

retroperitoneum The space behind the peritoneum.

somatomedins Proteins produced in the liver, skeletal muscle, and other tissues that are stimulated by growth hormone.

somatostatin A hormone released by the hypothalamus that inhibits the secretion of growth hormone; also called growth hormone release–inhibiting hormone.

somatotropin Hormone that stimulates growth in many tissues, especially of long bones in the extremities; also called growth hormone.

testes The male reproductive glands.

testosterone The major androgen produced by the testes.

tetany Painful muscle spasms that result from several conditions including a low blood calcium level.

tetraiodothyronine (T$_4$) One of the two major hormones produced by the thyroid gland; it is essential for normal growth and development in children as well as regulation of body metabolism.

thymosins Hormones that affect early production and differentiation of lymphocytes.

thymus A gland that is larger in children but shrinks with age; it secretes thymosins, which are important in early immunity by affecting production and differentiation of lymphocytes.

thyroglobulin A protein to which thyroid hormones are bound.

thyroid gland A large endocrine gland that is located at the base of the neck and produces and excretes hormones that influence growth, development, and metabolism.

thyroid-stimulating hormone (TSH) A hormone that controls the release of thyroid hormone from the thyroid gland; also called thyrotropin.

thyrotropin A hormone that controls the release of thyroid hormone from the thyroid gland; also called thyroid-stimulating hormone.

thyroxine-binding globulin A protein synthesized in the liver that binds to hormones T_3 and T_4.

triiodothyronine (T_3) One of the two major hormones produced by the thyroid gland; it is essential for normal growth and development in children as well as regulation of body metabolism.

vasopressin A hormone secreted by the posterior pituitary gland that constricts blood vessels and raises the blood pressure; also called antidiuretic hormone.

zona fasciculata One of three divisions of the adrenal cortex; it produces corticosteroids.

zona glomerulosa One of three divisions of the adrenal cortex; it produces mineralocorticoids.

zona reticularis One of three divisions of the adrenal cortex; it secretes a few relatively weak male sex hormones, or androgens.

■ Case Study Answers

1. What is the hormone that is influencing the sympathetic nervous system during this time of stress?

   Answer: Adrenaline, or epinephrine, is a hormone produced and secreted by the adrenal glands that mediates the fight-or-flight response of the sympathetic nervous system in times of stress.

2. What is the name of the organ known as the "master gland," and why is it called that?

Answer: The pituitary gland, or hypophysis, is sometimes called the master gland because it secretes hormones that regulate the function of many other glands in the body.

3. What two primary hormones are vital for controlling the body's metabolism and blood glucose level, and where are they produced?

   Answer: Insulin and glucagon are vital for controlling the body's metabolism and blood glucose level. They are produced in the pancreas, in a specialized group of cells known as islets of Langerhans.

4. What is diabetes mellitus?

   Answer: Diabetes mellitus is a disorder that results from impaired production of insulin by the pancreas. The disorder, which is caused by a combination of heredity and environmental factors, primarily affects the metabolism of carbohydrates.

5. Why is oral glucose helpful for this patient?

   Answer: In any patient with an altered mental status, the possibility of the presence of hypoxia and a low blood glucose level must be considered first and oxygen should be applied immediately. In this case, because the patient was responsive enough to tell you that she has type 1 diabetes, skipped a meal, and has been ill for the past 24 hours, you were able to presume that she has hypoglycemia even before testing her blood glucose level with a glucose monitor.

6. Why is it so urgent that the patient's condition is managed?

   Answer: The brain needs a constant source of glucose. Without glucose, the patient's mental status quickly becomes altered as the brain loses its source of energy. Without rapid intervention, the patient's condition could quickly deteriorate, and permanent brain damage could result. In this case, the patient's glucose level was low, but the condition was quickly recognized and glucose was administered, rapidly improving the patient's condition.

The Urinary System

Learning Objectives

1. Describe the three major functions of the urinary system. (p 242)
2. Describe the location and structural features of the kidneys. (p 242-244)
3. Describe how the kidneys function in maintaining normal blood volume and pressure. (p 243, 246-247)
4. Name the parts of a nephron. (p 244-245)
5. Describe how the kidneys help to maintain normal blood pH and electrolyte balance. (p 244, 247-248)
6. Describe the characteristics of normal urine and how it is formed. (p 245-248)
7. State the hormones that affect kidney function. (p 249)

Introduction

The urinary system has three major functions: (1) excretion (the removal of organic wastes from body fluids), (2) elimination (the discharge of these wastes into the environment), and (3) homeostatic regulation of the volume and solute concentration of blood plasma. In addition to removing waste products generated by cells throughout the body, the urinary system has several more essential homeostatic functions that will be discussed later in this chapter. The urinary system consists of two kidneys, two ureters, a urinary bladder, and a urethra Figure 12-1. These structures are contained in the abdominal and pelvic cavities and are closely entwined with the gastrointestinal and reproductive systems.

Pathophysiology

Bacterial infection of the bladder and its urinary contents (cystitis) is common, especially in adult women. Cystitis results in frequent, painful, and sometimes bloody urination. Although this condition causes discomfort, most patients are easily treated with oral bladder relaxants and antibiotics.

The Kidneys

The kidneys are smooth, bean-shaped organs with a reddish-brown color Figure 12-2. In adults, the kidneys are each enclosed in a tough, fibrous capsule. They are about 12 centimeters in length by 6 centimeters wide and 3 centimeters thick. The kidneys lie on either side of the vertebral column in depressions on the upper posterior wall of the abdominal cavity. Their upper border is near the twelfth thoracic vertebra, and their lower border is near the third lumbar vertebra, with the left kidney being about 1.5 to 2 centimeters higher than the right one.

The kidneys are positioned behind the parietal peritoneum, against the deep muscles of the back (in the retroperitoneal space behind the abdominal cavity). They are surrounded and held in position by connective and adipose tissue. Each kidney has a convex lateral surface and a concave medial side, resulting in a medial depression leading to a

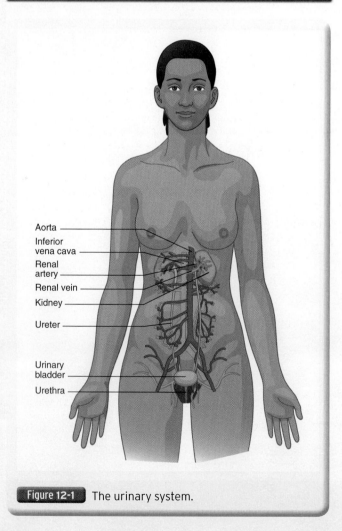

Figure 12-1   The urinary system.

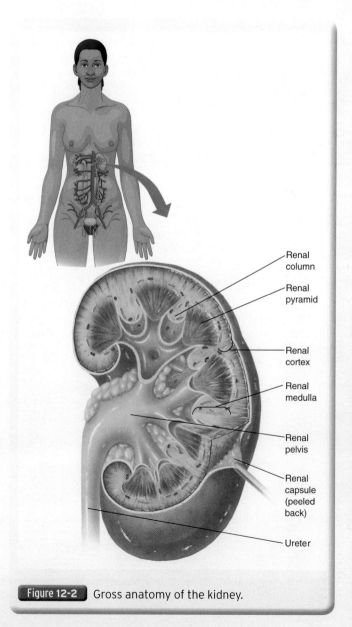

Figure 12-2   Gross anatomy of the kidney.

hollow renal sinus. This chamber's entrance is called the hilum, through which pass blood vessels, nerves, lymphatic vessels, and the ureter.

Inside the renal sinus, the renal pelvis (a funnel-shaped sac) exists, expanded from the superior end of the ureter. Several large urinary tubes, called calyces, enter the renal pelvis from kidney tissue. These tubes are subdivided into major calyces and minor calyces. Small elevations (renal papillae) project into the renal sinus from the renal pelvis walls, and tiny openings leading into the minor calyces pierce each projection.

Each kidney has an inner renal medulla and an outer renal cortex. The renal medulla is made of conical tissue called renal pyramids, and has striations. The renal cortex encloses the medulla, dipping into it between the renal pyramids to form renal columns. The cortex appears to have granules due to tiny tubules associated with the functional units of the kidneys, the nephrons.

The kidneys help to maintain homeostasis by regulating the composition, pH, and volume of the extracellular fluid. This is accomplished by their removal of metabolic wastes from the blood and diluting them with water and electrolytes. This process forms urine, which the kidneys excrete. The other important functions of the kidneys include:

- Secretion of the hormone erythropoietin, which helps to control red blood cell production
- Helping with the activation of vitamin D
- Helping to maintain blood volume and pressure via secretion of the enzyme renin

The kidneys are supplied with blood from the renal arteries, which arise from the abdominal aorta. These arteries transport large volumes of blood. While a person rests, the renal arteries carry between 15% and 30% of the total cardiac output into the kidneys.

The renal arteries branch off inside the kidneys into interlobar arteries, arcuate arteries, and interlobular arteries. The final branches of the interlobular arteries lead to the nephrons, and are called afferent arterioles **Figure 12-3**. Corresponding, in general, with the arterial pathways, the venous blood returns through a similar series of vessels. The renal vein then joins the inferior vena cava. Venous blood returns through a series of vessels that correspond generally to arterial pathways.

Pathophysiology

The kidneys are important in the regulation of the body's fluid balance and blood pressure. They perform these vital functions in conjunction with complex hormone-driven mechanisms. Fluid balance is controlled by the effects of antidiuretic hormone on the kidney. The blood pressure effects are influenced by the renin-angiotensin system, of which the kidneys are an important part.

Case Study | PART 1

At 2:00 PM, you are dispatched to a downtown bus stop for a 24-year-old man on a city transit bus who is in extreme distress from low back pain. You initially think that the patient may have injured himself; however, you quickly determine that there is no traumatic injury. Your general impression is a slender man in his 20s who is pale and very restless. He can barely sit still for a moment.

As you begin your primary assessment, you note that the patient clearly is alert and has an open airway and no breathing problems. You quickly apply a nonrebreathing mask, and then assess the patient's pulse. The patient tells you that he hopes he is not passing a kidney stone, a problem he has had previously. He says the only thing that brought him any pain relief then was a painkiller he received in the emergency department.

Recording Time: 0 Minutes	
Appearance	Pale, diaphoretic skin
Level of consciousness	Alert (oriented to person, place, and day)
Airway	Appears patent
Breathing	Regular
Circulation	Pale, diaphoretic skin; regular, strong distal pulse; no obvious external hemorrhage

1. List four types of common urinary disorders.
2. What is a kidney stone, and why is it so painful?

Pathophysiology

The nephron is not only essential in excreting waste products into the urine, but in maintenance of normal electrolyte and acid balance in the body. Various parts of the nephron are selectively permeable to electrolytes, hydrogen, and bicarbonate. Balancing these substances helps maintain homeostasis.

The Nephrons

There are about 1 million nephrons in a kidney, each consisting of a renal corpuscle and a renal tubule. Fluid moves through the renal tubules as it moves toward exiting the body. A glomerulus is a tangled cluster of blood capillaries that comprises a renal corpuscle. The first step in urine formation is the filtering of fluid via the glomerular capillaries Figure 12-4. The glomerulus is surrounded by a sac-like structure called a glomerular capsule. It is located at

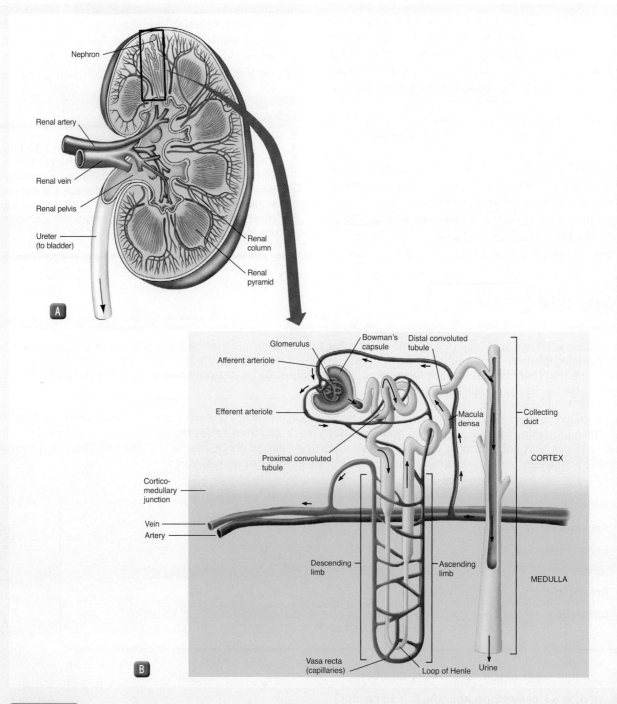

Figure 12-3   The main branches of a renal artery and renal vein. **A.** Blood flow within the kidney. **B.** Blood flow through a nephron.

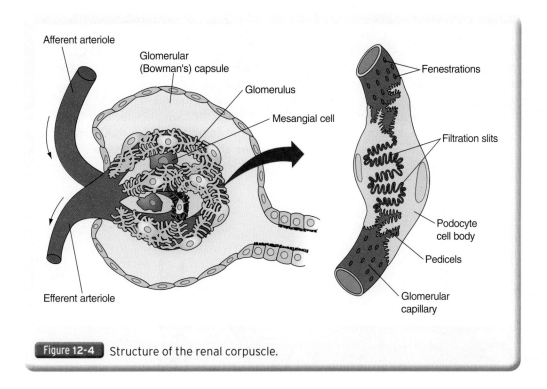

Figure 12-4 Structure of the renal corpuscle.

the proximal end of a renal tubule and receives filtered fluid from the glomerulus. The renal tubule then leads away from the glomerular capsule, coiling into the proximal convoluted tubule.

The proximal convoluted tubule dips toward the renal pelvis to form the descending limb of the nephron loop, also called the loop of Henle. It then curves toward the renal corpuscle to form the ascending limb of the nephron loop. This returns to the renal corpuscle region, coiling tightly to become the distal convoluted tubule. Therefore, the loop of Henle has a horseshoe shape. These tubules, from several nephrons, merge to form collecting ducts in the renal cortexes. They pass into the renal medulla, resulting in tubes that empty into the minor calyces through openings in the renal papillae.

Glomerular capillaries arise from afferent arterioles, with blood (minus filtered fluids) entering an efferent arteriole. Efferent arterioles are smaller in diameter than afferent arterioles. The efferent arterioles resist blood flow slightly and back up into the glomeruli, increasing glomerular capillary pressure. Efferent arterioles branch into complex, interconnected capillary networks, each called a peritubular capillary. This structure surrounds the renal tubule. Blood in this capillary system is under low pressure, and eventually enters the venous system of the kidney.

The distal convoluted tubule contacts the afferent and efferent arterioles while passing between them. The densely packaged, narrow distal tubule epithelial cells form the macula densa. Enlarged smooth muscle cells

(juxtaglomerular cells), along with the macula densa, constitute the juxtaglomerular apparatus (juxtaglomerular complex).

Pathophysiology

Pyelonephritis is a bacterial infection of the renal pelvis, medulla, and cortex. It can be quite severe and may require hospitalization and intravenous antibiotics.

Pathophysiology

Renal failure can occur when a condition interferes with kidney function. People with severe, acute or chronic renal failure may require the use of an artificial kidney in a process called hemodialysis.

■ Formation of Urine

Glomerular filtration initiates urine formation. The plasma is filtered by the glomerular capillaries, with most of this fluid reabsorbed into the bloodstream via the colloid osmotic pressure of the plasma. Using two capillaries in series, the nephrons use this process to help produce urine. The first capillary bed filters instead of forming interstitial fluid, with the filtrate moving into the renal tubule to form urine.

Every 24 hours, glomerular filtration produces 180 liters of fluid—this is more than four times the amount of total body water. The rate at which blood is filtered through the glomerula is called the glomerular filtration rate. Two other processes contribute to urine formation. Tubular reabsorption moves substances from the tubular fluid into the blood, within the peritubular capillary **Figure 12-5**. The kidney reclaims the correct amounts of water, electrolytes, and glucose as required by the body. Tubular secretion moves substances from the blood in the peritubular capillary into the renal tubule. Some substances that the body must excrete, such as hydrogen ions and some toxins, are removed more quickly than through filtration. Urine is the final product of these processes.

The composition of urine is modified during its transit through the loop of Henle to the distal convoluted tubes. In maintaining the body's fluid balance, capillary blood pressure affects a change in volume by increasing filtration and urine output when there is an increase in blood pressure.

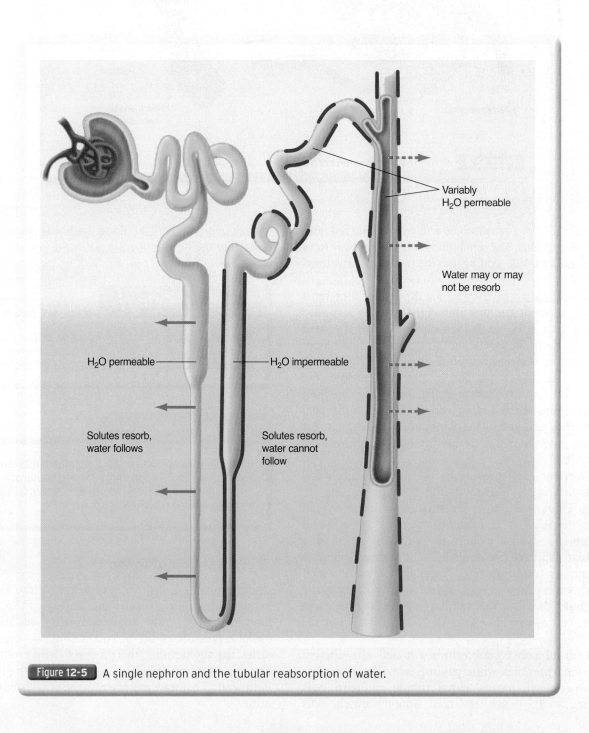

Variably H$_2$O permeable

Water may or may not be resorb

H$_2$O permeable

H$_2$O impermeable

Solutes resorb, water follows

Solutes resorb, water cannot follow

Figure 12-5 A single nephron and the tubular reabsorption of water.

When the blood pressure is lowered, there is increased water retention.

Of the water that the kidney reabsorbs, 99% is taken up via a passive, nonenergy-requiring process. Electrolytes, such as chloride and sodium, are actively transported, requiring energy. As urine flows through the various levels of the nephron, fluid and solids (solute) move about. This process is called the countercurrent multiplier mechanism and involves flow from the tubules into the vasa recta, surrounding vessels that lead

Case Study | PART 2

Your partner obtains a set of baseline vital signs, and you continue with the secondary assessment, including the focused history and physical examination. The patient is unable to sit still on the stretcher because of the pain.

A patient history shows a 24-year-old man who weighs 70 kg. The SAMPLE history shows:

- **S**igns and symptoms: Extreme pain in the low back, left kidney area, and posterior flank
- **A**llergies to medications: Sulfa drugs and peanuts
- **M**edications taken: Tylenol
- **P**ast pertinent medical history: The patient has a history of kidney stones and passed a stone about 2 years ago.
- **L**ast food/fluid intake: Tuna sandwich and chips for lunch at noon
- **E**vents prior to onset: The patient was sitting on the bus when his pain started.

The OPQRST history shows:

- **O**nset of symptoms: The pain came on suddenly.
- **P**rovoking factors: The patient forgot to carry his water bottle with him today.
- **Q**uality of discomfort: The patient describes a sharp, stabbing pain in the left flank area but no pain on palpation of the abdominal quadrants.
- **R**adiating/related signs/symptoms/relief: The patient states that the pain is in the left flank area and nothing provides relief. This pain is similar to the pain felt with the last stone, but worse.
- **S**everity of complaint: On a scale of 1 to 10, with 10 being the worst pain he has ever experienced, the patient says the pain is a 10.
- **T**ime: The pain began in the past 20 minutes and continues to get worse.

Recording Time: 4 Minutes	
Appearance	Still very uncomfortable
Level of consciousness	Alert (oriented to person, place, and day)
Airway	Open and patent
Breathing	Normal
Circulation	Pale, diaphoretic skin
Pulse	108 beats/min, strong and regular
Blood pressure	160/92 mm Hg
Respirations	20 breaths/min, regular
Spo$_2$	99%
Pupils	Equal and reactive
Electrocardiogram	Sinus tachycardia with no ectopy

3. Name the structures of the urinary tract and their functions.

4. Why can't the patient find a comfortable position?

from the arterioles in the glomerulus and vice versa. This process allows the body to produce either concentrated or dilute urine, depending on its needs at the time. Urine production varies between 0.6 and 2.5 liters per day. Urine production of 50 to 60 mL per hour is normal, with output of less than 30 mL per hour possibly indicating kidney failure.

Pathophysiology

Several types of central nervous system disease results in decreased production of antidiuretic hormone (ADH). Decreased production of ADH can result in a condition known as diabetes insipidus, in which the patient produces large volumes of dilute urine and experiences intense thirst.

Clinical Tip

Urinalysis is the laboratory evaluation of urine. Urinalysis involves two steps. In the first step, chemically coated paper is dipped into urine and evaluated for numerous chemical parameters. In the second step, a sample of urine is evaluated under a microscope for the presence of specific types of cells, debris, and other chemical residues such as uric acid crystals Table 12-1 .

Table 12-1	Characteristics of Normal Urine
Feature	**Description**
Color	Yellow or amber but varies with concentration and diet
Appearance	Clear to slightly hazy
Volume	1 to 2 L in 24 hours but varies significantly
pH	pH: 4.5 to 8.0
Specific gravity:	1.015 to 1.025

Pathophysiology

Urethritis is a bacterial infection of the urethra that commonly results from sexually transmitted diseases such as gonorrhea. The most prevalent disease of this type, nonspecific nongonococcal urethritis, is caused by organisms of the Chlamydia family.

Pathophysiology

Kidney stones can form in the kidney and may become trapped anywhere along the urinary tract. A common location of entrapment is within the ureter Figure 12-6 . This blockage causes backflow of urine into the kidney, stretching of the capsule, and spasm of the ureter. A patient with a kidney stone (urolithiasis) often has severe pain, nausea, and vomiting. Patients frequently describe the pain associated with a kidney stone as the worst they have ever experienced.

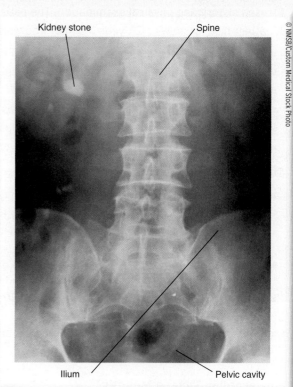

Kidney stone   Spine

© NMSB/Custom Medical Stock Photo

Ilium   Pelvic cavity

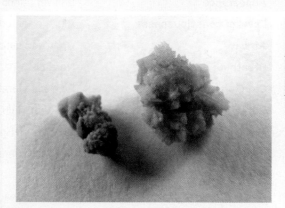

© remik44992/ShutterStock, Inc.

Figure 12-6 Kidney stones. **A.** Radiograph of a kidney stone. **B.** Kidney stones removed surgically.

Hormonal Regulation of Kidney Function

Several hormones affect the function of the kidneys Figure 12-7. Renin is produced by cells of the juxtaglomerular apparatus when the blood pressure is low. Renin contributes, through a series of steps, to the production of angiotensin II, a form of kinin that causes vasoconstriction and sympathetic activation and acts on the cells of the adrenal gland to increase the production of aldosterone. Aldosterone is a steroid hormone produced by the adrenal glands. It increases the rate of sodium and water resorption from the tubules to the blood. Increased aldosterone concentrations result in retention of sodium and chloride, while decreased concentrations result in increased urinary losses of these ions.

Antidiuretic hormone (ADH) is produced by the hypothalamus and is stored in the posterior lobe of the pituitary gland. ADH regulates the permeability of the distal convoluted tubules and the collecting ducts. In the presence of ADH, these structures are more permeable to water, resulting in relatively concentrated urine. A lack of ADH results in production of a large volume of very dilute urine by leading to decreased permeability of the distal convoluted tubules.

The Ureters

The ureters are a pair of thick-walled, hollow tubes that carry urine from the kidneys to the urinary bladder. Each ureter is about 30 centimeters long, descending behind the parietal peritoneum to run parallel to the vertebral column. It joins the urinary bladder from underneath. The wall of each ureter has three layers, the mucous coat, muscular coat, and fibrous coat. Urine is propelled by the muscular walls of the ureters. A flap-like fold of mucous membrane covers the opening through which urine flows from each ureter into the bladder. These folds keep urine from backing up and flowing back into ureters from the bladder.

The Urinary Bladder

The urinary bladder is a hollow, muscular organ that stores urine and forces it into the urethra. It is found in the pelvic cavity behind the pubic symphysis, beneath the parietal peritoneum. The wall of the bladder has many folds when it is empty, but these smooth out as it fills. The bladder's internal floor has a triangular area (trigone), which has an opening at each of its three angles. Figure 12-8 shows the male and female urinary bladders and related structures. The urinary bladder wall has four layers, and its cellular thickness changes based on

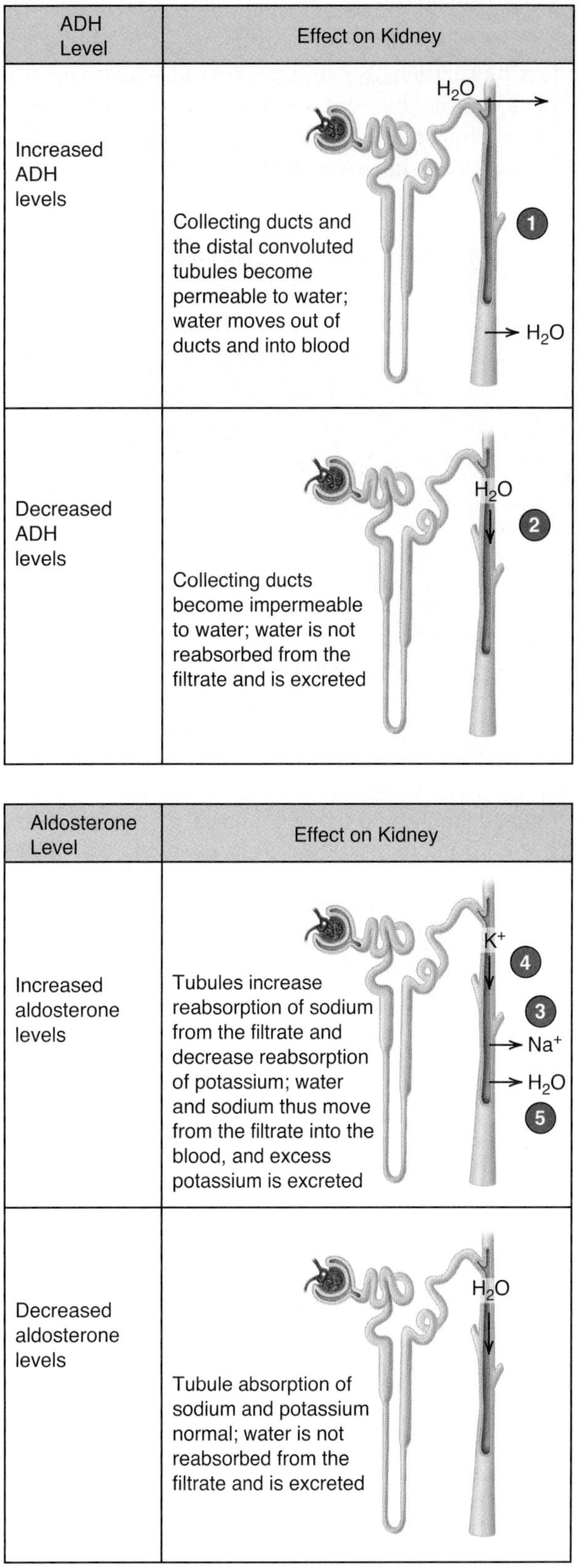

ADH Level	Effect on Kidney
Increased ADH levels	Collecting ducts and the distal convoluted tubules become permeable to water; water moves out of ducts and into blood
Decreased ADH levels	Collecting ducts become impermeable to water; water is not reabsorbed from the filtrate and is excreted

Aldosterone Level	Effect on Kidney
Increased aldosterone levels	Tubules increase reabsorption of sodium from the filtrate and decrease reabsorption of potassium; water and sodium thus move from the filtrate into the blood, and excess potassium is excreted
Decreased aldosterone levels	Tubule absorption of sodium and potassium normal; water is not reabsorbed from the filtrate and is excreted

Figure 12-7 How hormones regulate kidney function.

how much urine it holds. Its layers are the mucous coat, submucous coat, muscular coat, and serous coat. The smooth muscle fibers of the muscular coat are interlaced, comprising the detrusor muscle, part of which surrounds the neck of the bladder to form the internal urethral sphincter. This muscle is innervated with parasympathetic nerve fibers that function in the micturition reflex. The mucous coat of the urinary bladder is lined with transitional epithelium.

Micturition (urination) is the process of expelling urine from the urinary bladder. The detrusor muscle contracts along with the abdominal wall and pelvic floor muscles, and the external urethral sphincter relaxes. The micturition reflex center in the spinal cord sends parasympathetic motor impulses to the detrusor muscle, causing it to rhythmically contract.

The urinary bladder may hold up to 1,000 mL of urine before stimulating pain receptors, but the urge to urinate usually occurs once it contains around 150 mL. The external urethral sphincter is under conscious control, allowing the micturition reflex to occur once the person decides to urinate. The detrusor muscle contracts and urine flows through the urethra.

■ The Urethra

Urine drains from the bladder to the outside of the body via the urethra, which has a tubular construction. The urethra is lined with mucous membrane and a thick layer of smooth muscle tissue. The wall of the urethra has many mucous glands (urethral glands), which secrete mucus into the urethral canal.

Case Study | PART 3

En route to the hospital, an IV line is inserted and serial vital signs are obtained. Because the patient's vital signs have remained stable, you contact medical control for authorization to administer an analgesic. You receive and confirm an order for 5 mg of morphine via IV push and administer the medication.

The patient feels nauseous, so you also administer an antiemetic. The patient is unable to find a comfortable position on the stretcher during transport to the hospital. You are checking back with medical control for another 5 mg of morphine at this point.

Recording Time: 20 Minutes	
Appearance	The pain medications have not eased his pain.
Level of consciousness	Alert (oriented to person, place, and day), restless, and severely distressed due to the pain
Airway	Open and patent
Breathing	Normal but rapid
Circulation	Pale, warm, and a little moist
Pulse	112 beats/min, strong and regular
Blood pressure	130/80 mm Hg
Respirations	24 breaths/min, regular
Spo$_2$	100%

5. What additional questions about the urinary system should be asked?

6. What physical finding might lead you to suspect that the patient is experiencing a urinary tract infection rather than kidney stones?

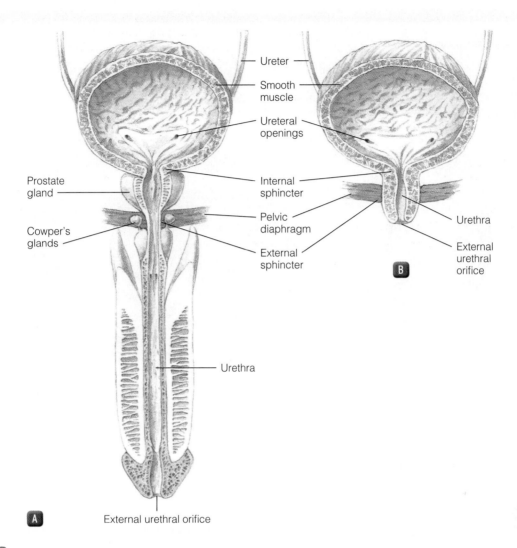

Ureter

Smooth muscle

Ureteral openings

Prostate gland

Internal sphincter

Pelvic diaphragm

Cowper's glands

External sphincter

Urethra

External urethral orifice

B

Urethra

A External urethral orifice

Figure 12-8 Longitudinal sections of the urinary bladder, urethra, and related structures. **A.** Male. **B.** Female.

The male urethra consists of three parts. The prostatic urethra travels through the prostate gland Figure 12-9. The membranous urethra runs from the prostate gland to the base of the penis. The urethral sphincter surrounds the membranous urethra. The spongy urethra lies within the corpus spongiosum of the penis and terminates at the external urethral orifice, the narrowest portion of the entire urethra.

The female urethra is only about 4 cm long and is fused with the anterior wall of the vagina. The urethra ends between the clitoris and the vagina.

Pathophysiology

Enlargement of the prostate gland is common in men older than age 50 years. If the enlargement is significant, the prostate gland can impinge on the prostatic portion of the urethra, resulting in difficulty initiating micturition, a need for frequent urination, and production of urine in small amounts. If the prostate gland becomes very large, it can completely obstruct urinary flow, resulting in an uncomfortable condition known as acute urinary retention.

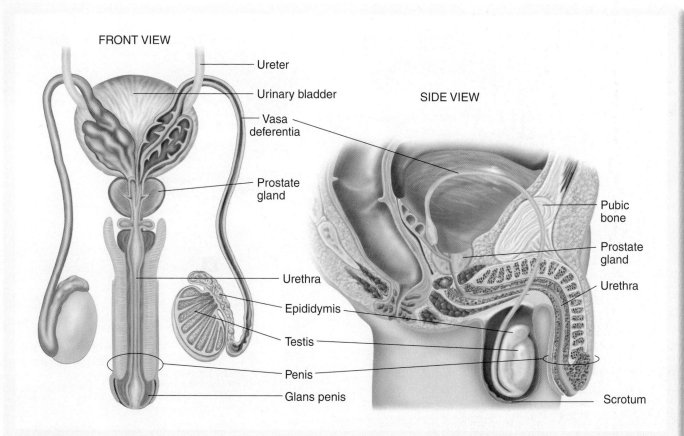

FRONT VIEW

Ureter

Urinary bladder

Vasa deferentia

Prostate gland

Urethra

Epididymis

Testis

Penis

Glans penis

SIDE VIEW

Pubic bone

Prostate gland

Urethra

Scrotum

Figure 12-9   Diagram of the male reproductive system showing the relationship between the urinary and reproductive structures including the course of the urethra through the prostate gland.

Case Study | **PART 4**

On arrival at the hospital, the patient is still in pain but is only now able to settle down and sit still. Apparently, the two doses of morphine have relieved some of the pain and have begun to make him drowsy. He tells you he definitely will not forget to drink fluids again.

Prep Kit

Chapter Summary

- The urinary system removes waste products from the blood by a complex filtration process that results in the production of urine.

- The urinary system consists of two kidneys, two ureters, a urinary bladder, and a urethra.

- The urinary system also has several essential homeostatic functions.

- The kidneys are smooth, bean-shaped organs that filter blood and excrete body wastes in the form of urine.

- The kidneys help to maintain homeostasis by regulating the composition, pH, and volume of the extracellular fluid.

- The nephrons are the functional units of the kidney and where urine is formed.

- Urine formation is initiated by glomerular filtration. The plasma is filtered by the glomerular capillaries, with most of this fluid reabsorbed into the bloodstream via the colloid osmotic pressure of the plasma.

- Several hormones, such as renin, angiotensin II, and aldosterone, affect the function of the kidneys.

- Urine volume and concentration are affected by antidiuretic hormone (ADH) and aldosterone hormone in differing ways.

- Aldosterone is produced by the adrenal glands and increases the rate of sodium and water reabsorption from the distal tubules to the blood.

- ADH, which is produced by the hypothalamus and stored in the posterior lobe of the pituitary gland, regulates the permeability of the distal convoluted tubules and the collecting ducts.

- The ureters are a pair of thick-walled, hollow tubes that carry urine from the kidneys to the urinary bladder.

- The urinary bladder is a hollow, muscular organ in the midline of the lower abdominal area that stores urine until it is excreted.

- The urethra is a hollow, tubular structure that drains urine from the bladder to the outside of the body.

Vital Vocabulary

acute urinary retention A complete obstruction of urinary flow sometimes caused by enlargement of the prostate gland.

afferent arteriole The structure of the kidney that supplies blood to the glomerulus.

aldosterone One of two main hormones responsible for adjustments to the final composition of urine; increases the rate of active reabsorption of sodium and chloride ions into the blood and decreases reabsorption of potassium.

angiotensin II A form of kinin that plays a role in blood pressure maintenance by causing vasoconstriction and sympathetic activation and by stimulating the adrenal gland to increase the production of aldosterone.

antidiuretic hormone (ADH) A hormone released by the pituitary gland that causes the kidney to reabsorb more water into the blood and excrete less urine.

calyces Large urinary tubes that enter the renal pelvis from kidney tissue.

clitoris In females, a small, cylindrical mass of erectile tissue and nerves located at the anterior junction of the labia minora, similar to the glans penis of the male.

countercurrent multiplier mechanism A process by which the body produces either concentrated or diluted urine, depending on the body's needs.

cystitis A bacterial infection of the bladder and its urinary contents.

detrusor muscle Surrounding the neck of the bladder to form the internal urethral sphincter, this muscle functions in the micturition reflex.

diabetes insipidus A condition often caused by pituitary dysfunction that is associated with production of large volumes of dilute urine and in which patients experience intense thirst.

distal convoluted tubule One of two complex sections of a nephron, it empties urine into a collection duct that then carries it to the calyces.

efferent arteriole Structure of the kidney that drains blood from the glomerulus.

external urethral orifice The narrow opening at the end of the male urethra.

glomerular capsule A sac-like structure that surrounds the glomerulus, from which it receives filtered fluid.

glomerular filtration The process that initiates urine formation.

glomerular filtration rate The rate at which blood is filtered through the glomerula.

glomerulus A tangled cluster of blood capillaries that comprises a renal corpuscle.

hemodialysis A procedure in which an artificial kidney external to the body is used to purify the blood.

hilum The point on the medial side of each kidney where the renal artery and nerves enter and the renal vein and ureter exit.

juxtaglomerular apparatus Structure formed at the site where the efferent arteriole and distal convoluted tubule meet; also called a juxtaglomerular complex; plays an important role in regulating fluid balance.

juxtaglomerular cells A group of cells located in the afferent arterioles of the glomerulus that play a part in regulating the volume status of the body.

kidney stones Solid crystalline masses formed in the kidney that may become trapped anywhere along the urinary tract.

kidneys Two retroperitoneal organs that excrete the end products of metabolism as urine and regulate the body's salt and water content.

loop of Henle U-shaped portion of the renal tubule that extends from the proximal to the distal convoluted tubule.

macula densa Specialized tubular cells in the juxtaglomerular area that play a part in regulating the volume status of the body.

membranous urethra One of three parts of the male urethra; it extends from the prostate gland to the base of the penis.

micturition Urination; the process of expelling urine from the urinary bladder.

nephrons The structural and functional units of the kidney that form urine, composed of the glomerulus, the glomerular capsule, the proximal convoluted tubule, the loop of Henle, and the distal convoluted tubule.

nonspecific nongonococcal urethritis An infection of the urethra caused by organisms of the Chlamydia family.

peritubular capillary One of many complex, interconnected capillary networks that branch off of efferent arterioles.

plasma A sticky, yellow fluid that carries the blood cells and nutrients and transports cellular waste material to the organs of excretion; normally makes up 55% of the total blood volume.

prostate gland A small gland that surrounds the male urethra at the section where it emerges from the urinary bladder; it secretes a fluid that is part of the ejaculatory fluid.

prostatic urethra One of three parts of the male urethra; it travels through the prostate gland.

proximal convoluted tubule One of two complex sections of a nephron; it includes an enlargement at the end called the glomerular capsule.

pyelonephritis Inflammation of the kidney linings.

renal arteries The vessels that supply the kidneys with blood; they arise from the abdominal aorta.

renal corpuscle The initial blood-filtering component of the nephron.

renal cortex The outer portion of each kidney; it forms renal columns and has tiny tubules associated with the nephrons.

renal failure Loss of kidney function that occurs secondary to injury or illness.

renal medulla The inner portion of each kidney; it is made of conical renal pyramids and has striations.

renal papillae The tips of each renal pyramid, which extend into the medulla and are encircled by the opening of a minor calyx.

renal pelvis A funnel-shaped sac inside the renal sinus that is subdivided into major and minor calyces (tubes).

renal pyramids Parallel cone-shaped bundles of urine-collecting tubules that are located in the medulla of the kidneys.

renal sinus Cavity formed by the hilum that is filled with fat and connective tissue.

renal tubule The portion of the nephron containing the tubular fluid filtered through the glomerulus.

renal vein The blood vessel connecting the kidneys to the inferior vena cava.

renin A hormone produced by cells in the juxtaglomerular apparatus when the blood pressure is low.

renin-angiotensin system System located in the kidney that helps to regulate fluid balance and blood pressure.

spongy urethra One of the three parts of the male urethra; it lies within the corpus spongiosum of the penis and terminates at the external urethral orifice.

tubular reabsorption The process that moves substances from the tubular fluid into the blood, within the peritubular capillary.

tubular secretion The process that moves substances from the blood in the peritubular capillary into the renal tubule.

ureters A pair of thick-walled, hollow tubes that carry urine from the kidneys to the urinary bladder.

urethra A hollow, tubular structure that drains urine from the bladder to outside of the body.

urethritis A bacterial infection of the urethra.

urinalysis The laboratory evaluation of urine.

urinary bladder A hollow, muscular sac in the midline of the lower abdominal area that stores urine until it is excreted.

urinary system The organs that control the discharge of certain waste materials filtered from the blood and excreted as urine.

urine The final product of tubular reabsorption and secretion; it is a clear, yellow fluid that carries wastes out of the body.

urolithiasis A condition characterized by the presence of a kidney stone.

vagina A canal in a female reproductive system extending from the uterus to the external orifice.

vasa recta A series of peritubular capillaries that surround the loop of Henle, into which water moves after passing through the descending and ascending limbs of the loop of Henle.

■ Case Study Answers

1. List four types of common urinary disorders.

Answer: Bladder infection, kidney stones, kidney failure, and pyelonephritis.

2. What is a kidney stone, and why is it so painful?

Answer: Kidney stones, or calculi, are solid crystalline masses formed of minerals in the kidneys. Pain occurs when the stones move from the kidney into the urinary tract. The onset of pain often is acute, and the pain is experienced in waves. The sharp edges of the stone can cut into the muscle walls of the ureters and urethra, causing great pain. Most of the pain is believed to be associated with stretching of the walls of the ureter with peristaltic waves and urinary obstruction. People have said that the pain from kidney stones is the worst they have ever known. Kidney stones can become lodged in the ureters and urethra and obstruct urinary flow, causing a backpressure and possible damage to the nephrons.

3. Name the structures of the urinary tract and their functions.

Answer: Kidneys, ureters, urinary bladder, and urethra. The kidneys are smooth, bean-shaped organs that filter blood and excrete body wastes in the form of urine. The ureters, a pair of thick-walled, hollow tubes, carry urine from the kidneys to the urinary bladder. The urinary bladder is a hollow, muscular sac in the midline of the lower abdomen that stores urine until it is excreted. The urethra is a hollow, tubular structure that drains urine from the bladder.

4. Why can't the patient find a comfortable position?

Answer: The patient is in extreme pain and is unable to find a position that alleviates the pain. Often you will find patients squirming around as you approach them. Generally, urolithiasis is not improved by any particular position. Analgesia is the appropriate treatment.

5. What additional questions about the urinary system should be asked?

Answer: To determine the severity of the condition, the patient should be asked whether he is having any difficulty urinating (dysuria), if it hurts to urinate, how frequently he is urinating, and whether there is any blood in the urine.

6. What physical finding might lead you to suspect that the patient is experiencing a urinary tract infection rather than kidney stones?

Answer: If the patient has evidence of an infection, such as a fever, it is possible that he has a urinary tract infection rather than kidney stones. Although urinary tract infections occur more commonly in women, men also experience them.

Learning Objectives

1. List the essential and accessory reproductive organs of the male and female, describing the general function of each. (p 257-266)

2. Name the hormones necessary for the formation of gametes. (p 258)

3. Describe the difference between spermatogenesis and oogenesis. (p 258, 264)

4. Describe the three layers of the uterine wall. (p 259)

5. Briefly describe the life cycle of an oocyte. (p 259-260)

6. Describe the menstrual cycle in terms of changes in hormone levels and the condition of the endometrium. (p 259-260)

7. Define the following terms: diploid, haploid, gametes, endometrium, genetic disease, homologous chromosomes, autosomes, sex chromosomes, genes, alleles, genotype, phenotype, homozygous, and heterozygous. (p 259, 269-274)

8. Identify and describe the structures that constitute the external genitalia in both sexes. (p 261, 265)

9. Name the parts of a sperm cell. (p 264)

10. Beginning with fertilization, describe the major developmental changes during gestation. (p 266-268)

11. Describe the structure and function of the placenta and umbilical cord. (p 266-268)

12. State the length of an average gestation period. (p 267)

13. Describe the stages of labor. (p 268)

14. Describe the difference between fetal circulation/respiration and adult circulation/respiration. (p 268-269)

15. Describe the major changes that take place in an infant at birth. (p 268-269)

16. Discuss the difference between dominant and recessive traits. (p 272-273)

17. List some important genetic diseases found in out of hospital care. (p 274)

18. Explain how genes can cause disease. (p 274-275)

Skidplate: © Photodisc; Cells © ImageSource/age fotostock

Introduction

The reproductive system is the only body system that is not essential to survival of a person, but is needed to ensure the continued existence of the human species. The reproductive systems of both males and females contain organs and glands that create sex cells and transport them to areas where fertilization can occur. The male and female reproductive systems are functionally very different. Male sex cells are called sperm. Female sex cells are called oocytes or eggs. The reproductive system is linked with genetics. Sex cells carry genetic instructions via 23 chromosomes. Other types of cells in the body carry 46 chromosomes. When sex cells from a male and female unite during fertilization, the 23 chromosomes from each partner unite to form 46 chromosomes. Certain reproductive organs secrete hormones needed for development and maintenance of secondary sex characteristics and for reproduction.

The Human Reproductive System

The human reproductive system includes all of the male and female structures responsible for sexual reproduction. This organ system is integrally linked with genetics, the branch of biology dealing with heredity and inherited traits, both normal and abnormal. As scientific knowledge advances, it has become increasingly clear that a hereditary component accompanies many human diseases. The patient's family medical history has been a routine part of the prehospital evaluation for many years.

The Female Reproductive System

The female reproductive organs produce and maintain the egg cells (oocytes), which are the female sex cells. The organs also transport them to the site of fertilization, provide a nurturing environment for the developing fetus, give birth to a child, and produce female sex hormones. The principal

Case Study | PART 1

At 10:00 AM, your unit is dispatched to the interstate highway for a woman in labor. The patient's husband greets you as you arrive and anxiously yells, "Come quick, I think the baby is coming!" You grab the OB kit and ask the husband whether this is his wife's first pregnancy, whether it is her first delivery, and the baby's due date. You also ask him about any prenatal care she has received and whether there are any known complications. The husband tells you that this is his wife's third pregnancy and second delivery; her first pregnancy ended in a miscarriage. She has had good prenatal care, and there is no reason to believe there would be any complications. The baby was due 4 days ago. Apparently, the couple had been sent home from the hospital yesterday and was planning on returning this morning so that labor could be induced.

As you approach the car, you note that the patient is screaming in pain and is lying across the front seat. The baby's head is crowning and about to deliver, so you quickly open the OB kit, drape the patient, and apply the appropriate standard precautions. Your partner times the contractions at 1 minute apart and lasting 45 seconds. Because birth is imminent, you plan to deliver the baby at the scene and then move the patient onto your stretcher for transport. You determine that extra personnel would be helpful, especially if there are problems with the newborn, so your partner alerts dispatch to send an engine company to assist with manpower and law enforcement for traffic control.

Recording Time: 0 Minutes	
Appearance	Working hard at labor
Level of consciousness	Alert (oriented to person, place, and day)
Airway	Appears patent
Breathing	Regular
Circulation	Flushed with beads of sweat on her forehead

1. What are the major organs of the female reproductive system?

2. What are the layers of the uterine wall, including the functional wall?

organs of the female reproductive system (besides the ovaries) are the fallopian tubes, uterus, vagina, and the components of the external genitalia Figure 13-1 . The primary sex organs (gonads) are the two ovaries, which produce female sex cells and sex hormones. The accessory sex organs are the internal and external reproductive organs. As in males, a variety of accessory glands release secretions into the female reproductive tract.

The Ovaries

The ovaries are oval-shaped, solid structures about 3.5 centimeters long, 2 centimeters wide, and 1 centimeter thick. They lie in shallow depressions in the lateral pelvic cavity wall. Ovarian tissues consist of an inner medulla and an outer cortex. The medulla is made up of loose connective tissue with many blood and lymphatic vessels as well as nerve fibers. The cortex has more compact tissue with a granular appearance because of masses of ovarian follicles. The ovary's free surface is covered with cuboidal epithelium above a layer of dense connective tissue. Two ligaments, the suspensory ligament and the ovarian ligament, as well as a fold of peritoneum, the mesovarium, hold the ovaries in place. The ovaries perform three main functions: (1) production of immature female gametes (oocytes), (2) secretion of female sex hormones (including estrogens and progestins), and (3) secretion of inhibin (involved in the feedback control of pituitary follicle-stimulating hormone production). The precursors to mature eggs, oocytes are also produced in the ovaries. These undergo a maturation process, termed oogenesis, resulting in an ovum, the mature egg.

During the reproductive years of a woman's life, the pituitary gland releases hormones at roughly monthly intervals. These hormones, follicle-stimulating hormone (FSH) and luteinizing hormone (LH), stimulate one oocyte to undergo meiosis, the process of cell division that results in the formation of a mature ovum. A mature ovum is released into one of the fallopian tubes during ovulation and is then ready for fertilization by a sperm Figure 13-2 .

During meiosis, an immature diploid oocyte undergoes a series of two cell divisions to form a final haploid ovum. During this process, the number of chromosomes is reduced from 46 (the diploid number) to 23 (the haploid number). As a result, a final ovum contributes half of the total genetic information to the zygote, or fertilized ovum.

The Fallopian Tubes

Fallopian tubes are long, slender tubes that pass medially to the uterus, penetrating its wall, and opening into the uterine cavity. Fertilization of the ovum by a sperm usually takes place here.

Each fallopian tube opens directly into the peritoneal cavity in an expanded area called the infundibulum. The opening of the fallopian tube is the ostium, which is surrounded by long, thin processes called fimbriae. The fimbriae help direct an oocyte into the fallopian tube following ovulation. Once inside the tube, movement of cilia (hairs) on the cell surfaces results in passage of an oocyte toward the uterus.

Pathophysiology

In an ectopic pregnancy, the egg becomes implanted at a location other than within the uterus, most often within the fallopian tubes. An ectopic pregnancy often is referred to as a tubal pregnancy.

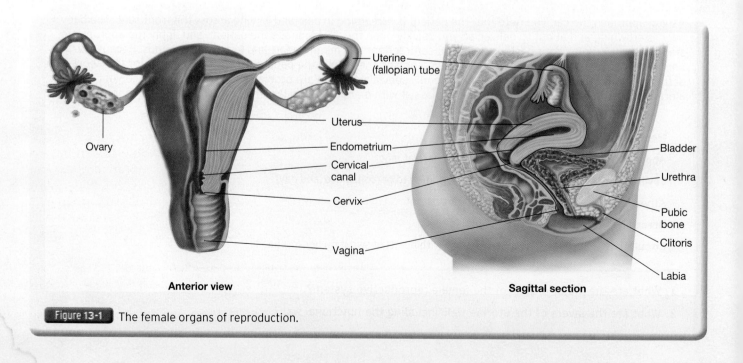

Anterior view

Sagittal section

Figure 13-1 The female organs of reproduction.

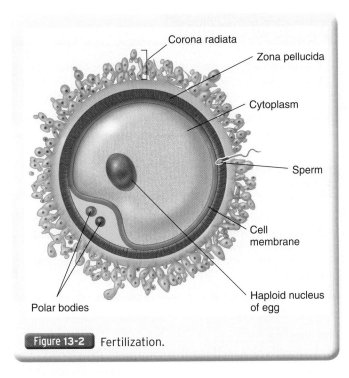

Corona radiata

Zona pellucida

Cytoplasm

Sperm

Cell membrane

Haploid nucleus of egg

Polar bodies

Figure 13-2 Fertilization.

Clinical Tip

It is crucial that a woman becomes aware of a pregnancy as soon as possible because the embryonic period is a time of high susceptibility to teratogens, external substances that may cause birth defects.

Pathophysiology

Pregnancy tests, whether performed on serum or urine, assay for human chorionic gonadotropin (hCG). A negative urine test result reliably excludes pregnancy; however, a positive urine pregnancy test result is nonspecific. Sometimes, contaminants in the urine, such as infectious material, cause a false-positive result. Thus, a positive urine pregnancy test result should always be confirmed by a blood pregnancy test. False-positive readings are rare when the blood test is used. When an ectopic pregnancy is suspected, quantitative blood hCG levels may be obtained, in which a total amount of hCG is measured. Blood progesterone levels also are helpful when an ectopic or otherwise abnormal pregnancy is suspected. However, these levels are not obtained with a normal pregnancy.

The Uterus

The uterus is a pear-shaped and hollow organ with muscular walls. If the oocyte is fertilized to become a zygote, the uterus receives the developing embryo, sustaining its development.

In a normal pregnancy, the fetus implants in the uterus. The uterus is located in the anterior pelvic cavity, superior to the vagina, usually bending over the urinary bladder. The uterine body (corpus) is the largest portion of the uterus. The fundus is the rounded portion of the corpus, and is superior to the attachment of the fallopian tubes. It ends at a constriction known as the isthmus of the uterus. The cervix is the inferior portion of the uterus, extending from the isthmus to the vagina. The cervix surrounds the cervical orifice, where the uterus opens to the vagina.

The uterine wall is thick, with three layers. The endometrium is the inner mucosal layer, covered with columnar epithelium and many tubular glands. Controlled by estrogen, the uterine glands, blood vessels, and epithelium change with the phases of the monthly menstrual cycle. The myometrium is the thickest portion of the uterine wall, making up the muscular middle layer, with bundles of smooth-muscle fibers. During the female reproductive cycle and during pregnancy, the endometrium and myometrium change greatly. The perimetrium is the outer serosal layer covering the body of the uterus and part of the cervix.

The uterus is supported and held in place by suspensory ligaments, which stabilize its position. These include the following:

- The broad ligaments. These attach to the entire body of the uterus laterally, and superiorly to the fallopian tubes.
- The uterosacral ligaments. These extend from the lateral uterus surfaces to the anterior face of the sacrum; they keep the body of the uterus from moving inferiorly and anteriorly.
- The round ligaments. These arise on the lateral margins of the uterus just posterior and inferior to the attachments of the fallopian tubes; they extend through the inguinal canal to end in the connective tissues of the external genitalia, primarily restricting posterior movement of the uterus.
- The lateral ligaments. These extend from the base of the uterus and vagina to the lateral walls of the pelvis; they tend to prevent inferior movement of the uterus, with additional support provided by the pelvic floor muscles and fascia.

During the menstrual cycle, an ovum matures, forming a graafian follicle, or developed ovum. At ovulation, this follicle ruptures through the surface of the ovary. If fertilization occurs, the fertilized egg, or embryo, proceeds through the fallopian tube to implant in the uterus. If fertilization does not occur, a series of hormonal changes causes the remnants of the follicle, called the corpus luteum, to be sloughed, along with the uterine lining.

The menstrual cycle is a recurring cycle, beginning at menarche, which is the time of the first menstrual cycle, and ending at menopause, the cessation of menstruation. During each cycle, the lining of the uterus proliferates in preparation for pregnancy. If pregnancy does not occur, this functional layer is shed during menstruation. The average menstrual cycle is 28 days, with day 1 being the first day of menstrual flow. The length of menstruation varies greatly among women. Gonadotropin-releasing hormone (GnRH) from the hypothalamus, follicle-stimulating hormone and luteinizing hormone from the pituitary, and estrogen and progesterone from the ovaries stimulate the uterine lining at different stages during the menstrual cycle. **Figure 13-3** shows the endometrial lining during the various phases of the of the female reproductive cycle.

Pathophysiology

Cancer of the cervix is relatively common in women. A pap smear, performed during a routine gynecologic examination, may detect cervical cancer early. Many physicians recommend annual pap smears in women following the first menstrual cycle.

Pathophysiology

During pregnancy, the enlarging uterus may place strain on the ligaments that hold it in place, resulting in abdominal pain. Pain from stretching of the round ligaments is a relatively common occurrence, especially as the pregnancy progresses.

Pathophysiology

Endometritis is a severe infection of the endometrium that can occur following delivery of a newborn. Failure to recognize or treat this disease can result in death of the mother.

Clinical Tip

A missed menstrual period often is the first indication of pregnancy. The third week of embryonic development coincides with the first missed menstrual period. Thus, by the time pregnancy is suspected, the embryo has already undergone 2 weeks of development.

The Vagina

The vagina (birth canal) is a fibromuscular tube, about 7.5 to 9 centimeters long, extending from the cervix to the outside of the body (the external female genitalia). It conveys uterine secretions, receives the erect penis during intercourse, and provides the open channel for offspring. The vagina extends up and back into the pelvic cavity, and lies posterior to the urinary bladder and urethra, but anterior to the rectum. It is attached to these other structures by connective tissues. The hymen is a thin membrane of connective tissue and epithelium

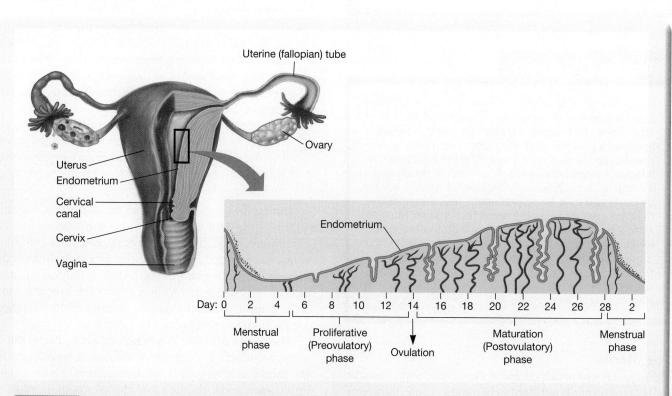

Figure 13-3 Endometrial changes during the female reproductive cycle.

that partially covers the vaginal orifice. It has a central opening that allows uterine and vaginal secretions to pass to the outside of the body. The three major functions of the vagina include: (1) serving as a passageway for the elimination of menstrual fluids, (2) receiving the penis during sexual intercourse, and (3) holding the spermatozoa prior to their passage into the uterus. The vagina forms the interior portion of the birth canal, through which the fetus passes during delivery.

The vaginal wall has three layers:

- Inner mucosal layer. Layer of stratified squamous epithelium with no mucous glands.
- Middle muscular layer. Layer of mostly smooth muscle fibers; helps to close the vaginal opening.
- Outer fibrous layer. Layer of dense connective tissue and elastic fibers.

Pathophysiology

Vaginitis is a nonspecific term for infection within the vagina. Often, infection is sexually transmitted. Yeast infections, however, are relatively common and are not sexually transmitted.

The External Genitalia

The external accessory organs of the female reproductive system include the labia majora, labia minora, clitoris, and vestibular glands **Figure 13-4**. They surround the openings of the urethra and vagina, composing the vulva.

The labia majora enclose and protect the other external reproductive organs. They are made up of rounded folds of adipose tissue and thin smooth muscle covered by skin. They lie close together, with a cleft that includes the urethral and vaginal openings separating the labia longitudinally. They merge at their anterior ends to form a medial, rounded elevation called the mons pubis, overlying the pubic symphysis.

The labia minora lie between the labia majora and are flattened, longitudinal folds composed of connective tissue. They have a rich blood supply and, therefore, a pinkish appearance. They merge posteriorly with the labia majora. Anteriorly, they converge to form the hood-like covering of the clitoris.

The clitoris projects from the anterior end of the vulva between the labia minora. It is usually about 2 centimeters long and 0.5 centimeters in diameter. It corresponds to the penis in males, with a similar structure. It is made up of two columns of erectile tissue (the corporus cavernosus) and forms a glans at its anterior end that has many sensory nerve fibers.

The labia minora encloses the vestibule, into which the vagina opens posteriorly. The urethra opens into the vestibule in the midline, about 2.5 centimeters posterior to the glans of the clitoris. One vestibular gland lies on each side of the vaginal opening. Under the vestibule's mucosa, on either side, is a mass of vascular erectile tissue (the vestibular bulb).

The erectile tissues of the clitoris and vaginal entrance respond to sexual stimulation. Parasympathetic nerve impulses release nitric oxide to dilate the erectile tissues, increase blood inflow, and swell the tissues. The vagina expands and elongates. If sexual stimulation is sufficiently intense, parasympathetic impulses cause the vestibular glands to secrete mucus into the vestibule, moistening and lubricating the surrounding tissues and lower vagina. This facilitates insertion of the penis.

The clitoris responds to local stimulation, culminating in an orgasm if stimulation is sufficient. Just before orgasm, the outer one third of the vagina is engorged with blood. This increases friction on the penis, with orgasm initiating reflexes directed by the sacral and lumbar spinal cord. The muscles of the perineum and walls of both the uterus and fallopian tubes contract rhythmically. This helps transport sperm through the female reproductive tract toward the upper part of the fallopian tubes.

Pathophysiology

During examination of a sexual assault victim (typically in the hospital emergency department), the health care provider looks for wounds about the perineum. The presence or absence of any wounds should be documented in the medical record.

The Mammary Glands

Breasts contain the organs of milk production, the mammary glands. Mammary glands actually are modified sweat glands. In both male and female breasts, there is an external raised nipple that is surrounded by the pigmented areola. In the female breast, areolar glands produce secretions that protect the nipple and areola during nursing.

The female mammary gland contains 15 to 20 glandular lobes covered by a large amount of fatty tissue **Figure 13-5**. This superficial fat gives the breast its form. The lobes

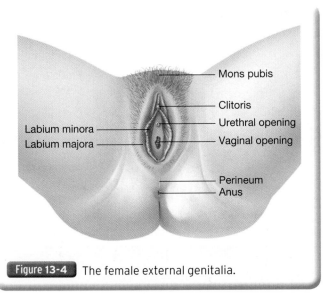

Figure 13-4 The female external genitalia.

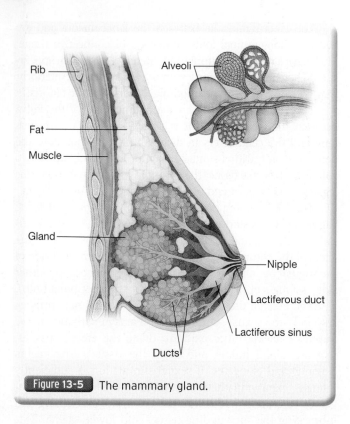

Rib

Fat

Muscle

Gland

Alveoli

Nipple

Lactiferous duct

Lactiferous sinus

Ducts

Figure 13-5 The mammary gland.

produce milk, which is stored in the lactiferous sinuses and expressed from the nipple. The mammary glands are supported by a group of mammary ligaments that extend from the fascia over the pectoralis major muscles to the skin over the mammary glands. These ligaments extend inward to help support the weight of the breast.

The Male Reproductive System

Sperm cells are produced and maintained by the male reproductive organs, which also transport these cells to outside of the body, as well as secreting male sex hormones. The primary sex organs (gonads) of the male consist of the two testes, in which sperm cells and male sex hormones are formed. The accessory sex organs are the internal and external reproductive organs **Figure 13-6**.

Pathophysiology

Breast cancer is a leading cause of death in women. Monthly self-examinations, combined with mammography screening in certain persons, may help increase the rate of early diagnosis.

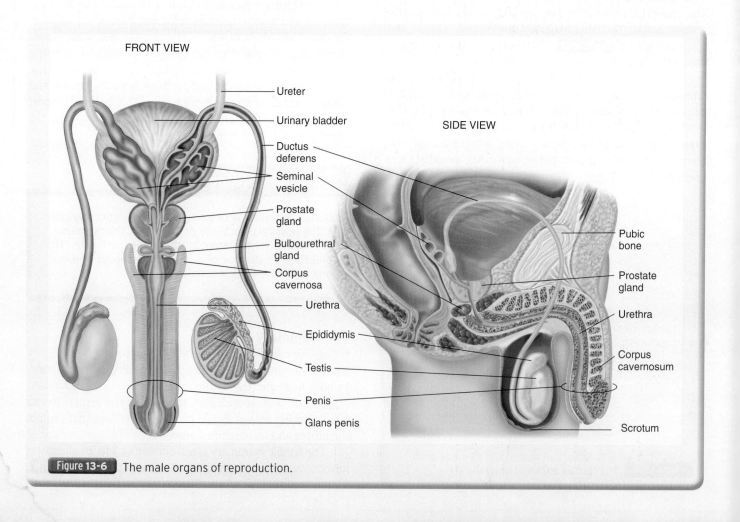

FRONT VIEW

Ureter

Urinary bladder

Ductus deferens

Seminal vesicle

Prostate gland

Bulbourethral gland

Corpus cavernosa

Urethra

Epididymis

Testis

Penis

Glans penis

SIDE VIEW

Pubic bone

Prostate gland

Urethra

Corpus cavernosum

Scrotum

Figure 13-6 The male organs of reproduction.

Case Study | PART 2

After three sets of contractions, the baby's head delivers. You suction the baby's mouth and nose just before you assist with the delivery of the shoulders. The delivery continues with no complications, and as the newborn boy begins to cry, your partner hands you a towel to dry him off and notes the time of birth. Once it is clear that the baby is healthy, an Apgar score, a newborn assessment score, is obtained and there is time to get a full set of baseline vital signs on the mother while you prepare to let the father cut the cord.

The vital signs are all within normal range and just then the medic unit arrives on the scene. The medics perform some additional assessment on the mother, obtaining a SAMPLE history and asking the appropriate OPQRST questions for this presenting medical patient. The patient is a 26-year-old woman who weighs 80 kg. The SAMPLE history shows:

- **S**igns and symptoms: Active labor with crowning (imminent birth)
- **A**llergies to medications: No known drug allergies
- **M**edications taken: Prenatal vitamins
- **P**ast pertinent medical history: Third pregnancy and second delivery, her first pregnancy ended in a miscarriage; good prenatal care with no complications expected
- **L**ast food/fluid intake: Eggs and toast for breakfast about 3 hours ago
- **E**vents prior to onset: On the way to the hospital with active labor

The OPQRST history shows:

- **O**nset of symptoms: Regular contractions began naturally today
- **P**rovoking factors: 4 days past due date
- **Q**uality of discomfort: Similar to last childbirth
- **R**adiating/related signs/symptoms: Contractions are within 1 minute of each other and last 45 seconds
- **S**everity of complaint: 10 on a scale of 1 to 10
- **T**ime: Approximately 2 hours

The newborn's Apgar results 1 minute after birth are:

- **A**ppearance/color = 1
- **P**ulse rate = 2
- **G**rimace/reflex = 2
- **A**ctivity/muscle tone = 1
- **R**espiratory effort = 2
- Total = 8

Recording Time: 15 Minutes	
Appearance	Exhausted but very happy
Level of consciousness	Alert (oriented to person, place, and day)
Airway	Open and patent
Breathing	Normal and rapid
Circulation	Flushed and moist
Pulse rate	98 beats/min and regular
Blood pressure	128/66 mm Hg
Respirations	22 breaths/min, nonlabored
Pupils	Equal and reactive
Spo$_2$	100%

3. What is the embryonic period of gestation and why is it a critical time?

4. In genetics, how is the gender of a fetus determined?

The Testes

The testes are oval-shaped structures about 5 centimeters long and 3 centimeters in diameter. They are located within the cavity of the scrotum. Two internal compartments, one for each testis, are separated by a wall of connective tissue. A layer of cutaneous muscle, the dartos muscle, contracts during cold weather, causing the skin of the scrotum to become firm and wrinkled. Combined with the actions of the cremaster muscle, which pulls the testicles close to the body, contraction of the scrotum maintains a steady temperature around the testes. If the testes are too warm or too cold, normal production of sperm, spermatogenesis, cannot occur.

Each testicle contains specialized cells and ducts; some of these produce male hormones, such as testosterone, and others develop sperm. The hormones are absorbed directly into the bloodstream from the testicles. Spermatozoa (sperm cells) are male gametes that are produced in the seminiferous tubules of the testes in a process known as spermatogenesis Figure 13-7. This process takes approximately 64 days and results in the formation of mature, haploid sperm, each containing 23 chromosomes. Spermatogenesis is the male equivalent of oogenesis and is under the influence of hormones, primarily testosterone, that are produced in the testes. Mature sperm contain a head, neck, and tail. The tail of the sperm moves in a whip-like motion, propelling the sperm deeper into the female reproductive tract in an attempt to fertilize an ovum.

Ducts and Glands

Spermatozoa leave the testes through efferent ductules, which form long, coiled tubes on the back of the testes, called the epididymides. The epididymides control the composition

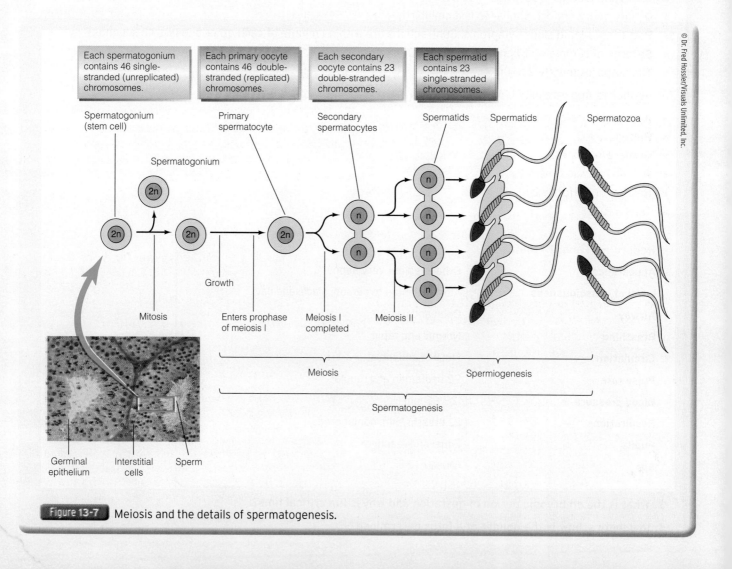

Figure 13-7 Meiosis and the details of spermatogenesis.

of the fluid that is produced by the seminiferous tubules. They also absorb and recycle damaged spermatozoa, while also absorbing cellular debris. Spermatozoa undergo a final maturation process in the epididymides, and then flow into the vas deferens. The vas deferens is surrounded by several structures, including the testicular artery and venous plexus, lymph vessels, nerves, connective tissue, and the cremaster muscle, which together constitute the spermatic cord. The spermatic cord passes obliquely through the inferior abdominal wall via the inguinal canal, into the abdominal cavity.

The prostate gland is a male sex gland. It is chestnut-shaped and located at the base of the urethra. The prostate secretes a viscous fluid that becomes part of semen. At the prostate gland, the vas deferens dilates, forming a pouch called the ampulla. The ampulla joins the seminal vesicles, a pair of pouches from which a sugar and protein ejaculatory fluid is secreted, to form the ejaculatory duct. Sperm and ejaculatory fluid combine in the seminal vesicles to form semen. The prostate gland and the bulbourethral glands, located on either side of the prostate gland, produce the remaining secretions that become part of semen. Semen flows from the ejaculatory duct into the urethra, a hollow tube that drains from the bladder and provides the pathway by which semen is released from the penis during sexual intercourse.

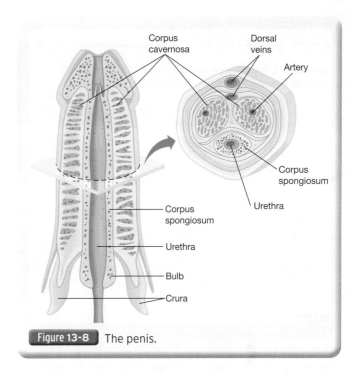

Figure 13-8   The penis.

The glans of the penis is the expanded distal end that surrounds the external urethral orifice. This structure covers the ends of the corpora cavernosa and opens as the external urethral orifice. Skin in this area is thin and hairless, with sensory receptors for sexual stimulation. At birth, a loose fold of skin, the foreskin, covers the glans. It often is removed surgically after birth in a procedure known as circumcision.

Blood vessels and nerves of the penis run on the dorsal side. During erection, both the corpora cavernosa and the corpus spongiosum fill with blood, causing an increase in penis length and diameter. As erectile tissues are filled, venous drainage is temporarily blocked, resulting in continued erection.

Pathophysiology

Enlargement of the prostate gland is common with increasing age. Unfortunately, cancer of the prostate gland is a frequent cause of death in men. A blood test, prostate-specific antigen (PSA), aids physicians in making an early diagnosis. Many doctors routinely perform this test in men older than age 50 years. If you have not been tested, ask about it!

Pathophysiology

Vasectomy is a form of birth control in which the vas deferens on each side is surgically cut and tied off. It is possible, although complicated, to have a surgical procedure to reverse the procedure by reconnecting the tubes.

The Penis

The penis is the male external reproductive organ, through which the urethra passes. When erect, it stiffens and enlarges, enabling insertion into the vagina during sexual intercourse **Figure 13-8** . The penis is divided into three regions: the root, body, and glans. The root of the penis is the fixed portion that attaches the penis to the body wall. The shaft (or body) of the penis is the tubular, movable portion of the organ. It contains three columns of erectile tissue. It has two dorsal corpora cavernosa and one ventral corpus spongiosum. At the base of the penis, the corpus spongiosum expands to form the bulb of the penis; the corpora cavernosa expand to form the crus of the penis. Dense connective tissue surrounds each column in a capsule. The penis is enclosed by a layer of connective tissue, a thin layer of subcutaneous tissue, and skin.

Pathophysiology

Testicular torsion occurs when the testicle becomes twisted about the spermatic cord. This condition results in severe and sudden pain, nausea, and vomiting. Because the blood supply to the involved testicle is impaired, failure to diagnose and treat this condition in a timely manner may result in loss of the testis. Testicular torsion should be suspected in any person with an acute onset of scrotal pain, especially when accompanied by nausea and vomiting.

Pathophysiology

Erection is primarily controlled by the parasympathetic nervous system, but the sympathetic nerves also play a role by controlling ejaculation of semen. Sympathetic fibers take over control of an erection in people with damage to the spinal cord who have lost parasympathetic stimulation. Persistent erection in a patient with a spinal cord injury is referred to as a priapism.

The Perineum

As in the female genitalia, the area between the urethral opening and the anus is the perineum. It includes skin, the external genitalia, the anus, and underlying tissues. The perineum is divided into the urogenital triangle, containing the base of the penis, and the anal triangle, containing the anal opening. In both sexes, the perineum supports the distal structures of the reproductive and excretory systems.

■ Pregnancy

Typically, fertilization occurs when sperm and an ovum meet in the fallopian tube. If fertilization occurs, the zygote that results moves through the fallopian tube toward the uterus. At the same time, it undergoes progressive cell divisions

Figure 13-9. When the zygote contains approximately 32 cells, it usually implants into the uterine wall. Implantation occurs approximately 7 days after fertilization. Once the zygote is implanted into the lining of the uterus, pregnancy begins. The inner group of cells (the embryoblast) becomes the embryo; the outer group of cells (the trophoblast) becomes the placenta.

The placenta is attached to the endometrium on one side and surrounds the embryo on the other side. It is highly vascular and, via the umbilical cord, is the means by which the fetus absorbs oxygen, nutrients, and other substances from the pregnant woman. The placenta also transmits carbon dioxide and other waste products from the fetus to the pregnant woman. The placenta is expelled during the third stage of labor.

Pregnancy is divided into three trimesters. The first trimester extends from the last menstrual period through week 12 of the pregnancy. Major events in the first trimester include a positive pregnancy test result (blood hCG) at 8 to 10 days, a palpable uterine fundus at the pubic symphysis at week 12, and audible fetal heart tones noted on Doppler ultrasound.

■ Gestation

Gestation refers to the process of fetal development following fertilization of an egg. The process of gestation is stimulated by production of the hormone human chorionic

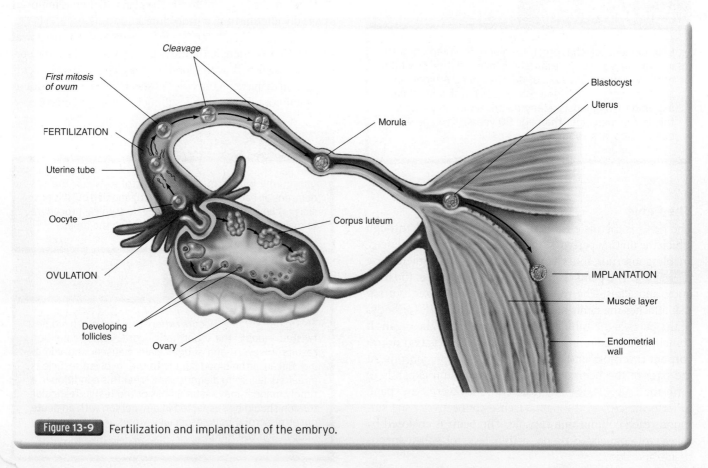

Figure 13-9   Fertilization and implantation of the embryo.

gonadotropin (hCG) by the trophoblast. This hormone stimulates the corpus luteum to produce progesterone, which is essential for normal continuation of the pregnancy. During the first week of gestation, a fertilized egg moves along the fallopian tube, dividing continuously, and implants into the uterine wall.

The normal human gestation period is 266 days following implantation of the fertilized egg into the uterine wall Figure 13-10 .

During the second week of gestation, the placenta and membranes that will surround and protect the embryo continue to develop. Collectively, these amniotic membranes form the amniotic sac. Amniotic fluid is produced by the filtration of maternal and fetal blood through blood vessels in the placenta and by excretion of fetal urine into the amniotic sac. Amniotic fluid is swallowed by the fetus and removed by the placenta where it passes into the mother's blood. The placenta connects to the fetus via the umbilical cord Figure 13-11 .

All major organ systems begin to develop during the embryonic period (weeks 3 through 8) Figure 13-12 . After the 8th week of gestation, the placenta takes over production of progesterone and the corpus luteum is absorbed into the placental tissue. From the embryonic period until delivery, organ systems undergo continuing maturation and development.

The second trimester extends from weeks 13 through 27. The major events are a palpable uterine fundus between the pubic symphysis and the umbilicus at week 16, the first fetal movements (quickening) at weeks 16 through 18 in a woman who has had one or more previous pregnancies, and fetal heart tones that become audible with a fetoscope at weeks 17 through 20. In addition, female and male fetal external genitalia may be distinguished by ultrasound at week 18. In a woman's first pregnancy, first fetal movements (quickening) are noted at weeks 18 through 20, and the uterine fundus is palpable at the umbilicus at week 20. At weeks 25 through 27, the lungs become capable of respiration and produce surfactant, a liquid protein substance that coats the alveoli in the lungs. Infants born at the end of the second trimester have a 70% to 80% chance of survival.

The third trimester extends from week 28 until term, or week 40. The major events of the third trimester include the presence of a papillary light reflex in the fetus, descent of the fetal head to the pelvic inlet (lightening), and rupture of the fetal membranes. Once the membranes have ruptured, the fetus must be delivered within 24 hours because of the risk of infection. At the end of the third trimester, the fetus typically weighs 7.0 to 7.5 lb (3,300 g).

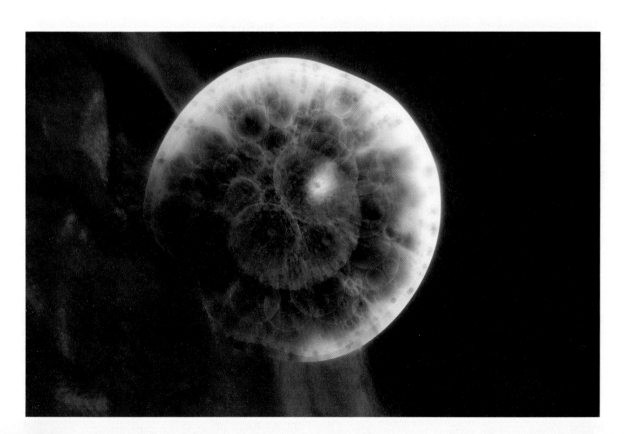

© 3D4Medical/Science Source

Figure 13-10   Implantation of the preembryo cells onto the uterine wall.

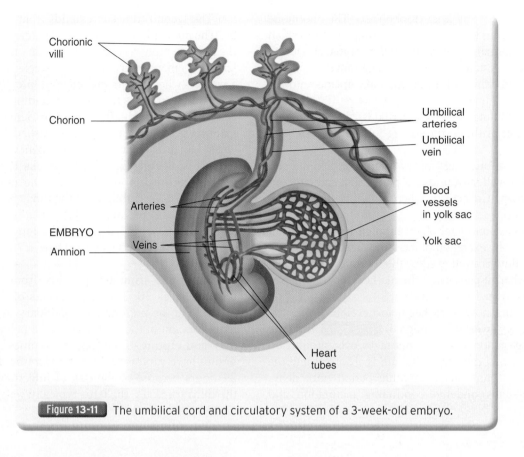

Figure 13-11 The umbilical cord and circulatory system of a 3-week-old embryo.

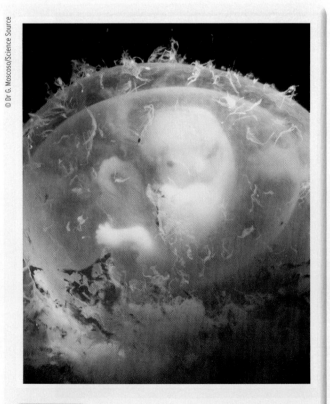

Figure 13-12 All major organ systems begin to develop during the embryonic period.

Labor

Scientists are still uncertain exactly what initiates labor. The most likely explanation is a combination of maternal and fetal stimuli. The average duration of labor is 13 hours in the first pregnancy and about 8 hours in subsequent pregnancies. Labor consists of three stages. During the first stage, the uterine wall begins to contract and the cervix dilates. The birth of the baby occurs in the second stage. During the third stage, the placenta is expelled.

Birth

Birth places a major stress on the newborn. During fetal life, the lungs are fluid-filled and nonfunctioning. All oxygen and carbon dioxide exchange takes place through the placenta. The fetus is attached to the placenta by the umbilical cord. Oxygenated blood from the mother's circulation travels through the placenta and via the umbilical vein to the fetus' liver and from there through the inferior vena cava to the right atrium of the fetus' heart. Blood then passes through the foramen ovale, an opening in the fetus' atrial wall between the right and left atria, into the left atrium. From the left atrium, the blood circulates to the left ventricle and through the head and upper body parts. The returning blood flows through the superior vena cava into the right atrium, and then flows at low pressure into the right ventricle and through the pulmonary artery to the descending aorta.

The pulmonary artery and descending aorta are connected via a ductus arteriosus in the fetus, allowing this pathway of blood flow to occur. From the descending aorta, blood circulates through the lower body parts. The blood that flows through the umbilical arteries back to the placenta carries the fetal waste. In the placenta, the fetal waste diffuses into the mother's bloodstream for eventual excretion.

At birth, several changes occur. The foramen ovale and ductus arteriosus close partially or completely, so that blood no longer flows from the right atrium to the left atrium and from the pulmonary artery to the descending aorta. Vascular changes occur as a result of decreased right atrial pressure from occlusion of the placental circulation and increased left atrial pressure from increased pulmonary venous return from the lungs. Circulation through the newborn's lungs begins with the first breath.

Genetics

Genetics is the study of heredity, the transmission of characteristics from parents to their offspring. Many principles of heredity are similarly applicable to all living organisms, making it possible to apply knowledge gained from one plant or animal to humans. Developmentally, there are remarkable similarities among the homologous chromosomes (the chromosomal contents or genomes) of different species.

Case Study PART 3

You wrap up the newborn in towels and a blanket and allow the mother to hold him. As the stretcher is brought to the side of the vehicle, you and the paramedic crew gently lift the mother and newborn onto the stretcher. In this way, the delivery of the placenta can easily be managed while you are en route to the hospital, rather than waiting for it to deliver on the scene. As you load the stretcher into the ambulance, you can hear the baby's father calling his mother-in-law on his cell phone with the good news. Once in the ambulance, the newborn is reassessed and another Apgar score is obtained.

The Apgar score 5 minutes after birth is:

- **A**ppearance/color = 2
- **P**ulse rate = 2
- **G**rimace/reflex = 2
- **A**ctivity/muscle tone = 2
- **R**espiratory effort = 2
- Total = 10

Recording Time: 20 Minutes	
Appearance	Excited, exhausted, and happy
Level of consciousness	Alert (oriented to person, place, and day)
Airway	Open and patent
Breathing	Normal and slightly rapid
Circulation	Pale, clammy, and bleeding has subsided
Pulse	100 beats/min and regular
Blood pressure	110/70 mm Hg
Respirations	22 breaths/min, nonlabored
Pupils	PEARRL
SpO_2	100%

5. What are two major circulation changes that occur in the infant at birth?

6. At this point, what stage of labor is occurring?

7. In reference to genetic diseases, what is the "carrier state?"

Not all observable characteristics of an organism are attributable to inheritance. Environmental factors may affect inherited traits and conditions. These factors include nutrition, exposure to toxins or pathogens, and physical activity. Environmental factors hold great importance for polygenic traits (those determined by more than one gene) such as height, skin color, and intelligence.

Genetic material is carried on chromosomes in the nucleus of each cell. Other than when cells are actively dividing, the chromosomes are indiscrete, contained within bundles of DNA and protein called chromatin Figure 13-13.

Genes, Nucleic Acids, and Chromosomes

Genes are the fundamental units of heredity. In the form of nucleic acids located in the cell's nucleus, genes store and release information on how to build and control cells. Nucleic acids are complex chemicals contained in the chromosomes. Human chromosomes contain deoxyribonucleic acid (DNA), which carries the so-called genetic code, or sets of thousands of different genes that code for proteins that carry out various body functions. In mature cells, ribonucleic acid (RNA) is made from DNA in the cell's nucleus. RNA then moves to the cytoplasm of the cell where it serves as a template for the production of proteins. The central dogma of life is the hypothesis ascribed to Francis Crick in 1958 that says that "DNA leads to RNA, which leads to proteins, which leads to cells."

Diploid and Haploid Cells

Each parent contributes one copy of each gene to his or her children. Body cells contain two sets of chromosomes, one contributed by each parent and, thus, two sets of genes. During fertilization, the two sets of genes are brought together, resulting in an equal complement of genes from each parent. The interaction of both sets of genes determines the characteristics of a person. As previously noted, environment also may play a significant role in the expression of genetic information.

The total number of chromosomes in a mature human cell, 46 chromosomes, is the diploid number (two sets). Each sex cell, or gamete, contains one half of the total chromosome complement of a mature cell, or 23 chromosomes. The number of chromosomes in each sex cell is the haploid number Figure 13-14. The union of the haploid sperm and haploid egg results in the formation of a zygote (fertilized ovum), which contains a diploid number of chromosomes.

Autosomal and Sex-Linked Traits

Both body cells and sex cells contain two different types of chromosomes. Autosomes carry genes that code for numerous body proteins independent of sex. Each person, regardless of sex, has the same number of autosomes. Sex chromosomes, on the other hand, code for proteins that

Pathophysiology

In a procedure called amniocentesis, a sample of the amniotic fluid sometimes is obtained by placing a needle, using ultrasound or CT scan guidance, into the uterus and withdrawing a small portion of amniotic fluid. The fluid can then be analyzed for various chemical abnormalities. In addition, the fetus sheds cells into the fluid. Using special preparations, the chromosomes in these fetal cells may be studied to detect genetic diseases, such as Down syndrome.

determine sex, as well as for other proteins. Each sex has different sex chromosomes.

There are two sex chromosomes, X and Y. Each ova contains one X chromosome and each spermatocyte contains either an X or a Y chromosome. Once fertilized, the zygote can have two X chromosomes (XX), resulting in a female embryo, or an X and a Y chromosome (XY), resulting in a male embryo.

Traits are classified by the type of chromosome on which they reside. Autosomal-linked traits reside in genes located on autosomes. Generally, there are no differences in inheritance between the sexes. Sex-linked traits reside in genes located on the sex chromosomes. Because the two sexes have different normal complements of sex chromosomes, certain traits are more likely to be passed on to either male or female offspring, depending on the parental genes.

Alleles and Dominant and Recessive Traits

Each single gene contributed by one parent for any particular characteristic is called an allele. For many inherited features, there may be more than one potential allele. Each parent contributes one gene (allele) for each inherited characteristic, and it is the combination of both maternal and paternal alleles that results in the final outcome.

In genetics, alleles and inherited traits are either recessive or dominant. For a recessive trait to be expressed, a person must receive the same recessive allele from each parent. On the other hand, for a dominant trait to be expressed, a person need only receive one dominant allele. For genes located on autosomes, it does not matter which parent donates the dominant allele; however, for sex chromosomes, it is a different matter.

Letters are used to indicate various alleles. The dominant allele is written in upper case letters, the recessive in lower case. Each gamete carries one allele. The fertilized egg has two alleles, one from each parental gamete.

Depending on whether or not a particular trait is inherited as dominant or as recessive, and on the alleles contributed by each parent, the final appearance of a person may or may not demonstrate the trait. For example, if a trait is

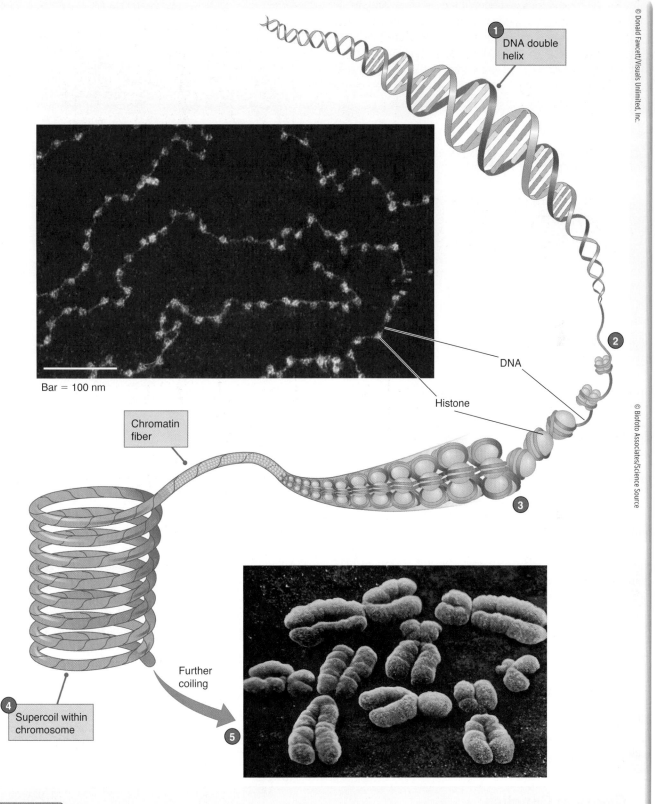

Figure 13-13 Chromatin and chromosomes. Proteins and DNA comprise the chromatin within a cell. When coiled and condensed, chromatin forms chromosomes.

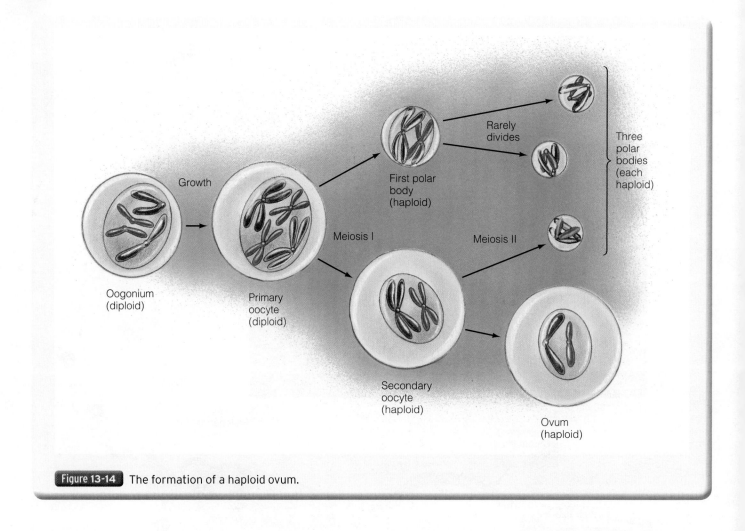

Figure 13-14 The formation of a haploid ovum.

autosomal recessive, a person must have two recessive alleles (one from each parent) to have the trait. If a person inherits one recessive allele from one parent and a dominant allele from the other parent, he or she will not demonstrate the recessive trait clinically.

Genotype and Phenotype

A phenotype is an observable characteristic of an organism that results from genetic composition and environmental factors. The genotype is the genetic composition for the same trait. In a dominant trait, if either or both dominant alleles are present in the genotype, the trait is observable. A recessive characteristic, however, will only be visible clinically when the genotype contains two recessive alleles for that particular trait.

Classical Genetics

In the mid 19th century, an Austrian monk, Gregor Mendel, performed the first experiments in "classical genetics." In fact, this branch of genetics is commonly referred to as mendelian genetics, or Mendel's Laws of Heredity. Mendel studied the color of the flowers in pea plants and discovered that

when he crossed plants with red flowers with plants with white flowers, all the resulting offspring had red flowers. He called these plants the first generation, or F_1 Figure 13-15.

He then crossed two F_1-generation plants. The second-generation (F_2) plants produced red flowers and white flowers, with a predictable ratio of three red-flowered plants to one white-flowered plant Figure 13-16.

On the basis of these experiments, Mendel proposed a theory of inheritance that has since been verified many times. Mendel suggested that color in these plants is determined by one gene, with two potential alleles (R and r). The dominant allele (R) codes for red flowers while the recessive allele (r) codes for white flowers. Only one R allele is necessary for a plant to have red flowers. However, two r alleles are necessary for a plant to have white flowers.

Mendel reasoned that the red-flowered parent plants of the F_1 generation must have two R alleles, while the white-flowered plants had two r alleles. Despite demonstrating a red phenotype (appearance), the resultant F_1 generation plants all had an Rr genotype. Because the R allele was dominant over the r allele, any plant with even one R allele in its genotype demonstrated a red phenotype.

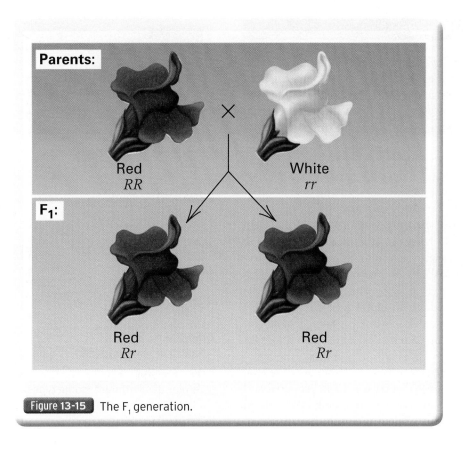

Figure 13-15 The F$_1$ generation.

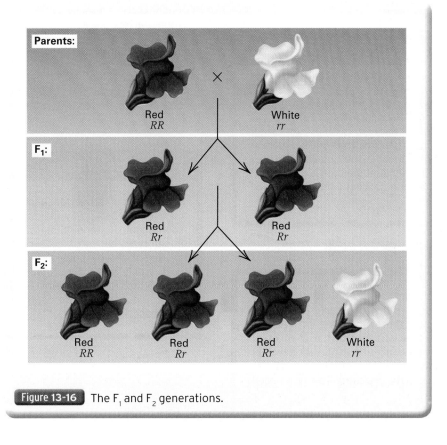

Figure 13-16 The F$_1$ and F$_2$ generations.

Genetic Diseases

An organism that has two identical alleles for a trait, such as *rr* or *RR*, is identified as being homozygous for that trait. An organism that has two different alleles for a trait, such as *Rr*, is identified as being heterozygous for the trait. Whether a heterozygote expresses a trait clinically (phenotypically) depends on whether the trait is dominant or recessive. A recessive trait will not be expressed phenotypically unless two of the same recessive alleles are present, such as *rr*. However, if the trait is dominant, it will be expressed whether the alleles are homozygous (*RR*) or heterozygous (*Rr*).

A genetic disease is a hereditary condition that occurs when a genotypic abnormality results in an observable phenotypic finding. In some autosomal-recessive conditions, a person may carry only one abnormal allele and be perfectly healthy. This often is referred to as the carrier state. The carrier may pass the disease on if he or she mates with another carrier.

Many human genetic diseases involve a single gene and are inherited in mendelian patterns (eg, autosomal-dominant inheritance) **Table 13-1**.

Although many diseases involve just one gene, several diseases involve many genes that have a small, yet equal and additive effect. This genetic component, combined with an environmental component, makes a person susceptible to inheriting certain conditions. This form of inheritance is called multifactorial. An inherited disease caused by the combined actions of two or more genes is called a polygenic disease.

Table 13-1 Autosomal and X-Linked Conditions

Autosomal dominant
Diabetes (some types)
Familial hypercholesterolemia
Huntington disease (chorea)
Marfan syndrome
Myotonic dystrophy
Neurofibromatosis
Osteogenesis imperfecta

Autosomal recessive
Alpha-thalassemia
Albinism
Beta-thalassemia
Cystic fibrosis
Dwarfism
Hypothyroidism
Premature senility
Sickle cell anemia
X-linked recessive
Muscular dystrophy
Hemophilia A and B
Testicular feminization syndrome

Mitochondrial
Cardiac dysrhythmias (some types)
Cardiomyopathy (some types)
Hereditary optic neuropathy

Multifactorial
Cancer
Cleft lip
Cleft palate
Clubfoot
Congenital heart disease
Coronary artery disease
Epilepsy
Hyperlipoproteinemia
Rheumatic fever
Type 1 diabetes
Type 2 diabetes

Pathophysiology

An abnormality in a gene results in defective RNA and, thus, a defective protein. Errors at any step of this process result in genetic diseases.

Mitochondria in human cells contain their own independent complement of DNA and genes.

Developmentally, this is believed to stem from when they were independent organisms that finally incorporated into human cells. Although the number of genes carried only in the mitochondrial genome is small, heritable defects have been noted recently that account for several human diseases.

Pathophysiology

Many human autosomal-linked traits or diseases are the result of a single dominant or recessive gene on an autosome. Diagrams, such as those illustrated for Mendel's pea plants, can help clinicians predict the chances of certain inherited diseases (genetic diseases) developing in a child. The medical process of advising couples of the possibility that genetic disease will occur is called genetic counseling.

Pathophysiology

There are numerous mechanisms by which the genes carried on DNA may become abnormal. The body spontaneously repairs many of these defects. Even if not repaired, most cells containing abnormal DNA are destroyed by body defense mechanisms. Disease occurs only when abnormalities are either missed by the normal repair systems or the abnormality is not severe enough to cause death in utero, yet still results in disease.

Pathophysiology

Several common human diseases are caused by defects in genes that reside on either the X or Y chromosome (more commonly, on the X chromosome). These diseases are called <u>sex-linked diseases</u>. Unlike autosomal-linked conditions, sex-linked diseases will not be passed equally to male and female offspring. If a dominant condition is linked to the Y chromosome, then female offspring will not inherit it because they will not receive a Y chromosome from either parent. X-linked diseases are far more common than Y-linked diseases. In a male human (XY), only one X-linked allele is necessary to cause disease, whether the allele is dominant or recessive, because there is no counterbalancing allele on the Y chromosome. The Y chromosome is essentially "neutral" in determining the final outcome. A mother has a 50% chance of passing a recessive sex-linked condition on to each son **Figure 13-17** .

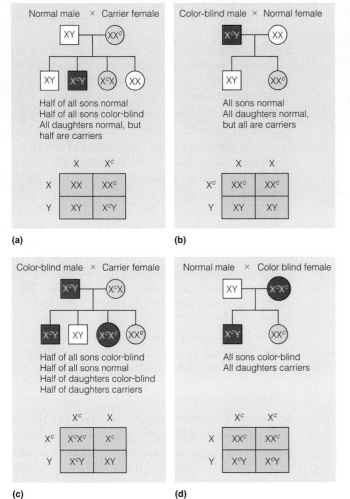

Figure 13-17 Inheritance of color blindness. Four possible genetic ways a sex-linked recessive gene such as color blindness can be passed to offspring. Males are indicated by boxes and females by circles. In this scheme, green boxes and circles represent men and women with color blindness. Light blue boxes represent men and women who are carriers. White boxes and circles represent men and women without the color blindness gene. The notation X^c indicates an X chromosome carrying the gene for color blindness.

Case Study | PART 4

En route to the hospital, both patients are monitored and serial vital signs taken. The newborn is kept warm and reassessed. Medical control directs you to proceed to the labor and delivery unit on arrival at the hospital to meet the patient's obstetrician. Within a few minutes, the mother states she is having more contractions and the placenta is delivered. You carefully examine it to make sure it is complete and place it in a plastic bag for further examination at the hospital.

Prep Kit

Chapter Summary

- The reproductive system consists of the structures responsible for sexual reproduction and is integrally linked with genetics. The genetic material is carried on chromosomes in the nucleus of each cell.

- The reproductive system is the only body system that is not essential to survival of a person, but is needed to ensure the continued existence of the human species.

- The ovaries are the female reproductive organs and produce the precursor to the mature egg, or oocyte, and hormones that regulate female reproductive function.

- Within the ovaries, oocytes undergo a maturation process, oogenesis, resulting in production of an ovum, or egg.

- The fallopian tubes serve as a passage for the movement of an ovum from the ovary and for sperm from the uterus distally.

- The uterus allows the implantation, growth, and nourishment of a fetus during pregnancy.

- The cervix is the part of the uterus that extends into the vagina.

- The uterine wall consists of three layers: the perimetrium, the myometrium, and the endometrium.

- The average menstrual cycle is 28 days.

- Typically, fertilization occurs when a sperm and ovum meet in the fallopian tube. If fertilization occurs, the zygote moves proximally through the fallopian tube toward the uterus, while undergoing progressive cell divisions.

- The placenta surrounds the embryo and, via the umbilical cord, is the means by which the fetus absorbs oxygen and nutrients. The placenta also allows excretion of carbon dioxide and other waste products from the fetus.

- The vagina is a muscular tube that forms the lower part of the female reproductive tract. It is the female organ of copulation and receives the male penis during sexual intercourse.

- The muscular walls of the vagina are able to expand, allowing the vagina to stretch greatly during childbirth.

- The external female genitalia are referred to as the vulva. A pair of skin folds, the labia minora, border the vestibule, a space into which the vagina and the urethra open.

- The clitoris is located in the anterior margin of the vestibule. The labia minora unite over the clitoris.

- Lateral to the labia minor are two prominent, rounded folds of skin, the labia majora.

- The breasts contain the mammary glands, the organs of milk production.

- The scrotum is the pouch of skin and muscle that contains the testes. The dartos muscle contracts during cold weather, causing the skin of the scrotum to become firm and wrinkled.

- The cremaster muscle pulls the testicles close to the body to maintain a steady temperature around the testes.

- The testes are the male reproductive organs and produce sperm and testosterone. Spermatozoa are produced in the testes through a process known as spermatogenesis.

- The penis is the male external reproductive organ, through which the urethra passes. The seminal vesicles produce most of the fluid portion of semen. The prostate gland and the bulbourethral glands produce the remaining secretions that become part of semen.

- Gestation refers to the process of fetal development following fertilization of the egg. During the first week of gestation, the fertilized egg moves proximally through the fallopian tube, dividing continuously, and implants into the uterine wall. The normal human gestation period is 266 days following implantation of the fertilized egg into the uterine wall.

- The first trimester extends from the first day of the last menstrual period through week 12 of the pregnancy. The second trimester extends from weeks 13 through 27. The third trimester extends from week 28 to term, or week 40.

- The average duration of labor is 13 hours for the first pregnancy and 8 hours for subsequent pregnancies.

- In the first stage of labor, the uterine wall contracts and the cervix dilates. In the second stage, the baby is born. In the third stage, the placenta is expelled.

- During fetal life, the lungs are fluid-filled and nonfunctioning. All oxygen and carbon dioxide exchange takes place through the placenta. The fetus is attached to the mother's placenta by the umbilical cord.

- At birth several changes occur, including partial or complete closure of the foramen ovale so that blood no longer flows from the right atrium to the left atrium and closure of the ductus arteriosus so that blood no longer flows from the pulmonary artery to the aorta. Circulation through the newborn's lungs begins with the first breath.

- Genetics is the study of heredity, the transmission of characteristics from parents to their offspring.

- A mature cell contains 23 pairs of chromosomes. One half of the chromosomes come from each parent via the sex cells.

- Developmentally, there are remarkable similarities between the chromosomal contents, or genomes, of different species (homologous chromosomes). Environmental factors also can strongly influence the expression of genetic information.

- Genes are the fundamental units of heredity that store and release information on how to build and control the cells. Human chromosomes contain DNA, or sets of thousands of different genes that code for proteins that carry out various body functions.

- In mature cells, RNA is made from DNA in the nucleus of the cell. RNA then moves to the cytoplasm of the cell where it serves as a template for the production of proteins.

- Each parent contributes one copy of each gene. Body cells contain two sets of chromosomes, one contributed by each parent. Body cells contain a diploid number of chromosomes. Each cell contains 46 chromosomes. Sex cells from each parent contain half that amount.

- Autosomes carry genes that code for numerous body proteins in both sexes. Each person has the same number of autosomes.

- Sex chromosomes code for proteins that determine sex, as well as for other proteins. The two sex chromosomes are the X and Y chromosomes. Each gamete from the father contains one or the other chromosome, and each gamete from the mother contains one X chromosome.

- A zygote with two X chromosomes (XX) results in a female embryo. A zygote with an X and a Y chromosome (XY) results in a male embryo.

- Autosomal-linked traits reside in genes located on autosomes. Sex-linked traits, on the other hand, reside in genes located on the sex chromosomes.

- Each single gene contributed by one parent for a characteristic is called an allele. For many inherited features, there may be more than one potential allele.

- Alleles and inherited traits are classified as either recessive or dominant. For a recessive trait to be expressed, a person must receive the same recessive allele from each parent. For a dominant trait to be expressed, a person need only receive one dominant allele. For genes located on autosomes, it does not matter which parent donates the dominant allele.

- The phenotype is the observable characteristic of an organism that results from genetic composition and environmental factors.

- The genotype is the genetic composition for the same trait. In a dominant trait, if either or both dominant alleles are present in the genotype, the trait is expressed.

- A recessive characteristic will only be visible clinically when the genotype contains two recessive alleles for that particular trait.

- Gregor Mendel performed the first experiments in classical genetics and proposed the theory of inheritance based on his studies of flower color in pea plants.

- An organism that has two identical alleles for a trait is identified as being homozygous for that trait.

- An organism that has two different alleles for a trait is identified as being heterozygous for the trait. Whether a heterozygote expresses a trait clinically depends on whether the trait is dominant or recessive.

- A genetic disease is a hereditary condition that occurs when a genotypic abnormality results in an observable phenotypic finding.

■ Vital Vocabulary

allele Variant form of a gene, which can be identical or slightly different in DNA sequence.

amniocentesis A procedure of extracting amniotic fluid from the uterus using a needle and ultrasound or CT scan guidance.

amniotic fluid Fluid produced by the filtration of maternal and fetal blood through blood vessels in the placenta and by excretion of fetal urine into the amniotic sac.

amniotic membranes The placenta and membranes that surround and protect the developing embryo.

amniotic sac The sac formed from the amniotic membranes that surround and protect the developing embryo.

ampulla A pouch in the vas deferens at the prostate gland.

areola The pigmented ring around the nipple in the breast.

areolar glands Glands that produce secretions that protect the nipple and areola during nursing.

autosomes The chromosomes that do not carry genes that determine sex.

breast cancer Cancer in one or both breasts.

breasts Structures that contain the organs of milk production.

broad ligaments One of several ligaments that support the uterus.

bulb of the penis The area of the corpus spongiosum that expands at the base of the penis.

bulbourethral glands Glands that lie inferior to the prostate gland and secrete a lubricating fluid that prepares the penis for sexual intercourse.

carrier state An autosomal-recessive condition with only one abnormal allele and no disease state that could be passed on if the carrier mates with another carrier.

cervix The narrowest portion (lower third of the neck) of the uterus that opens into the vagina.

chromatin Protein matter in which chromosomes are contained within a cell.

chromosomes Structures formed from condensed DNA fibers and protein; they are thread-like and are contained within the nucleus of the cells.

cilia The hairlike microtubule projections on the surface of a cell that can move materials over the cell surface.

circumcision Surgical removal of the foreskin of the glans of the penis.

clitoris In females, a small, cylindrical mass of erectile tissue and nerves located at the anterior junction of the labia minora, similar to the glans penis of the male.

corpus cavernosus The erectile tissue found in the clitoris and penis.

corpus luteum Yellow body; a temporary glandular structure created from enlarged follicular cells because of the release of luteinizing hormone.

corpus spongiosum Erectile tissue that surrounds the male urethra.

cremaster muscle The muscle that contracts and pulls the testicles close to the body during cold weather.

crus of the penis Area at the base of the penis formed by the expanded corpora cavernosa.

dartos muscle A layer of cutaneous muscle within the scrotum that contracts during cold weather, causing the skin to become firm and wrinkled.

deoxyribonucleic acid (DNA) Nucleic acid that carries the genetic code; sets of thousands of different genes that code for proteins that carry out various body functions.

diploid Cells that carry two of each of the 23 chromosomes—one from the father and one from the mother.

ectopic pregnancy A pregnancy in which the ovum implants somewhere other than the uterine endometrium.

efferent ductule The pathway by which spermatozoa leave the testes.

ejaculatory duct A structure formed by the vasa deferentia uniting with the duct of a seminal vesicle; this type of duct passes through the prostate gland to empty into the urethra.

embryo A fertilized egg.

embryoblast The inner group of cells within a zygote that develops to become the embryo.

embryonic period The period of gestation between weeks 3 and 8 in which all major organ systems begin to develop.

endometrium The inner layer of the uterine wall.

epididymides Tightly coiled tubes connected to ducts within a testis; they become the vas deferens.

estrogen A hormone released from the ovaries that stimulates the uterine lining during the menstrual cycle.

fallopian tubes The two hollow tubes or ducts that extend from the uterus to the region of the ovary and serve as a passageway for the ova and sperm.

fetoscope A device used for listening to fetal heart tones.

fimbriae Long thin finger-like processes at the end of the fallopian tubes that surround the ostium.

follicle-stimulating hormone (FSH) A hormone released from the pituitary gland at roughly monthly intervals that helps to stimulate one oocyte to undergo meiosis.

foramen ovale An opening between the two atria that is present in the fetus but normally closes shortly after birth.

foreskin A loose fold of skin that covers the glans of the penis.

fundus The top portion of the uterus.

gamete Sex cell; in humans, sperm and ovaries.

genes The fundamental units of heredity that store and release information on how to build and control cells.

genetic counseling The medical process of advising couples of the possibility that certain inherited diseases may develop in their child.

genetic diseases Diseases that develop as a result of an abnormality in a gene.

genetics The study of heredity.

genomes Chromosomal contents.

genotype The genetic composition for a given trait.

gestation The process of fetal development following fertilization.

glans The portion of the corpus spongiosum that extends to form a cap over the tip of the penis.

gonadotropin-releasing hormone (GnRH) A hormone released from the hypothalamus that stimulates the uterine lining during the menstrual cycle.

graafian follicle A mature or developed ovum.

haploid Cells that carry genetic instructions via 23 individual chromosomes.

heredity The passing of traits and qualities from parents to offspring, primarily through DNA or RNA.

heterozygous An organism that has two different alleles for a trait.

homologous chromosomes Chromosomes of the same numbered pair from the opposite parent.

homozygous An organism that has two identical alleles for a trait.

human chorionic gonadotropin (hCG) A hormone that stimulates the corpus luteum to produce progesterone during the first 8 weeks of gestation.

hymen A fold of mucous membrane that partially covers the entrance to the vaginal opening.

infundibulum The space formed in the peritoneum by the distal end of the fallopian tubes.

inguinal canal The canal through which the spermatic cord passes through the inferior abdominal wall and into the abdominal cavity.

labia majora Two prominent, rounded folds of skin lateral to the labia minora of the female external genitalia.

labia minora A pair of skin folds in the female external genitalia that border the vestibule.

lactiferous sinuses The area in the mammary glands in which milk is stored.

luteinizing hormone (LH) A hormone released from the pituitary gland at roughly monthly intervals that helps to stimulate one oocyte to undergo meiosis.

mammary glands The organs of milk production in the breasts.

mammary ligaments Structures that support the mammary glands.

mammography screening Radiographic screening of the breasts for early detection of cancer.

meiosis The process of cell division that occurs during the formation of a mature ovum or spermatocyte.

menarche The beginning phase of a woman's life cycle of menstruation.

menopause The ending phase of a woman's life cycle of menstruation.

menstrual cycle The entire monthly cycle of menstruation from start to finish, lasting approximately 28 days.

menstruation The sloughing and discharge of the functional layer of the endometrium; monthly flow of blood.

mesovarium The peritoneal fold that helps to hold the ovaries in place.

mons pubis A rounded pad of fatty tissue that overlies the pubic symphysis and is anterior to the urethral and vaginal openings.

myometrium A thick muscular middle layer of the uterine wall.

nipple An external raised protuberance on the breast surrounded by the pigmented areola.

nucleic acids Large organic molecules, or macromolecules, that carry genetic information or form structures within cells, and include DNA and RNA.

oocytes The precursors to a mature egg, formed in the ovaries.

oogenesis The process of egg cell formation, which begins at puberty.

ostium The opening in the infundibulum formed by the fallopian tubes.

ovarian ligament One of the two ligaments that help to hold the ovaries in place.

ovaries The female reproductive organs that produce egg precursors, or oocytes.

ovulation The release of a mature ovum into the fallopian tube from the ovary.

penis The male external reproductive organ through which the urethra passes.

perimetrium A serous membrane coating that makes up the outside layer of the uterine wall.

perineum The area between the urethral opening and the anus.

phenotype The observable characteristics of an organism that result from genetic composition and environmental factors.

placenta The organ that develops from trophoblastic cells of the zygote and attaches to the endometrium on one side and surrounds the embryo on the other side.

polygenic disease The genetic component of a multifactorial disease.

pregnancy The condition that begins when the developing offspring implants into the uterine lining; it consists of three trimesters (each about 3 months long).

progesterone A hormone released from the ovaries that stimulates the uterine lining during the menstrual cycle.

prostate gland A male sex gland that secretes an alkaline viscous ejaculatory fluid.

prostate-specific antigen (PSA) A blood test used in the diagnosis of prostate cancer.

ribonucleic acid (RNA) Nucleic acid made from DNA in the nucleus of the cell; it moves to the cytoplasm of the cell where it serves as a template for the production of proteins.

round ligaments One of several ligaments that supports the uterus.

scrotum The pouch of skin and subcutaneous tissue hanging from the lower abdominal region, posterior to the penis.

semen Seminal fluid ejaculated from the penis and containing sperm.

seminal vesicles Storage sacs for sperm and seminal fluid, which empty into the urethra at the prostate.

seminiferous tubules Highly coiled structures inside each lobule of a testis; they form a network of channels, then ducts, which join the epididymis.

sex chromosomes The X and Y chromosomes, which determine sex.

sex-linked diseases Disease resulting from defects on either the X or the Y chromosome.

sperm cells Male gametes that are produced in the testicles; also called spermatozoa.

spermatic cord A cord composed of the testicular artery, venous plexus, lymph vessels, nerves, connective tissue, and the cremaster muscle.

spermatogenesis The process by which sperm cells are formed.

spermatozoa Male gametes that are produced in the testicles; also called sperm.

surfactant A liquid protein substance that coats the alveoli in the lungs.

suspensory ligament One of the two ligaments that help to hold the ovaries in place.

testes The male reproductive organs that produce sperm and secrete male hormones; also called testicles.

testicular torsion Twisting of the testicle on the spermatic cord, from which it is suspended; associated with scrotal pain and swelling, and is a medical emergency.

testosterone The most important male hormone (androgen).

trimesters Three segments of time, each made up of approximately 3 months, that comprise the length of a pregnancy.

trophoblast The outer group of cells in a zygote that develop to become the placenta.

tubal pregnancy An ectopic pregnancy in which the oocyte has been abnormally implanted within the fallopian tube.

ultrasound A special device that uses sound waves to determine the location and shape of internal tissues and organs.

umbilical cord The connection between the placenta and the fetus.

uterosacral ligaments One of several ligaments that supports the uterus.

uterus In females, the muscular organ where the fetus grows; found between the urinary bladder and the rectum; also called the womb.

vagina The lower portion of the birth canal, which also serves as a passage for menstrual flow and as the receptacle of the penis during sexual intercourse.

vaginitis An inflammation of the vagina that is caused by an infection.

vas deferens The spermatic duct of the testicles.

vasectomy A form of birth control in which the vas deferens on each side is surgically cut and tied.

vestibular gland One of two glands that lie on each side of the vaginal opening; it secretes mucus into the vestibule to moisten and lubricate the vagina for insertion of the penis.

vestibule The space into which the vagina and the urethra open.

vulva The female external genitalia; includes the labia majora, labia minora, clitoris, and vestibular glands.

zygote A large fertilized egg cell produced after contacting a male sperm cell; the first cell of a future offspring, it contains 23 chromosomes from the father and 23 chromosomes from the mother.

■ Case Study Answers

1. What are the major organs of the female reproductive system?

   Answer: The two ovaries are located one on each side of the lower abdominal quadrants and are suspended by a peritoneal fold and two ligaments. The fallopian tubes are hollow tubes that serve as a passage for movement of the ovum and sperm and often are the location of fertilization. The uterus is a pear-shaped organ located in the midline of the lower abdomen. It is held in place by several ligaments and allows the implantation, growth, and nourishment of a fetus during pregnancy. The vagina is a muscular tube that forms the lower part of the female reproductive tract and is the organ of copulation. Mammary glands are the organs of milk production and are supported by a group of mammary ligaments.

2. What are the layers of the uterine wall, including the functional wall?

   Answer: The uterine wall consists of three layers. From the outside to the inside are the perimetrium, myometrium, and endometrium. The endometrium has two layers; the deep layer is connected to the myometrium and the functional layer lines the cavity. During the menstrual cycle, the functional layer undergoes menstrual changes and sloughing.

3. What is the embryonic period of gestation and why is it a critical time?

Answer: The embryonic period includes weeks 3 to 8 of gestation. During this time, all major organ systems begin to develop. The embryonic period is a time of high susceptibility to drugs, alcohol, viruses, or external substances that may cause birth defects before the pregnancy is realized.

4. In genetics, how is the gender of a fetus determined?

Answer: Sex chromosomes code for proteins that determine sex. A zygote with two X chromosomes (XX) develops into a female embryo. A zygote with an X and a Y chromosome (XY) develops into a male embryo.

5. What are two major circulation changes that occur in the infant at birth?

Answer: Circulation through the lungs of the infant begins with the first breath and closure (at least partially) of the foramen ovale and ductus arteriosus occurs.

6. At this point, what stage of labor is occurring?

Answer: The patient has completed the second stage of labor with the delivery of the newborn and is about to begin the third stage, which is delivery of the placenta. The first stage of labor involves contractions of the uterine wall and dilation of the cervix.

7. In reference to genetic diseases, what is the "carrier state?"

Answer: In some autosomal-recessive conditions, a person with one abnormal allele may not be affected; however, the person is a carrier and may pass the disease on to offspring if he or she mates with another carrier.

Special Sensory Systems

Learning Objectives

1. Explain the general purposes of sensations. (p 283)
2. Name the parts of the sensory pathway and the general functions of each part. (p 283-292)
3. Describe the characteristics of sensations. (p 283-292)
4. Name the parts of the eye and explain their function in sight. (p 283-285)

5. Describe the pathways for the senses of smell and taste and explain how these senses are interrelated. (p 285-286, 290-291)
6. Name the parts of the ear and explain their function in hearing. (p 286-289)
7. Describe the physiology of balance, or equilibrium. (p 288-290)
8. Explain referred pain and its importance to out of hospital care. (p 292)

Introduction

The special sensory systems of the body consist of special nerve receptors that perceive light, sound, taste, odors, position, and sensations from the skin or areas outside of the body. Although the specific mechanisms of each system are different, they all share a common principle. Sensations are detected by receptors, which then convert them into nerve signals. These signals return to the brain either directly via one of the cranial nerves or indirectly via the spinal cord. After being processed in the brain, the signals can be consciously appreciated.

Vision

The eyes are the organs of sight, and work along with accessory organs, including the eyelids, lacrimal apparatus, and extrinsic muscles. All of these organs are housed within the orbital cavity (or orbit) of the skull. Each orbit also contains blood vessels, fat, connective tissues, and nerves. Each eyelid has skin, muscle, connective tissue, and conjunctiva layers. The eyelid is the thinnest portion of skin on the body, covering the lid's outer surface while being fused to its inner lining near the margin of the lid. The eyelids are moved by the orbicularis oculi muscle, and the levator palpebrae superioris muscle.

The lacrimal apparatus contains the lacrimal gland, which secretes tears. It also has a series of ducts carrying tears into the nasal cavity Figure 14-1. Tears are actually secreted continuously, exiting through tubules flowing downward and medially across the eye. Tears produced in the lacrimal gland drain through the punctum lacrimale, a small opening at the corner of each eye, into lacrimal ducts. The tears flow into the lacrimal sac and then into the nasolacrimal duct, emptying into the nasal cavity.

The six extrinsic muscles move the eye in many directions, with each muscle associated with one primary action. The extrinsic muscles are shown in Figure 14-2.

The eye is globe shaped, approximately 1 inch in diameter, and fits within the orbit Figure 14-3. In an adult, more than 80% of the eyeball is protected within this bony orbit. The orbit is composed of the adjacent bones of the face and skull and forms the base of the floor of the cranial cavity. The frontal lobes of the brain are directly above the orbit. Between and below the orbits are the nasal bones and the sinuses, respectively.

The eyeball, or globe, keeps its global shape as a result of the pressure of the fluid contained within its two chambers,

Case Study | PART 1

At 12:00 PM, your unit is dispatched to an auto body shop for a possible burn injury in which the patient is in extreme pain. Two men meet you as you pull up outside the shop and quickly explain that they were working on a personal project during their lunch break when one of their coworkers started to scream in pain. He had attempted to operate an arc welder without the proper protective equipment and may have flash burned his eyes.

You determine that the scene is safe, and as you hurry into the shop and approach the patient, you note that he is screaming and appears to be in a tremendous amount of pain. You begin your primary assessment and determine that the patient is alert, has an open airway, and is breathing adequately. He has no obvious external or internal bleeding. His skin is red, possibly from the exposure to the light, but the condition of the skin is normal. The patient is sitting near the welding unit, and he tells you that he did not use the face shield. The patient then cries out, "Please help me.... I can't see!"

Recording Time: 0 Minutes	
Appearance	Male with flushed skin
Level of consciousness	Alert (oriented to person, place, and day)
Airway	Appears patent
Breathing	Regular
Circulation	Strong, rapid, regular pulse, no obvious bleeding

1. What parts of the eye may be immediately affected by this type of injury?

2. How do the eyes perceive light?

the anterior chamber and the posterior chamber. The clear, jellylike fluid near the back of the eye is called the vitreous humor. If the globe is ruptured and the vitreous humor leaks out, it cannot be replaced or replenished. In front of the lens is a clear fluid called the aqueous humor. If the aqueous humor is lost through a penetrating injury to the eye, it will gradually be replenished.

A delicate transparent membrane, the conjunctiva, covers the inner surface of the eyelids and the outer surface of the sclera, but not the iris. These surfaces are kept moist by fluid produced by the lacrimal glands. Humans blink unconsciously many times per minute. This action sweeps fluid from the lacrimal glands over the surface of the eye, cleaning it. The white of the eye, the sclera, extends over

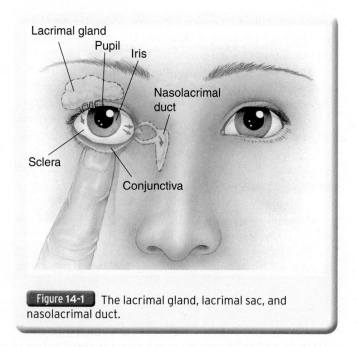

Figure 14-1   The lacrimal gland, lacrimal sac, and nasolacrimal duct.

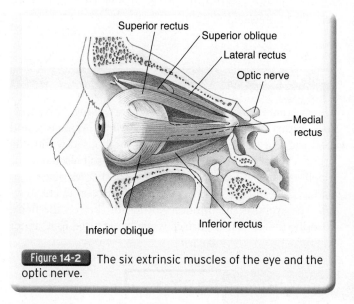

Figure 14-2   The six extrinsic muscles of the eye and the optic nerve.

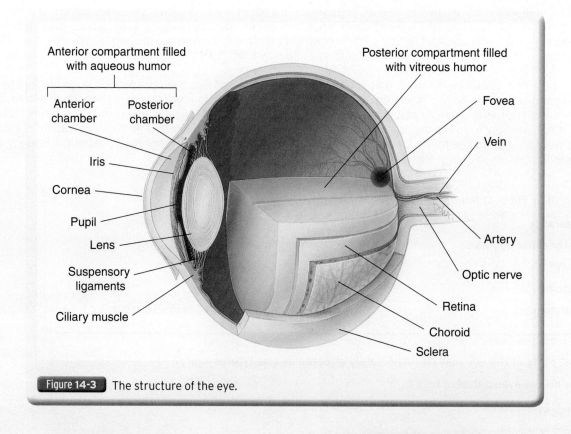

Figure 14-3   The structure of the eye.

the surface of the globe. This extremely tough, fibrous tissue helps maintain the eye's globular shape and protects the more delicate inner structures. On the front of the eye, the sclera is replaced by a clear, transparent membrane called the cornea that allows light to enter the eye. A circular muscle lies behind the cornea with an opening in its center. Like the shutter in a camera, this muscle adjusts the size of the opening to regulate the amount of light that enters the eye. This circular sphincter muscle and surrounding tissue together are called the iris. The iris is pigmented, giving the eye its characteristic brown, green, or blue color.

The opening in the center of the iris, which allows light to move to the back of the eye, is called the pupil. Normally, the pupil appears black. Like the opening in a camera, the pupil becomes smaller in bright light and larger in dim light. The pupil also becomes smaller and larger when the person is looking at objects near at hand and farther away; these adjustments occur almost instantaneously. Normally, the pupils in both eyes are equal in size. Some people are born with pupils that are not equal; however, in unconscious patients, unequal pupil size may indicate serious injury or illness to the brain or eye.

Behind the iris is the lens. Between the iris and the lens is the posterior chamber. Like the lens of a camera, this lens focuses images on the light-sensitive area at the back of the globe, called the retina. Think of the retina as the film in the camera. Within the retina are numerous nerve endings, which respond to light by transmitting nerve impulses through the optic nerve that passes through the optic foramen into the brain. In the brain, the impulses are interpreted as vision.

Light rays enter the eyes through the pupil and are focused by the lens. The image formed by the lens is cast on the retina, where sensitive nerve fibers that form the optic nerve are located. The optic nerve transmits the image to the brain, where it is converted into conscious images in the visual cortex.

Pathophysiology

Cataracts occur when opacities develop in the lens of the eye, obscuring vision. If the cataract is severe enough, the lens may be removed surgically and replaced with an artificial lens.

Pathophysiology

A patient's cornea may be damaged by trauma or infection, such as from a herpes virus. A cornea transplant is one of the oldest and most successful transplant procedures performed. If a patient's vision is severely impaired, an ophthalmologist may replace the injured cornea with a cornea from a cadaver donor. EMS providers sometimes are required to determine whether a dead patient is a potential organ donor.

Pathophysiology

Perforating injuries of the globe can threaten the patient's vision. You should assume a perforating injury of the globe is present based on the history of the incident or if a jelly-like material is seen in the vicinity of the eye, regardless of whether the patient has an obvious wound.

Pathophysiology

Blockage of the lacrimal duct can be caused by a foreign body, congenital defect, or infection and results in painful swelling of the eyelids and upper part of the face. Although this condition may be uncomfortable, it usually is not a threat to vision.

Pathophysiology

Conjunctivitis (pink eye) is an inflammation of the conjunctivae **Figure 14-4**. It usually is caused by bacteria, viruses, or allergies and is often highly contagious. You should always use appropriate personal protection equipment when treating or coming into contact with a patient who has possible conjunctivitis.

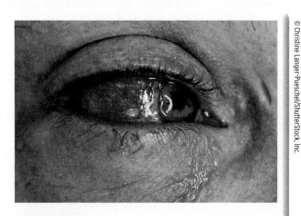

© Christine Langer-Pueschel/ShutterStock, Inc.

Figure 14-4 Conjunctivitis.

■ Taste

Taste buds, or taste receptors, in the mouth and tongue are responsible for gustation, the sense of taste. The taste buds number more than 10,000. Most are found on the surface of the tongue, with tiny elevations called papillae **Figure 14-5**.

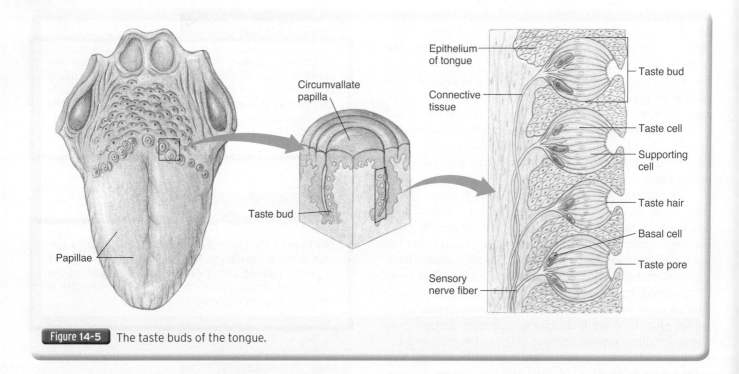

Figure 14-5   The taste buds of the tongue.

In addition, about 1,000 taste buds are found in the roof of the mouth and the throat walls. Each taste bud has up to 150 taste cells (gustatory cells), which are replaced every 3 days. The spherical taste buds have openings called taste pores, and tiny projections called taste hairs. The taste hairs are the sensitive parts of the taste receptor cells. Stimulation triggers an impulse on a nearby nerve fiber, traveling to the brain.

Chemicals must dissolve in the saliva before they can be tasted. Although taste cells in taste buds are similar in appearance, there are five types:

- Those that sense sweetness (such as sugar)
- Those that sense sourness (such as lemons)
- Those that sense saltiness (such as table salt)
- Those that sense bitterness (such as caffeine)
- Those that sense umami or deliciousness (responding to specific amino acids and related chemicals such as monosodium glutamate [MSG])

Other sensations that may be sensed are alkaline and metallic sensations.

Flavors are tasted because of combinations of the primary sensations. The sense of smell also influences the flavors that are tasted. Though taste cells are spread over the tongue, they are, in general, concentrated in the following areas of the tongue:

- Tip of the tongue: Sweetness
- Sides of the tongue: Sourness
- Front and sides: Saltiness
- Back of the tongue: Bitterness and umami (savory and pleasant)

Taste sensations, like smell sensations, also adapt rapidly. Sensory impulses from the tongue travel to the medulla oblongata via the facial, glossopharyngeal, and vagus nerves. They then move to the thalamus and gustatory cortex (located in the parietal lobe of the cerebrum) where they are converted into sensations that can be perceived. The taste buds sense salt and sweet individually.

Hearing, Position, and Balance

Hearing

The ear is divided into outer (external), middle, and inner parts Figure 14-6 . The external ear consists of the pinna, the ear canal (external auditory canal), and the exterior portion of the tympanic membrane, or eardrum. The middle ear consists of the inner portion of the tympanic membrane and the ossicles. The inner ear consists of the cochlea and semicircular canals.

The large outside portion of the ear, the auricle (pinna) traps sound waves. Waves of sound pass through the external auditory canal (ear canal), hitting the tympanic membrane (eardrum). Vibrations are transmitted to the ossicles, three small bones on the inner side of the tympanic membrane. Vibrations then pass to the cochlear duct through the oval window. Movement of the oval window causes fluid within the cochlea, the shell-shaped structure in the inner ear that contains the organ of Corti, to vibrate. At the organ of Corti, vibration stimulates hair movements that form nerve impulses that travel to the brain via the auditory nerve. The brain then converts these impulses into sound Figure 14-7 .

Case Study | PART 2

You reassure the patient that you and your partner will do everything you can to help him. As you question the patient about the accident, your partner obtains the patient's vital signs. The patient tells you that he did not fall to the ground nor did he have a period of altered level of consciousness. You decide to proceed with a secondary assessment, including the focused history and physical exam of this patient.

The patient is a 22-year-old man who weighs 90 kg. His SAMPLE patient history reveals:

- **S**igns and symptoms: Extreme pain in his eyes
- **A**llergies to medications: Penicillin and sulfa drugs
- **M**edications taken: No prescribed or over-the-counter medications, but the patient often uses recreational drugs
- **P**ast pertinent medical history: The patient has a history of a fractured tibia from a skiing accident last winter.
- **L**ast food/fluid intake: Breakfast
- **E**vents prior to onset: The patient was rushing to do a personal project with the auto body shop's equipment during his lunch hour.

His OPQRST patient history reveals:

- **O**nset of symptoms: Very sudden
- **P**rovoking/palliative factors: The patient failed to put on a protective face shield while using the arc welder.
- **Q**uality of discomfort: The patient describes a sharp, burning pain in his eyes.
- **R**adiating/related signs/symptoms/relief: The patient states that the pain is in his eyes and the skin around his eyes and that his vision is very blurry.
- **S**everity of complaint: On a scale of 1 to 10, with 10 being the worst pain he has ever experienced, the patient says the pain is a 10.
- **T**ime: The pain began at the time of the accident, about 20 minutes ago.

Recording Time: 5 Minutes	
Appearance	Nervous and in a lot of pain
Level of consciousness	Alert (oriented to person, place, and day)
Airway	Open and clear
Breathing	Normal rate and depth
Circulation	Strong and rapid pulse with no obvious bleeding. There are superficial burns to the face and neck, warm and moist skin
Pulse	96 beats/min, strong and regular
Blood pressure	140/80 mm Hg
Respirations	20 breaths/min, regular
Pupils	Equal and reactive to ambient light
Spo$_2$	99%

3. Describe the location of the optic nerves.

4. How are tears produced?

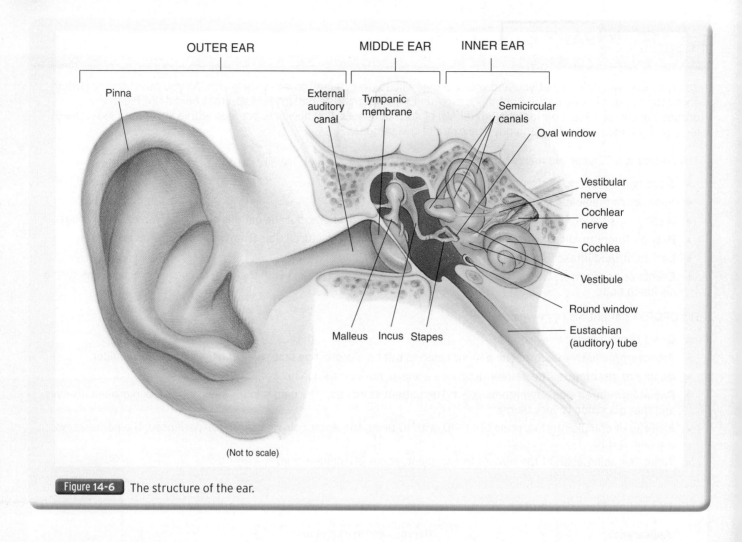

OUTER EAR   MIDDLE EAR   INNER EAR

Pinna

External auditory canal

Tympanic membrane

Semicircular canals

Oval window

Vestibular nerve

Cochlear nerve

Cochlea

Vestibule

Round window

Eustachian (auditory) tube

Malleus   Incus   Stapes

(Not to scale)

Figure 14-6   The structure of the ear.

Position and Balance

The sensation of balance involves two different mechanisms: the kinetic labyrinth system and the static labyrinth system. The kinetic labyrinth system senses movements of the head. The system consists of three semicircular canals in the bony labyrinth of the ear, each at right angles to the other. Movements of the head cause the endolymph, the fluid inside each canal, to stimulate hairs lying on the cupula, a cap of gelatinous tissue in the crista, a small rise in each canal. The head and the endolymph move at different rates. Thus, the brain senses the differences between movements of the cupula, indicating head movement, and movements of the endolymph.

The static labyrinth system senses the position of the head relative to gravity or linear acceleration/deceleration. Two membranous pouches in the membranous labyrinth of the ear, the utricle and the saccule, contain a specialized patch of tissue, the macula. Hair cells of the macula lay below the otolithic membrane, a gelatinous mass of protein and otolith, small particles of calcium carbonate. This mass moves in response to gravity, acceleration, or

deceleration. The hairs of the macula bend, stimulating the nerve. The stimulus is converted in the brain to a sensation of motion.

The special sensory receptors for equilibrium are the utricle, saccule, macula, and cristae in the semicircular ducts. There are two kinds of equilibrium, dynamic equilibrium and static equilibrium. In dynamic equilibrium, when the head and body move or rotate, the motion is detected, aiding in balance. The organs of dynamic equilibrium are the three semicircular canals in the labyrinth. Inside these canals is a swelling near the end called an ampulla, housing the sensory organs of the semicircular canals. Each of these organs is called a crista ampullaris, containing sensory hair cells extending upward into a gelatinous mass (the cupula). **Figure 14-8** shows the crista ampullaris within the ampulla.

When the head or body turns rapidly, the hair cells of the crista ampullaris are stimulated, but the endolymph inside the canals remains stationary. The hair cells within the cupula are bent, sending signals to the brain. The cerebellum can predict consequences of rapid

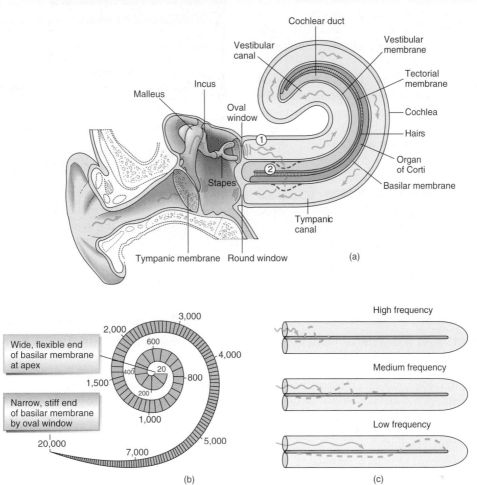

The numbers indicate the frequencies with which different regions of the basilar membrane maximally vibrate.

Figure 14-7 The transmission of sound waves through the cochlea.

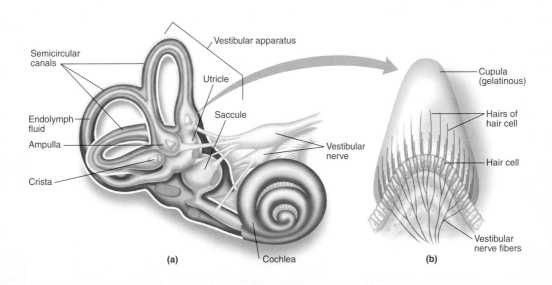

Figure 14-8 The crista ampullaris is located within the ampulla of each semicircular canal.

body movements and trigger the skeletal muscles to maintain balance. Additionally, mechanoreceptors associated with the neck joints communicate with the brain about position changes, and the eyes assist in maintaining balance.

In static equilibrium, the position of the head is sensed while the head and body are still, maintaining stability. When the head is upright, the hairs project upward into the gelatinous material. When the head bends forward, backward, or to one side, the hairs bend to signal nerve fibers. Nerve impulses travel into the central nervous system via the vestibulocochlear nerve, and the brain controls the skeletal muscles to maintain balance. **Figure 14-9** shows how the maculae respond to changes in head position.

Pathophysiology

Numerous conditions, including ear problems, may result in vertigo (the sensation of spinning) or in dizziness. It is nearly impossible to differentiate the cause of the discomfort, especially in the field, without sophisticated medical tests.

Smell

Olfactory receptor cells line the upper posterior region of the nose. These cells are the first to detect odor. The sense of smell works closely with the sense of taste. Odorant molecules

Case Study PART 3

You cover the patient's eyes with a sterile, moist dressing and pad. You then bring the stretcher to the patient's side and have him lie down on the stretcher for the 20-minute ride to the hospital.

En route to the hospital, you conduct a reassessment and apply oxygen via a nonrebreathing mask. You also contact medical control for an order to administer analgesia. Medical control orders morphine to help alleviate the patient's intense pain.

During the reassessment, you find:

    Head: Superficial burns to the face, no blisters

    Neck: Superficial burns

    Chest: No scars, patches or a medical alert chain or bracelet

    Lung sounds: Clear in all fields (unremarkable)

    Upper extremities: Unremarkable

    Lower extremities: Unremarkable

Recording Time: 10 Minutes	
Appearance	Still in obvious pain and anxious about eyes being covered
Level of consciousness	Alert (oriented to person, place, and day) but very frightened
Airway	Open and patent
Breathing	Normal rate and depth
Circulation	Strong, rapid pulse and no obvious bleeding
Pulse	90 beats/min, strong and regular
Blood pressure	132/74 mm Hg
Respirations	20 breaths/min, regular
Spo_2	99%

5. **What are the two types of fluid found within the globe and how might this type of injury affect them?**

6. **Would the use of analgesia be appropriate for this patient?**

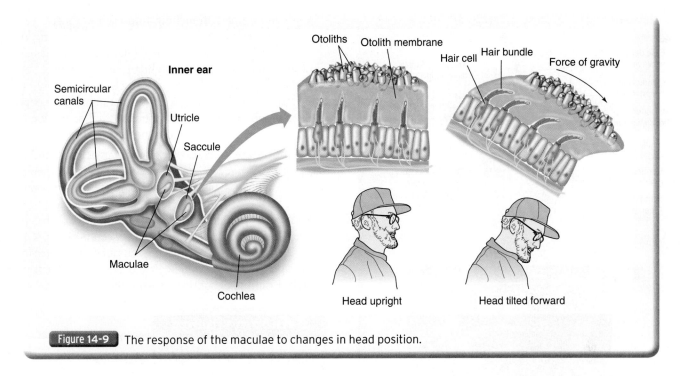

Figure 14-9 The response of the maculae to changes in head position.

stimulate varieties of olfactory recep- tor proteins to differentiate between odors. These molecules must partially condensate from gases to fluids before receptors can detect them. From here, axons of the olfactory receptor cells pass through the cribriform plate to the olfactory bulbs. These bulbs ana- lyze odor impulses, which are trans- mitted along the olfactory tracts to the limbic system **Figure 14-10**. Most smells are interpreted in the olfactory cortex of the temporal lobes of the brain, and at the lower frontal lobes, in front of the hypothalamus.

Olfactory stimulation occurs as biochemical pathways are activated, allowing an influx of sodium ions, triggering an action potential. There are several hundred types of olfactory receptor cells. They can bind to several types of odorant molecules, and vice versa. Because the olfactory organs are high up in the nasal cavity, faint odors may be difficult to perceive. The sense of smell is more intense with a new odor at first, fading over time.

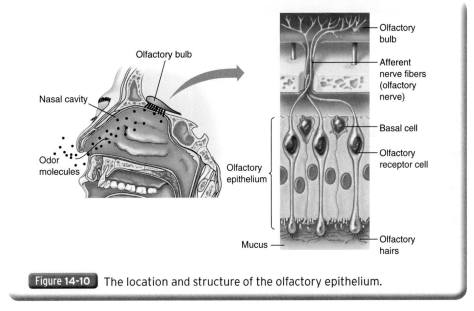

Figure 14-10 The location and structure of the olfactory epithelium.

Pathophysiology

The senses of smell and taste complement each other. The ability to taste is limited severely when the nasal passages are blocked or olfaction is otherwise impaired.

■ Touch

The skin's touch receptors sense pressure, pain, and tempera- ture. Afferent peripheral nerves transmit these impulses to the spinal cord, and then to the brain. At this point, the person becomes consciously aware of the sensation on the skin.

Touch and pressure senses are derived from the follow- ing three types of receptors **Figure 14-11**:

- Free nerve endings. Common in epithelial tissues with free ends extending between epithelial cells; they con- trol the sensation of itching.
- Meissner (tactile) corpuscles. Oval, yet flattened con- nective tissue cells inside connective sheaths, with two

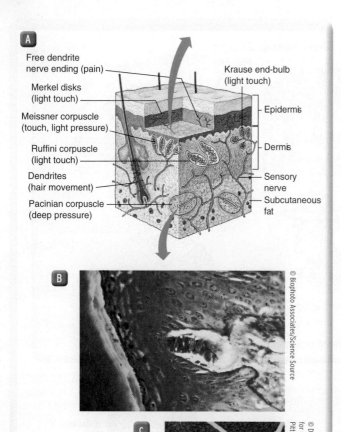

A.

Free dendrite
nerve ending (pain)

Merkel disks
(light touch)

Meissner corpuscle
(touch, light pressure)

Ruffini corpuscle
(light touch)

Dendrites
(hair movement)

Pacinian corpuscle
(deep pressure)

Krause end-bulb
(light touch)

Epidermis

Dermis

Sensory
nerve

Subcutaneous
fat

© Biophoto Associates/Science Source

B.

© Donna Beer Stolz, Ph.D., Center
for Biologic Imaging, University of
Pittsburgh Medical School

C.

Pacinian corpuscle

Figure 14-11 Touch and pressure senses are derived from different receptors in the skin. **A.** The position of various receptors in tissue layers. **B.** Meissner corpuscle. **C.** Pacinian corpuscle.

or more fibers branching into each corpuscle to end in small knobs; located in hairless skin (fingertips, lips, palms, soles, external genitalia, and nipples), they respond to objects that lightly touch the skin.

- Pacinian (lamellated) corpuscles. Relatively large structures of connective tissue, common in deeper dermal and subcutaneous tissues as well as tendons and ligaments; they respond to heavy pressure.

Temperature is sensed via warm receptors and cold receptors. Warm receptors are most sensitive to temperatures above 77°F (25°C), becoming unresponsive to temperatures above 113°F (45°C). At this temperature, pain receptors are stimulated to produce a burning sensation. Cold receptors are most sensitive to temperatures between 50°F (10°C) and 68°F (20°C) to produce a freezing sensation. These receptors work rapidly and sensation begins to fade away after approximately 1 minute of continuous stimulation.

Pathophysiology

Certain conditions result in excess skin sensitivity, especially to touch or to cold. The general term for this phenomenon is <u>hyperesthesia</u>.

Referred Pain

Referred pain is pain that may seem to be coming from a different area of the body than the one actually being stimulated. Heart pain, for example, may appear to be occurring in the shoulder or upper left arm. Embryonic development explains this type of referred pain. The heart originates in the neck, as do the arms, resulting in embryologic nerve distribution patterns in which the heart and arms receive pain nerve fibers from the same spinal cord segments. Because of this, the location of the pain does not always indicate the cause of distress.

Case Study **PART 4**

You administer the morphine and try to keep the patient calm by asking him questions about his family. The patient asks you, "Will I lose my eyesight?" You distinctly remember your EMS instructor saying, "Don't make promises you cannot keep." So you tell him the injury is serious and will require an examination by an eye specialist to determine if there is any long-term damage.

Prep Kit

Chapter Summary

- The special sensory systems of the body consist of nerve receptors that perceive light, sound, taste, odors, and sensations from the skin or areas outside of the body.

- The eyes lie within the bony orbits and are held in place by loose connective tissue and several muscles.

- The optic nerve enters the globe posteriorly, through the optic foramen.

- The parts of the eye include the globe, sclera, iris, pupil, lens, cornea, anterior chamber, aqueous humor, posterior chamber, conjunctiva, vitreous humor, and retina.

- Tears are produced in the lacrimal gland, and then drain through the punctum lacrimale into the lacrimal ducts, into the lacrimal sacs, and through the nasolacrimal ducts.

- The retina is a delicate, 10-layered structure of nervous tissue that receives light impulses, which generate nerve signals that are conducted to the brain.

- The mouth and tongue contain taste receptors, which sense salt and sweet sensations separately.

- The five primary taste types are sweetness, sourness, saltiness, bitterness, and umami, or deliciousness.

- The ear is divided into the outer (external), middle, and inner parts.

- Sound waves enter the ear through the auricle and travel through the external auditory canal to the tympanic membrane, where the vibration against the membrane sets up vibrations in the ossicles.

- The vibrations of the ossicles are transmitted to the cochlear duct at the oval window, causing fluid within the cochlea to vibrate. Vibration stimulates hairs at the organ of Corti, forming nerve impulses that travel to the brain via the auditory nerve.

- The sensation of balance consists of static equilibrium and dynamic equilibrium.

- In static equilibrium, the position of the head is sensed while the head and body are still, maintaining stability.

- In dynamic equilibrium, when the head and body move or rotate, the motion is detected, aiding in balance.

- Sensations of smell are detected by olfactory receptor cells lining the nasal cavity, where they then pass through the cribriform plate to the olfactory bulb.

From the olfactory bulb, odor impulses travel along the olfactory tract to the olfactory cortex of the brain.

- The special sense of touch is interrelated with the function of the peripheral nervous system. Receptors on the skin detect when something is touched.

Vital Vocabulary

ampulla An expansion at the end of each semicircular canal containing a crista ampullaris.

anterior chamber The anterior area of the globe between the lens and the cornea that is filled with aqueous humor.

aqueous humor The clear, watery fluid in the anterior chamber of the globe.

auricle The large outside portion of the ear through which sound waves enter the ear; also called the pinna.

cataracts Clouding in the lens of the eye or its surrounding transparent membrane; normally a result of aging.

cochlea The shell-shaped structure within the inner ear that contains the organ of Corti.

cochlear duct A canal within the cochlea that receives vibrations from the ossicles.

conjunctiva A thin, transparent membrane that covers the sclera and internal surfaces of the eyelids.

conjunctivitis An inflammation of the conjunctivae that usually is caused by bacteria, viruses, or allergies and should be considered highly contagious; also called pink eye.

cornea The transparent anterior portion of the eye that overlies the iris and pupil.

crista A small elevation in each ear canal.

crista ampullaris The sensory organ in a semicircular canal that aids with dynamic equilibrium.

cupula A cap of gelatinous tissue in the ear that is involved in the sensation of balance and movement.

dynamic equilibrium Maintenance of balance when the head and body are suddenly moved or rotated.

ear canal The cavity leading from the exterior atmosphere to the tympanum; also called the external auditory canal.

eardrum A thin membrane that separates the middle ear from the inner ear and transmits vibrations to the ossicles; also called the tympanic membrane.

endolymph Fluid in the membranous labyrinth of the ear.

external auditory canal The area in which sound waves are received from the auricle before they travel on to the eardrum; also called the ear canal.

external ear One of three anatomic parts of the ear; it contains the pinna, the ear canal, and the exterior portion of the tympanic membrane.

extrinsic muscles Muscles that do not originate in the body part to which they insert.

eyelid Thin fold of skin that covers and protects the eye.

eyes The organs of sight.

globe The eyeball.

gustation The sense of taste.

hyperesthesia Any of several conditions that result in excess skin sensitivity, especially to touch or to cold.

inner ear One of three anatomic parts of the ear; it consists of the cochlea and semicircular canals.

iris The sphincter muscle and surrounding tissue behind the cornea that dilate and constrict the pupil, regulating the amount of light that enters the eye; pigment in this tissue gives the eye its color.

kinetic labyrinth system One of two mechanisms involved in the sensation of position, balance, and movement, it senses movements of the head.

lacrimal apparatus The structures in which tears are secreted and drained from the eye.

lacrimal ducts Ducts located on the nasal border of the eyelids through which tears from the lacrimal sacs pass.

lacrimal gland The structure in which tears are produced.

lacrimal sac Sac in the eye into which tears are drained from the lacrimal glands.

lens The transparent part of the eye through which images are focused on the retina.

macula Specialized patches of tissue within the utricle and saccule that aid in the sensation of motion.

middle ear One of three anatomic parts of the ear; it consists of the inner portion of the tympanic membrane and the ossicles.

nasolacrimal duct The passage through which tears drain from the lacrimal sacs into the nasal cavity.

olfactory bulbs Structures in the forebrain that are needed to perceive odors; the cranial nerve for smell.

olfactory cortex The area in the brain that receives odor impulses and perceives them as smell.

olfactory tracts Passageways for odor impulses to travel from the olfactory bulb to the olfactory cortex.

optic foramen The opening in the bony orbit behind the eyeball through which the optic nerve passes to the eyeball.

optic nerve Either of the second cranial nerves that enter the eyeball posteriorly, through the optic foramen.

orbit The bony cavity that contains the eyeball and its associated muscles, vessels, and nerves.

organ of Corti The organ that is the primary receptor for sound, and is made up of thousands of individual cilia, each with their own associated nerve.

ossicles The three small bones in the inner ear that transmit vibrations to the cochlear duct at the oval window.

otolith Small calcium carbonate stones within the gelatinous protein of the otolithic membrane of the inner ear that aid in the sensation of motion.

otolithic membrane A membrane within the inner ear that contains otolith and aids in the sensation of motion.

oval window An oval opening between the middle ear and the vestibule.

pinna The large outside portion of the ear through which sound waves enter the ear; also called the auricle.

posterior chamber The posterior area of the globe between the lens and the iris.

punctum lacrimale Small opening in the corner of the eye through which tears drain from the lacrimal gland into the lacrimal ducts.

pupil The circular opening in the center of the eye, through which light passes to the lens.

retina A delicate, 10-layered structure of nervous tissue located in the rear of the interior of the globe that receives light and generates nerve signals that are transmitted to the brain through the optic nerve.

saccule An enlarged region of the membranous labyrinth of the inner ear that contains a specialized patch of tissue that aids in the sensation of position and motion.

sclera The white part of the eye.

static equilibrium The maintenance of balance when the head and body are motionless.

static labyrinth system One of two mechanisms involved in the sensation of balance and movement, it evaluates the position of the head relative to gravity or linear acceleration/deceleration.

taste buds Receptors in the tongue and mouth that sense salt and sweet sensations separately; also called taste receptors.

taste hairs Hair-like projections of the gustatory cells of the taste buds.

taste receptors Receptors in the tongue and mouth that sense salt and sweet sensations separately; also called taste buds.

touch receptors Receptors located in various areas of the skin to detect the sense of touch.

tympanic membrane A thin membrane that separates the middle ear from the inner ear and transmits vibrations to the ossicles; also called the eardrum.

utricle An enlarged portion of the labyrinth of the inner ear that contains a specialized patch of tissue that aids in the sensation of position and motion.

vestibule The central part of the labyrinth, behind the cochlea and in front of the semicircular canals.

visual cortex The area in the brain where signals from the optic nerve are converted into visual images.

vitreous humor A jelly-like substance found in the posterior compartment of the eye between the lens and the retina.

■ Case Study Answers

1. What parts of the eye may be immediately affected by this type of injury?

Answer: The extent of injury will vary greatly, depending on whether the eyelids were partially or completely closed at the time of the burn. Closed eyelids may have helped protect the outer membranes (the conjunctiva and cornea) of the eyeball from the heat and flash of the arc welder. If the eyelids were open, the conjunctiva, cornea, sclera, iris, and pupils may have been directly affected. In this patient, the retina, which receives light and generates nerve signals to the brain, is likely to be the area of the eye injured and the immediate cause of the loss of vision.

2. How do the eyes perceive light?

Answer: The cornea, which is the membrane that covers the iris and pupil, admits light rays through the pupil. The lens focuses the light rays, which are then cast into the back of the globe onto the retina (a 10-layered structure of nervous tissue continuous with the optic nerve), where nerve signals are generated and conducted to the brain via the optic nerve.

3. Describe the location of the optic nerves.

Answer: The optic nerves are the second set of the twelve pairs of cranial nerves. From the midbrain, the optic nerve passes through an opening called the optic foramen and enters the back of the globe.

4. How are tears produced?

Answer: Tears are produced in the lacrimal gland. From the lacrimal gland, tears drain through the punctum lacrimale into the lacrimal ducts, into the lacrimal sacs, and through the nasolacrimal ducts.

5. What are the two types of fluid found within the globe and how might this type of injury affect them?

Answer: Aqueous humor is a watery fluid that fills the anterior portion of the globe between the cornea and the lens. Vitreous humor is a clear jelly-like material that fills the posterior portion of the globe behind the lens. It is unlikely that either of these fluids will be affected by this type of injury. Penetrating injuries are the type of injuries that directly affect the fluid within the eyes.

6. Would the use of analgesia be appropriate for this patient?

Answer: Burns in any location can be extremely painful, and eye injuries are especially painful. In addition to the pain, the patient is probably extremely anxious about the prospect of a permanent loss of vision. Analgesia is definitely indicated for the care of this patient. His mental status is good, he experienced no loss of consciousness or other associated traumatic injury, and he has no underlying illness that would contraindicate the use of analgesia. Analgesia such as morphine would help to reduce the pain and anxiety associated with this type of injury.

Learning Objectives

1. Define nutrition. (p 297)
2. Describe the two groups of nutrients. (p 297)
3. Define kilocalories. (p 297)
4. Describe the metabolic roles of fats, glucose, and proteins. (p 298-299, 301)
5. Describe the functions of catabolism and anabolism. (p 300-301)
6. State what the products of cellular respiration are and how the body disposes of them. (p 302-306)

7. State the different ways heat is generated and lost in the body. (p 306)
8. State the normal range of body temperature. (p 306)
9. State why the hypothalamus is the thermostat of the body. (p 306)
10. Describe the fluid compartments and the name for the water in each. (p 306-307)
11. Explain how fluid moves between the compartments. (p 306-307)
12. Explain how fluid is taken in by the body and exits the body. (p 306-307)

Introduction

Typical meals contain carbohydrates, lipids, proteins, water, electrolytes, and vitamins. The digestive system handles each of these components differently. Digestion involves breaking down large organic molecules before absorption can occur. Water, electrolytes, and vitamins can be absorbed without preliminary breakdown, but may require special transport mechanisms. Discussion of the various types of nutrients is essential in understanding their actions within the digestive system.

The study of nutrients and how the body uses them is known as nutrition. Nutrients include carbohydrates, lipids, proteins, vitamins, minerals, and water. They are grouped as follows:

- **Macronutrients.** Those required in large amounts (carbohydrates, lipids, and proteins); they provide energy and have other specific functions. Potential energy is expressed in calories (units of heat).

- **Micronutrients.** Those required in much smaller amounts (vitamins and minerals); they do not directly provide energy, but allow biochemical reactions that extract energy from macronutrients.

Digestion and Absorption of Nutrients

A calorie is the amount of heat needed to raise the temperature of a gram of water by 1°C. The calorie used to measure food energy is greater, by 1,000 times. The term *calorie* when used to measure food energy is equivalent to 1,000 actual calories. Though referred to commonly as a calorie, it is actually a kilocalorie of energy.

Cellular oxidation causes the following calorie releases:

- 1 gram of carbohydrate yields about 4 calories.
- 1 gram of protein yields about 4 calories.
- 1 gram of fat yields about 9 calories.

Case Study | PART 1

At 8:30 PM, your unit is dispatched to a local assisted-living group home where you often respond to EMS calls. A staff member meets you at the door with a police officer. Apparently an elderly resident could not be located for most of the afternoon. When he did not arrive for dinner, the police were contacted to assist in locating the resident. After a search of the premises, the resident was found sitting on a bench behind the building. The temperature outside was 28°F, and the man was not wearing a coat, hat, or gloves, and he appeared to be confused. The patient was moved inside the building and covered with a blanket.

The scene is determined to be safe and you have taken the appropriate standard precautions so you begin the primary assessment. The patient's mental status is verbal and he knows his name but is confused about the day of the week and his exact location. His airway is open and clear and his breathing is slow and shallow. Your partner sets up a nonrebreathing mask while you assess the patient's circulation. There is no external life-threatening bleeding, he has a slow radial pulse, and his skin is cold, pale, and dry.

You ask your partner to retrieve the thermometer to check the patient's temperature because he is cold to the touch. In the meantime you consider other causes of an altered mental status. The plan of action is to obtain a baseline set of vital signs and check his blood glucose level. You also need to do a secondary assessment as well as obtain his medical history.

Recording Time: 0 Minutes	
Appearance	Looking pale and acting confused
Level of consciousness	Verbal (oriented to person, confused about the place and day)
Airway	Appears patent
Breathing	Slow and shallow
Circulation	No external bleeding; skin is cold, pale, and dry

1. What is the normal range of body temperature?

2. What structure is considered the thermostat of the body?

Digestion breaks down nutrients so they can be absorbed and transported via the bloodstream. Essential nutrients are those that human cells cannot synthesize (such as certain amino acids).

Carbohydrates include sugars and starches, and are organic compounds. Energy from carbohydrates mostly is used to power cellular processes. They are ingested in forms that include grains, vegetables, glycogen (from meats), disaccharides (from cane sugar, beet sugar, and molasses), and monosaccharides (from fruits and honey). Digestion breaks carbohydrates down into monosaccharides (which include fructose, galactose, and glucose) for easy absorption. Liver enzymes convert fructose and galactose into glucose, which is the form of carbohydrate most commonly oxidized for use as cellular fuel.

Cellulose is a complex carbohydrate not digestible by humans. It provides bulk (fiber, or roughage) that helps the muscular digestive system walls to push food through its tubes. Many cells get their energy by oxidizing fatty acids, though neurons require continuous glucose to survive. The central nervous system can be seriously injured by even short term lack of glucose. When carbohydrates are not consumed sufficiently, the liver may convert amino acids (from proteins) into glucose.

Some excess glucose is changed to glycogen, which is stored in the liver and muscles. Glucose can be rapidly mobilized from glycogen, but only a certain amount of glycogen can be stored. Excess glucose is usually converted into fat and stored in adipose tissue. For energy, the body first metabolizes glucose, then glycogen into glucose, and lastly, fats and proteins.

Carbohydrates are used by cells to synthesize vital biochemicals such as ribose and deoxyribose, which are needed to produce the nucleic acids RNA and DNA. They are also needed to synthesize the disaccharide lactose (milk sugar) during breast milk secretion. Physically active people need more fuel than less active people, but eating excess carbohydrates may cause obesity and increase the risk for cardiovascular disease. Carbohydrate intake differs for each person, but current estimates are that between 125 and 175 grams of carbohydrates should be consumed daily to avoid protein breakdown as well as metabolic disorders that result from the utilization of excess fat.

Lipids include fats, fat-like substances, and oils. They supply energy for body processes and building of certain structures. Lipids include fats, cholesterol, and phospholipids. The most common lipids found in the diet are fats known as triglycerides. They are found in both plant and animal-based foods. Saturated fats are found mostly in meats, eggs, milk, animal fat (lard), palm oil, and coconut oil. These fats, when consumed excessively, can increase the risk of cardiovascular disease. Unsaturated fats exist in nuts, seeds, and plant oils. Monounsaturated fats are found in olive, peanut, and canola oils, and they are the healthiest type of fats. Cholesterol is found in animal products, including liver, egg yolk, whole milk, butter, cheese, and meats. It is not present in foods of plant origin.

Lipids have many functions, but mostly they supply energy. Triglyceride molecules must first undergo hydrolysis (breakdown in the presence of water) before they can release energy. When this occurs, fatty acids and glycerol are released, absorbed, and transported in lymph and blood to the tissues. Some fatty acid portions react to form molecules of acetyl coenzyme A via reactions known as beta oxidation. Excess amounts of this coenzyme convert into ketone bodies such as acetone, and can be reconverted as needed.

Certain fatty acids cannot be synthesized by the liver. These are known as essential fatty acids. For example, linoleic acid, needed for phospholipid synthesis, cell membrane formation, and transport of lipids, is an essential fatty acid found in corn, cottonseed, and soy oils. Another essential fatty acid is arachidonic acid.

Free fatty acids are used by the liver to synthesize triglycerides, phospholipids, and lipoproteins. Lipids are less dense than proteins; therefore, the proportion of lipids in a lipoprotein increases as the density of the particle decreases. The reverse is also true. Very low-density lipoproteins (VLDLs) have a relatively high concentration of triglycerides. Low-density lipoproteins (LDLs) have a relatively lower concentration of triglycerides. High-density lipoproteins (HDLs) have a relatively high concentration of proteins and a low concentration of triglycerides.

The liver controls cholesterol in the body. It synthesizes cholesterol and releases it into the bloodstream, or removes it from the bloodstream to be excreted via bile, or to produce bile salts. Cholesterol does not create energy but provides structural materials for cell membranes, as well as being important in the synthesis of certain sex hormones and adrenal hormones. Triglycerides are stored in adipose tissue, and may be hydrolyzed into free fatty acids and glycerol when blood lipid concentration drops, such as during fasting.

Lipids vary in how they may be required for health. Fat intake must be enough to carry the fat-soluble vitamins. Lipids also make foods taste more appetizing. It is recommended that lipid intake not exceed 30% of daily calories.

Proteins are created from amino acids, and include enzymes, plasma proteins, muscle components (actin and myosin), hormones, and antibodies. After digestion breaks proteins down into amino acids, they can also be used to supply energy. They are transported to the liver, where deamination occurs, which is the loss of their nitrogen-containing portions. They are then converted to form the waste urea, excreted in urine.

Foods rich in protein include meats, fish, poultry, cheese, nuts, milk, eggs, and cereals, and in lesser amounts, legumes (including beans and peas). All except nine of the required amino acids can be synthesized by an adult's body. Essential amino acids are those that the body cannot synthesize on its own. The body requires all of these amino acids for proper growth and tissue repair.

The three classes of proteins are complete, incomplete, and partially complete proteins. Complete proteins (found in milk, meats, and eggs) have adequate amounts of the essential amino acids. Incomplete proteins (such as those in corn) have too little tryptophan and lysine to maintain human tissues or support growth and development. A partially complete protein (such as gliadin, found in wheat) does not have enough lysine to promote growth, but does have enough to maintain life.

Proteins supply the essential amino acids and provide nitrogen and other elements. Protein requirements differ based on body size, metabolism, activity levels, and other factors. Nutritionists recommend a daily protein intake of 0.8 grams per kilogram of body weight; therefore, most average adults should consume 50 to 80 grams of protein per day.

Vitamins are other organic compounds that are required for normal metabolism. Body cells cannot synthesize adequate amounts of vitamins, so they must come from foods. They are classified by their solubility. Fat-soluble vitamins include A, D, E, and K. Water-soluble vitamins include the B vitamin group and vitamin C Table 15-1.

Bile salts in the small intestine promote absorption of fat-soluble vitamins. They can accumulate in various tissues and intake must be controlled. For example, when too much vitamin A is consumed, the body receives too much beta carotene, and the skin may appear orange in color. Table 15–1 explains the fat-soluble vitamins, including their adult recommended daily allowance (RDA).

The water-soluble vitamins include the B vitamins and vitamin C. The B vitamins consist of compounds essential for normal metabolism, and help to oxidize carbohydrates, lipids, and proteins. They are often present together in foods, hence they are referred to as the vitamin B complex. Cooking and food processing destroy some of these vitamins. Vitamin C (ascorbic acid) is one of the least stable vitamins. It is found in many plant foods, and is necessary for the body to produce collagen, convert folate to dihydropholic acid, and metabolize certain amino acids. Vitamin C also promotes synthesis of hormones from cholesterol and is vital for iron absorption.

Minerals are inorganic elements essential for human metabolism. Humans obtain minerals from plant foods, or from animals that have eaten plants. Minerals are most concentrated in the bones and teeth, and make up about 4% of body weight. Certain minerals are often incorporated into organic molecules, such as phosphorus (found in phospholipids), iron (in hemoglobin), and iodine (in thyroxine). Others are part of inorganic compounds, such as calcium phosphate (in bone). Still others are free ions (sodium, chloride, and calcium) in blood.

Minerals make up part of every cell's structure, and are present in enzymes, affect osmotic pressure, and are required for nerve impulse conduction. Other functions that rely on minerals include blood coagulation, muscle fiber contraction, and pH of body fluids. The minerals calcium and phosphorus make up almost 75% (by weight) of the body's mineral elements. These are called major minerals.

Trace elements are essential minerals that are found in very small amounts. Each makes up less than 0.005% of adult body weight.

When a person's diet lacks essential nutrients, malnutrition results. This may be caused by either undernutrition or overnutrition. Causes can include lack of food, poor-quality food, overeating, or taking too many vitamin supplements.

Table 15-1   Fat-Soluble Vitamins

Vitamin	Source	Adult RDA	Characteristics	Functions
A	Liver, fish, whole milk, butter, eggs, leafy green vegetables, yellow and orange vegetables, and fruits	4,000 to 5,000 international units (IU)	Several forms; synthesized from carotenes; stored in liver; stable in heat, acids, and bases; unstable in light	Necessary for synthesis of visual pigments, mucoproteins, and mucopolysaccharides; for normal development of bones and teeth; and for maintenance of epithelial cells
D	Produced when skin is exposed to ultraviolet light; also exists in milk, egg yolk, fish liver oils, and fortified foods	400 IU	A group of steroids; resistant to heat, oxidation, acids, and bases; stored in liver, skin, brain, spleen, and bones	Promotes absorption of calcium and phosphorus, as well as development of teeth and bones
E	Oils from cereal seeds, salad oils, margarine, shortenings, fruits, nuts, and vegetables	30 IU	A group of compounds; resistant to heat and visible light; unstable in presence of oxygen and ultraviolet light; stored in muscles and adipose tissues	An antioxidant; prevents oxidation of vitamin A and polyunsaturated fatty acids; may help maintain stability of cell membranes
K	Leafy green vegetables, egg yolk, pork liver, soy oil, tomatoes, cauliflower	55 to 70 micrograms	Occurs in several forms; resistant to heat, but destroyed by acids, bases, and light; stored in the liver	Required for synthesis of prothrombin, which functions in blood clotting

Overeating, as well as insufficient exercise, results in the body becoming overweight, and potentially obese (defined as having a body mass index of 30 or more). A person's body mass index (BMI) is used to determine adequate weight, being overweight, or being obese. BMI is calculated by dividing a person's weight in kilograms (1 kilogram = 2.2 pounds) by height in meters squared (1 foot = 0.3 meters). For example, a person who is 5 feet 6 inches tall is equivalent to 1.65 meters tall. If this person weighs 180 pounds, that is equivalent to 82 kilograms. By dividing 82 kilograms by 1.65 meters squared, a BMI of 29 is found, which is considered overweight but not obese.

After digestion, individual cells are supplied these nutrients and use them in various processes. The term that encompasses all of the processes occurring within the cell is known as cellular metabolism.

■ Cellular Metabolism

Metabolism consists of the chemical changes that take place inside living cells. As a result of metabolism, organisms grow, maintain body functions, release or store energy, produce and eliminate waste, digest nutrients, or destroy toxins. These reactions alter the chemical nature of a substance, maintaining homeostasis. Numerous conditions can affect this vital balance, resulting in disease.

Two major types of metabolic reactions control how cells use energy. The buildup of larger molecules from smaller molecules is called anabolism. The breakdown of larger molecules into smaller ones is called catabolism. Each of these actions requires the use of energy.

Case Study | PART 2

After obtaining a set of baseline vital signs, you notice that the patient is not shivering. You use the hypothermia thermometer to determine that the patient has a temperature of 92°F. Your partner has checked the patient's blood glucose level and found it to be 100 mg/dL, within normal limits.

You consider other reasons why the patient could have an altered mental status because you do not want to focus only on the obvious. You complete the trauma exam on your 72-year-old male patient who weighs 90 kg. You obtain a SAMPLE history from a family member over the phone. The SAMPLE history shows:

- **S**igns and symptoms: Cold to the touch
- **A**llergies to medications: Allergy to penicillin
- **M**edications taken: ASA, antihypertensive
- **P**ast pertinent medical history: Under physician care for hypertension, TIA 3 years ago, old shoulder dislocation
- **L**ast food/fluid intake: Grilled cheese sandwich and fries for lunch about 7 hours ago
- **E**vents prior to onset: Not clear if he was confused and went outdoors or if confusion is a result of being outdoors

Recording Time: 10 Minutes	
Appearance	Still confused and cold
Level of consciousness	Verbal (oriented to person, confused about place and day)
Airway	Open and patent
Breathing	Shallow and rapid
Circulation	Pale, dry, and cold
Pulse	60 beats/min and regular
Blood pressure	128/66 mm Hg
Respirations	24 breaths/min, nonlabored
Pupils	Equal and reactive
Spo$_2$	97%

3. What are the products of cellular respiration?

4. How does the body dispose of the products of cellular respiration?

Anabolism

Anabolism is the process of building complex molecules in the body from simpler materials. When a person is healthy and has adequate nutrition, simple nutrients (such as amino acids, fats, and glucose) are used by the body to build the basic chemicals that support cellular functioning and sustain life.

Anabolism supplies biochemicals needed for cells to grow and repair themselves. An example of anabolism is when simple sugar molecules called monosaccharides are linked to form a chain, making up molecules of glycogen (a carbohydrate). This anabolic process is called dehydration synthesis. As the links in this chain are formed, an OH (hydroxyl group) is removed from one molecule while an H (hydrogen atom) from another is removed. Together the OH and H produce a water molecule (H_2O). The monosaccharides are then joined by a shared oxygen atom, resulting in growth of the chain.

Dehydration synthesis, which links glycerol and fatty acid molecules in adipose (fat) cells, results in formation of fat molecules (triglycerides). This occurs when three hydrogen atoms are removed from a glycerol molecule. An OH group is removed from each of three fatty acid molecules. This creates three water molecules and one fat molecule. Oxygen atoms are then shared between the glycerol and fatty acid portions.

Cells also use dehydration synthesis to join amino acid molecules, eventually leading to formation of protein molecules. As two amino acids unite, one OH molecule is removed from one of them, while one H molecule is removed from the NH_2 group of another. This leads to formation of one water molecule. The amino acid molecules are then joined by a bond created between a nitrogen atom and a carbon atom (called a peptide bond).

A dipeptide is formed from two amino acids bound together, and a polypeptide is formed from many amino acids bound into a chain. Polypeptides usually have specialized functions. When a polypeptide has more than 100 molecules, it is considered to be a protein. Certain protein molecules include more than one polypeptide.

Catabolism

Catabolism can be defined as the metabolic breakdown of stored carbohydrates, fats, or proteins to provide energy. It occurs continuously to differing degrees. Excessive catabolism leads to wasting of tissues. An example of catabolism is the process of hydrolysis, which is actually the opposite of dehydration synthesis. This involves the decomposition of carbohydrates, lipids, and proteins.

Hydrolysis splits a water molecule; for example, hydrolysis of sucrose (a disaccharide) gives off glucose and fructose (two monosaccharides) as the water molecule splits. The equation is as follows:

$$C_{12}H_{22}O_{11} + H_2O \rightarrow C_6H_{12}O_6 + C_6H_{12}O_6$$
(Sucrose) (Water) (Glucose) (Fructose)

As shown in the equation, inside the sucrose molecule, the bond between the simple sugars breaks. The water molecule supplies a hydrogen atom to one of the sugar molecules while supplying a hydroxyl group to the other.

Both dehydration synthesis and hydrolysis are reversible, and are summarized in the following equation:

Hydrolysis → Disaccharide + Water ↔ Monosaccharide + Monosaccharide ← Dehydration synthesis

During digestion, hydrolysis breaks down carbohydrates into monosaccharides. It also breaks down fats into glycerol and fatty acids, nucleic acids into nucleotides, and proteins into amino acids.

Control of Metabolic Reactions

Nerve, muscle, and blood cells are specialized to carry out distinctive chemical reactions; however, every type of cell performs basic chemical reactions. These include the buildup and breakdown of carbohydrates, lipids, nucleic acids, and proteins. Enzymes coordinate hundreds of rapid chemical changes to control metabolic reactions.

Enzymes and Their Actions

As mentioned earlier, an enzyme is a protein that catalyzes biochemical reactions. Enzymes are among the most important of all the body's proteins. They catalyze the reactions that sustain life. Nearly everything that occurs in the human body relies on a specific enzyme. In the body, enzymes assist in the digestion of food, metabolism of drugs, formation of proteins, and in many other types of reactions. Enzymes make metabolic reactions possible inside cells by controlling temperature conditions that otherwise would be too mild for them to occur.

Enzymes are complex molecules. They lower the activation energy needed for metabolic reactions to occur. This speeds up the rates of the reactions in a process called catalysis. Enzyme molecules that are not used in the reactions they catalyze are recycled. Activation energy is defined as the excess energy that must be added to an atomic or molecular system to allow a particular process to take place.

Enzymes catalyze very specific reactions. Each enzyme acts on a substrate, which is a particular chemical affected by the enzyme. Enzymes are often named after their substrates using the suffix -ase. For example, a lipid is catalyzed by an enzyme called a lipase. Another enzyme, called a catalase, breaks down hydrogen peroxide into water and oxygen. Hydrogen peroxide is a toxic substance that forms as a byproduct of certain metabolic reactions.

Every cell contains hundreds of different enzymes, each of which recognizes a specific substrate. Enzyme molecules have three-dimensional shapes (conformations) that allow them to identify their substrates. The coiled and twisted polypeptide chain of each enzyme fits the shape of its substrate. The active site of an enzyme molecule combines with portions of substrate molecules temporarily. This forms an enzyme–substrate complex.

When enzyme–substrate complexes are formed, some chemical bonds within the substrates are distorted or strained. Requiring less energy as a result, the enzyme is released as it was originally configured. Enzyme-catalyzed reactions can be summarized as follows:

$$\text{Substrate molecules} + \text{Enzyme molecule} \rightarrow \text{Enzyme-substrate complex} \rightarrow \text{Product (changed substrates)} + \text{Enzyme molecule}$$

These reactions are often reversible. Sometimes, the same enzyme catalyzes the reaction in both directions. The reactions occur at differing rates, based on the number of molecules of the enzyme and its substrate. Some enzymes process a few substrate molecules every second, whereas others can process thousands in the same length of time.

Pathophysiology

The term <u>basal metabolic rate (BMR)</u> refers to the baseline metabolic rate of the body, or the rate at which the body uses energy while at rest. Calculation of BMR requires fairly sophisticated laboratory equipment. BMR is a piece of information that is sometimes useful in specialized clinical settings, such as exercise physiology labs or by endocrine and metabolism specialists. BMR describes the number of kilocalories metabolized per square meter of body surface area per hour. Kilocalories (C) are a unit of heat measurement. Each kilocalorie (1 C) is the amount of heat needed to raise the temperature of 1 kg of water from 14.5°C to 15.5°C. (C is always capitalized to distinguish it from a "small calorie" (c).)

Altering of Enzymes

Enzymes are most often proteins that can change due to exposure to heat, electricity, chemicals, radiation, or fluids that have extreme pH levels. Many enzymes are inactive at 45°C (111°F), and most of them are denatured at 55°C (131°F). Denaturing is defined as changing or altering some of the structures of the enzyme. Poisons such as potassium cyanide achieve their effects by denaturing enzymes. The poison stops the cells from being able to release energy from nutrient molecules.

Some enzymes must combine with a nonprotein component in order to be active. These nonprotein components are referred to as cofactors, and may be an element's ion (such as calcium, magnesium, copper, iron, or zinc). Cofactors may also be small (non-protein) organic molecules called coenzymes. The human body converts many vitamins into essential coenzymes. Coenzyme A, which is involved in cellular respiration, represents one such example.

Chemical Energy

Performing work and changing or moving matter requires energy. Most metabolic processes use chemical energy.

Other forms of energy include heat, light, electrical energy, mechanical energy, and sound.

Chemical Energy Release

When the bonds between the atoms of molecules are broken, chemical energy is released. When a substance is burned, for example, bonds break and energy escapes as both light and heat. During the process of oxidation, cells "burn" molecules of glucose to release chemical energy that fuels the process of anabolism; however, oxidation is different from the burning of substances that exist outside cells.

Inside the cells, enzymes reduce the activation energy which is the amount of energy needed for oxidation as part of cellular respiration. Energy is released in the bonds of nutrient molecules. The cells then transfer about 40% of the released energy to special energy-carrying molecules. The remaining energy escapes as heat, helping the body to remain at normal temperature.

Cellular Respiration

<u>Cellular respiration</u>, which is also called <u>aerobic metabolism</u>, is a process through which energy is released from organic compounds. This process requires three types of reactions: glycolysis, the citric acid cycle, and the electron transport chain. In cellular respiration, glucose and oxygen are needed. The products of these reactions include carbon dioxide, water, and energy. Therefore, in cellular respiration, the presence of oxygen is vital to produce a significant amount of energy. With low oxygen levels, the above reactions do not occur and the cell reverts to <u>anaerobic metabolism</u>. Less energy is produced during anaerobic metabolism than during aerobic metabolism, and lactic acid waste products are produced.

Glycolysis

<u>Glycolysis</u> is a process that involves a series of enzymatically catalyzed reactions in which glucose is broken down to yield lactic acid or pyruvic acid. The breakdown releases energy as <u>adenosine triphosphate (ATP)</u> **Figure 15-1**. The six-carbon sugar glucose is broken down in the cytosol; it becomes 2 three-carbon pyruvic acid molecules, gaining two ATP molecules and releasing high-energy electrons.

Glycolysis begins the process of <u>cellular respiration</u>. It occurs in the cytosol (the liquid portion of the cytoplasm). Glycolysis does not require oxygen and is occasionally referred to as the anaerobic phase. If oxygen is present in the right amounts, pyruvic acid, which is generated by glycolysis, can enter the more energy-efficient pathways of aerobic respiration. These pathways are located in the <u>mitochondria</u>.

Aerobic reactions yield as many as 36 ATP molecules per glucose molecule. Completely decomposed glucose molecules can produce up to 38 molecules of ATP.

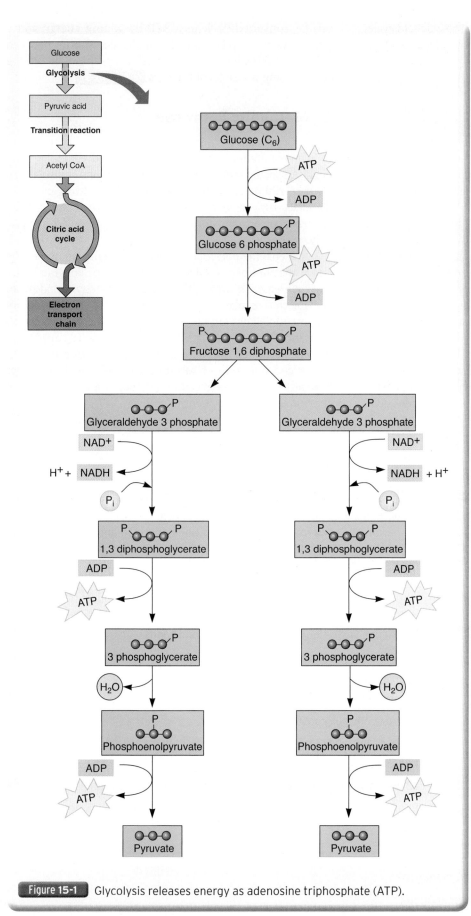

Figure 15-1 Glycolysis releases energy as adenosine triphosphate (ATP).

Most result from the aerobic phase, with only two resulting from glycolysis. Approximately half of the released energy is used for ATP synthesis, while the rest becomes heat. The oxidation of glucose also produces carbon dioxide (which is exhaled) and water (which is absorbed into the internal body environment). The volume of water produced by metabolism is lower than the requirements of the body, so drinking water is necessary for survival.

■ Citric Acid Cycle

The citric acid cycle is also called the tricarboxylic acid cycle or the TCA cycle. It is a sequence of enzymatic reactions involving the metabolism of carbon chains of glucose, fatty acids, and amino acids to yield carbon dioxide, water, and high-energy phosphate bonds (ATP) **Figure 15-2** . The three-carbon pyruvic acids enter the mitochondria, each losing a carbon. They then combine with a coenzyme to form a two-carbon acetyl coenzyme A, and release more high-energy electrons; then, each acetyl coenzyme A combines with a four-carbon oxaloacetic acid to form a six-carbon citric acid.

A series of reactions removes two carbons, synthesizes one ATP, and releases more high-energy electrons. When food is ingested, large macromolecules are broken down to simple molecules. Proteins are broken down into amino acids, carbohydrates are broken down into simple sugars (glucose), and fats are broken down into both glycerol and fatty acids. The breakdown of simple molecules to acetyl coenzyme A is accompanied by the production of limited amounts of ATP (via glycolysis) and high-energy electrons.

Glucose, through glycolysis, is converted into pyruvic acid. Glycerol and amino acids are also broken down into pyruvic acid. Actually, all of these processes result, in differing ways, in acetyl coenzyme A. Complete oxidation of acetyl coenzyme A to H_2O and CO_2 produces high-energy electrons, which yield greater amounts of ATP via the electron transport chain. In the tricarboxylic acid cycle, the process of oxidation provides more molecules of ATP.

Electron Transport Chain

In the electron transport chain, the high-energy electrons still contain most of the chemical energy of the original glucose molecule. Special carrier molecules bring them to enzymes that store most of the remaining energy in more ATP molecules; heat and water are also produced. Oxygen is the final electron acceptor in this step; therefore, the overall process is termed aerobic metabolism.

For cellular respiration, glucose and oxygen are required. This process produces carbon dioxide, water, and energy. Nearly half of the energy is recaptured as high-energy electrons stored in the cells through the synthesis of ATP.

Each ATP molecule has a chain of three chemical groups. These groups are called phosphates. Some of the energy is recaptured in the bond of the end phosphate. When energy is later needed, the terminal phosphate bond breaks to release the stored energy. Cells use ATP for many functions, including active transport and the synthesis of needed compounds.

When an ATP molecule has lost its terminal phosphate, it becomes an ADP (adenosine diphosphate) molecule. ADP can be converted back into ATP by adding energy and a third phosphate. ATP and ADP molecules shuttle between the energy-releasing reactions of cellular respiration and the energy-using reactions of the cells Figure 15-3 .

Metabolic Pathways

A number of steps are involved in each of the processes of cellular respiration, anabolic reactions, and catabolic reactions. A specific sequence of enzymatic actions controls each of these reactions; therefore, the enzymes are organized in the exact same sequence as the reactions they control. Each sequence of enzyme-controlled reactions is called a metabolic pathway.

An enzyme-controlled reaction usually increases its rate if the number of substrate molecules or enzyme molecules increases; however, the rate is often determined by an enzyme that regulates one of the reaction's steps. Regulatory enzyme molecules are limited, and when the substrate concentration exceeds a certain level, the enzyme supply can become saturated. When this occurs, increasing the number or concentration of substrate molecules will no longer have any effect on the reaction rate. Because of this, just one enzyme can control the entire pathway.

Case Study PART 3

You place the patient on your stretcher, cover him with blankets, and start warm IV fluids because his lungs are clear. As the stretcher is loaded into the ambulance, the paramedic reviews the ECG that has been obtained and finds no irregularities at this point. There is concern about the altered mental status with the history of a TIA so a rapid neurologic exam is conducted, followed by reassessment including a new set of vital signs.

Recording Time: 15 Minutes

Appearance	Some color is starting to return to his face and hands
Level of consciousness	Verbal (oriented to person and place, but still confused about the day)
Airway	Open and patent
Breathing	Normal at this point
Circulation	Pale, dry, and still cool to touch
Pulse	64 beats/min and regular
Blood pressure	110/70 mm Hg
Respirations	22 breaths/min and nonlabored
Pupils	PEARRL
Sp$_{O_2}$	98%

5. What is hyperthermia and how is it managed?

6. What is hypothermia and how is it managed?

A rate-limiting enzyme is usually the first enzyme in a series. Being first is critical because if a rate-limiting enzyme were located somewhere else in the chemical pathway, an intermediate chemical could accumulate. Fats and proteins, as well as glucose, can be broken down to release energy needed to synthesize ATP. In all three cases, aerobic respiration is still the final result of these breakdown processes. The most common point of entry is into the citric acid cycle as acetyl coenzyme A.

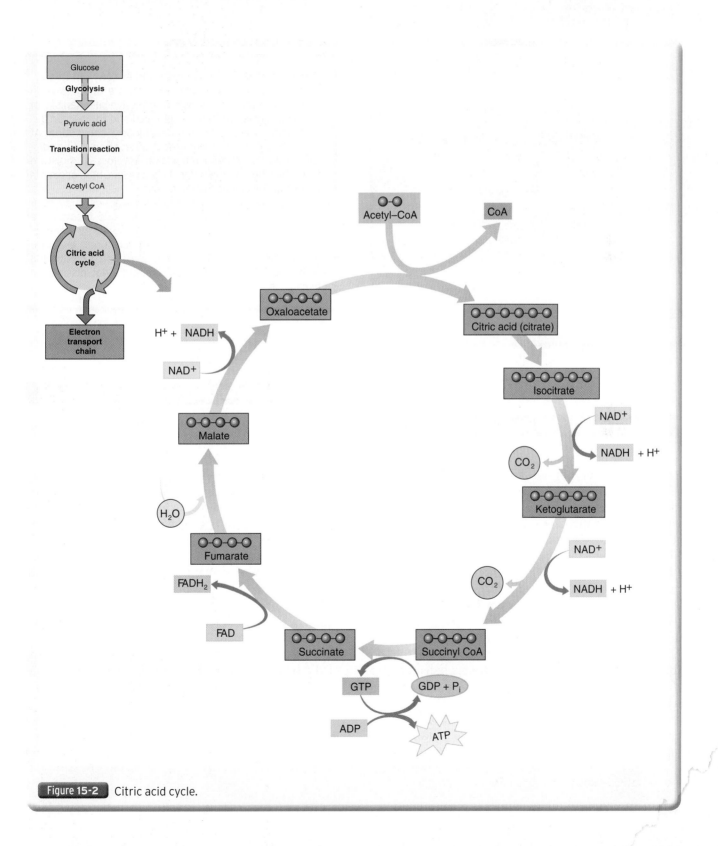

Figure 15-2 Citric acid cycle.

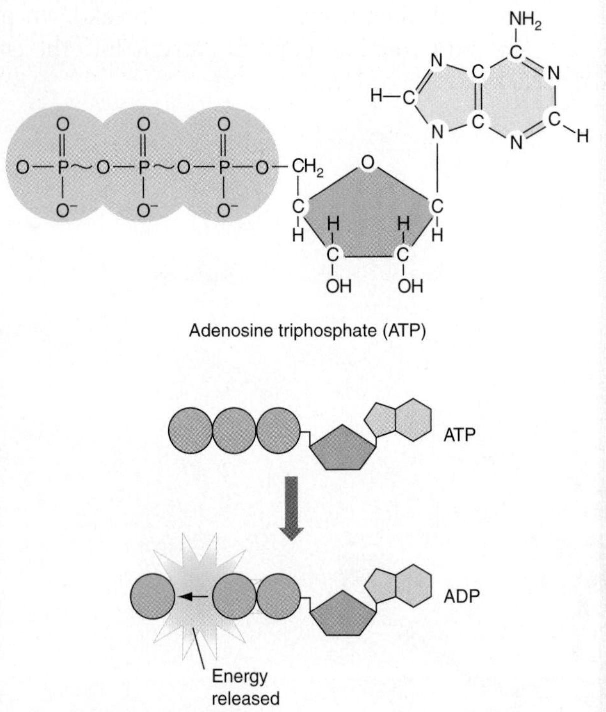

Adenosine triphosphate (ATP)

ATP

ADP

Energy
released

Figure 15-3 Adenosine triphosphate and adenosine diphosphate molecules.

Body Temperature

One major role of metabolic processes is thermoregulation, or maintenance of normal body temperature (98.6°F, or 37.0°C). Peripheral processes of heat regulation are under the primary control of the hypothalamus in the brain, the body's thermostat. Thermolysis refers to normal bodily means of heat loss and gain. Heat is generated by muscular activity and through metabolic reactions in the body. As the body temperature increases, changes occur in each organ system. If a person is exposed to a hot environment gradually, the body acclimates, or becomes used to the heat. Heat is dissipated from the body by four mechanisms: radiation, conduction, convection, and evaporation. When radiation occurs, heat is transmitted through space, such as with warmth from a radiant heater or fireplace. Conduction is the transmission of heat from warmer to cooler objects by direct contact, such as touching a cold surface or lying on a cold floor. Convection is the transfer of heat by circulation of heated particles, such as occurs with wind chill, cold-water exposure, or cooling

soup by blowing on it. Evaporation occurs when heat at the surface is lost because of vaporization of liquid, such as from sweating or spraying water mist on the body to keep cool. Heat also is lost during breathing, mostly from evaporation.

Pathophysiology

Extremes of body temperature, either too high (hyperthermia) or too low (hypothermia), are dangerous. In humans, conduction is not an effective mechanism of heat loss unless clothing is removed and the person lies on a cool surface. Clothing also hinders convection. At room temperature, 75% of heat dissipation is by radiation and convection. Evaporation, the loss of moisture from the skin and the lungs during respiration, accounts for about 25% of normal heat loss.

As the ambient temperature approaches body temperature, radiation is no longer effective to dissipate heat. The body may actually gain heat by conduction and convection. At high temperatures, evaporation becomes the only effective method of dissipating heat. High humidity seriously impairs heat dissipation because evaporation occurs slowly.

Body Fluid Balance

There are two types of body fluids: extracellular fluid is fluid outside of cells and intracellular fluid is fluid inside cells. There is a delicate balance in body fluid that is essential to maintain homeostasis. Extracellular fluid comprises approximately 25% of total body fluid. It is made up of intravascular fluid (plasma), which is fluid inside the blood vessels, and interstitial fluid which is fluid outside of the blood vessels. Intracellular fluid is inside individual cells and represents about 75% of all body fluid. Depending on gender and age, the total body fluid of the average adult is 50% to 70% of body weight. This percentage is higher in infants.

Fluid balance maintains homeostasis despite inconsistencies in the body's intake and output of water from day to day. Significant loss of fluid from any compartment of the body can interfere with homeostasis and result in shock. The body has several ways to maintain fluid balance. Decreased body fluid triggers the release of antidiuretic hormone (ADH) by the pituitary gland. This causes retention of fluid by the kidneys—more water is kept by the body and less is excreted as urine. The result is increased fluid volume in the body. Thirst is also a major mechanism in fluid balance. When body fluid levels become decreased, the sensation of thirst stimulates a person to take in more fluids. Increased body fluid levels, on the other hand, suppress thirst and increase excretion of fluid by the kidneys as urine.

Another way that the body maintains fluid balance is by moving water within and between the extracellular and intracellular compartments. Osmotic forces and hormonal stimuli cause water movement. Without proper fluid balance, alterations in the levels of fluids and electrolytes within the body may cause disease and even be life threatening.

Case Study **PART 4**

En route to the hospital, serial vital signs are obtained and the patient's ECG is monitored. The patient begins to talk about his family and what he did before he retired from the railroad. He is still not clear as to why he was sitting outdoors without the proper clothing. For this reason, the potential for other causes of altered mental status are still included in your differential diagnosis. This patient requires transport so he can be evaluated by a physician and tested for drug or alcohol use and possibly to obtain a CT scan of his brain. His daughter is planning on meeting you at the emergency department. You decide to check his body temperature one more time before arrival at the emergency department to see if he started to warm up.

Prep Kit

Chapter Summary

- The study of nutrients and how the body uses them is known as nutrition.

- The body requires macronutrients (those needed in large amounts), which include carbohydrates, lipids, and proteins. The body also requires micronutrients (those needed in smaller amounts), which include vitamins and minerals.

- Metabolism is the sum of all chemical processes that take place in the body, resulting in storage or expenditure of energy.

- Anabolism is the build up of energy reservoirs and molecules in the body—the constructive component of metabolism.

- Catabolism is the breakdown of energy in the body—the destructive component of metabolism.

- Once glucose, amino acids, and fats are absorbed from the gastrointestinal tract, they are metabolized by the body to produce energy. Some glucose is stored in the liver as glycogen, which is broken down when necessary to raise the blood glucose level.

- Glucose, fat, and proteins generate energy via cellular respiration, which is a biochemical process resulting in the production of energy in the form of adenosine triphosphate (ATP) molecules.

- Cellular respiration (aerobic metabolism) occurs normally in the presence of oxygen.

- With low oxygen levels, the cell reverts to anaerobic metabolism, in which lactic acid as a waste product is produced as well as less energy.

- Thermoregulation is under primary control of the hypothalamus in the brain, the body's "thermostat." Thermolysis refers to normal bodily means of heat dissipation or loss.

- Heat is dissipated from the body by the following four mechanisms: radiation, conduction, convection, and evaporation.

- The average adult has a body water content of 50% to 70% of the total body weight.

- Body fluid is divided into intracellular fluid, which is found within individual cells, and extracellular fluid, which is found outside cell membranes.

- Extracellular fluid is further divided into intravascular fluid (plasma) and extravascular or interstitial fluid.

- Loss of fluid volume from any area of the body can result in disruption of homeostasis and shock. Normally, the total volume of water in the body as well as its distribution in the body compartments remains relatively constant.

- When the fluid volume drops, the pituitary gland secretes antidiuretic hormone (ADH), signaling the kidney tubules to reabsorb more water back into the blood and excrete less urine.

- Thirst also regulates fluid intake. A decrease in body fluids results in the sensation of thirst, stimulating a person to drink more.

- When too many fluids enter the body, thirst decreases, ADH secretion decreases, the kidneys are activated, and more urine is excreted, eliminating the excess fluid.

- The body also maintains fluid balance by shifting water from one compartment to another.

Vital Vocabulary

adenosine triphosphate (ATP) A form of energy created by cellular respiration.

aerobic metabolism A biochemical process that occurs in the presence of oxygen and results in the production of energy in the form of ATP; also called cellular respiration.

anabolism The synthesis of larger molecules from smaller ones.

anaerobic metabolism An alternate form of metabolism that occurs when oxygen levels are low and less energy is produced than during aerobic respiration; lactic acid is produced as a waste product during this process.

antidiuretic hormone A hormone secreted by the posterior pituitary lobe of the pituitary gland; constricts blood vessels and raises the blood pressure, and also is responsible for adjustments to the final composition of urine by causing ducts in the kidney to become more permeable to water; also called vasopressin.

basal metabolic rate (BMR) The rate at which nutrients are consumed by the body at rest.

calorie The amount of heat needed to raise the temperature of one gram of water by 1°C.

catabolism The breakdown of larger molecules into smaller molecules.

cellular metabolism Process within a cell where nutrients are broken down from complex to simpler forms or where complex forms are built from simpler blocks.

cellular respiration A biochemical process resulting in the production of energy in the form of adenosine triphosphate; also called metabolism.

extracellular fluid Fluid found outside of the cell membranes in which most of the body's supply of sodium is contained, representing approximately 15% of the total body weight.

fluid balance The process of maintaining homeostasis through equal intake and output of fluids.

glycogen A long polymer from which glucose is converted in the liver.

glycolysis A process that involves a series of enzymatically catalyzed reactions in which glucose is broken down to yield lactic acid or pyruvic acid.

hydrolysis The splitting of a molecule by adding water.

hyperthermia Elevated body temperature.

hypothalamus A small region of the brain that is the primary link between the endocrine system and the nervous system; contains several control centers for emotions and body functions including thermoregulation; it produces antidiuretic hormone.

hypothermia Low body temperature.

interstitial fluid The fluid located outside of the blood vessels in the spaces between the body's cells.

intracellular fluid Fluid found within individual cells, representing approximately 45% of total body weight.

intravascular fluid The noncellular portion of blood found within the blood vessels; also called plasma.

kilocalorie A unit of heat measurement, abbreviated as C.

metabolism The chemical processes that provide the cells with energy from nutrients.

minerals Inorganic elements essential for human metabolism.

mitochondria The metabolic center or powerhouse of the cell; small and rod-shaped organelles.

nutrients Carbohydrates, lipids, proteins, vitamins, minerals, and water.

substrate The target of enzyme action.

thermolysis Normal bodily means of heat dissipation from the body.

thermoregulation The maintenance of normal body temperature (98.6°F, or 37.0°C).

trace elements Essential minerals found in very small amounts; including chromium, cobalt, copper, fluorine, iodine, iron, manganese, selenium, and zinc.

vitamins Organic compounds required for normal metabolism.

■ Case Study Answers

1. What is the normal range of body temperature?

   Answer: One major role of metabolic processes is thermoregulation, or maintenance of normal body temperature (98.6°F, or 37.0°C).

2. What structure is considered the thermostat of the body?

   Answer: The body's thermostat is the structure called the hypothalamus.

3. What are the products of cellular respiration?

   Answer: Cellular respiration, which is also called aerobic metabolism, is a process that releases energy from organic compounds. This process includes three series of reactions: glycolysis, the citric acid cycle, and the electron transport chain. In cellular respiration, glucose and oxygen are both needed. The products of these reactions include carbon dioxide, water, and energy. Therefore, in cellular respiration, the presence of oxygen is vital to the production of a significant amount of energy.

4. How does the body dispose of the products of cellular respiration?

   Answer: The products of cellular respiration are removed from the cells by the bloodstream. Carbon dioxide is exhaled through the lungs, and water is removed by the kidneys.

5. What is hyperthermia and how is it managed?

   Answer: Hyperthermia is an abnormally warm body temperature. When the body's thermostat fails to adequately manage the temperature and the patient is in a hot environment, the body temperature will quickly increase, ultimately killing brain cells. Management consists of rapidly reducing the body temperature while monitoring the progress and transporting to the emergency department.

6. What is hypothermia and how is it managed?

   Answer: Hypothermia is an abnormally low body temperature. When the body's thermostat fails to adequately manage the temperature and the patient is in a cold environment, the body temperature will quickly decrease, ultimately killing brain cells. Management consists of beginning the rewarming process from the core of the body outward. It is important not to reheat too fast because the patient may go into ventricular fibrillation. The typical medications and interventions used to manage a cardiac arrest are not effective when the patient is hypothermic. It will be necessary to warm up the patient before the medications or interventions such as defibrillation are helpful.

Biological Roots

One of the major challenges of an anatomy and physiology course is mastering new terminology. One of the best ways to learn and remember technical terms is to first learn their component parts—that is, their roots. But studying common Latin and Greek roots for biological terms before you begin your study can also help. Spend a few minutes early in your course studying these common roots. They will not only help you understand new terms, but also make them easier to remember.

a-, an- [Gk. an-, not, without, lacking]: anaerobic, abiotic, anemia

ad- [L. ad-, toward, to]: adrenalin

amphi- [Gk. amphi-, two, both, both sides of]: amphibian

ana- [Gk. ana-, up, up against]: anaphase, anabolic, anatomy

andro- [Gk. andros, an old man]: androgen

anti- [Gk. anti-, against, opposite, opposed to]: antibiotic, antibody, antigen, antidiuretic hormone

arthro- [Gk. arthron, a joint]: arthropod, arthritis

auto- [Gk. auto-, self, same]: autoimmune, autotroph

bi-, bin- [L. bis, twice; bini, two-by-two]: binary fission, binocular vision, bicarbonate

bio- [Gk. bios, life]: biology, biomass, biome, biosphere, biotic

blasto-, -blast [Gk. blastos, sprout; pertains to embryo]: blastula, trophoblast, osteoblast

broncho- [Gk. bronchos, windpipe]: bronchus, bronchi, bronchiole, bronchitis

carb- [L. carbo, coal]: carbon, carbohydrate

carcino- [Gk. karkin, a crab, cancer]: carcinogen

cardio- [Gk. kardia, heart]: cardiac, myocardium, electrocardiogram

cat- [Gk. kata, down, downward]: catabolic

chloro- [Gk. chloros, green]: chlorophyll, chloroplast, chlorine

chromo- [Gk. chroma, color]: chromosome, chromatin

coelo, -coel [Gk. koilos, hollow, cavity]: coelom

com-, con-, col-, co- [L. cum, with, together]: coenzyme, covalent

cranio- [Gk. kranios, L. cranium, skull]: cranial, cranium

cuti- [L. cutis, skin]: cutaneous, cuticle

cyto-, cyte [Gk. kytos, vessel or container; now, "cell"]: cytoplasm, cytokinesis, erythrocyte, leukocyte

de- [L. de-, away, off, removal, separation]: deciduous, decomposer, dehydration

derm-, dermato- [Gk. derma, skin]: dermis, epidermis, ectoderm, endoderm, mesoderm

di- [Gk. dis, twice, two, double]: disaccharide, dioxide

dia- [Gk. through, passing through, thorough, thoroughly]: diabetes, dialysis, diaphragm

diplo- [Gk. diploos, two-fold]: diploid

eco- [Gk. oikos, house, home]: ecology, ecosystem, economy

ecto- [Gk. ektos, outside]: ectoderm

endo- [Gk. endon, within]: endoderm, endometrium

epi- [Gk. epi, on, upon, over]: epidermis, epididymis, epiglottis, epithelium

equi- [L. aequus, equal]: equilibrium

eu- [Gk. eus, good; eu, well, true]: eukaryote

ex, exo-, ec-, e- [Gk., L. out, out of, from, beyond]: emission, ejaculation, excretion, exergonic, exhale, exocytosis, exoskeleton

extra- [L. outside of, beyond]: extracellular, extraembryonic

-fer [L. ferre, to bear]: fertile, fertilization, conifer

gam-, gameto- [Gk. gamos, marriage; now usually in reference to gametes (sex cells)]: gamete

gastro- [Gk. gaster, stomach]: gastric, gastrin, gastrovascular cavity

gen- [Gk. gen, born, produced by; Gk. genos, race, kind; L. genus, generare, to beget]: polygenic genotype, geneology, glycogen, pyrogen, heterogenous

gluco-, glyco- [Gk. glykys, sweet; now pertaining to sugar]: glucose, glycogen, glycolysis, glycoprotein

hemo-, hemato-, -hemia, -emia [Gk. haima, blood]: hematology, hemoglobin, hemophilia

hepato- [Gk. hepar, hepat-, liver]: hepatitis, hepatic portal system

hetero- [Gk. heteros, other, different]: heterogeneous, heterozygote

histo- [Gk. histos, web of a loom, tissue; pertains to biological tissues]: histology, histamine, antihistamine

homo-, homeo- [Gk. homos, same; Gk. homios, similar]: homeostasis, homogeneous, homologous, homozygote

hydro- [Gk. hydor, water; pertains either to water or to hydrogen]: dehydration, carbohydrate

hyper- [Gk. hyper, over, above, more than]: hyperthyroid, hypertonic hypo- [Gk. hypo, under, below, beneath, less than]: hypodermic, hypoglycemia, hypothalamus, hypothesis, hypotonic

ion- [Gk. ion, small]: ion, ionic

inter- [L. inter, between, among, together, during]: interbreed, intercellular, intercostal

intra-, intro- [L. intra, within]: intracellular, intrauterine, intravenous

-itis [L., Gk. -itis, inflammation of]: arthritis, bronchitis, dermatitis

leuko-, leuco- [Gk. leukos, white]: leukocyte, leukemia

libra- [L. libra, balance]: equilibrium

lip- [Gk. lipos, fat]: lipid, liposuction, liposome

-logy [Gk. -logia, the study of, from logos, word]: anthropology, biology, embryology

-lysis, lys-, lyso-, -lyze, -lyte [Gk. lysis, a loosening, dissolution]: hydrolysis, analysis, catalysis

macro- [Gk. makro-, great, large]: macromolecule, macrophage

mega, megalo-, megaly [Gk. megas, large, great, powerful]: acromegaly

-mere, -mer, mero- [Gk. meros, part]: centromere, polymer

meso-, mes- [Gk. mesos, middle, in the middle]: mesoderm

meta-, met- [Gk. meta, after, beyond; denotes change]: metabolism, metastasis

micro- [Gk. mikros, small]: microbe, microscope

mono- [Gk. monos, one, single]: mononucleosis, monosaccharide

myo- [Gk. mys, mouse, muscle]: myocardium, myoglobin, myosin

neuro- [Gk. neuron, nerve sinew, tendon]: neuron, neurotransmitter

-oma [Gk. -oma, tumor, swelling]: carcinoma, glaucoma, hematoma, sarcoma

oo- [Gk. oion, egg]: oogenesis, oogonium

-osis [Gk. -osis, a state of being, condition]: arteriosclerosis

osteo-, oss- [Gk. osteon, bone; L. os, ossa, bone]: ossification, osteoblast, periosteum

patho-, -pathy, -path [Gk. pathos, suffering; refers to disease or the treatment of disease]: pathogen, pathology, pathological

peri- [Gk. peri, around]: pericardial, periosteum

phago-, -phage [Gk. phagein, to eat]: phagocyte, phagocytosis, bacteriophage

plasm-, -plasm, -plast, -plasty [Gk. plasm, something molded or formed]: plasma, plasma membrane, plasmid, cytoplasm, nucleoplasm, chloroplast

-pod [Gk. pod, foot]: cephalopod, pseudopod

poly- [Gk. poly-, polys, many]: polygenic, polymer, polypeptide

pro- [Gk. pro, before]: prokaryote

prot- [Gk. protos, first, original]: protein, proton, protista

-rrhea [Gk. rhoia, flow]: rhinorrhea

-some, somat- [Gk. soma, body; Gk. somat-, of the body]: chromosome, ribosome

-stat, -stasis, stato- [Gk. stasis, stand]: metastasis, thermostat, electrostatic, hydrostatic

sub- [L. sub, under, below]: subatomic, subdural

sym-, syn- [Gk. syn, with together]: symbiont, symbiosis, symmetry, synapsis

taxo-, -taxis [Gk. taxis, to arrange, put in order; refers to ordered movement]: taxonomy, chemotaxis

tomo-, -tome, -tomy, [Gk. tome, a cutting; Gk. tomos, slice]: atom [can't be cut], anatomy

tropho-, -troph, -trophy [Gk. trophe, nutrition]: trophic level, trophoblast, atrophy, autotroph, heterotroph

ur-, -uria [Gk. ouron, urine]: uracil, urea, ureter, phenylketonuria

Glossary

abducens nerve   The cranial nerve (VI) that supplies the lateral rectus muscle of the eyeball (lateral movement).

abduction   Motion of a limb away from the midline.

abrasion   An injury in which the involved body part has lost its outer layer of skin or mucous membrane because it has been rubbed or scratched off.

absolute refractory period   The early phase of repolarization in which the cell contains such a large concentration of ions that it cannot be stimulated to depolarize.

absorptive cells   Cells that produce digestive enzymes and absorb digested food.

accessory nerve   The cranial nerve (XI) that provides motor innervation to the muscles of the soft palate and the pharynx and to the sternocleidomastoid and trapezius muscles; also referred to as the spinal accessory nerve.

acetabulum   The depression on the lateral pelvis where its three component bones join, articulates with the femoral head.

acetylcholine   A chemical neurotransmitter that serves as a mediator in both the sympathetic and parasympathetic nervous system.

acetylcholinesterase   An enzyme that causes muscle relaxation by helping to break down acetylcholine.

Achilles tendon   The strong tendon that joins the muscles in the posterior leg to the calcaneus.

acids   Electrolytes that dissociate in water to release hydrogen ions.

acquired immune deficiency syndrome (AIDS)   The disease process that occurs following infection with the human immunodeficiency virus (HIV).

acromegaly   A disorder caused by chronic overproduction of growth hormone by the pituitary gland that is characterized by a gradual and permanent enlargement of the flat bones (the lower jaw) and of the hands and feet, abdominal organs, nose, lips, and tongue; also called gigantism.

acromioclavicular (AC) joint   The point at which the clavicle attaches to the acromion process.

acromioclavicular (AC) separation   An injury caused by distraction of the clavicle away from the acromion process of the scapula.

acromion process   The tip of the shoulder and the site of attachment for both the clavicle and shoulder musculature.

actin   The component that makes up most of the thin protein filaments of the myofibrils.

action potentials   An electrochemical event associated with cell membrane depolarization that occurs when a cell or tissue has been activated by a stimulus.

activation energy   The amount of energy required to start a reaction.

active transport   A method used to move compounds across a cell membrane to create or maintain an imbalance of charges, usually against a concentration gradient and requiring the expenditure of energy.

acute urinary retention   A complete obstruction of urinary flow sometimes caused by enlargement of the prostate gland.

adaptive (specific) defense   Immunity; it targets specific pathogens and acts more slowly than innate defenses.

addisonian crisis   Acute adrenocortical insufficiency.

adduction   Motion of a limb toward the midline.

adductor brevis   The short muscle that adducts the thigh.

adductor longus   The long muscle that adducts the hip.

adenohypophysis   One of the two portions of the pituitary gland, it produces hormones that are not neurohormones; also called the anterior pituitary.

adenosine triphosphate (ATP)   The major source of energy created by cellular respiration for all chemical reactions of the body.

adipose (fat) tissue   A type of connective tissue that contains large amounts of fat.

adrenal cortex   The outer layer of the adrenal gland, it produces hormones that are important in regulating the water and salt balance of the body.

adrenal glands   Endocrine glands located on top of the kidneys that release epinephrine and norepinephrine when stimulated by the sympathetic nervous system.

adrenaline   A naturally occurring hormone that also may be given as a cardiac drug and has alpha and beta effects; also called epinephrine.

adrenergic   Description of a neuron that secretes the neurotransmitter norepinephrine.

adrenergic receptors   A type of receptor that is associated with the sympathetic nerves and is stimulated by epinephrine and norepinephrine.

adrenocorticotropic hormone (ACTH)   Hormone that targets the adrenal cortex to secrete cortisol.

adventitia   The muscular layer of the wall of the alimentary canal.

aerobic metabolism   A biochemical process that occurs in the presence of oxygen and results in the production of energy in the form of ATP; also called cellular respiration.

afferent arteriole   The structure of the kidney that supplies blood to the glomerulus.

afferent nerves   Nerves that send information to the brain; also called sensory nerves.

afterload   The pressure in the aorta against which the left ventricle must pump blood.

agonist   A prime mover; a muscle that contracts to provide most of a desired movement.

agranulocytes   Leukocytes that lack granules.

albinism   A condition of the skin resulting from the inability to synthesize melanin.

albumins   The smallest of plasma proteins; they make up about 60% of these proteins by weight.

aldosterone   One of two main hormones responsible for adjustments to the final composition of urine; increases the rate of active reabsorption of sodium and chloride ions into the blood and decreases reabsorption of potassium.

alimentary canal   The mouth, pharynx, esophagus, stomach, small intestine, large intestine, rectum, and anus.

allele   Variant form of a gene, which can be identical or slightly different in DNA sequence.

allergens   Antigens; chemicals that stimulate B cells to produce antibodies or allergies.

alpha cells   Cells located in the islets of Langerhans that secrete glucagon.

alpha effect   Stimulation of alpha receptors that results in vasoconstriction.

alpha receptors   One of two adrenergic receptors classified into two structural and functional categories; alpha receptors are further subdivided into alpha-1 and alpha-2 receptors.

alveolar arch   The ridges between the teeth, which are covered with thickened connective tissue and epithelium; also called alveolar ridges.

alveolar ducts   Ducts formed from division of the respiratory bronchioles in the lower airway; each duct ends in clusters known as alveoli.

alveoli   Tiny sacs of lung tissue in which gas exchange takes place.

alveolocapillary membrane   The very thin membrane, consisting of only one cell layer, that lies between the alveolus and capillary, through which respiratory exchange between the alveolus and the blood vessels occurs. Also known as the pulmonary capillary membrane.

amniocentesis   A procedure of extracting amniotic fluid from the uterus using a needle and ultrasound or CT scan guidance.

amniotic fluid   Fluid produced by the filtration of maternal and fetal blood through blood vessels in the placenta and by excretion of fetal urine into the amniotic sac.

amniotic membranes   The placenta and membranes that surround and protect the developing embryo.

amniotic sac   The sac formed from the amniotic membranes that surround and protect the developing embryo.

ampulla (prostate gland)   A pouch in the vas deferens at the prostate gland.

ampulla   An expansion at the end of each semicircular canal containing a crista ampullaris.

ampulla of Vater   Opening in the duodenum into which the common bile duct and the pancreatic duct drain.

amputation   Completely cutting or tearing off of a body part.

anabolic steroids   Synthetic androgens used to increase muscle mass.

anabolism   The synthesis of larger molecules from smaller ones.

anaerobic metabolism   An alternate form of metabolism that occurs when oxygen levels are low and less energy is produced than during aerobic respiration; lactic acid is produced as a waste product during this process.

anal canal   The short tube at the end of the rectum that contains two circular sphincters (internal and external), which help regulate the passage of stool.

anal triangle   The area within the pelvis that contains the anus.

anaphylaxis   An extreme systemic form of an allergic reaction involving two or more body systems.

anatomic planes   Imaginary surfaces used as references to identify parts of the body.

anatomic position   The position of reference in which the patient stands facing you, arms at the side, with the palms of the hands forward.

anatomy   The study of the structure of an organism and its parts.

androgens   Male sex hormones.

androstenedione   A steroid sex hormone secreted by the adrenal cortex, testes, and ovaries.

anemia   A lower than normal hemoglobin or erythrocyte level.

angiotensin II   A form of kinin that plays a role in blood pressure maintenance by causing vasoconstriction and sympathetic activation and by stimulating the adrenal gland to increase the production of aldosterone.

anion   An ion that contains an overall negative charge.

antagonists   Muscles working in opposition to each other.

antecubital fossa   The anterior surface at the bend of the elbow.

anterior   The front surface of the body; the side facing forward in the anatomic position.

anterior chamber   The anterior area of the globe between the lens and the cornea that is filled with aqueous humor.

anterior descending (LAD) coronary artery   One of the two branches of the left main coronary artery.

anterior pituitary (lobe)   One of the two portions of the pituitary gland; it produces hormones that are not neurohormones; also called the adenohypophysis.

anterior spinothalamic tracts   Ascending fiber tracts that carry information to the brain about light touch, pressure, and tickling and itching sensations.

anterior triangle   The area of the neck that is bordered by the sternocleidomastoid muscle, the anterior midline of the neck, and the inferior border of the mandible.

antibodies   Immunoglobulins; proteins secreted by certain immune cells that react against foreign antigens in the body by binding to the antigens, making them more visible to the immune system.

antidiuretic   hormone (ADH) A hormone released by the pituitary gland that causes the kidney to reabsorb more water into the blood and excrete less urine.

antidiuretic hormone (ADH)   A hormone secreted by the posterior pituitary lobe of the pituitary gland; constricts blood vessels and raises the blood pressure, and also is responsible for adjustments to the final composition of urine by causing ducts in the kidney to become more permeable to water; also called vasopressin.

antigen-presenting cell   An accessory cell, which may be a macrophage, B cell, or other type of cell that has processed antigen fragments on its surface.

antigens   Substances or molecules that, when taken into the body, stimulate an immune system response and cause formation of specific protective proteins called antibodies.

anulus fibrosus   A ring of fibrous or fibrocartilaginous tissue that is part of the intervertebral disk.

anus   The distal orifice of the alimentary canal, where stool passes from the body.

aorta   The principal artery leaving the left side of the heart and carrying freshly oxygenated blood to the body; the largest artery in the body.

aortic arch   One of the three described portions of the aorta; the section of the aorta between the ascending and descending portions that gives rise to the right brachiocephalic (innominate), left common carotid, and left subclavian arteries.

aortic valve   The semilunar valve that regulates blood flow from the left ventricle to the aorta.

apocrine glands   Coiled tubular glands that usually open into hair follicles of the axillae and genitalia, as well as around the anus.

aponeuroses   Broad sheets of fibers that may attach to bones or to the coverings of other muscles.

appendicitis   Inflammation of the appendix.

appendicular region   A division of the skeletal system that includes the extremities and their attachments to the body.

appendicular skeleton   The portion of the skeletal system that comprises the arms, legs, pelvis, and shoulder girdle.

appositional growth   The formation of new bone on the surface of a bone.

aqueous humor   The clear, watery fluid in the anterior chamber of the globe.

arachnoid   The middle membrane of the three meninges that enclose the brain and spinal cord.

areola   The pigmented ring around the nipple in the breast.

areolar glands   Glands that produce secretions that protect the nipple and areola during nursing.

arrector pili muscle   Muscle attached at the base of the hair that pulls the hair perpendicular to the surface of the skin in cold or threatening situations.

arteries   The muscular, thick-walled blood vessels that carry blood away from the heart.

arterioles   Subdivisions of arteries that are thinner and have muscles in their walls that are innervated by the sympathetic nervous system.

arteriosclerosis   A pathologic disease in which the arterial walls become thickened and inelastic.

asbestosis   A disease of the lungs caused by inhalation of asbestos particles.

ascending aorta   The first of three portions of the aorta; originates from the left ventricle and gives rise to two branches, the right and left main coronary arteries.

ascending colon   One of four portions of the colon; it extends upward from the cecum.

ascending reticular activating system   Several structures located throughout the brainstem that are responsible for maintenance of consciousness.

ascending tracts   Fibers that carry sensory information from the periphery to the brain; also called afferent tracts.

asthma   A chronic inflammatory lower airway disease resulting in intermittent wheezing and excess mucus production.

atherosclerosis   A disorder characterized by the formation of plaques of material, mostly lipids and cholesterol, on the inner arterial walls.

atlas   The first cervical vertebra (C1), which provides support for the head.

atomic number   A whole number representing the number of positively charged protons in the nucleus of an atom.

atomic weight   The total number of protons and neutrons in the nucleus of an atom.

atoms   The smallest complete units of an element that have the element's properties; they vary in size, weight, and interaction with other atoms.

atria   The upper chambers of the heart; they receive blood returning to the heart.

atrioventricular (AV) node   A specialized structure located in the AV junction that slows conduction through the AV junction.

atrioventricular valves   The mitral and tricuspid valves through which blood flows from the atria to the ventricles.

auditory ossicles   The three small bones in the middle ear: the malleus, incus, and stapes.

auricle   The large outside portion of the ear through which sound waves enter the ear; also called the pinna.

autoantibodies   Antibodies produced by the body in reaction to any of its own cells or cell products.

autocrine   Denoting self-stimulation through cellular production of a factor and a specific receptor for it.

autoimmunity   An abnormal immune response in which the body attacks its own tissues.

automaticity   A state in which the cardiac cells are at rest, waiting for the generation of a spontaneous impulse from within.

autonomic nervous system   A subdivision of the nervous system that operates without conscious control and regulates the function of the internal organs, glands, and smooth muscle; comprised of the sympathetic and parasympathetic nervous systems.

autosomes   The chromosomes that do not carry genes that determine sex.

avulsion   A wound in which flaps of skin and tissue are torn loose or pulled off completely.

axial region   A division of the skeletal system that includes the head, neck, and trunk.

axial skeleton   The part of the skeleton comprising the skull, spinal column, and rib cage.

axilla   The armpit.

axillary nerve   One of the major nerves emanating from the brachial plexus; it supplies the deltoid and teres minor muscles, enabling arm abduction and lateral rotation.

axillary nodes   A large collection of lymph nodes located in the axilla (armpit).

axillary vein   The vein that is formed from the combination of the basilic and cephalic veins; it drains into the subclavian vein.

axis   The second cervical vertebra, the point that allows the head to turn.

axons   Long, slender filaments projecting from a nerve cell that conduct impulses to adjacent cells.

B lymphocytes (B cells)   Lymphocytes that produce and secrete antibodies that bind and destroy foreign antigens; they exist in the blood, lymph nodes, bone marrow, intestinal lining, and spleen.

baroreceptors   Receptors in the blood vessels, kidneys, brain, and heart that respond to changes in pressure in the heart or main arteries to help maintain homeostasis.

basal ganglia   (basal nuclei) Structures located deep within the cerebrum, diencephalon, and midbrain that play an important role in coordination of motor movements and posture.

basal lamina   A thin, noncellular layer of ground substance lying under epithelial surfaces that separates the epidermis from the areolar tissue of the adjacent dermis.

basal metabolic rate (BMR)   The rate at which nutrients are consumed in the body.

basement membrane   The noncellular layer in an epithelial cell that anchors the overlying epithelial tissues.

bases   Electrolytes that release ions that bond with hydrogen ions.

basilar artery   The artery that is formed when the left and right vertebral arteries unite after entering the brain through the foramen magnum.

basilic vein   One of the two major veins of the arm; it combines with the cephalic vein to form the axillary vein.

basophils   White blood cells that work to produce chemical mediators during an immune response; make up approximately 1% of leukocytes.

Battle sign   Bruising over the mastoid process, usually from a basilar skull fracture.

Bell palsy   A condition caused by damage, either through trauma or infection, to the facial nerve, resulting in an inability to move the facial muscles on the affected side.

beta cells   Cells located in the islets of Langerhans that secrete insulin.

beta effect Stimulation of beta receptors that results in increased inotropic, dromotropic, and chronotropic states.

beta receptors One of two adrenergic receptors classified into two structural and functional categories; beta receptors are further subdivided into beta-1, beta-2, and beta-3 receptors.

beta-blockers A common class of cardiac drugs that blocks beta effects, causing a decrease in the workload of the heart by reducing the speed of contraction, as well as reducing blood pressure.

beta-endorphins Proteins produced in the hypothalamus and anterior pituitary that have the same effects as opiate drugs such as morphine but are 80 times more potent.

bicarbonate ions Ions related to carbonic acid; they are formed from carbon dioxide transport mechanisms.

biceps femoris Located in the posterior compartment of the leg; flexes and laterally rotates the knee and extends the hip.

bile A digestive enzyme produced in the liver and stored in the gallbladder.

bilirubin A waste product of red blood cell destruction that undergoes further metabolism in the liver.

black lung disease A disease of the lung caused by consistent inhalation of coal dust.

blood The fluid tissue that is pumped by the heart through the arteries, veins, and capillaries and consists of plasma and formed elements or cells, such as red blood cells, white blood cells, and platelets.

body cavities Hollow areas within the body that contain organs and organ systems.

bone marrow Specialized tissue found within bone that manufactures most erythrocytes.

brachial plexus The plexus of spinal nerves that consists of nerves C5 to T1 and innervates the shoulder and upper extremity.

brain The controlling organ of the body and center of consciousness; functions include perception, control of reactions to the environment, emotional responses, and judgment.

brainstem The area of the brain between the spinal cord and cerebrum, surrounded by the cerebellum; controls functions that are necessary for life, such as respiration.

breast cancer Cancer in one or both breasts.

breasts Structures that contain the organs of milk production.

broad ligaments One of several ligaments that support the uterus.

bronchial arteries Arteries that branch off of the thoracic aorta and supply the lung tissues with blood.

bronchial veins Veins that return deoxygenated blood to the heart from the lungs.

bronchioles Fine subdivisions of the bronchi that give rise to the alveolar ducts; made of smooth muscle and dilate or constrict in response to various stimuli.

bronchodilator Medication that is designed to improve lung function by widening the bronchial tubes.

bronchospasm Severe constriction of the bronchial tree.

bruit An abnormal whooshing sound indicating turbulent blood flow within a narrowed blood vessel; usually heard in the carotid arteries.

bruxism Grinding together of the upper and lower teeth.

bulb of the penis The area of the corpus spongiosum that expands at the base of the penis.

bulbourethral glands Glands that lie inferior to the prostate gland and secrete a lubricating fluid that prepares the penis for sexual intercourse.

bulging disk A ballooning of an intervertebral disk without frank herniation.

bundle of His The portion of the electric conduction system in the interventricular septum that conducts the depolarizing impulse from the atrioventricular junction to the right and left bundle branches.

burns The result of heat or other thermal injury to the skin.

bursae Small fluid-filled sacs located between a tendon and a bone help lubricate two surfaces that are rubbing against each other.

calcaneus The heel bone.

calcitonin A hormone produced by the parafollicular cells of the thyroid gland that is important in the regulation of calcium levels in the body.

callus The zone of repair in which a mass of exudates and connective tissue forms around a break in a bone and converts to bone during healing.

calmodulin An intracellular protein to which calcium binds, resulting in muscle contraction.

calorie The amount of heat needed to raise the temperature of one gram of water by 1°C.

calyces Large urinary tubes that enter the renal pelvis from kidney tissue.

canaliculi A minute canal in a bone.

cancellous bone Bone that is made up of a lacy network of bony rods called trabeculae.

capillaries Thin-walled vessels that allow oxygen and nutrients to pass out into the cells and allow carbon dioxide and waste products to pass from the cells into the capillaries.

carbaminohemoglobin The bonding of carbon dioxide with hemoglobin.

carbohydrates Substances (including sugars and starches) that provide much of the energy required by the body's cells, as well as help to build cell structures.

carbonic anhydrase An enzyme in red blood cells that speeds reaction of carbon dioxide and water, resulting in carbonic acid.

carboxypeptidase A pancreatic enzyme that digests proteins.

cardiac conduction system A group of complex electrical tissues within the heart that initiate and transmit stimuli that result in contractions of myocardial tissue.

cardiac cycle A heartbeat; each cardiac cycle consists of ventricular contraction (systole) and relaxation (diastole).

cardiac muscle Muscle that is found only in the heart, providing the contractions needed to propel the blood through the circulatory system.

cardiac muscle tissue Striated involuntary muscle that has the capacity to generate and conduct electrical impulses.

cardiac output The amount of blood pumped by the heart per minute, calculated by multiplying the stroke volume by the heart rate per minute.

cardiac tamponade Restriction of cardiac contraction, failing cardiac output, and shock, caused by the accumulation of fluid or blood in the pericardium.

cardiac veins Veins that branch out and drain blood from the myocardial capillaries to join the coronary sinus.

carina A ridgelike projection of tracheal cartilage located where the trachea bifurcates into the right and left mainstem bronchi.

carotid bifurcation The point of division at which the common carotid artery branches at the angle of the mandible into the internal and external carotid arteries.

carotid canals An opening in the cranial vault through which the carotid arteries enter.

carotid sinus A slight dilation in the carotid bifurcation that contains structures that are important in the regulation of blood pressure.

carotid triangle Area of the anterior triangle of the neck that contains the carotid artery and internal jugular vein.

carpal tunnel syndrome (CTS) Compression of the median nerve within the carpal canal at the wrist.

carpals The bones of the wrist; they include the scaphoid, lunate, triquetrum, pisiform, trapezium, trapezoid, capitate, and hamate bones.

carrier state An autosomal-recessive condition with only one abnormal allele and no disease state that could be passed on if the carrier mates with another carrier.

cartilage The support structure of the skeletal system that provides cushioning between bones; also forms the nasal septum and portions of the outer ear.

catabolism The breakdown of larger molecules into smaller molecules.

catalysts Atoms or molecules that can change the rate of a reaction without being consumed during the process.

cataracts Clouding in the lens of the eye or its surrounding transparent membrane; normally a result of aging.

cation An ion that contains an overall positive charge.

cauda equina Numerous individual nerve roots that extend from the spinal cord at the level of the second lumbar vertebra.

CD4 antigen A protein found on the surface of helper T cells that is adversely affected by exposure to HIV.

cecum The first part of the large intestine, into which the ileum opens.

cell-mediated immunity The immune process by which T cell lymphocytes and macrophages attack and destroy pathogens or foreign substances; the process involves recognizing antigens, then secreting cytokines (specifically lymphokines) that attract other cells or stimulate the production of cytotoxic cells that kill the infected cells.

cell membrane The cell wall; a selectively permeable layer of cells that surrounds intracellular contents and controls movement of substances into and out of the cell.

cells The basic building blocks of life, made up of protoplasm (cytoplasm); specialized for particular functions.

cellular immune response Cell-mediated immunity; it occurs when T cells attach to foreign, antigen-bearing cells such as bacterial cells, and interact with direct cell-to-cell contact.

cellular metabolism Process within a cell where nutrients are broken down from complex to simpler forms or where complex forms are built from simpler blocks.

cellular respiration A biochemical process resulting in the production of energy in the form of adenosine triphosphate; also called metabolism.

central disk herniation The most serious disk rupture that occurs when nuclear material protrudes straight back into the spinal canal, potentially compressing neurologic elements and causing neurologic injury.

central nervous system The brain and spinal cord.

centrioles Organelles that are essential in cell division.

cephalic vein One of the two major veins of the arm that combine to form the axillary vein.

cerebellar peduncles One of three bands of nerve fibers through which the cerebellum communicates with other regions of the central nervous system.

cerebellum The part of the brain that is located dorsal to the pons and is responsible for coordination and balance.

cerebral arteries The arteries that supply blood to large portions of the cerebral cortex of the brain.

cerebral cortex The largest portion of the brain, it controls the higher thought processes; also called the cerebrum.

cerebrospinal fluid (CSF) Fluid produced in the ventricles of the brain that flows in the subarachnoid space and bathes the meninges.

cerebrum The largest portion of the brain that controls the higher thought processes, including control of movement, hearing, balance, speech, visual perception, emotions, and personality; also called the cerebral cortex.

cervical nodes A large collection of lymph nodes located in the neck.

cervical vertebrae The seven smallest vertebrae, found in the neck.

cervix The narrowest portion (lower third of the neck) of the uterus that opens into the vagina.

chemical digestion Digestion of food by enzymes in the stomach and small bowel.

chemistry The study of the composition of matter and changes in its composition.

chemoreceptors Sense organs that monitor the levels of oxygen and carbon dioxide and the pH of the cerebrospinal fluid and blood and provide feedback to the respiratory centers to modify the rate and depth of breathing based on the body's needs at any given time.

chemotaxis The movement of additional white blood cells to an area of inflammation in response to the release of chemical mediators.

chief cells Cells in the stomach mucosa that produce pepsinogen, an important enzyme in the digestion of food.

cholecystitis Symptoms from cholelithiasis; also called a gallbladder attack.

cholecystokinin A hormone produced in the intestine that stimulates the production of pancreatic secretions and gallbladder contractions and inhibits gastric motility.

cholelithiasis The presence of gallstones.

cholinergic A term used to describe the fibers in the parasympathetic nervous system that release a chemical called acetylcholine.

chondroblasts Cells that produce cartilage.

chordae tendineae Thin bands of fibrous tissue that attach to the valves in the heart and prevent them from inverting.

choroid plexus Specialized cells within hollow areas in the ventricles of the brain that produce cerebrospinal fluid.

chromatin Protein matter in which chromosomes are contained within a cell.

chromosomes Structures of DNA fibers and protein contained within the cell's nucleus carrying genetic information; human cells contain 23 chromosomes.

chronic bronchitis A chronic inflammatory condition affecting the bronchi that is associated with excess mucus production that results from overgrowth of the mucous glands in the airways.

chronic obstructive pulmonary disease (COPD) A progressive and irreversible disease of the airway marked by decreased inspiratory and expiratory capacity of the lungs.

chronotropic effect The effect on the rate of contraction of the heart.

chyme The name given to the substance that leaves the stomach once food is digested; it is a combination of all of the eaten foods with added stomach acids.

chymotrypsin A pancreatic enzyme that digests proteins.

cilia The hairlike microtubule projections on the surface of a cell that can move materials over the cell surface.

circadian rhythms Associated with environmental day and night cycles; these rhythms help the body to distinguish day from night.

circle of Willis An interconnection of the anterior, middle, and posterior cerebral arteries and the anterior communicating artery, which forms an important source of collateral circulation to the brain.

circulatory system The complex arrangement of tubes, including the arteries, arterioles, capillaries, venules, and veins, that moves blood, oxygen, nutrients, carbon dioxide, and cellular waste throughout the body.

circumcision Surgical removal of the foreskin of the glans of the penis.

circumflex coronary artery One of the two branches of the left main coronary artery.

clavicle The collarbone; it is lateral to the sternum and anterior to the scapula.

clitoris In females, a small, cylindrical mass of erectile tissue and nerves located at the anterior junction of the labia minora, similar to the glans penis of the male.

closed fracture A fracture in which the bone ends have not been exposed by a break through the skin.

coagulation The formation of a blood clot.

coccyx The tailbone.

cochlea The shell-shaped structure within the inner ear that contains the organ of Corti.

cochlear duct A canal within the cochlea that receives vibrations from the ossicles.

collecting ducts The thoracic duct and right lymphatic duct.

colon A portion of the gastrointestinal system extending from the small intestine to the rectum that maintains water balance by absorbing and excreting water; also called the large intestine.

colonoscope A fiberoptic scope used in the visual examination of the colon.

columnar epithelium Rows of tall, thin epithelial cells.

common peroneal nerve A major nerve of the leg, providing sensation to the lateral leg and dorsum of the foot and motor activity to hip extensors, knee flexors, ankle dorsiflexors, and toe extensors.

compact bone Bone that is mostly solid, with few spaces.

compartment syndrome Accumulation of blood or fluid in a fascial compartment, typically following trauma, resulting in compression of blood vessels and tissue damage secondary to ischemia and, if not recognized and promptly treated, death of muscle and loss of the limb.

compartments Anatomic spaces within the body that are enclosed by fascia.

compounds Molecules made up of different bonded atoms.

compression fracture A fracture of a vertebral body associated with collapse of the body.

concentration gradient The natural tendency for substances to flow from an area of higher concentration to an area of lower concentration, within or outside the cell.

conchae Three bony ridges contained within the lateral walls of the nasopharynx.

conductivity The ability of cardiac cells to conduct electrical impulses.

conjunctiva A thin, transparent membrane that covers the sclera and internal surfaces of the eyelids.

conjunctivitis An inflammation of the conjunctivae that usually is caused by bacteria, viruses, or allergies and should be considered highly contagious; also called pink eye.

Conn syndrome A condition that results in excess secretion of aldosterone, most commonly caused by a benign tumor.

contractility The strength of heart muscle contraction.

cornea The transparent anterior portion of the eye that overlies the iris and pupil.

coronal suture The point where the parietal bones join together with the frontal bone.

coronary arteries Arteries that arise from the aorta shortly after it leaves the left ventricle and supply the heart with oxygen and nutrients.

coronary artery disease The condition that results when either atherosclerosis or arteriosclerosis is present in the arterial walls of the coronary arteries.

coronary sinus Veins that collect blood that is returning from the walls of the heart.

corpus cavernosus The erectile tissue found in the clitoris and penis.

corpus luteum Yellow body; a temporary glandular structure created from enlarged follicular cells because of the release of luteinizing hormone.

corpus spongiosum Erectile tissue that surrounds the male urethra.

corticospinal tracts Descending tracts that coordinate movements, especially of the hands.

corticosteroids Any of several steroids secreted by the adrenal gland.

cortisol The most important corticosteroid secreted by the zona fasciculata of the adrenal cortex, it has many effects on the body.

costochondritis Inflammation of the costal cartilage, which attaches the ribs to the sternum.

countercurrent multiplier mechanism A process by which the body produces either concentrated or diluted urine, depending on the body's needs.

covalent bond A chemical bond where atoms complete their outer electron shells by sharing electrons.

cranial cavity The hollow portion of the skull.

cranial nerves The 12 pairs of nerves that arise from the base of the brain.

cranium The bones that encase and protect the brain, including the parietal, temporal, frontal, occipital, sphenoid, and ethmoid bones.

creatine phosphate An organic compound in muscle tissue that can store and provide energy for muscle contraction.

cremaster muscle The muscle that contracts and pulls the testicles close to the body during cold weather.

crenation Shrinkage of a cell that results when too much water leaves the cell through osmosis.

crepitus A grinding sound or sensation.

cribriform plates Horizontal bones perforated with numerous foramina for the passage of the olfactory nerve filaments from the nasal cavity.

crista A small elevation in each ear canal.

crista ampullaris The sensory organ in a semicircular canal that aids with dynamic equilibrium.

crista galli A prominent bony ridge in the center of the anterior fossa to which the meninges are attached.

crus of the penis Area at the base of the penis formed by the expanded corpora cavernosa.

crypts Tubular glands located in the colon, which contain many mucus-producing goblet cells.

cuboidal epithelium Rows of square-shaped epithelial cells.

cupula A cap of gelatinous tissue in the ear that is involved in the sensation of balance and movement.

curare An agent that blocks transmission of neural motor impulses at the neuromuscular junction.

Cushing syndrome A condition caused by excessive production of cortisol by the adrenal glands resulting in obesity, abnormal hair growth, high blood pressure, emotional disturbances, and cushingoid facies or the so-called "moonface."

cusps The flaps that comprise the heart valves.

cystic duct The route through which the gallbladder releases bile.

cystitis A bacterial infection of the bladder and its urinary contents.

cytoplasm The gel-like material inside a cell. It makes up most of the cell's volume, and suspends the cell's organelles; also called protoplasm.

cytosol The clear liquid portion of the cytoplasm.

dartos muscle A layer of cutaneous muscle within the scrotum that contracts during cold weather, causing the skin to become firm and wrinkled.

decomposition reaction A reaction that occurs when bonds with a reactant molecule break, forming simpler atoms, molecules, or ions.

deep peroneal nerve A component and branch of the common peroneal nerve that innervates the muscles that dorsiflex the ankle and extend the toes.

degenerative disk disease A progressive form of arthritis that causes deterioration of the intervertebral disk.

dendrites Components of the neurons that receive impulses from the axon and contain vesicles for release of neurotransmitters.

deoxyribonucleic acid (DNA) The genetic material found on the chromosomes in the cell's nucleus.

depolarization The rapid movement of electrolytes across a cell membrane that changes the cell's overall charge. This rapid shifting of electrolytes and cellular charges is the main catalyst for muscle contractions and neural transmissions.

dermatome An area of skin that corresponds to the sensory distribution of a specific cranial or spinal nerve.

dermis The inner layer of the skin, containing hair follicles, sweat glands, nerve endings, and blood vessels; located immediately above the hypodermis.

descending aorta One of the three portions of the aorta; it is the longest portion and extends through the thorax and abdomen into the pelvis.

descending colon One of four portions of the colon; it extends from the splenic flexure to the sigmoid colon.

descending tracts Fibers that carry motor impulses from the brain to the fibers of the peripheral nervous system; also called efferent tracts.

desmosomes Cell structures specialized for cell-to-cell adhesion.

detrusor muscle Surrounding the neck of the bladder to form the internal urethral sphincter, this muscle functions in the micturition reflex.

diabetes insipidus A condition often caused by pituitary dysfunction that is associated with production of large volumes of dilute urine and in which patients experience intense thirst.

diabetes mellitus A disease that results from impaired production of insulin by the pancreas.

diapedesis A process whereby leukocytes leave blood vessels to move toward tissue where they are needed most.

diaphragm A large dome-shaped muscle that forms the undersurface of the thorax, separating the chest from the abdominal cavity. Contraction of the diaphragm (and the chest wall muscles) brings air into the lungs. Relaxation allows air to be expelled from the lungs.

diaphysis The shaft of a long bone.

diencephalon The part of the brain between the brainstem and the cerebrum that includes the thalamus and hypothalamus.

diffusion A process where molecules move from an area of higher concentration to an area of lower concentration.

digestion The mechanical and chemical breakdown of foods and the absorption of resulting nutrients by the body's cells.

digestive system The body system that carries out the processes of mechanical and chemical digestion; also called the gastrointestinal system.

diploid Cells that carry two of each of the 23 chromosomes—one from the father and one from the mother.

disaccharidases Enzymes that break down sugars.

displaced fracture A fracture in which bone fragments are separated from one another and are not in anatomic alignment.

distal (nephron) One of two complex sections of a nephron; it empties urine into a collection duct that then carries it to the calyces.

distal Farther from the trunk or nearer to the free end of an extremity.

diverticuli Weakened areas (outpouchings) in the walls of the colon.

diverticulitis Inflammation of the diverticuli.

dorsal The posterior surface of the body, including the back of the hand.

dorsal root One of two roots of a spinal nerve that passes posteriorly into the spinal cord and contains the dorsal root ganglion.

dorsal root ganglion A ganglion on the dorsal root of each spinal nerve.

dorsalis pedis artery A continuation of the anterior tibial artery at the foot.

dromotropic effect Related to the effect of the heart's conduction rate.

duodenojejunal flexure The sharp bend in the small intestine between the duodenum and the jejunum.

duodenum The first of three sections of the small intestine; it extends posteriorly from the stomach and forms a 180° arch within the retroperitoneal portion of the abdomen.

dura mater The outermost of the three meninges that enclose the brain and spinal cord; it is the toughest membrane.

dwarfism A condition resulting in abnormally small bones caused by a hormonal growth deficiency.

dynamic equilibrium Maintenance of balance when the head and body are suddenly moved or rotated.

dysrhythmias   Disturbances in cardiac rhythm.

ear canal   The cavity leading from the exterior atmosphere to the tympanum; also called the external auditory canal.

eardrum   A thin membrane that separates the middle ear from the inner ear and transmits vibrations to the ossicles; also called the tympanic membrane.

ectopic pregnancy   A pregnancy in which the ovum implants somewhere other than the uterine endometrium.

efferent arteriole   Structure of the kidney that drains blood from the glomerulus.

efferent ductule   The pathway by which spermatozoa leave the testes.

efferent nerves   Nerves that carry commands from the brain to peripheral muscles; also called motor nerves.

ejaculatory duct   A structure formed by the vasa deferentia uniting with the duct of a seminal vesicle; this type of duct passes through the prostate gland to empty into the urethra.

ejection fraction   The percentage of blood that leaves the heart each time it contracts.

electrical potential   An electrical charge difference that is created by the difference in sodium and potassium concentration across the cell membrane at any given instant.

electrocardiogram (ECG)   A graphic recording of the electrical activity of the heart.

electrolytes   Salt or acid substances that become ionic conductors when dissolved in a solvent (ie, water); chemicals dissolved in the blood.

electrons   Single, negatively charged particles that revolve around the nucleus of an atom.

eleidin   Granules within the stratum lucidum that are formed from keratohyaline and are eventually transformed to keratin.

elements   Fundamental substances, such as carbon, hydrogen, and oxygen, that compose matter.

embolus   A piece of clot that travels from one part of the body to another, potentially becoming an obstruction to blood flow.

embryo   A fertilized egg.

embryoblast   The inner group of cells within a zygote that develops to become the embryo.

embryonic period   The period of gestation between weeks 3 and 8 in which all major organ systems begin to develop.

emphysema   The infiltration of any tissue by air or gas; a chronic obstructive pulmonary disease characterized by distention of the alveoli and destructive changes in the lung parenchyma.

endocarditis   Infection of a heart valve.

endochondral growth   The growth of cartilage in the physis (epiphyseal plate) which is eventually replaced by bone.

endocrine cells   Cells in the stomach mucosa that produce regulatory hormones.

endocrine glands   Glands that produce and secrete hormones into the bloodstream.

endocrine system   The complex message and control system that integrates many body functions, including the release of hormones.

endocytosis   The uptake of material through the cell membrane by a membrane-bound droplet or vesicle formed within the cell's protoplasm.

endolymph   Fluid in the membranous labyrinth of the ear.

endometrium   The inner layer of the uterine wall.

endomysium   The delicate connective tissue surrounding individual muscular fibers.

endoplasmic reticulum   A series of membranes in which proteins and fats are manufactured.

endosteum   A layer that lines the inner surfaces of bone.

enzymes   Substances designed to speed up the rate of specific biochemical reactions.

eosinophils   White blood cells with a major role in allergic reactions and bronchoconstriction during an asthma attack; make up approximately 1% to 3% of leukocytes.

epicardium   The layer of the serous pericardium that lies closely against the heart; also called the visceral pericardium.

epicondylitis   An inflammation of the muscles of the elbow joint; more commonly known as tennis elbow.

epidermis   The superficial, outer layer of the skin that contains numerous nerve vessels, but no nerve endings; acts as the body's first line of defense.

epididymides   Tightly coiled tubes connected to ducts within a testis; they become the vas deferens.

epiglottis   A leaf-shaped cartilaginous structure that closes over the trachea during swallowing.

epimysium   A layer of connective tissue that closely surrounds skeletal muscles.

epinephrine   Hormone produced by the adrenal medulla that has a vital role in the function of the sympathetic nervous system; also called adrenaline.

epiphyses   The growth plate of a long bone.

epithalamus   Part of the diencephalon with functions related to emotions, circadian rhythms, and connecting the limbic system with other parts of the brain.

erythroblastosis fetalis   A serious condition that results when a pregnant woman's blood type is incompatible with the fetus' blood type and antibodies from the mother enter the fetal circulation and destroy the fetus' red blood cells.

erythrocytes   Disk-shaped cells that carry oxygen to the tissues; also known as red blood cells.

erythropoiesis   The process by which red blood cells are made.

esophageal hiatus   An opening in the diaphragm through which the esophagus passes.

esophageal sphincters   Two muscular rings (upper and lower) that regulate the movement of material into and out of the esophagus.

esophagus   A collapsible tube that extends from the pharynx to the stomach; contractions of the muscle in the wall of the esophagus propel food and liquids to the stomach.

estrogen   A hormone released from the ovaries that stimulates the uterine lining during the menstrual cycle; it is one of three major female hormones.

ethmoid bone   The main supporting structure of the nasal cavities; it also forms part of the eye orbits.

exchange reaction   A chemical reaction where parts of the reacting molecules are shuffled around to produce new products.

excitability   A property of cardiac cells that provides the cells with the ability to respond to electrical impulses.

exocrine glands   Glands that secrete chemicals for elimination.

exocytosis   The release of secretions from cells that have been accumulated in vesicles.

exophthalmos   Protrusion of the eyes from the normal position within the socket.

expiration   Exhalation.

expiratory reserve volume   Supplemental air; additional air that is expelled from the lungs due to forced exhalation.

extension   The bending of a joint resulting in the distal segment moving away from the proximal segment. Typically results in straightening of the limb at the joint.

extensor muscles   Groups of muscles that cause extension.

external acoustic meatus   An opening in the temporal bone that contains the ear canal.

external auditory canal   The area in which sound waves are received from the auricle before they travel on to the eardrum; also called the ear canal.

external ear   One of three anatomic parts of the ear; it contains the pinna, the ear canal, and the exterior portion of the tympanic membrane.

external nares   The external openings to the nasal cavity; also called the nostrils.

external rotation   Rotating an extremity at its joint away from the midline.

external urethral orifice   The narrow opening at the end of the male urethra.

extracellular   Substances located outside of the cell membrane.

extracellular fluid (ECF)   Fluid found outside of the cell membranes in which most of the body's supply of sodium is contained, representing approximately 15% of the total body weight.

extraocular movements   Movement of the eyes in various directions.

extrinsic muscles   Muscles that do not originate in the body part to which they insert.

eyelid   Thin fold of skin that covers and protects the eye.

eyes   The organs of sight.

facial nerve   The cranial nerve (VII) that supplies motor activity to all muscles of facial expression, the sense of taste to the anterior two thirds of the tongue, and cutaneous sensation to the external ear, tongue, and palate.

facial skeleton   The maxillae, zygomatic bones, nasal bones, vomer, inferior nasal conchae, lacrimal bones, palatine bones, and mandible.

facilitated diffusion   The process whereby a carrier molecule moves substances in or out of cells from areas of higher to lower concentration.

fallopian tubes   The two hollow tubes or ducts that extend from the uterus to the region of the ovary and serve as a passageway for the ova and sperm.

fascia   A layer of fibrous connective tissue outside the epimysium that separates individual muscles and individual muscle groups.

feedback inhibition   Negative feedback resulting in the decrease of an action in the body.

femoral arteries   The principal arteries of the thigh, a continuation of the external iliac artery. They supply circulation to the thigh, external genitalia, anterior abdominal wall, and knee.

femoral nerve   The branch of the lumbosacral plexus that innervates the muscles that flex the hip and extend the knee.

femoral vein   A continuation of the saphenous vein that drains into the external iliac vein.

femur   The thighbone; the longest and one of the strongest bones in the body.

fetoscope   A device used for listening to fetal heart tones.

fibrin   A white insoluble protein formed from fibrinogen in the clotting process.

fibrinogen   A plasma protein that is important for blood coagulation.

fibroblasts   Cells that secrete proteins and collagen to form connective tissue between broken bone ends and at other sites of injury throughout the body.

fibula   The long bone on the lateral aspect of the lower leg.

fimbriae   Long thin finger-like processes at the end of the fallopian tubes that surround the ostium.

first-degree burns   Burns involving only the epidermis; also called superficial burns.

flagella   Tail-like microtubule structures capable of motion to propel the cell.

flat bones   Types of bone that are relatively thin and flattened.

flatus   Gas within the colon.

flexion   The bending of a joint resulting in the distal segment moving toward the proximal segment.

flexor muscles   Groups of muscles that cause flexion when contracted.

flexor reflex   A withdrawal reflex in the flexor muscles of the limbs that contracts in response to an unpleasant stimulus.

fluid balance   The process of maintaining homeostasis through equal intake and output of fluids.

follicle-stimulating hormone (FSH)   A hormone released from the pituitary gland at roughly monthly intervals that helps to stimulate one oocyte to undergo meiosis.

follicles   Small cavity glands within the thyroid gland that contain thyroglobulin.

fontanelles   Areas in the infant's skull where the sutures between the skull bones have not yet closed.

foramen magnum   A large opening at the base of the skull through which the spinal cord exits the brain.

foramen ovale   An opening between the two atria that is present in the fetus but normally closes shortly after birth.

foramina   Small openings, perforations, or orifices in the bones of the cranial vault.

forced expiratory vital capacity   The volume of air exhaled from the lung following a forceful exhalation.

foreskin   A loose fold of skin that covers the glans of the penis.

fossa ovalis   A depression between the right and left atria that indicates where the foramen ovale had been located in the fetus.

Fowler position   The position in which the patient is sitting up with the knees bent or straight.

fracture   A break in the continuity of a bone.

frontal bone   The bone that forms the forehead and part of the roof of the nasal cavity.

frontal lobe   The portion of the brain that is important in voluntary motor actions and personality traits.

frontal (coronal) plane   An imaginary plan dividing the body into anterior and posterior halves.

full-thickness burns   Burns that involve the hypodermis and possibly bone, muscle, or internal organs; also called third-degree burns.

functional residual capacity   Expiratory reserve volume plus residual volume.

fundus   The bottom of a hollow organ. In the stomach, it is the portion that balloons superior to the cardiac portion to act as a temporary storage area.

fundus (uterus)   The top portion of the uterus.

gallbladder   A saclike organ located on the lower surface of the liver that acts as a reservoir for bile.

gallstones   Rigid stones formed by digestive enzymes within the gallbladder.

gamete   Sex cell; in humans, sperm and ovaries.

ganglia   Collections of nerve cell bodies located outside the central nervous system.

ganglionic synapse   The separation between two nerves (preganglionic and postganglionic neurons), that serves to connect the central nervous system and the organs innervated.

gap junctions   Conduction areas between cells (eg, in visceral smooth muscle) that interconnect individual muscle cells.

gastric inhibitory peptide   A hormone that inhibits both gastric secretion and motility.

gastric pits   Numerous pits in the stomach mucosa; also called invaginations.

gastrin   A hormone produced by the endocrine cells of the stomach that increases stomach secretions as well as the rate of gastric emptying.

gastritis   Irritation of the stomach often caused by overproduction of stomach acid by the parietal cells.

gastrointestinal (GI) system   System composed of structures and organs involved in the consumption, digestion, and elimination of food; also called the digestive system or gastrointestinal tract.

genes   The fundamental units of heredity that store and release information on how to build and control cells.

genetic counseling   The medical process of advising couples of the possibility that certain inherited diseases may develop in their child.

genetic diseases   Diseases that develop as a result of an abnormality in a gene.

genetics   The study of heredity.

genomes   Chromosomal contents.

genotype   The genetic composition for a given trait.

gestation   The process of fetal development following fertilization.

gigantism   A disorder caused by chronic overproduction of growth hormone by the pituitary gland that is characterized by a gradual and permanent enlargement of the flat bones (the lower jaw) and of the hands and feet, abdominal organs, nose, lips, and tongue; also called acromegaly.

girdles   Bony structures that attach the limbs to the body (hip and shoulder).

glands   A cell, group of cells, or an organ that selectively removes, concentrates, or alters materials in the blood and secretes them back into the body.

glans   The portion of the corpus spongiosum that extends to form a cap over the tip of the penis.

glenoid fossa   The part of the scapula that forms the socket in the ball-and-socket joint of the shoulder.

globe   The eyeball.

glomerular capsule   A saclike structure that surrounds the glomerulus, from which it receives filtered fluid.

glomerular filtration   The process that initiates urine formation.

glomerular filtration rate   The rate at which blood is filtered through the glomerula.

glomerulus   A tangled cluster of blood capillaries that comprises a renal corpuscle.

glossopharyngeal nerve   The cranial nerve (IX) that supplies motor fibers to the pharyngeal muscle, provides taste sensation to the posterior portion of the tongue, and carries parasympathetic fibers to the parotid gland.

glottis   The vocal cords and the opening between them.

glucagon   Hormone produced by the pancreas that is vital to the control of the body's metabolism and blood glucose level; glucagon stimulates the breakdown of glycogen to glucose.

glucocorticoids   Hormones secreted by the zona fasciculata of the adrenal glands that play an important role in metabolism and inhibit inflammation.

gluconeogenesis   A process that stimulates both the liver and the kidneys to produce glucose from noncarbohydrate molecules.

glycogen   A long polymer from which glucose is converted in the liver; also called animal starch.

glycolysis   A process that involves a series of enzymatically catalyzed reactions in which glucose is broken down to yield lactic acid or pyruvic acid.

goblet cells   Cells that produce a protective mucous lining.

goiter   Enlarged visible mass in the anterior part of the neck caused by enlargement of the thyroid gland.

Golgi apparatus   A set of membranes in the protoplasm involved in the formation of sugars and complex proteins.

gonadotropin-releasing hormone (GnRH)   A hormone released from the hypothalamus that influences the release of luteinizing hormone and follicle-stimulating hormone; stimulates the uterine lining during the menstrual cycle.

gonads   The reproductive glands.

graafian follicle   A mature or developed ovum.

granulocytes   A type of leukocyte that has large cytoplasmic granules that are easily seen with a simple light microscope.

gross anatomy   The study of body parts that are visible to the naked eye, such as bones, muscles, and organs.

growth hormone (GH)   A hormone that stimulates growth in most tissues, especially of long bones in the extremities; also called somatotropin.

growth hormone release–inhibiting hormone   A hormone released by the hypothalamus that inhibits the secretion of growth hormone; also called somatostatin.

growth hormone–releasing hormone   A hormone released by the hypothalamus that stimulates the secretion of growth hormone.

gustation   The sense of taste.

gyri   The numerous folds in the cerebrum, which greatly increase the surface area of the cortex.

hair   Threadlike, keratin-containing appendage of the outer layer of the skin.

hair follicles   Tubelike structures in which hairs develop; they extend from the skin surface into the dermis.

hair shafts   The portions of hair that extend above the skin.

haploid   Cells that carry genetic instructions via 23 individual chromosomes.

hapten   A substance that normally does not stimulate an immune response but can be combined with an antigen and at a later point initiate an antibody response; found in certain drugs, dust particles, animal dander, and various chemicals.

hard palate   The floor of the nasal cavity.

haustra   Recesses in the colon caused by contractions of the teniae coli.

haversian systems   Units of compact bone consisting of a tube (haversian canal) with the laminae of bone that surrounds them.

heart   A hollow muscular organ that pumps blood throughout the body.

heartburn   Sensation often caused by the back flow of stomach acid into the esophagus; also called reflux esophagitis.

helper T cells   Cells that aid other white blood cells in carrying out cell-mediated immune functions, including maturation of B cells into plasma cells and memory B cells, and activation of cytotoxic T cells and macrophages.

hematocrit   The percentage of blood volume made up by red blood cells.

hematopoiesis   The process of blood cell production in the bone marrow; also called hemopoiesis.

hemodialysis   A procedure in which an artificial kidney external to the body is used to purify the blood.

hemoglobin   An iron-containing protein within red blood cells that has the ability to bind to oxygen.

hemorrhoidal plexus   Large veins that line the inside of the anal canal.

hemorrhoids   Abnormal dilation of veins in the hemorrhoidal plexus.

hemostasis   Control of bleeding by formation of a blood clot.

hemothorax   An abnormal accumulation of bloody fluid within the pleural space following trauma.

heparin   A substance found in large amounts in basophils that inhibits blood clotting.

hepatic flexure   The first turn (sharp left turn near the inferior border of the liver) in the large intestine at the end of the ascending colon and beginning of the transverse colon.

hepatic portal system   A specialized part of the venous system that drains blood from the liver, stomach, intestines, and spleen.

hepatic veins   The veins to which blood empties after liver cells in the sinusoids of the liver extract nutrients, filter the blood, and metabolize various drugs.

hepatoportal system   A specialized portion of the circulatory system that directs blood from the stomach and intestine through the liver for processing.

heredity   The passing of traits and qualities from parents to offspring, primarily through DNA or RNA.

herniated disk   A tear in the anulus fibrosus that results in leakage of the nucleus pulposus, most commonly against exiting nerve roots.

heterozygous   An organism that has two different alleles for a trait.

hiatal hernia   A weakening in the esophageal hiatus that allows the stomach to move above the diaphragm and may result in acid reflux, causing heartburn.

hilum (lymph node)   An indented region of a lymph node where blood vessels and nerves are attached.

hilum (lung)   The point of entry for the bronchi, vessels, and nerves into each lung.

hilum (kidney)   The point on the medial side of each kidney where the renal artery and nerves enter and the renal vein and ureter exit.

histamine   A chemical found in mast cells that, when released, causes vasodilation, capillary leaking, and bronchiole constriction.

holocrine glands   Glands that secrete sebum; also called sebaceous glands.

homeostasis   A tendency to constancy or stability in the body's internal environment.

homologous chromosomes   Chromosomes of the same numbered pair from the opposite parent.

homozygous   An organism that has two identical alleles for a trait.

hormone-sensitive lipase   An enzyme that is activated by glucagon; it breaks triglycerides down into free fatty acids and glycerol.

hormones   Substances formed in specialized organs or glands and carried to another organ or group of cells in the same organism; regulate many body functions, including metabolism, growth, and body temperature.

human chorionic gonadotropin (hCG)   One of the three major female hormones that stimulates the corpus luteum to produce progesterone during the first 8 weeks of gestation.

human immunodeficiency virus (HIV)   A virus that may lead to acquired immunodeficiency syndrome (AIDS); cells in the immune system are killed or damaged so that the body is unable to fight infections and certain cancers.

humerus   The supporting bone of the upper arm.

humoral immune response   When antibodies react to destroy antigens or antigen-containing particles.

hydrochloric acid   An acid produced by parietal cells in the stomach that aids in digestion.

hydrogen bond   The attraction of the positive hydrogen end of a polar molecule to the negative nitrogen or oxygen end of another polar molecule.

hydrolysis   The splitting of a molecule by adding water.

hydroxyapatite   A mineral compound containing calcium and phosphate that, along with collagen, comprises the structural element of bone.

hymen   A fold of mucous membrane that partially covers the entrance to the vaginal opening.

hyoid bone   The bone that supports the tongue and its muscles.

hyperesthesia   Any of several conditions that result in excess skin sensitivity, especially to touch or to cold.

hyperextension   When a body part is extended to the maximum level or beyond the normal range of motion.

hyperflexion   When a body part is flexed to the maximum level or beyond the normal range of motion.

hyperkalemia   An excessive amount of potassium in the blood.

hypernatremia   A serum sodium level of greater than 145 mEq/L.

hyperosmolar hyperglycemic nonketotic coma (HHNC)   A diabetic emergency that occurs from a relative insulin deficiency, resulting in hyperglycemia, hyperosmolarity, and an absence of significant ketosis.

hyperparathyroidism   A condition that results in a loss of calcium from the bones, as well as increases in serum calcium levels, caused by excess secretion of parathyroid hormones.

hyperthermia   Elevated body temperature.

hyperthyroidism   Overactivity of the thyroid gland, which results in increased metabolic rates, weight loss, rapid pulse rate, elevated blood pressure, diarrhea, and at times, abnormal protrusion of the eyes.

hyperventilation   Deep, rapid breathing; it lowers blood carbon dioxide levels.

hypocalcemia   Potentially life-threatening low blood calcium levels resulting from loss of parathyroid function.

hypodermic   Referring to under the skin.

hypodermis   The layer of tissue immediately beneath the dermis; also called the subcutaneous layer.

hypoglossal nerve   The cranial nerve (XII) that provides motor function to the muscles of the tongue and throat.

hypoglycemia   Abnormally low blood glucose level.

hypokalemia   A low concentration of potassium in the blood.

hyponatremia   A serum sodium level that is less than 135 mEq/L.

hypophysis   The gland that secretes hormones that regulate the function of many other glands in the body; also called the pituitary gland.

hypothalamic-pituitary axis   The part of the neuroendocrine system that involves interactions of the hypothalamus and the pituitary gland.

hypothalamic-pituitary-adrenal axis   A major part of the neuroendocrine system that controls reactions to stress; regulates the secretion of corticosteroids.

hypothalamo-hypophyseal portal system   A specialized set of blood vessels that carry releasing factors from the hypothalamus to the anterior pituitary.

hypothalamus   The inferior portion of the diencephalon of the brain that is the primary link between the endocrine and nervous systems; it controls many body functions, including emotional activity, pulse rate, digestion, sexual development, body temperature, hunger, thirst, and the regulation of the sleep cycle.

hypothermia   Low body temperature.

hypoxia   A deficiency of oxygen reaching the tissues.

ileocecal junction   The junction between the ileum and large intestine.

ileum (gastrointestinal system)   The last portion of the small intestine, which extends from the jejunum to the ileocecal valve at the beginning of the large intestine.

ilium (musculoskeletal system)   One of three bones that fuse to form the pelvic ring.

immune system   The body system that includes all of the structures and processes designed to mount a defense against foreign substances and disease-causing agents.

immunity   Physiologically, refers to the body's ability to protect itself from infectious disease.

immunoglobulins   See antibodies.

incision   A smooth cut, usually made by a sharp object such as a scalpel.

infection   The invasion of a host or tissue by pathogenic organisms such as bacteria, viruses, or parasites that produces illness that may or may not have clinical manifestations.

infectious disease   A disease that is caused by infection or one that is capable of being transmitted to another person with or without direct contact.

inferior   Below a body part or nearer to the feet.

inferior nasal conchae   Scroll-shaped bones attached to the lateral nasal cavity walls that support the mucous membranes.

inferior vena cava   One of the two largest veins in the body; carries blood from the lower extremities and the pelvic and the abdominal organs to the heart.

inflammatory response   A reaction by tissues of the body to irritation or injury, characterized by pain, swelling, redness, and heat.

infundibulum (reproductive system)   The space formed in the peritoneum by the distal end of the fallopian tubes.

infundibulum (nervous system)   The stalk that connects the hypothalamus to the pituitary gland.

inguinal canal   The canal through which the spermatic cord passes through the inferior abdominal wall and into the abdominal cavity.

inguinal nodes   A large collection of lymph nodes located in the groin.

inhibiting factors   Compounds that travel from the hypothalamus to the pituitary gland in a specialized set of blood vessels; also called releasing factors.

innate (nonspecific) defense   An immune response that is predictable each time the body is exposed to a particular challenge. One that protects the body from pathogens involving mechanical barriers, chemical barriers, natural killer cells, inflammation, phagocytosis, fever, or species resistance.

inner ear   One of three anatomic parts of the ear; it consists of the cochlea and semicircular canals.

inorganic   Not having both carbon and hydrogen atoms.

inotropic effect   The effect on the contractility of muscle tissue, especially cardiac muscle.

insertion   A moveable part of the body to which a skeletal muscle is fastened at a moveable joint.

inspiration   Inhalation.

inspiratory capacity   Tidal volume plus inspiratory reserve volume.

inspiratory reserve volume   Additional air that enters the lungs due to forced inspiration.

insulin   Hormone produced by the pancreas that is vital in the control of the body's metabolism and blood glucose level.

integument   Skin, the covering of the body surface.

integumentary system   The body's external surface, including the skin, nails, hair, and sweat and oil glands.

intercalated disks   Branching fibers in cardiac muscle that allow action potentials to pass from cell to cell.

interior nares   The posterior opening from the nasopharynx into the pharynx.

internal auditory meatus   A short canal through which auditory and facial nerves pass.

internal rotation   Rotating the segment of the extremity distal to the joint toward the midline.

interstitial fluid   The fluid located outside of the blood vessels in the spaces between the body's cells.

intervertebral disk   A mass of fibrocartilage between each vertebral body of the spine, composed of the anulus fibrosus and the nucleus pulposus.

intervertebral foramen   Openings between successive vertebrae through which nerves exit the vertebral column.

intervertebral foramina   The opening between each vertebra through which the spinal (peripheral) nerves pass from the spinal cord.

intracellular fluid (ICF) Fluid found within individual cells, containing most of the body's supply of potassium and representing approximately 45% of total body weight.

intracellular membrane Substances, such as the organelles, that are found inside the cell membrane.

intravascular fluid The noncellular portion of blood found within the blood vessels; also called plasma.

intrinsic automaticity The ability of a muscle to generate its own electrical activity.

intrinsic factor The chemical substance produced by parietal cells in the stomach that is important in the absorption of vitamin B_{12}.

invaginations Numerous pits in the stomach mucosa; also called gastric pits.

ion channels Protein-lined pores or transport channels, specifically sized for each substance, which allow electrolyte movements among the cells.

ions Atoms that either gain or lose electrons.

iris The sphincter muscle and surrounding tissue behind the cornea that dilate and constrict the pupil, regulating the amount of light that enters the eye; pigment in this tissue gives the eye its color.

ischemia Insufficient oxygen at a particular tissue site often associated with obstruction of arterial blood flow to the site.

ischium One of the three bones that fuse to form the pelvic ring.

islets of Langerhans A specialized group of cells in the pancreas where insulin and glucagon are produced.

isotope One of two (or more) forms of an element having the same number of protons and electrons, but different numbers of neutrons; they may or may not be radioactive.

isthmus A band of tissue that connects the two lobes of the thyroid gland.

jaundice A yellowing of the skin and sclera of the eyes because of excessive concentrations of bilirubin in the blood.

jejunum The middle portion of the small intestine; it has thicker walls and more folds than the other portions of the small intestine.

joint The point where two or more bones come together, allowing movement to occur.

jugular veins The two main veins that drain the head and neck.

juxtaglomerular apparatus Structure formed at the site where the efferent arteriole and distal convoluted tubule meet; also called a juxtaglomerular complex; plays an important role in regulating fluid balance.

juxtaglomerular cells A group of cells located in the afferent arterioles of the glomerulus that play a part in regulating the volume status of the body.

keratin A protein in the skin that is responsible for the strength and permeability of the epidermis.

keratinocytes The cells in the epidermis that produce a protein called keratin.

keratohyalin A precursor of keratin that is located in the stratum granulosum of the epidermis.

kidney stones Solid crystalline masses formed in the kidney that may become trapped anywhere along the urinary tract.

kidneys Two retroperitoneal organs that excrete the end products of metabolism as urine and regulate the body's salt and water content.

kilocalorie A unit of heat measurement, abbreviated as C.

kinetic labyrinth system One of two mechanisms involved in the sensation of position, balance, and movement, it senses movements of the head.

kyphosis Outward curve of the thoracic spine.

labia majora Two prominent, rounded folds of skin lateral to the labia minora of the female external genitalia.

labia minora A pair of skin folds in the female external genitalia that border the vestibule.

laceration A wound with a smooth or jagged edge, resulting from a tearing, scraping, or sharp cutting action.

lacrimal apparatus The structures in which tears are secreted and drained from the eye.

lacrimal bones Bones that make up part of the eye orbits and contain the tear sacs.

lacrimal ducts Ducts located on the nasal border of the eyelids through which tears from the lacrimal sacs pass.

lacrimal gland The structure in which tears are produced.

lacrimal sac Sac in the eye into which tears are drained from the lacrimal glands.

lacteal A capillary and lymph channel contained in each villus.

lactic acid A metabolic end product of the breakdown of glucose that accumulates when metabolism proceeds in the absence of oxygen.

lactiferous sinuses The area in the mammary glands in which milk is stored.

lambdoid suture The point where the occipital bones attach to the parietal bones.

lamellae Thin sheets or layers into which bone tissue is organized.

large intestine A portion of the gastrointestinal system that extends from the small intestine to the rectum and maintains water balance by absorbing and excreting water; also called the colon.

larynx A complete structure formed by the epiglottis, thyroid cartilage, cricoid cartilage, arytenoid cartilage, corniculate cartilage, and cuneiform cartilage; the voice box.

lateral In anatomy, parts of the body that lie farther from the midline; also called outer structures.

lateral malleolus An enlargement of the distal end of the fibula, which forms the lateral wall of the ankle joint.

lateral spinothalamic tracts Ascending tracts that carry information to the brain about pain and temperature.

lens The transparent part of the eye through which images are focused on the retina.

leukemia A cancerous condition in which certain white blood cell lines begin to grow abnormally fast and invade other tissues.

leukocytes White blood cells that are responsible for fighting infection.

ligaments Bands of fibrous tissue that connect bones to bones; they support and strengthen a joint.

limbic system Structures within the cerebrum and diencephalon that influence emotions, motivation, mood, and sensations of pain and pleasure.

lingual tonsils One of three sets of lymphatic organs that comprise the tonsils, they are located on the posterior margin of the tongue and help protect the body from bacteria introduced into the mouth and nose.

lingula A small portion of the left lung that is the equivalent of the middle lobe in the right lung.

lipases Pancreatic enzymes that break down fat.

lipids   Fats, fat-like substances (cholesterol and phospholipids), and oils that supply energy for body processes and building of certain structures.

liver   A large abdominal organ that lies in the right upper quadrant immediately below the diaphragm; it produces bile, stores glucose for immediate use by the body, and produces many substances that help regulate immune responses.

lobes   Subdivisions within each hemisphere of the cerebrum; each lobe shares the name of the bone of the skull that overlies it.

long bone   Type of bone that is longer than it is wide.

longitudinal fissure   The crevasse that separates the right and left hemispheres of the cerebrum.

loop of Henle   U-shaped portion of the renal tubule that extends from the proximal to the distal convoluted tubule.

lordosis   Inward curve of the lumbar spine just above the buttocks; an exaggerated form of lordosis results in the condition known as swayback.

lower limbs   The femurs, tibias, fibulas, patellae, tarsals, metatarsals, and phalanges.

lumbar puncture   A needle insertion through the vertebral canal into the subarachnoid space to obtain a specimen of cerebrospinal fluid.

lumbar vertebrae   The five vertebrae of the lower back.

lumbosacral plexus   A combination of the lumbar plexus, the sacral plexus, and the coccygeal root.

lumen   The inside opening of a vessel such as an artery, vein, capillary, or hollow structure.

lungs   The two primary organs of breathing.

lunula   A whitish, crescent-shaped structure at the base of the nail body.

luteinizing hormone (LH)   A hormone released from the pituitary gland at roughly monthly intervals that helps to stimulate one oocyte to undergo meiosis.

lymph   A thin plasma-like liquid formed from interstitial or extracellular fluid that bathes the tissues of the body.

lymph nodes   Round or bean-shaped structures interspersed along the course of the lymph vessels, which filter the lymph and serve as a source of lymphocytes.

lymph nodules   Tissue that is denser than diffuse lymphatic tissue, found in the loose connective tissue of the digestive, respiratory, and urinary systems.

lymph sinuses   Spaces inside lymph nodes that comprise complex channels through which lymph moves.

lymphadenitis   Inflammation of a lymph node caused by infection.

lymphadenopathy   Any swelling of the lymph nodes, with or without pain.

lymphangitis   An infection that spreads beyond the local area into a lymphatic vessel causing red streaks to run from the infected area proximally.

lymphatic capillaries   Vessels of the lymphatic system that carry fluid away from the tissues and toward one of the great lymph vessels.

lymphatic duct   One of two great lymph vessels; it empties into the subclavian vein.

lymphatic pathways   Tiny tubes formed from lymphatic capillaries that merge to form larger vessels.

lymphatic system   A passive circulatory system that transports a plasma-like liquid called lymph, a thin fluid that bathes the tissues of the body.

lymphatic trunks   Structures that drain lymph from lymphatic vessels and join either the thoracic duct or the right lymphatic duct.

lymphatic vessels   Thin-walled vessels through which lymph circulates in the body, they travel close to the major arteries and veins.

lymphocytes   The white blood cells responsible for a large part of the body's immune protection.

lymphokines   Cytokines produced by T cells that recruits mast cells and other nonspecific inflammatory mediators to aid in destruction of antigens.

lysis   The process of disintegration or breakdown of cells that occurs when excess water enters the cell through osmosis.

lysosomes   Membrane-bound vesicles that contain a variety of enzymes functioning as a cell's digestive system.

macrophages   Cells that develop from the monocytes that provide some of the body's first line of defense in the inflammatory process.

macula   Specialized patches of tissue within the utricle and saccule that aid in the sensation of motion.

macula densa   Specialized tubular cells in the juxtaglomerular area that play a part in regulating the volume status of the body.

mainstem bronchi   The part of the lower airway below the larynx through which air enters the lungs.

mammary glands   The organs of milk production in the breasts.

mammary ligaments   Structures that support the mammary glands.

mammography screening   Radiographic screening of the breasts for early detection of cancer.

mandible   The bone of the lower jaw; the only moveable bone in the face.

mast cells   Cells resembling basophils that are formed in response to allergens. When allergens attach to antigens on the mast cell surface, the cells release potent inflammatory mediators resulting in allergic symptoms or potentially anaphylaxis.

mastication   Chewing.

mastoid process   A prominent bony mass at the base of the skull behind the ear.

maxillae   The bones that make up the upper jaw.

McBurney point   An anatomic landmark in the right lower quadrant of the abdomen that typically represents the location of pain associated with appendicitis.

meatus   A passage located below each turbinate.

mechanical digestion   Chewing of food.

medial   Parts of the body that lie closer to the midline; also called inner structures.

medial malleolus   The distal end of the tibia, which forms the medial side of the ankle joint.

median nerve   The nerve in the brachial plexus that innervates the pronator muscles of the forearm, as well as those that flex the wrist, fingers, and thumb.

mediastinum   The space between the lungs, in the center of the chest, that contains the heart, trachea, mainstem bronchi, part of the esophagus, and large blood vessels.

medulla (endocrine system)   The inner portion of the adrenal glands, which produces epinephrine and norepinephrine.

medulla (nervous system)   The inferior portion of the midbrain, which serves as a conduction pathway for both ascending and descending nerve tracts.

medullary cavity   The internal cavity of the diaphysis of a long bone that contains bone marrow.

medullary respiratory center The dorsal and ventral respiratory groups in the medulla oblongata as well as the respiratory group of the pons.

meiosis A specialized form of cell division that occurs during the formation of a mature ova and sperm.

melanin The dark pigment in skin that protects the skin from the sun's ultraviolet rays.

melanocytes Epidermal cells that contribute to skin color by producing a dark pigment called melanin.

melatonin A hormone secreted by the pineal gland that functions as a biologic clock, helping to regulate the circadian rhythms.

membranous urethra One of three parts of the male urethra; it extends from the prostate gland to the base of the penis.

memory T cells The form into which T cells differentiate when activated by an antigen; memory T cells remain within the body, ready to respond to a second challenge.

menarche The beginning phase of a woman's life cycle of menstruation.

meninges A set of three tough membranes, the dura mater, arachnoid, and pia mater, that encloses the entire brain and spinal cord.

meningitis An inflammation of the meninges and cerebrospinal fluid, usually caused by infection.

menisci Shock-absorbing fibrocartilage pads within some synovial joints.

menopause The ending phase of a woman's life cycle of menstruation.

menstrual cycle The entire monthly cycle of menstruation from start to finish, lasting approximately 28 days.

menstruation The sloughing and discharge of the functional layer of the endometrium; monthly flow of blood.

merocrine (eccrine) glands Sweat glands that produce a solution containing salt and urea that is secreted directly onto the surface of the skin through sweat pores.

mesenteric angina Pain caused by partial occlusion of the mesenteric artery from atherosclerosis.

mesenteric infarction Blockage of a mesenteric artery, resulting in necrosis of a portion of the bowel.

mesenteries Parts of the peritoneum that hold the abdominal organs in place and provide a passageway for blood vessels and nerves to the organs.

mesovarium The peritoneal fold that helps to hold the ovaries in place.

metabolism The chemical processes that provide the cells with energy from nutrients.

metacarpals The bones of the palms of the hand.

metaphysis The area of a long bone where the diaphysis and epiphysis converge; where the physis (epiphyseal plate) is located.

metastasize The spreading of a disease from one part of the body to another, especially with many forms of cancer.

metatarsals The bones on the soles of the feet; they form the foot arches.

microorganisms Organisms of microscopic size.

microscopic anatomy The study of tissue structure and/or cellular structure or organization, often visible only through a microscope.

microtubules Hollow filamentous structures that make up various components of the cell.

micturition Urination; the process of expelling urine from the urinary bladder.

midaxillary line An imaginary line drawn through the midportion of the axilla to the waist that is parallel to the midline.

midclavicular line An imaginary line drawn through the midpoint of the clavicle that is parallel to the midline.

middle ear One of three anatomic parts of the ear; it consists of the inner portion of the tympanic membrane and the ossicles.

midsagittal plane An imaginary vertical line drawn from the middle of the forehead through the nose and the umbilicus (navel) to the floor; also called the midline.

mineralocorticoids Hormones produced in the zona glomerulosa of the adrenal cortex that are important in the regulation of water and salt balance in the body.

minerals Inorganic elements essential for human metabolism.

mitochondria Small, rod-like organelles that function as the metabolic center of the cell and produce adenosine triphosphate (ATP).

mitosis The division of chromosomes in a cell nucleus.

mitral valve The valve in the heart that separates the left atrium from the left ventricle.

molecule Particles made up of two or more joined atoms.

monocytes Granulocytes that migrate out of the blood and into the tissues in response to an infection.

mononuclear phagocytic system Phagocytic cells that remove foreign particles from the lymph and blood.

mons pubis A rounded pad of fatty tissue that overlies the pubic symphysis and is anterior to the urethral and vaginal openings.

motility The motion that results in the passage of substances through the digestive tract.

motor end plate The flattened end of a motor neuron that transmits neural impulses to a muscle.

motor nerves Nerves that carry commands from the brain to the muscle; also called efferent nerves.

motor neurons Specialized nerve cells that deliver an impulse to muscle cells, causing them to contract.

motor unit A motor neuron and the muscle fibers that it controls.

mucosa The innermost lining of the lumen of each portion of the alimentary canal; rich in glands, lymphatic tissue, and blood vessels.

mucus Related to digestion, it is a thick liquid that binds food particles and lubricates them during swallowing.

multiunit smooth muscle One of the two types of smooth muscle, it is formed into sheets of muscle (as in the walls of blood vessels), small bundles of muscles (as in the iris of the eye), or single cells (as in the capsule of the spleen).

murmur An abnormal heart sound, heard as "whooshing," indicating turbulent blood flow within the heart.

muscarinic receptors Receptors at the target tissue that are stimulated by acetylcholine and can also be stimulated in the laboratory by the compound extracted from muscarine mushrooms.

muscle Fibers that contract causing movement; three types of muscle are present in the body: skeletal muscle, smooth muscle, and cardiac muscle.

muscle fasciculus A bundle of skeletal muscle cells bound together by connective tissue and forming one of the constituent elements of a muscle.

muscle impulse One that passes in many directions over a muscle fiber membrane after stimulation by acetylcholine.

musculocutaneous nerve A nerve in the upper extremity that innervates muscles that flex the shoulder and elbow.

musculoskeletal system The bones and voluntary muscles of the body.

myelin sheath   A membrane formed by Schwann cells, which cover the axons of certain neurons.

myelinated nerves   An axon surrounded by a membrane sheath produced by Schwann cells.

myocardial infarction   Blockage of one or more of the arteries that supply oxygen to the heart, resulting in death to a portion of the myocardium.

myocardium   The heart muscle.

myofibrils   Threadlike structures that extend from one end of the muscle fiber to the other.

myoglobin   An iron-containing red pigment, similar to hemoglobin, that is found in muscle fibers.

myometrium   A thick muscular middle layer of the uterine wall.

myosin   The component that makes up most of the thick protein filaments of the myofibrils.

nail   A flattened structure at the end of each finger and toe made of keratin from the epidermis.

nail bed   The portion of the nail over which the nail body lies.

nasal bones   The thin, delicate bones that join to form the bridge of the nose.

nasal cavity   The chamber inside the nose that lies between the floor of the cranium and the roof of the mouth.

nasal septum   The rigid partition composed of bone and cartilage that separates the right and left nostrils.

nasolacrimal duct   The passage through which tears drain from the lacrimal sacs into the nasal cavity.

nasopharynx   The nasal cavity (the portion of the pharynx that lies above the level of the roof of the mouth); formed by the union of the facial bones.

negative feedback   The concept that once the desired effect of a hormone has been achieved, further production of the hormone is inhibited until it is needed again; also called feedback inhibition.

nephrons   The structural and functional units of the kidney that form urine, composed of the glomerulus, the glomerular capsule, the proximal convoluted tubule, the loop of Henle, and the distal convoluted tubule.

nerve fibers   Groups of nerve cells that are bundled together.

nerve impulse   Electrochemical changes transmitted by neurons to other neurons and to cells outside the nervous system.

nerve   Nervous tissue that connects the nervous system with body parts or organs.

nervous system   The system that controls virtually all activities of the body, both voluntary and involuntary.

nervous tissues   Neurons and neuroglia.

neuroeffector cells   The target tissues of the autonomic nervous system.

neuroglia   One of two basic types of neural tissue, neuroglia support, protect, defend, and aid in the repair of injury of neural tissue, and regulate composition of nervous system interstitial fluid.

neurohormones   Hormones secreted by the posterior pituitary.

neurohypophysis   One of the two portions of the pituitary gland; it is an extension of the central nervous system and secretes hormones called neurohormones; also called the posterior pituitary.

neuromuscular blockers   A group of drugs derived from curare that are used in anesthesia to induce muscle relaxation.

neuromuscular junction   The junction between a motor neuron and a muscle fiber; one type of a synapse.

neurons   The basic nerve cells of the nervous system, containing a nucleus within a cell body and extending one or more processes; they exist in masses to form nervous tissue.

neurotransmitters   Chemicals produced by neurons that stimulate electrical reactions in adjacent cells.

neutrons   Uncharged or "neutral" particles in the nucleus of an atom.

neutrophils   White blood cells that are one of the three types of granulocytes; they have multi-lobed nuclei that resemble a string of baseballs held together by a thin strand of thread; they destroy bacteria, antigen-antibody complexes, and foreign matter.

nicotinic receptors   Receptors in the postganglionic neuron that can be stimulated in the laboratory by the alkaloid nicotine.

nipple   An external raised protuberance on the breast surrounded by the pigmented areola.

nodes of Ranvier   Regions between individual Schwann cells in myelinated neurons, between which action potentials jump.

nondisplaced fracture   A fractured bone that has not moved from its normal position.

nonspecific nongonococcal urethritis   An infection of the urethra caused by organisms of the Chlamydia family.

nonstriated   Smooth muscle tissue.

norepinephrine   A hormone produced by the adrenal glands that is vital in the function of the sympathetic nervous system.

norepinephrine (medication)   A naturally occurring hormone with a greater stimulatory effect on alpha receptors that also may be given as a cardiac drug.

norepinephrine   A neurotransmitter secreted by the autonomic nervous system.

normal flora   Bacteria that is located in the colon to help in the digestion of food, as well as other sites in the body, such as the vagina, skin, oral and nasal cavities to help maintain homeostasis.

nuclear envelope   The membrane that surrounds the nucleus of the cell.

nucleic acids   Large organic molecules, or macromolecules, that carry genetic information or form structures within cells, and include DNA and RNA.

nucleoli   Rounded, dense structures in the protoplasm that contain RNA and synthesize proteins.

nucleus pulposus   The gelatinous mass that makes up the center of each intervertebral disk.

nucleus   The nerve center, or central body, of the cell, embedded within the protoplasm.

nutrients   Carbohydrates, lipids, proteins, vitamins, minerals, and water.

oblique fracture   A fracture that forms an angle to the shaft of the bone.

obturator nerve   A nerve emanating from the lumbosacral plexus that innervates muscles that adduct the thigh and rotate it medially.

occipital bone   The bone that forms the back and base of the cranium.

occipital condyles   Articular surface on the occipital bone where the skull articulates with the atlas on the vertebral column.

occipital lobe   The portion of the brain that is responsible for the processing of visual information.

oculomotor nerve   The cranial nerve (III) that innervates the muscles that cause motion of the eyeballs and upper lid.

olfactory bulb   The portion of the olfactory nerve formed by the olfactory tract that lies on the cribriform plate of the ethmoid bone and is penetrated by nerve fibers that provide information about smell from the nose.

olfactory cortex   The area in the brain that receives odor impulses and perceives them as smell.

olfactory nerve   The cranial nerve (I) that transmits information about the sense of smell.

olfactory tract   The part of the olfactory nerve that arises at the base of the brain.

olfactory tracts   Passageways for odor impulses to travel from the olfactory bulb to the olfactory cortex.

omental bursa   A cavity created by a double fold of mesentery, which extends inferiorly from the stomach.

oocytes   The precursors to a mature egg, formed in the ovaries.

oogenesis   The process of egg cell formation, which begins at puberty.

open fracture   A fracture in which a bone end has penetrated the skin; also called a compound fracture.

optic chiasm   Location where approximately half of the nerve fibers from each eye cross over to the opposite side of the brain.

optic foramen   The opening in the bony orbit behind the eyeball through which the optic nerve passes to the eyeball.

optic foramina   The openings through which the optic nerves pass to reach each eyeball.

optic nerve   The cranial nerve (II) that transmits visual information to the brain. This is the only of the cranial nerves considered to be part of the central nervous system.

optic tracts   The parts of the optic nerve that arise at the base of the brain, forming the optic chiasm.

orbit   The bony cavity in the frontal skull that contains the eyeball and its associated muscles, vessels, and nerves.

organ of Corti   The organ that is the primary receptor for sound, and is made up of thousands of individual cilia, each with their own associated nerve.

organ system   A group of organs that have a common purpose, such as the skeleton and muscles.

organelles   The internal structures within the cell that carry out specific functions for the cell.

organic   Having both carbon and hydrogen atoms.

organism   Any individual living thing; made up of various organ systems.

organs   Different types of tissues working together to perform a particular function.

origin   A relatively immovable part of the body where a skeletal muscle is fastened at a moveable joint.

oropharynx   A tubular structure that forms the posterior portion of the oral cavity, extending vertically from the back of the mouth to the esophagus and trachea.

osmoreceptors   Specialized neurons in the brain that regulate the secretion of antidiuretic hormone.

osmosis   The movement of a solvent, such as water, from an area of low solute concentration to one of high concentration through a selectively permeable membrane to equalize concentrations of a solute on both sides of the membrane.

osmotic pressure   The measure of the tendency of water to move by osmosis across a membrane.

ossicles   Small bones in the inner ear.

ossification   The formation of bone by osteoblasts.

osteoblasts   Bone-forming cells.

osteoclasts   Large, multinucleated cells that dissolve bone tissue and play a major role in bone remodeling.

osteocyte   An osteoblast that becomes surrounded by bony matrix; a mature bone cell.

osteogenesis imperfecta   A genetic bone disease that results in fragile bones.

osteomalacia   An abnormal softening of bones because of a loss of calcium.

osteomyelitis   Inflammation of the bone and muscle caused by infection.

osteons   Units within a compact bone in which blood vessels are located; also called the haversian system.

osteoporosis   A reduction in the quantity of bony tissue.

ostium   The opening in the infundibulum formed by the fallopian tubes.

otoliths   Small calcium carbonate stones within the gelatinous protein of the otolithic membrane of the inner ear that aid in the sensation of motion.

otolithic membrane   A membrane within the inner ear that contains otolith and aids in the sensation of motion.

oval window   An oval opening between the middle ear and the vestibule.

ovarian ligament   One of the two ligaments that help to hold the ovaries in place.

ovaries   The female reproductive organs that produce egg precursors, or oocytes.

ovulation   The release of a mature ovum into the fallopian tube from the ovary.

oxygen debt   The amount of oxygen that liver cells need to convert lactic acid into glucose, as well as the amount needed by muscle cells to restore adenosine triphosphate and creatine phosphate levels.

oxyhemoglobin   The combination of oxygen that diffuses into the blood and the hemoglobin molecule.

oxytocin   A hormone that causes the smooth muscles of the pregnant uterus to contract and milk to be released from the breasts of lactating women.

P wave   The first wave in the ECG complex, representing depolarization of the ventricles.

palatine bones   Irregularly shaped bones found in the posterior part of the nasal cavity.

palatine tonsils   One of three sets of lymphatic organs that comprise the tonsils. They are located in the back of the throat, on each side of the posterior opening of the oral cavity, and help protect the body from bacteria introduced into the mouth and nose.

palmar arches   The two arches formed from the radial and ulnar vessels within the hand, creating the superficial and deep palmar arches.

pancreas   A flat, solid organ that lies below and behind the liver and the stomach, and which is a digestive gland that secretes digestive enzymes into the duodenum through the pancreatic duct; considered both an endocrine gland and an exocrine gland.

pancreatic duct   The duct through which digestive enzymes pass on their way through the common hepatic duct to the duodenum at the ampulla of Vater.

papillary muscles   Specialized muscles that attach the ventricles to the cusps of the valves by muscular strands called chordae tendineae.

paracrine Relating to a kind of hormone function in which the effects of the hormone are restricted to the local environment.

parafollicular cells Cells located between the follicles in the thyroid gland that produce the hormone calcitonin.

paranasal sinuses The sinuses, or hollowed sections of bone in the front of the head, that are lined with mucous membrane and drain into the nasal cavity; the frontal and maxillary sinuses.

parasympathetic-blocking drug A drug that blocks acetylcholine at the neuroeffector synapse.

parasympathetic nervous system The part of the autonomic nervous system that relaxes the body.

parathyroid glands Four glands that are embedded in the posterior portion of the thyroid, they produce and secrete parathyroid hormone.

parathyroid hormone Hormone produced and secreted by the parathyroid glands; it maintains normal levels of calcium in the blood and normal neuromuscular function.

parietal bones Bones that form the upper sides and roof of the cranium.

parietal cells Cells in the gastric mucosa that produce hydrochloric acid.

parietal layer One of two layers of the serous pericardium; it is separated from the visceral pericardium by a small amount of pericardial fluid.

parietal lobe The portion of the brain that is the site for reception and evaluation of most sensory information, except smell, hearing, and vision.

parietal peritoneum A smooth membrane of connective tissue that lines the abdominal cavity.

parietal pleura The membrane that lines the walls of the pleural cavity.

parietal portion The portion of the serous membrane that lines the walls of the trunk cavities.

parotid glands One pair of the three sets of salivary glands.

partial pressure The amount of pressure each gas contributes to diffusion.

partial pressure of carbon dioxide (Paco$_2$) A measurement of the percentage of carbon dioxide in the blood.

partial pressure of oxygen (Pao$_2$) A measurement of the percentage of oxygen in the blood.

partial-thickness burns Burns that involve the epidermis and a portion of the dermis; also called second-degree burns.

patella The kneecap.

pathogen A disease-causing agent, which may be a virus, bacterium, fungus, or protozoan.

pathophysiology The study of body functions of a living organism in an abnormal state.

pectineus muscles Deep muscles of the medial compartment that adduct, flex, and internally rotate the thigh.

pectoral girdle The scalpulae and clavicles.

pectoralis major The largest muscle of the chest wall; it adducts and internally rotates the shoulder.

pedicles The feet of each vertebra in the vertebral arch.

pelvic girdle The hip bones.

pelvis The attachment of the lower extremities to the body, consisting of the sacrum and two pelvic bones.

penetrating wound Wound made by a sharp instrument that passes through the skin, affecting all tissues in its path.

penis The male external reproductive organ through which the urethra passes.

pepsin The enzyme formed from the exposure of pepsinogen to hydrochloric acid in the stomach that is important in the initial breakdown of proteins.

pepsinogen An enzyme produced by the chief cells in the stomach that is converted to pepsin by hydrochloric acid

peptic ulcer disease A condition in which parts of the stomach and duodenal lining are eroded by stomach acid.

peptidases Enzymes that break down proteins.

peptides Protein molecules consisting of amino acids held together by peptide bonds.

pericardial cavity The region around the heart.

pericardial effusion A condition, often caused by trauma, in which the pericardial sac fills with too much fluid, impairing the heart's ability to expand and contract properly.

pericardial fluid A serous fluid that fills the space between the visceral pericardium and the parietal pericardium and helps to reduce friction.

pericardial sac A thick, fibrous membrane that surrounds the heart; also called the pericardium.

pericardial tamponade A condition that occurs as fluid accumulates around the heart, which restricts the heart's stroke volume.

pericardiocentesis A life-saving procedure to correct cardiac tamponade, in which a needle is inserted into the pericardial sac to remove excess fluid that is restricting the heart from expanding and contracting properly.

pericarditis Infection or inflammation of the pericardial membranes, resulting in severe chest pain.

pericardium The thick, fibrous membrane and serous membranes that surround the heart; also called the pericardial sac.

perimetrium A serous membrane coating that makes up the outside layer of the uterine wall.

perimysium The connective tissue sheath that surrounds a muscle and forms sheaths for the bundles of muscle fibers.

perineum The area below the coccygeus and levator ani muscles, which forms the floor of the pelvis.

periosteum A double layer of connective tissue that lines the outer surface of the bone.

peripheral nerves Nerves that extend from the brain and spinal cord to supply motor function and convey sensory information to various areas of the body.

peripheral nervous system The portion of the nervous system that consists of 31 pairs of spinal nerves and 11 of the 12 pairs of cranial nerves; these nerves may be sensory, motor, or connecting nerves.

peristalsis The process of contraction of the smooth muscle in the wall of the alimentary tract that serves to propel food through the system.

peritoneum A two-layer smooth membrane of connective tissue that surrounds a group of digestive organs within the abdomen.

peritonitis Inflammation of the peritoneum, the protective membrane that lines the abdominal and pelvic cavities.

peritubular capillary One of many complex, interconnected capillary networks that branch off of efferent arterioles.

Peyer patches Intermittent patches of lymph nodes located in the ileum.

pH   The measure of acidity or alkalinity of a solution.

phagocytosis   The process of ingesting and destroying foreign matter by certain types of leukocytes.

phalanges   The small bones of the digits of the fingers and toes.

pharyngeal tonsils   One of three sets of lymphatic organs that comprise the tonsils, they are located near the internal opening of the nasal cavity and help protect the body from bacteria introduced into the mouth and nose. Also called adenoids.

pharynx   The cavity lying posterior to the mouth, connecting to the esophagus; the throat.

phenotype   The observable characteristics of an organism that result from genetic composition and environmental factors.

phlebitis   Inflammation of the wall of the vein, sometimes caused by an IV line, manifested by tenderness, redness, and slight edema along part of the length of the vein.

phospholipid   A type of lipid molecule that comprises the cell membrane.

physiology   The study of the body functions of the living organism.

physis   The major site of bone elongation, located at each end of a long bone between the epiphysis and metaphysis; also called the growth plate.

pia mater   The innermost of the three meninges that enclose the brain and spinal cord; it rests directly on the brain and spinal cord.

pineal body   Part of the epithalamus in the diencephalon.

pineal gland   Secretes the hormone melatonin in response to changes in light conditions.

pinna   The large outside portion of the ear through which sound waves enter the ear; also called the auricle.

pinocytosis   A process by which cells ingest the extracellular fluid and its contents.

pituitary gland   An endocrine gland, located in the sella turcia of the brain, that secretes hormones that regulate all major bodily functions.

placenta   The organ that develops from trophoblastic cells of the zygote and attaches to the endometrium on one side and surrounds the embryo on the other side.

plantar fasciitis   An irritation of the tough band of connective tissue extending from the calcaneus to the metatarsal head of each toe.

plasma   A sticky, yellow fluid that carries the blood cells and nutrients and transports cellular waste material to the organs of excretion; normally makes up 55% of the total blood volume.

plasma cells   Cells that produce antibodies (immunoglobulins) to destroy antigens or antigen-containing particles; plasma cells are formed from divided and differentiated B cells.

plasma proteins   The most abundant solutes (dissolved substances) in the plasma.

plasmin   A naturally occurring clot-dissolving enzyme, usually present in the body in its inactive form, plasminogen.

platelets   Tiny, disk-shaped cell fragments that are much smaller than the red or white blood cells; they are essential in the initial formation of a blood clot, the mechanism that stops bleeding.

pleura   The serous membranes covering the lungs and lining the thoracic cavity, completely enclosing a potential space known as the pleural space.

pleural cavity   The cavity formed by the inner borders of the rib cage and the diaphragm.

pleural effusion   Excessive accumulation of fluid within the pleural space.

pleural fluid   The small amount of lubricating fluid that fills the pleural space.

pleural space   A potential space between the visceral pleura and parietal pleura; it is described as "potential" because under normal conditions, the space does not exist.

plexuses   Complex networks made up by the combination of the main portions of the spinal nerves.

plicae circulares   Circular folds that run perpendicular to the long axis of the digestive tract and increase the surface area available for absorption.

pneumothorax   An abnormal accumulation of air within the pleural space.

polar molecule   A molecule that uses a covalent bond in which electrons are not shared equally; this results in a shape that has an uneven distribution of charges.

polarized state   The state of the resting cell, which normally has a net negative charge with respect to the outside of the cell.

polarized   When a cell is at rest, ions are actively transported into and out of the cell to create an electrochemical gradient across the cell membrane.

polygenic disease   The genetic component of a multifactorial disease.

pons   The mass of nerve fibers located below the midbrain and above the medulla oblongata that regulate sleep and respiration.

popliteal artery   A continuation of the femoral artery at the knee.

popliteal fossa   The space behind the knee.

popliteal vein   The vein that forms when the anterior and posterior tibial veins unite at the knee.

positive feedback   The concept that once the desired effect of a hormone begins, further production of the hormone is stimulated.

posterior chamber   The posterior area of the globe between the lens and the iris.

posterior   In anatomy, the back surface of the body.

posterior pituitary (lobe)   One of the two portions of the pituitary gland; it is an extension of the central nervous system and produces hormones called neurohormones; also called the neurohypophysis.

posterior triangle   The area of the neck containing the lymph nodes, brachial plexus, spinal accessory nerve, and a portion of the subclavian artery.

postganglionic neuron   The second of two nerves, separated by a ganglionic synapse, in a series between the central nervous system and the organs that are innervated.

postsynaptic terminal   The end of a nerve where electrical impulses are received from the synaptic cleft.

PR segment   The period between the beginning of the P wave (atrial depolarization) and the onset of the QRS complex (ventricular depolarization), signifying the time required for atrial depolarization and passage of the excitation impulse through the atrioventricular junction.

preganglionic neuron   The first of two nerves, separated by a ganglionic synapse, in a series between the central nervous system and the organs that are innervated.

pregnancy   The condition that begins when the developing offspring implants into the uterine lining; it consists of three trimesters (each about 3 months long).

presynaptic terminal   The end of a nerve where neurotransmitters are released into the synaptic cleft.

primary immune response   The activation of B or T cells after they first encounter the antigens for which they are specialized to react; the process continues for several weeks.

primary respiratory acidosis   A decrease in the blood pH secondary to insufficient exhalation of CO_2.

primary respiratory alkalosis   An increase in the blood pH secondary to excessive exhalation of CO_2.

prime mover   The muscle in a group of muscles that has the major role in movement.

progesterone   A hormone released by the ovaries that stimulates the uterine lining during the menstrual cycle; it is one of three major female hormones.

prolactin   A hormone that plays an important role in milk production in women.

prolactin-inhibiting hormones   Hormones released by the hypothalamus that influence the inhibition of prolactin.

pronation   Rotation of an extremity so that the palm faces downward.

prone position   Lying flat, and face down.

proprioception   Information about the body's position and of its parts in relation to itself, to one another, and to the pull of gravity.

prostaglandins   A group of hormone-like fatty acids that are produced in many body tissues, including the uterus, brain, and kidneys.

prostate gland   A small gland that surrounds the male urethra at the section where it emerges from the urinary bladder; it secretes an alkaline viscid ejaculatory fluid.

prostate specific antigen (PSA)   A blood test used in the diagnosis of prostate cancer.

prostatic urethra   One of three parts of the male urethra; it travels through the prostate gland.

proteins   Created from amino acids, they include enzymes, plasma proteins, muscle components (actin and myosin), hormones, and antibodies.

prothrombin   An alpha globulin made in the liver that is converted to thrombin.

protons   Single, positively charged particles inside the nucleus of an atom.

protoplasm   A viscous liquid matrix that supports all internal cellular structures and provides a medium for intracellular transport; also called cytoplasm.

proximal   Closer to the trunk.

proximal convoluted tubule   One of two complex sections of a nephron; it includes an enlargement at the end called the glomerular capsule.

pseudostratified epithelium   A single layer of epithelial cells of varying heights, all of which attach to the basement membrane, but all do not reach the free surface.

pubic arch   An angle formed by the anterior portion of the hip bone (pubis).

pubis   One of three bones that fuse to form the pelvic ring.

pulmonary circuit   The venules and veins, which send deoxygenated blood to the lungs to receive oxygen and unload carbon dioxide.

pulmonary embolism   A blood clot or foreign matter trapped within the pulmonary circulation.

pulmonary valve   The semilunar valve that regulates blood flow between the right ventricle and the pulmonary artery.

punctum lacrimale   Small opening in the corner of the eye through which tears drain from the lacrimal gland into the lacrimal ducts.

pupil   The circular opening in the center of the eye, through which light passes to the lens.

pyelonephritis   Inflammation of the kidney linings.

QRS complex   Deflections of the ECG produced by ventricular depolarization.

quadriceps femoris   Muscle contained in the anterior compartment of the thigh that extends the knee when contracted.

radial nerve   One of the major nerves in the upper extremity, it supplies muscles that extend the elbow, supinate the forearm, and extend the wrist, fingers, and thumb.

radioisotopes   Also known as radioactive isotopes or radionuclides, they are atoms with unstable nuclei.

radius   The shorter, lateral bone of the forearm.

range of motion (ROM)   The arc of movement of an extremity at a joint.

Raynaud phenomenon   Spasms that develop in the digital arteries, particularly following emotional stress or cold exposure, resulting in white and cool fingertips.

recovery position   When a patient is placed on his or her side to allow the easy drainage of fluids from the mouth; also called the left lateral recumbent position.

rectum   The distal portion of the large intestine, ending at the anal canal.

rectus abdominis   The linear muscle of the midline of the abdomen.

recumbent   Any position in which the patient is lying down or leaning back.

red blood cells   Cells that transport gases, including oxygen; also called erythrocytes.

reflux esophagitis   The back flow of stomach acid into the esophagus; also called heartburn.

regional anatomy   Study of anatomy associated with a particular body region; also called topographic anatomy.

relative refractory period   The latter phase of repolarization in which the cells are able to respond to a stronger-than-normal stimulus.

releasing factors   Compounds that travel from the hypothalamus to the pituitary gland in a specialized set of blood vessels; also called inhibiting factors.

remodeling   The ongoing process of cell renewal where some cells actively divide during life and others die and are replaced by new cells.

renal arteries   The vessels that supply the kidneys with blood; they arise from the abdominal aorta.

renal corpuscle   The initial blood-filtering component of the nephron.

renal cortex   The outer portion of each kidney; it forms renal columns and has tiny tubules associated with the nephrons.

renal failure   Loss of kidney function that occurs secondary to injury or illness.

renal medulla   The inner portion of each kidney; it is made of conical renal pyramids and has striations.

renal papillae   The tips of each renal pyramid, which extend into the medulla and are encircled by the opening of a minor calyx.

renal pelvis   A funnel-shaped sac inside the renal sinus that is subdivided into major and minor calyces (tubes).

renal pyramids   Parallel cone-shaped bundles of urine-collecting tubules that are located in the medulla of the kidneys.

renal sinus Cavity formed by the hilum that is filled with fat and connective tissue.

renal tubule The portion of the nephron containing the tubular fluid filtered through the glomerulus.

renal vein The blood vessel connecting the kidneys to the inferior vena cava.

renin A hormone produced by cells in the juxtaglomerular apparatus when the blood pressure is low.

renin-angiotensin system System located in the kidney that helps to regulate fluid balance and blood pressure.

repolarization The process by which ions are moved across the cell wall to return to a polarized state.

residual volume The volume of air remaining in the respiratory passages and lungs after maximal expiration.

respiratory areas Parts of the brain that control inspiration and expiration.

respiratory bronchioles Structures formed by the final branching of the bronchioles.

respiratory capacities The four capacities created by the combination of two or more of the respiratory volumes.

respiratory cycle One cycle of inspiration followed by expiration.

respiratory membrane Layers of an alveolus that separate air from blood in a capillary; it is where blood and alveolar air exchange gases. Also known as the pulmonary capillary membrane or the alveolar capillary membrane.

respiratory system All the structures of the body that contribute to the process of breathing, including the upper and lower airways and their component parts.

respiratory volumes Four distinct volumes involved in respiration: tidal volume, inspiratory reserve volume, expiratory reserve volume, and residual volume.

resting tidal volume The volume of air that leaves during a normal, resting expiration (about 500 mL).

restrictive lung disease A disease that limits the ability of the lungs to expand appropriately.

reticulospinal tracts Descending tracts that are involved in involuntary body movements.

retina A delicate, 10-layered structure of nervous tissue located in the rear of the interior of the globe that receives light and generates nerve signals that are transmitted to the brain through the optic nerve.

retroperitoneal organs The organs (kidneys, pancreas, and duodenum) and major blood vessels located in the retroperitoneal space.

retroperitoneal space An area behind the parietal peritoneum that contains the kidneys, pancreas, duodenum, and major blood vessels of the abdominal cavity.

retroperitoneum The space behind the peritoneum.

reversible reaction A chemical reaction where the products of the reaction can change back into the reactants they originally were.

rheumatic fever An inflammatory disease caused by streptococcal bacterial infection that can cause a stenosis of the mitral valve or aortic valve.

ribonucleic acid (RNA) Nucleic acid made from DNA in the nucleus of the cell; it moves to the cytoplasm of the cell where it serves as a template for the production of proteins.

ribosomes Organelles that contain RNA and protein.

ribs The 12 pairs of bones that primarily make up the thoracic cage, connecting posteriorly to the thoracic vertebrae.

rickets A disease caused by vitamin D deficiency.

right lymphatic duct The smaller of the two collecting ducts; it receives lymph from the right side of the head and neck, right upper limb, and right thorax.

rootlets Small nerves.

rotator cuff A special group of four muscles that forms a cap over the proximal humerus and ties the humerus to the scapula; it controls rotation at the shoulder joint.

round ligaments One of several ligaments that supports the uterus.

rugae Thick folds of the stomach wall.

saccule An enlarged region of the membranous labyrinth of the inner ear that contains a specialized patch of tissue that aids in the sensation of position and motion.

sacrum One of three bones (sacrum and two pelvic bones) that make up the pelvic ring; consists of five fused sacral vertebrae.

saddle joint Two saddle-shaped articulating surfaces oriented at right angles to each other so that complementary surfaces articulate with each other, such as is the case with the thumb.

sagittal (lateral) plane An imaginary plane dividing the body into left and right parts.

sagittal suture The point of the skull where the parietal bones join together.

saliva The fluid produced by the salivary glands that helps break down starches and other polysaccharides into simple sugars, washes the oral cavity, and helps weaken bacteria.

salivary amylase The primary enzyme in saliva.

salivary glands The glands that produce saliva to keep the mouth and pharynx moist; includes the parotid, sublingual, and submandibular glands.

saphenous vein The longest vein in the body, it drains the leg, thigh, and dorsum of the foot.

sarcolemma The thin transparent sheath surrounding a striated muscle fiber.

sarcomeres The repeating patterns of striation units that appear along each skeletal muscle fiber.

sarcoplasmic reticulum A system of membranes that transport materials in muscle cells.

sartorius muscle The longest muscle in the human body, it is located in the anterior compartment of the thigh and flexes both the hip and knee when it contracts.

scalene muscles Muscles of respiration that elevate the first two ribs during inspiration.

scapula The triangular-shaped bone that comprises the shoulder blade, which is an integral component of the shoulder girdle.

Schwann cells Nervous tissue that helps form the myelin sheath around certain neurons.

sciatic nerve The longest peripheral nerve in the body, formed by the combination of the common peroneal nerve and the tibial nerve.

sciatica Pain and muscle weakness that travels from the back, into the buttocks, and along the leg into the foot as a result of irritation of the sciatic nerve or a lumbar spinal nerve root.

sclera The white part of the eye.

scoliosis Sideways curvature of the spine.

scrotum   The pouch of skin and subcutaneous tissue hanging from the lower abdominal region, posterior to the penis.

sebaceous glands   Glands that produce sebum and are located in the dermis of the entire body, except for the palms and soles.

sebum   Material produced by sebaceous glands that contains a combination of fatty material and cellular debris.

second-degree burns   Burns that involve the epidermis and a portion of the dermis; also called partial-thickness burns.

secondary bronchi   Airway passages in the lungs that are formed from the division of the right and left mainstem bronchi.

secondary immune response   The appearance of concentrations of antibodies in the blood plasma, usually 5 to 10 days after exposure to antigens.

secretin   A hormone produced by the duodenum that inhibits gastric secretion and stimulates the production of alkaline pancreatic secretions.

segmentation   Alternating contraction and relaxation of smooth muscle in nonadjacent segments of the small intestine.

selective permeability   The ability of the cell membrane to selectively allow compounds into the cell based on the cell's current needs.

sella turcica   A depression in the middle of the sphenoid bone where the pituitary gland is located.

semen   Seminal fluid ejaculated from the penis and containing sperm.

semilunar valves   The two valves, the aortic and pulmonic valves, that divide the heart from the aorta and pulmonary artery.

seminal vesicles   Storage sacs for sperm and seminal fluid, which empty into the urethra at the prostate.

seminiferous tubules   Highly coiled structures inside each lobule of a testis; they form a network of channels, then ducts, which join the epididymis.

semipermeable   The property of the cell membrane that describes the ability to allow certain elements to pass through while not allowing others to do so.

sensory nerves   Nerves that carry sensations of touch, taste, heat, cold, pain, and other modalities from the body to the central nervous system.

septum   A solid, wall-like structure that separates the left atrium and ventricle from the right atrium and ventricle.

serosa   The outer lining of the bowel.

serous membranes   Membranes that line body cavities that lack openings to the outside.

serous pericardium   The inner membrane of the pericardium, which contains two layers called the visceral pericardium and the parietal pericardium.

serum osmolality   The number of osmotically active particles in serum.

sex cells   Germ (reproductive) cells; in males they are known as sperm and in females they are known as oocytes (eggs).

sex chromosomes   The X and Y chromosomes, which determine sex.

sex-linked diseases   Disease resulting from defects on either the X or the Y chromosome.

short bones   Types of bones that are as broad as they are long.

shoulder joint   A ball-and-socket joint consisting of the head of the humerus and the glenoid fossa.

sigmoid colon   One of four portions of the colon; it extends from the descending colon and forms an S-shaped tube that extends into the pelvis and ends as the rectum.

simple epithelium   A single layer of cells, all of which are in contact with the basement membrane of the epithelial cell.

sinoatrial (SA) node   The dominant pacemaker of the heart, located at the junction of the superior vena cava and the right atrium.

sinusitis   Inflammation of the paranasal sinuses.

sinusoids   A part of the hepatic portal system in which blood collects within the liver and the liver cells extract nutrients from the blood, filter the blood, and metabolize various drugs.

skeletal muscle   Striated muscles that are under direct volitional control of the brain; also called voluntary muscle.

skeletal muscle tissue   Voluntary muscle tissue attached to bones and composed of long thread-like cells that have light and dark striations.

skull   The structure at the top of the axial skeleton that houses the brain and consists of the 28 bones that comprise the auditory ossicles, the cranium, and the face.

sliding filament model   A method of action of muscle contraction involving how sarcomeres shorten, with thick and thin filaments sliding past each other toward the center of the sarcomere from both ends.

small intestine   The portion of the gastrointestinal system that consists of the duodenum, jejunum, and ileum and is the major site of food digestion and nutrient absorption.

smooth muscle   Nonstriated muscle that carries out much of the automatic work of the body, such as moving food through the digestive tract and dilating and constricting the pupils of the eye; also called involuntary muscle.

sodium-potassium exchange pump   A mechanism that uses active transport to move sodium out of the cells and potassium into the cells.

sodium-potassium pump   A molecular (ion-transporting) mechanism whereby sodium is actively moved out of a cell and potassium moved in.

solutes   Dissolved particles, such as salts, contained in a solvent.

somatic cells   All of the other cells in the human body besides the sex cells.

somatic nervous system   The part of the nervous system that regulates activities over which there is voluntary control.

somatomedins   Proteins produced in the liver, skeletal muscle, and other tissues that are stimulated by growth hormone.

somatostatin   A hormone released by the hypothalamus that inhibits the secretion of growth hormone; also called growth hormone release–inhibiting hormone.

somatotropin   Hormone that stimulates growth in many tissues, especially of long bones in the extremities; also called growth hormone.

species resistance   An innate (nonspecific) defense wherein one species is resistant to certain diseases that may affect other species.

sperm cells   Male gametes that are produced in the testicles; also called spermatozoa.

spermatic cord   A cord composed of the testicular artery, venous plexus, lymph vessels, nerves, connective tissue, and the cremaster muscle.

spermatogenesis   The process by which sperm cells are formed.

spermatozoa   Male gametes that are produced in the testicles; also called sperm.

sphenoid bone   The anterior portion of the base of the cranium.

sphincters   Rings of muscle that surround an opening, allowing for contraction or closing.

spinal cavity   The spinal column or vertebral canal, housing the spinal cord.

spinal cord An extension of the brain, composed of virtually all the nerves carrying messages between the brain and the rest of the body; it lies inside of and is protected by the spinal canal.

spinal nerves The 31 pairs of nerves responsible for sending and receiving sensory and motor messages to and from the central nervous system from a portion of the body.

spinal reflex arcs Automatic reactions to stimuli mediated by neuronal pathways within the spinal cord that occur without conscious thought.

spinal tap A needle insertion through the vertebral canal to the subarachnoid space to obtain a specimen of cerebrospinal fluid.

spindle fibers Microtubules radiating from the centrioles.

spinocerebellar tracts Ascending tracts that carry information regarding body position (proprioception) to the cerebellum.

spirometer A device used in pulmonary function testing that measures air entering and leaving the lungs over a specific period of time.

spleen The largest lymphatic organ; filters the blood via the actions of lymphocytes and macrophages.

splenectomy Surgical removal of the spleen.

splenic flexure The second sharp turn in the large intestine, connecting the transverse colon to the descending colon.

spongy urethra One of the three parts of the male urethra; it lies within the corpus spongiosum of the penis and terminates at the external urethral orifice.

squamous epithelia The flat sheets of cells that make up the epidermis.

squamous epithelium Flat sheets of epithelial cells.

ST segment The interval between the end of the QRS complex and the beginning of the T wave; often elevated or depressed with respect to the isoelectric line when there is significant myocardial ischemia.

static equilibrium The maintenance of balance when the head and body are motionless.

static labyrinth system One of two mechanisms involved in the sensation of balance and movement, it evaluates the position of the head relative to gravity or linear acceleration/deceleration.

sternum The breastbone in the center of the anterior chest.

steroid Molecules with four connected rings of carbon atoms, including cholesterol, estrogen, progesterone, testosterone, cortisol, and estradiol.

stomach An expandable organ that is located in the left upper quadrant, below the diaphragm.

stratified epithelium More than one layer of cells, only one of which is in contact with the basement membrane of the epithelial cell.

stratum corneum The outer layer of the epidermis, which contains about 25 layers of dead cells that continuously shed as new cells push upward.

stratum germinativum The innermost layer of epidermis.

stratum granulosum The layer of epidermis between the stratum lucidum and the stratum spinosum that is composed of flattened cells that contain granules of keratohyalin.

stratum lucidum The first inner layer of the epidermis, it is readily visible only in the thick epithelium of the palms of the hands and the soles of the feet.

stratum spinosum The layer of epidermis between the stratum granulosum and the stratum germinativum that contains cells known as keratinocytes, which synthesize the keratohyaline, a precursor of keratin.

striated Muscle tissue that has microscopic bands and may be either voluntary, such as leg muscles, or involuntary, such as cardiac muscle.

striations Areas of alternating, colored bands of skeletal muscle fiber.

stroke Brain damage typically resulting from a disruption of the circulation to the brain, causing abnormal neurologic findings.

stroke volume The volume of blood pumped forward with each ventricular contraction.

subarachnoid hemorrhage A hemorrhage into the brain tissue beneath the arachnoid membrane.

subarachnoid space The space located between the pia mater and the arachnoid in which the cerebrospinal fluid is contained.

subclavian artery The proximal part of the main artery of the arm, which supplies the brain, neck, anterior chest wall, and shoulder.

subclavian vein The proximal part of the main vein of the arm, which unites with the internal jugular vein and terminates at the superior vena cava.

subcutaneous layer The layer of soft tissue immediately below the dermis; also called the hypodermis.

sublingual glands One pair of the three sets of salivary glands; located beneath the tongue.

submandibular glands One pair of the three sets of salivary glands located beneath the mandible.

submucosa The lining next to the mucosa in the gastrointestinal system that contains blood vessels and lymphatic channels.

substantia nigra A layer of gray matter located in the midbrain.

substrate The target of enzyme action.

subthalamus The part of the diencephalon that is involved in controlling motor functions.

sulci Grooves located between the gyri in the cerebrum.

superficial burns Burns involving only the epidermis; also called first-degree burns.

superficial peroneal nerve The nerve in the leg that innervates the muscles of foot eversion.

superior Above a body part or nearer to the head.

superior oblique muscle The muscle that controls the downward gaze of the eyeball.

superior vena cava One of the two largest veins in the body; carries blood from the upper extremities, head, neck, and chest into the heart.

supination Turning the palms upward (toward the sky).

supine position The position in which the body is lying face up.

surface tension An effect that makes it difficult for the alveoli to inflate; it is caused by attraction of water molecules.

surfactant A mixture of lipids and proteins synthesized to reduce the tendency of alveolar collapse and to ease alveolar inflation.

suspensory ligament One of the two ligaments that help to hold the ovaries in place.

sutures Attachment points in the skull where the cranial bones join together.

sweat pores Pores in the skin through which sweat is secreted.

sympathetic pathway The part of the autonomic nervous system that is responsible for the body's response to shock and stress.

synapse The junction between nerve cells across which nervous stimuli are transmitted. Includes the synaptic cleft, presynaptic cell membrane with synaptic vesicles and axon terminal and postsynaptic cell membrane.

synaptic cleft The space between neurons where electrical impulses trigger the release of neurotransmitters, which in turn stimulate an electrical reaction in adjacent neurons.

synaptic vesicles Vesicles that contain neurotransmitters.

synergists Muscles that work together to accomplish a particular movement.

synovial fluid The small amount of liquid within a joint used as lubrication.

synthesis reaction A reaction that occurs when two or more reactants (atoms) bond to form a more complex product or structure.

systemic anatomy The study of anatomy associated with a particular organ system.

systemic circuit The arteries and arterioles, which send oxygenated blood and nutrients to the body cells while removing wastes.

systole The period of time when the atria or ventricles are contracting; also called atrial or ventricular systole.

T lymphocytes (T cells) Specialized lymphocytes that make up the majority of circulated blood lymphocytes. Once activated, they interact directly with antigens to produce the cellular immune response; they also stimulate B cells to produce antibodies.

T wave The upright, flat, or inverted wave following the QRS complex of the ECG, representing ventricular repolarization.

tachycardia A rapid pulse rate.

tachypnea A rapid respiratory rate.

talus A bone that articulates with the tibia, calcaneus, and navicular bones to form the lower part of the ankle joint.

tarsals The bones of the ankles; they include the medial cuneiform, intermediate cuneiform, lateral cuneiform, navicular, cuboid, talus, and calcaneus.

taste buds Receptors in the tongue and mouth that sense salt and sweet sensations separately; also called taste receptors.

taste hairs Hair-like projections of the gustatory cells of the taste buds.

taste receptors Receptors in the tongue and mouth that sense salt and sweet sensations separately; also called taste buds.

temporal bones Bones that form the lower sides and base of the cranium.

temporal lobe The portion of the brain that plays an important role in hearing and memory.

temporomandibular joint (TMJ) The joint between the temporal bone and the posterior condyle of the mandible that allows for movements of the jaw.

tendons Tough, ropelike cords of fibrous tissue that attach muscles to bones.

teniae coli A portion of the longitudinal muscle layer of the wall of the large intestine that encircles the colon.

tertiary bronchi Airway passages in the lungs that are formed from branching of the secondary bronchi.

testes The male reproductive organs that produce sperm and secrete male hormones; also called testicles.

testicular torsion Twisting of the testicle on the spermatic cord, from which it is suspended; associated with scrotal pain and swelling, and is a medical emergency.

testosterone The major androgen produced by the testes.

tetany Painful muscle spasms that result from several conditions, including a low blood calcium level.

tetraiodothyronine (T$_4$) One of the two major hormones produced by the thyroid gland; it is essential for normal growth and development in children as well as regulation of body metabolism.

thalamus The part of the diencephalon that processes most sensory input and influences mood and general body movements, especially those associated with fear or rage.

thermolysis Normal bodily means of heat dissipation from the body.

thermoregulation The maintenance of normal body temperature (98.6°F, or 37.0°C).

third-degree burns Burns that involve the hypodermis and possibly bone, muscle, or internal organs; also called full-thickness burns.

Thompson test A test used to evaluate the integrity of the Achilles tendon for possible rupture.

thoracic cage The ribs, thoracic vertebrae, and sternum.

thoracic duct One of two great lymph vessels; it empties into the superior vena cava.

thoracic vertebrae The 12 vertebrae located in the center of the vertebral column that (mostly) connect with the ribs.

thrombi Blood clots.

thrombin An enzyme that causes the conversion of fibrinogen to fibrin, which binds to the platelet plug, forming the final mature clot.

thrombocytes Incomplete cells important in blood clotting; also called platelets.

thymosins Hormones that affect early production and differentiation of lymphocytes.

thymus A gland that is larger in children but shrinks with age; it secretes thymosins, which are important in early immunity by affecting production and differentiation of lymphocytes.

thyroglobulin A protein to which thyroid hormones are bound.

thyroid gland A large endocrine gland that is located at the base of the neck and produces and excretes hormones that influence growth, development, and metabolism.

thyroid-stimulating hormone (TSH) A hormone that controls the release of thyroid hormone from the thyroid gland; also called thyrotropin.

thyrotropin A hormone that controls the release of thyroid hormone from the thyroid gland; also called thyroid-stimulating hormone.

thyroxine-binding globulin A protein synthesized in the liver that binds to hormones T$_3$ and T$_4$.

tibia The shin bone; the larger of the two bones of the lower leg.

tibial nerve The nerve in the leg that innervates the muscles that extend the hip, flex the knee, plantar flex the ankle, and flex the toes.

tibial veins A continuation of the veins of the feet that unite at the knee to form the popliteal vein, which then drains into the femoral vein.

tidal volume A measure of the depth of breathing; the volume of air that is inhaled or exhaled during a single respiratory cycle.

tinnitus The perception of sound in the inner ear with no external environmental cause; often reported as "ringing" in the ears, but may be roaring, buzzing, or clicking.

tissue plasminogen activator An important element of the fibrinolytic system; causes clots that have already formed to lyse or be disrupted; works by converting plasminogen to plasmin.

tissues Groups of similar cells that work together.

tonsils Three sets of lymphatic organs—the palatine tonsils, pharyngeal tonsils, and lingual tonsils—that are located in the back of the throat and nasopharynx and protect the body from bacteria introduced into the mouth and nose.

topographic anatomy   The study of anatomy associated with a particular body region; also called regional anatomy.

total lung capacity   Vital capacity plus residual volume.

touch receptors   Receptors located in various areas of the skin to detect the sense of touch.

trabeculae   Bony rods that make up a lacy network of cancellous bones and are oriented to increase weight-bearing capacity of long bones.

trace elements   Essential minerals found in very small amounts; including chromium, cobalt, copper, fluorine, iodine, iron, manganese, selenium, and zinc.

trachea   The conduit for all entry into the lungs; a tubular structure that is approximately 10 to 12 cm long and composed of a series of C-shaped cartilaginous rings; also called the windpipe.

tracts   Pathways within the spinal cord that contain nerves.

transient ischemic attack   An episode of neurologic impairment that lasts less than 24 hours and represents a warning sign of an impending stroke.

transitional epithelium   Tissue that changes in appearance due to tension; it lines the urinary bladder, ureters, and superior urethra.

transverse (axial) plane   An imaginary line where the body is cut into top and bottom parts.

transverse colon   One of four portions of the colon; it extends from the hepatic flexure across the abdomen to the splenic flexure.

transverse tubules   T-tubules; membranous channels extending inward and passing through muscle fibers.

Trendelenburg position   The position in which the body is supine with the head lower than the feet.

tricuspid valve   The heart valve that separates the right atrium from the right ventricle.

trigeminal nerve   The cranial nerve (V) that supplies sensation to the scalp, forehead, face, and lower jaw and innervates the muscles of mastication, the throat, and the inner ear.

triiodothyronine (T_3)   One of the two major hormones produced by the thyroid gland; it is essential for normal growth and development in children as well as regulation of body metabolism.

trimesters   Three segments of time, each made up of approximately 3 months, that comprise the length of a pregnancy.

trismus   Involuntary contraction of the mouth resulting in clenched teeth; occurs during seizures and head injuries.

trochlear nerve   The cranial nerve (IV) that innervates the superior oblique muscle of the eyeball, which controls a downward gaze.

trophoblast   The outer group of cells in a zygote that develop to become the placenta.

tropomyosin   An actin-binding protein that regulates muscle contraction and other actin-related mechanical function of the body.

troponin   A regulatory protein in the actin filaments of skeletal and cardiac muscle that attaches to tropomyosin.

true vocal cords   The inferior portion of the vocal cords that vibrate to produce sound.

trypsin   A pancreatic enzyme that aids in the digestion of proteins.

tubal pregnancy   An ectopic pregnancy in which the oocyte has been abnormally implanted within the fallopian tube.

tubular reabsorption   The process that moves substances from the tubular fluid into the blood, within the peritubular capillary.

tubular secretion   The process that moves substances from the blood in the peritubular capillary into the renal tubule.

tunica media   The middle and thickest layer of tissue of a blood vessel wall, composed of elastic tissue and smooth muscle cells that allow the vessel to expand or contract in response to changes in blood pressure and tissue demand.

turbinates   A set of bony convolutions formed by the conchae in the nasopharynx that help to maintain smooth airflow.

tympanic membrane   A thin membrane that separates the middle ear from the inner ear and transmits vibrations to the ossicles; also called the eardrum.

ulna   The longer, medial bone of the forearm.

ulnar nerve   The nerve in the arm that innervates muscles that flex the wrist and fingers and abduct and adduct the fingers and thumb.

ultrasound   A special device that uses sound waves to determine the location and shape of internal tissues and organs.

umbilical cord   The connection between the placenta and the fetus.

umbilicus   The navel, which serves as the central reference point in determining the location of organs in the abdominal quadrants.

unmyelinated axons   Neurons with no myelin sheath or white matter.

upper limbs   The humerus bones, radius bones, ulna bones, carpals, metacarpals, and phalanges.

ureters   A pair of thick-walled, hollow tubes that carry urine from the kidneys to the urinary bladder.

urethra   A hollow, tubular structure that drains urine from the bladder to outside of the body.

urethritis   A bacterial infection of the urethra.

urinalysis   The laboratory evaluation of urine.

urinary bladder   A hollow, muscular sac in the midline of the lower abdominal area that stores urine until it is excreted.

urinary system   The organs that control the discharge of certain waste materials filtered from the blood and excreted as urine.

urine   The final product of tubular reabsorption and secretion; it is a clear, yellow fluid that carries wastes out of the body.

urogenital triangle   The region within the pelvis that contains the structures of the urogenital system.

urolithiasis   A condition characterized by the presence of a kidney stone.

uterosacral ligaments   One of several ligaments that supports the uterus.

uterus   In females, the muscular organ where the fetus grows; found between the urinary bladder and the rectum; also called the womb.

utricle   An enlarged portion of the labyrinth of the inner ear that contains a specialized patch of tissue that aids in the sensation of position and motion.

uvula   A soft-tissue structure that resembles a punching bag; located in the posterior aspect of the oral cavity, at the base of the tongue.

vaccine   A substance that includes antigens that stimulate an immune response against a particular pathogen.

vagina   A canal in a female reproductive system extending from the uterus to the external orifice. The vagina allows for the discharge of menstrual flow, receives the penis during sexual intercourse, and serves as the birth canal.

vaginitis   An inflammation of the vagina that is caused by an infection.

vagus nerve   The cranial nerve (X) that provides motor functions to the soft palate, pharynx, and larynx and carries taste bud fibers from the posterior tongue, sensory fibers from the inferior pharynx, larynx, thoracic, and abdominal organs, and parasympathetic fibers to thoracic and abdominal organs.

vas deferens   The spermatic duct of the testicles.

vasa recta   A series of peritubular capillaries that surround the loop of Henle, into which water moves after passing through the descending and ascending limbs of the loop of Henle.

vasectomy   A form of birth control in which the vas deferens on each side is surgically cut and tied.

vasoconstriction   The contraction of blood vessels, which decreases their diameter.

vasodilation   The relaxation of blood vessels, which increases their diameter.

vasopressin   A hormone secreted by the posterior pituitary gland that constricts blood vessels and raises the blood pressure; also called antidiuretic hormone.

vasospasm   The action of a muscle contraction in a small blood vessel that occurs after it is cut or broken; this action can completely close the ends of a severed vessel.

veins   The blood vessels that bring blood back to the heart.

venous sinuses   Spaces between the membranes surrounding the brain that are the primary means of venous drainage from the brain.

ventilation   The process of exchanging air between the lungs and the environment; includes inhalation and exhalation.

ventral root   One of two roots of a spinal nerve that is formed from six to eight rootlets.

ventral   The anterior surface of the body.

ventricles (brain)   Specialized fluid-filled areas in the brain.

ventricles (heart)   The two lower chambers of the heart that pump blood out of the heart.

venules   Microscopic vessels that link capillaries to veins.

vermiform appendix   An appendage attached to the end of the cecum that contains large numbers of lymph nodules.

vertebral arch   The posterior portion of a vertebra, which contains the bony processes, facets, and pedicles.

vertebral canal   The bony canal formed by vertebrae that houses and protects the spinal cord.

vertebral column   The spine or primary support structure of the body that houses the spinal cord and the peripheral nerves.

vertebral foramen   A hole through which spinal nerves pass from the spinal cord.

vestibular folds   The superior portion of the vocal cords; also called the false vocal cords.

vestibular gland   One of two glands that lie on each side of the vaginal opening; it secretes mucus into the vestibule to moisten and lubricate the vagina for insertion of the penis.

vestibule (ear)   The central part of the labyrinth, behind the cochlea and in front of the semicircular canals.

vestibule (vagina)   The space into which the vagina and the urethra open.

vestibulocochlear nerve   The cranial nerve (VIII) that passes through the internal auditory meatus and transmits information important to the senses of hearing and balance.

vestibulospinal tracts   Descending tracts that are involved in involuntary body movements.

villi   Fingerlike projections in the plicae circulares.

visceral layer   The layer of the serous pericardium that lies closely against the heart; also called the epicardium.

visceral peritoneum   A smooth membrane of connective tissue that lies in immediate contact with the organs within the peritoneal cavity.

visceral pleura   The pleural membrane that covers the lungs.

visceral portion   The portion of a serous membrane that covers the outside of an internal organ.

visceral smooth muscle   Sheets of muscle found in the digestive, reproductive, and urinary tracts.

visual cortex   The area in the brain where signals from the optic nerve are converted into visual images.

vital capacity   The amount of air moved in and out of the lungs with maximum inspiration and exhalation.

vitamins   Organic compounds required for normal metabolism.

vitreous humor   A jelly-like substance found in the posterior compartment of the eye between the lens and the retina.

vomer bone   The flat bone making up the lower posterior nasal septum.

vulva   The female external genitalia; includes the labia majora, labia minora, clitoris, and vestibular glands.

whiplash   A layman's term for traumatic soft-tissue injury to the structures of the neck, associated with sudden flexion or extension.

white blood cells   Cells that protect the body against disease, particularly infectious disease; also called leukocytes.

white matter   Bundles of myelinated nerves.

wounds   Breaks in the integrity of the integumentary system.

Yergason test   Supination of the forearm against resistance to evaluate whether a patient has bicipital tendinitis.

zona fasciculata   One of three divisions of the adrenal cortex; it produces corticosteroids.

zona glomerulosa   One of three divisions of the adrenal cortex; it produces mineralocorticoids.

zona reticularis   One of three divisions of the adrenal cortex; it secretes a few relatively weak male sex hormones, or androgens.

zygomatic bones   Also known as the malar bones; they form the prominence of each cheek.

zygote   A large fertilized egg cell produced after contacting a male sperm cell; the first cell of a future offspring, it contains 23 chromosomes from the father and 23 chromosomes from the mother.

Index

maxillae, 58
McBurney point, 210, 220
meatus, 98, 110
mechanical barriers, innate (nonspecific)
   defenses, 155
mechanical digestion, 206, 207, 220
medial line, 6, 18
medial malleolus, 67
median nerve, 179–180, 187
mediastinum, 36, 40, 115, 143
medulla, 172, 187, 233, 239
medulla oblongata, 105
medullary cavity, 46
medullary respiratory center, 105, 110
meiosis, 27, 40, 258, 279
melanin, 195, 203
melanocytes, 195, 197f, 203
melatonin, 235, 239
membrane-associated proteins, 22f
membranous urethra, 251, 254
memory T cells, 158, 163
menarche, 259, 279
Mendel's Laws of Heredity, 272
meninges, 58, 172–174, 187
meningitis, 173, 187
menisci, 47
menopause, 259, 279
menstrual cycle, 259, 279
menstruation, 260, 279
merocrine (eccrine) glands, 198, 203
mesenteric angina, 131, 143
mesenteric infarction, 131, 143
mesenteries, 217, 220
mesovarium, 258, 279
messenger RNA (mRNA), 25
metabolic pathways, 304–306
metabolic reactions, control of, 301–302
metabolism, 300, 309
metacarpals, 64
metaphase, mitosis, 27
metaphysis, 46
metastasize, 148, 163
metatarsals, 68
micronutrients, 297
microorganisms, 160, 163
microscopic anatomy, 2, 18
microscopic lymphatic capillaries, 148
microtubules, 26, 40
micturition, 250, 254
midaxillary lines, 6, 8f, 18
midclavicular lines, 6, 8f, 18
middle ear, 286, 294
midsagittal plane (midline), 5, 6, 18
mineralocorticoids, 233, 239
minerals, 299, 309
mitochondria, 26, 40, 302, 309
mitosis, 27, 28f, 40
mitral valve, 116, 143
molecule, 11–12, 18
monocytes, 136, 143
mononuclear phagocytic system, 156, 163
monosaccharides, 14, 214
mons pubis, 261, 279
motility, 212, 220
motor end plate, 77–78, 94
motor nerves, 179, 187
motor neurons, 77, 94
motor unit, 94
mouth, 210
mRNA. See messenger RNA
mucosa, 207, 220
mucus, 23, 210, 215, 220
multiunit smooth muscle, 82, 94
murmur, heart, 120, 143
muscarinic receptors, 183, 187
muscarinic stimulation, 184
muscle fasciculus, 76, 94
muscle impulse, 80, 94
muscle tissues, 31–32, 31f

muscles, 76, 94
muscular anatomy, 83
   abdomen, 87
   anterior and posterior views, 84f
   face, 84, 85f
   head, 83–84, 85f
   lower extremity, 90–92, 90f–92f
   pelvic floor and perineum, 88–89, 89f
   shoulder and back, 84–86
   thorax, 87, 87f
   tongue muscles, 84, 86f
   upper extremity, 87–88, 87f–89f
muscular system, 3
musculocutaneous nerve, 179, 187
musculoskeletal system, 76, 94
myelin sheath, 167, 187
myelinated nerves, 167, 169f, 187
myocardial cell, 123
myocardial infarction, 119, 143
myocardial muscle, 31–32
myocardium, 31, 115, 143
myofibrils, 76, 94
myoglobin, 81, 94
myometrium, 259, 279
myosin, 77, 94

N

nail bed, 198, 203
nails, 198, 203
naloxone, 229
nares, 98
nasal bones, 58
nasal cavity, 55
nasal mucosa, 97
nasal septum, 58, 98, 110
nasolacrimal ducts, 98, 110, 283, 284f, 294
nasopharynx, 97, 98, 110
neck
   arteries of, 128–129, 129f
   venous circulation, 132, 132f
negative feedback, 225, 239
nematodes, 160
nephrons, 243–245, 244f, 254
nerve fibers, 167, 188
nerve impulse, 79, 94
nerves, 167, 180f, 188
nervous system, 3, 166–168, 167f, 188
   ANS, 182–184
   central nervous system, 168–169
      brainstem, 172
      cerebellum, 172
      cerebrum, 169–171
      diencephalon, 171
      meninges, 172–174
      spinal cord, 174–178
   peripheral nervous system, 178–179
      brachial plexus, 179–180
      cervical plexus, 179
      cranial nerves, 181–182
      lumbosacral plexus, 181
   subdivisions of, 167f
nervous tissues, 32–33, 40
neuroeffector cells, 183, 188
neuroglia, 32, 40, 167, 188
neurohormones, 226, 239
neurohypophysis, 225, 239
neuromuscular blockers, 179, 188
neuromuscular junction, 77, 79f, 94,
   179, 188
neurons, 32, 32f, 40, 166, 169f, 188
neurotransmitters, 77, 94, 167, 170f,
   183–184, 188
neutrons, 9, 18, 22, 40
neutrophils, 136, 143, 156, 163
nicotinic receptors, 183, 188
nodes of Ranvier, 167, 188
nondisplaced fracture, 52
nonelectrolytes, 14

nonspecific defenses. See innate (nonspecific)
   defenses
nonspecific nongonococcal urethritis, 248, 254
nonstriated involuntary muscles, 32
nonstriated muscle tissue, 31, 40
norepinephrine, 122, 143, 183, 184, 188, 233, 239
normal flora, 160, 163, 215, 220
nuclear chromatin, 26
nuclear envelope, 25–26, 40
nucleic acids, 15, 16f, 18, 270, 279
nucleoli, 26, 40
nucleolus, 25
nucleoplasm, 25
nucleus, 25, 40
nucleus pulposus, 59, 61f
nutrients, 297, 309
   digestion and absorption, 297–300
nutritional disorders, 38

O

oblique fracture, 53, 53f
obturator nerve, 181, 188
occipital bone, 55
occipital condyles, 61
occipital lobe, 171, 188
oculomotor nerve, 182, 188
olecranon bursitis, 64
olfactory bulbs, 182, 188, 291, 294
olfactory cortex, 291, 294
olfactory nerve, 182, 188
olfactory tracts, 182, 188, 291, 294
omental bursa, 217, 220
oocytes, 257, 279
oogenesis, 258, 279
open fracture, 52, 52f, 54
optic chiasm, 182, 188
optic foramen, 182, 188, 285, 294
optic nerve, 182, 182f, 188, 285, 294
optic tracts, 182, 188
oral digestion, 206, 208
orbits, 58, 283, 294
organ of Corti, 286, 294
organ system, 21, 33, 40
   body cavities, 35–37, 37f
   body regions, 33, 34f, 35
organelles, 14, 21, 22, 25–26, 40
organic chemicals, 14, 18
organic substances, 14–15
organism, 33, 40
organizational levels of body, 3f
origin, 81, 94
oropharynx, 97, 111
osmoreceptors, 226, 239
osmosis, 23, 41
osmotic pressure, 23–24, 41
ossicles, 55, 286, 294
ossification, 51
osteoblasts, 50
osteoclasts, 46
osteocytes, 50
osteogenesis imperfecta, 54
osteomalacia, 54
osteomyelitis, 54
osteons, 46
osteoporosis, 54
ostium, 258, 279
otolithic membrane, 288, 294
otoliths, 288, 294
oval window, 286, 294
ovarian ligament, 258, 279
ovaries, 234, 239, 258, 279
ovulation, 258, 279
oxygen, 14
   capillary function and, 125
   gas exchange, 106, 268
   red blood cells and, 134–136
oxygen debt, 81, 94
oxyhemoglobin, 107, 111
oxytocin, 226, 239

P

P wave, 124, 143
pain, referred, 292
palatine bones, 58
palatine tonsils, 152, 163
palmar arches, 129, 143
pancreas, 217, 220, 231–232, 232f, 239
pancreatic duct, 217, 220
pancreatic enzymes, 217
pap smear, 260
papillary muscles, 116, 143
paracrine, 224, 239
parafollicular cells, 229, 239
paranasal sinuses, 54
parasympathetic-blocking drug, 184, 188
parasympathetic nerve impulses, 210
parasympathetic nervous system, 183, 188
parathyroid glands, 230, 230f, 239
parathyroid hormone, 230, 239
parietal arteries, 130
parietal bones, 55
parietal cells, 211, 220
parietal layer, 115, 143
parietal lobe, 171, 188
parietal peritoneum, 217, 220
parietal pleura, 101, 111
parietal portion, 41
    of serous membrane line, 35
parotid glands, 210, 220
partial pressure of carbon dioxide (PaCO$_2$),
    106, 111
partial pressure of oxygen (PaO$_2$), 106, 111
partial-thickness burns, 200, 203
passive immunity, 158
patella, 67
patent foramen ovale, 120
pathogen, 154, 163
pathologic fracture, 53, 53f
pathologic parasympathetic, symptoms of, 184
pathophysiology, 2, 18
pectineus muscles, 90, 94
pectoral girdle, 63
pectoralis major, 83, 94
pedicles, 59
pelvic cavities, 37f
pelvic floor muscles, 88–89
pelvic fractures, 67
pelvic girdle, 65–67, 66f
pelvis, 65
    arteries of, 131, 131f
    venous circulation, 133
penetrating wound, 200, 203
penis, 265, 265f, 279
pepsin, 212, 220
pepsinogen, 211–212, 220
peptic ulcer disease, 212, 220
peptidases, 214, 220
peptide bond, 301
peptide hormones, 225f
peptides, 15, 18
perforating wounds, 285
pericardial cavity, 36, 41
pericardial effusion, 37, 41, 119, 143
pericardial fluid, 115, 143
pericardial sac, 36, 41, 115, 143
pericardial tamponade, 37, 41
pericardiocentesis, 119, 119f, 143
pericarditis, 119, 143
pericardium, 36, 41, 115, 143
perimetrium, 259, 279
perimysium, 76, 94
perineum, 88–89, 89f, 94, 266, 279
periosteum, 33, 45
peripheral chemoreceptors, 105
peripheral nerves, 32, 41, 179, 188
peripheral nervous system, 178–179, 188
    brachial plexus, 179–180
    cervical plexus, 179
    cranial nerves, 181–182

efferent neurons in, 182
    lumbosacral plexus, 181
    pathways of somatic and autonomic
        divisions of, 183f
peristalsis, 208, 220
peritoneum, 217, 220
peritonitis, 38, 41, 210, 220
peritubular capillary, 245, 254
permeability of cell membrane, 23–24
pernicious anemia, 212
peroneal nerve, 181
pesticides, 38
Peyer patches, 152, 214, 220
pH, 111
    of blood, 106
    scale, 13, 14f, 18
phagocytosis process, 24, 41, 136, 155, 156, 163
phalanges, 64
pharyngeal tonsils, 152, 163
pharynx, 97, 110
phenotype, 272, 279
phlebitis, 138, 143
phospholipid, 15, 18
phrenic nerves, 179f
physical agents, 38
physiology, 2, 18
physis, 46
pia mater, 173, 188
pineal body, 171, 188
pineal gland, 235, 235f, 239
pinna, 286, 294
pinocytosis, 24, 41
pituitary gland, 55, 225, 227f, 239, 258
pivot joints, 48
placenta, 266, 279
plane joints, 48
planes of body, 5, 5f, 5t
plantar arteries, 131
plantar fasciitis, 69
plaque formation, 127
plasma. See intravascular fluid
plasma cells, 157, 163
plasma membrane. See cell membranes
plasma proteins, 134, 143
plasmin, 137, 143
platelets, 135f, 137–138, 140, 143
pleura, 36, 41, 101, 101f, 111
pleural cavity, 101, 111
pleural effusion, 37, 41
pleural fluid, 36, 41
pleural membrane, 101
pleural space, 36, 41, 101, 101f, 111
plexus, 179, 188
plicae circulares, 214, 220
pneumothorax, 36, 41
polar molecule, 12, 18
polarized cell, 80, 94
polarized state, 123, 144
polygenic disease, 274, 279
polypeptides, 25, 301
polysaccharides, 14
polyunsaturated fat, 15
pons, 128, 144, 172, 188
popliteal artery, 131, 144
popliteal fossa, 33, 41
popliteal vein, 133, 144
positive feedback, 225, 239
posterior chamber, eye, 284, 294
posterior, definition, 6, 18
posterior pituitary (lobe), 225, 226, 239
posterior triangle, 33, 41
postganglionic neuron, 183, 188
postsynaptic terminal, 167, 188
potassium channels, 33
potassium ions, 122, 133
PR segment, 124, 144
preganglionic neuron, 183, 188
pregnancy, 266–269, 279
    birth, 268–269
    ectopic. See ectopic pregnancy

embryo implantation, 266f
    erythroblastosis fetalis, 138
    gestation, 266–267
    labor, 268
    ligament stretch during, 260
    trimesters, 266–267
    tubal. See tubal pregnancy
presynaptic terminal, 167, 188
primary hyperaldosteronism, 234
primary immune response, 158, 163
primary respiratory acidosis, 106, 111
primary respiratory alkalosis, 106, 111
prime mover, 82, 94
prions, 160
procainamide, 122
progesterone, 234, 239, 260, 279
prolactin, 229, 239
prolactin-inhibiting hormones, 229, 239
prolactin-releasing hormones, 229, 239
pronation, 8, 18
prone position, 8, 10f, 18
prophase, 27
proprioception, 178, 188
prostaglandins, 224, 239
prostate gland, 251, 254, 265, 279
prostate-specific antigen (PSA), 265, 279
prostatic urethra, 251, 254
proteins, 15, 18, 22, 298–299
prothrombin, 137, 144
protons, 9, 18, 22, 41
protoplasm, 21, 41
protozoans, 160
proximal convoluted tubule, 245, 254
proximal, definition, 6, 18
PSA. See prostate-specific antigen
pseudostratied columnar epithelium, 28, 28t,
    29f, 41
pubic arch, 65
pubis, 65
pulmonary circuit, 114
pulmonary circulation, 127, 144
pulmonary embolism, 138, 144
pulmonary function tests, 104
pulmonary valve, 116, 144
punctum lacrimale, 283, 294
pupil, 285, 294
pyelonephritis, 245, 254

Q

QRS complex, 124, 144
quadriceps femoris, 91, 94

R

radial nerve, 179, 188
radiation, 10, 11, 306
radioactive decay, 10–11
radioactivity, 10
radioisotopes, 10, 18
radius, 64
range of motion (ROM), 7, 9f, 18
Raynaud phenomenon, 130, 144
RBCs. See red blood cells
receptors, 183–184
recovery position, 8, 10f, 18
rectum, 215, 220
rectus abdominis, 83, 94
recumbent position, 8, 18
red blood cells (RBCs), 133–136, 135f, 140, 144
red pulp, blood capillaries of, 154
referred pain, 292
reflex arc, components of, 168f
reflux esophagitis, 211, 220
refractory period, 124
regional anatomy, 2, 18
relative refractory period, 124, 144
releasing factors, 225, 239
remodeling process, 27, 41
renal arteries, 243, 244f, 254